Aphasia and Related Cognitive-Communicative Disorders

G. Albyn Davis

Adjunct Professor, New York University
University of Massachusetts (Emeritus)

PEARSON

Boston Columbus Indianapolis New York San Francisco Upper Saddle River
Amsterdam Cape Town Dubai London Madrid Milan Munich Paris Montréal Toronto
Delhi Mexico City São Paulo Sydney Hong Kong Seoul Singapore Taipei Tokyo

MW

Vice President and Editor in Chief: *Jeffery W. Johnston*
Executive Editor and Publisher: *Stephen D. Dragin*
Editorial Assistant: *Anne-Marie Bono*
Director of Marketing: *Margaret Waples*
Marketing Manager: *Joanna Sabella*
Operations Specialist: *Michelle Klein*
Cover Designer: *Suzanne Behnke*
Cover Art: *oconner*
Full-Service Project Management: *Shylaja Gattupalli*
Composition: *Jouve India Private Limited*

Credits and acknowledgments borrowed from other sources and reproduced, with permission, in this textbook appear on appropriate page within text.

Library of Congress Cataloging-in-Publication Data

Davis, G. Albyn (George Albyn).
  Aphasia and related cognitive-communicative disorders / G. Albyn Davis, Adjunct Professor, New York University, University of Massachusetts (Emeritus). — First edition.
      pages cm
    ISBN-13: 978-0-13-261435-1
    ISBN-10: 0-13-261435-9
  1. Aphasia—Textbooks.   2. Language disorders—Textbooks.   I. Title.
    RC425.D3787 2013
    616.85'52—dc23

                                                                                2013016486

10 9 8 7 6 5 4 3 2 1

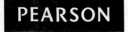

ISBN 10: 0-13-261435-9
ISBN 13: 978-0-13-261435-1

3/17/14

ABOUT THE AUTHOR

G. Albyn Davis is an adjunct professor of Communicative Sciences and Disorders at New York University and is professor emeritus for the University of Massachusetts at Amherst. He began his career as a speech-language pathologist at the Veterans Administration Medical Center in Pittsburgh and then directed a VA-funded training program in clinical aphasiology at the University of Memphis. While at Memphis, he co-developed PACE therapy for aphasia and began writing texts with *A Survey of Adult Aphasia*.

Dr. Davis has published articles and chapters ranging broadly from basic research to clinical essays, and he has presented his research internationally. He was an associate editor for the *Journal of Speech, Language, and Hearing Research*. He serves on the steering committee for the Clinical Aphasiology Conference (past chair) and served on the board of directors for the National Aphasia Association. He is also a clinical research advisor to the Adler Aphasia Center.

CONTENTS

PREFACE

This is my fifth textbook about aphasia and related disorders. This one was rewritten entirely with students in mind. The style is more relaxed, as if talking over a cup of coffee. I wanted this book to have my classroom voice. Space is devoted to walking the reader slowly through key theories and methods. I am hoping that this enhances learning and provides a foundation for disciplined curiosity.

The book is organized according to a logical progression. First, we try to understand a disorder. Our understanding then leads to assessment. Based on assessment, we treat the disorder. Running through these topics are some fundamentals that make the study of aphasia so fascinating, such as neurological foundations (Chapters 2, 7, 9, 12, and 13), psycholinguistic methodologies (Chapters 3, 8, 9, 11, and 13), and the pragmatics of linguistic communication (Chapters 4, 6, 10, 11, 12, and 13).

The book includes research doing its normal work of substantiating claims and therapies. Some studies are like figures or photos in that they illustrate a principle that should be remembered. An experimental procedure can make a cognitive theory or process seem more concrete or comprehensible. I invite the reader to use these moments to work on understanding. The memory, if needed, will be there. It's the way the mind works.

Part of a narrative is the identification of "characters" by naming names and telling where the work was done. While location of past work will remain accurate, individuals move on. I apologize for any location that becomes obsolete over the life of this edition.

I want to thank the members of the Adler Aphasia Center for their inspiration and the National Aphasia Association for allowing me to serve the aphasia public in a small way. My model audience was my students at the University of Memphis, University of Massachusetts, and Lehman College. I am currently enjoying the enthusiasm and grace of graduate students at New York University, including Melissa Chalef, who had the courage to critique my previous book for a class project, and Alvaro Heinig, who, among other things, discovered that I had been misspelling "gibberish" for 30 years. Also, I wish to thank everyone at Pearson Higher Education for overcoming my stressed out moments and being supportive and helpful. I would also like to thank the reviewers, including Barbara B. Shadden, University of Arkansas. Steve Dragin, executive editor, has been like a friend.

Finally, my wife, Betsy Elias, has been all of the above and my favorite golf partner.

Introduction to Acquired Language Disorders

Sanjay Gupta, CNN's medical expert, was reporting to Anderson Cooper early in 2012 about wounded Congresswoman Gabrielle "Gabby" Giffords's communication difficulties. Dr. Gupta described her symptoms astutely but did not hint that they have a name. A similar omission had occurred in a *20/20* story a couple of months earlier (Simon, 2012). Most of us hear about "aphasia" in adults for the first time as we pass through college on our way to becoming speech-language pathologists.

This chapter has one main goal and a subtext. The goal is to prepare the reader for what lies ahead by introducing the range of topics associated with the rehabilitation of persons with aphasia. The subtext is a foundation of thought that underlies studies of aphasia and related disorders.

Diagnosing Aphasia

Responding to the referral of someone with brain damage, a speech-language pathologist (SLP) evaluates oral motor function and communicative capacity. The SLP also determines whether the patient has aphasia. The nature of aphasia has not changed over the years, but scientific progress has influenced the way we talk about this disorder, including the way we define it. One of these influences pertains to how we view the relationship between language and cognition (Davis, 2012).

Aphasia can be defined as *a selective impairment of the cognitive system specialized for comprehending and formulating language, leaving other cognitive capacities relatively intact.* In addition to an obvious reference to cognition, the definition omits a frequently included reference to etiology. Other definitions are likely to add ". . . caused by brain damage" to a statement about language impairment. A cause is indeed an important diagnostic clue, and SLPs expect that people with aphasia will have damage to a particular part of the brain. Yet the cause does not comprise the dysfunction.

Let us put the definition to work for us. It implies that a diagnosis can be based on at least two comparisons. First, to identify impairment, we compare a client's language behavior to a norm. Then, to identify aphasia, we compare language functions to other cognitive functions. The relationship between language and cognition is not simple, and it is something to be dealt with throughout this text. There is one more thing to think about. Language comprehension and formulation utilize both auditory–oral codes (phonologic) and visual–written codes (orthographic), so that damaged language processes are manifested in both. The same syntax contributes to listening and reading. Thus, a third type of comparison is among modalities to distinguish aphasia from communicative disorders of a single modality. The following sections expand on these key diagnostic features of aphasia.

Language Disorder

The wife of someone with aphasia is usually quick to note that "although he doesn't talk, his mind is OK." Advocacy groups for aphasia place "disorder of language, not intellect" on buttons and banners. Both quotations characterize a pattern of impaired and retained mental faculties across the range of things people do every day. When someone has aphasia, many nonverbal skills, such as preparing a meal or driving a car, are unchanged. People with aphasia do not forget who everyone is. They know where they are. Their difficulty centers squarely on the use of words.

Brain pathology can cause other patterns of impairment and preservation known as "cognitive communication disorders" (Kimbarow, 2011). A review of 14,000 cases of brain pathology at the Mayo Clinic revealed that 11 percent fit the category of "other cognitive-language disorders" (Duffy, 2012). For one example, Robert Wertz (1985) wrote about the **language of confusion** of an individual whose speaking becomes twisted into incoherence by distraction, disorientation, failures of recollection, and extreme impatience and irritation. These problems are caused by traumatic brain injury (TBI).

TBI causes *amnesia*, a problem with remembering people, places, and events. Distinguishing amnesia from aphasia may help us to understand each. Someone with amnesia may not recognize a friend or recall a birthday party. Someone with aphasia, on the other hand, recognizes the friend and remembers the party, but has difficulty thinking of the friend's name or the names of memorable gifts. Frustrated, the person with aphasia says, "I know what I want to say, but I cannot think of the words," like the slogan on the button. Aphasia is a problem with words.

Dementias are similar to confusion because of their compromise of various intellectual skills. Dementias are linked to familiar and unfamiliar neuropathologies. Alzheimer's disease is the most well-known cause of dementia. Like Alzheimer's disease, other pathologies evolve slowly and grow worse relentlessly over months or years. Other mysterious progressive pathologies can target small regions of the brain. When these diseases are concentrated in language regions, a person can develop *primary progressive aphasia* (PPA).

Specific visuospatial or musical skills can be damaged by stroke, affecting artistic expression as well as orientation to everyday sights and sounds. A music lover may no longer be able to tolerate listening to the radio. This clinical population eludes neat labels and is usually identified with respect to general location of brain damage (i.e., **right hemisphere dysfunction**). The general pattern of deficits is the opposite of aphasia, namely, reduction of nonverbal functions with verbal functions relatively spared. For a long time, physicians did not refer these patients to SLPs. Nevertheless, talking with "right hemisphere patients" can be disconcerting. They have communicative difficulties that do not hinge on specific linguistic skills. They may not get the point of jokes, or they stray from the topic of a conversation.

To increase our confidence in a diagnosis of aphasia, we organize an evaluation partly around an informal comparison between verbal and nonverbal cognitive abilities. We ask patients to name things and if they can recall what happened to them. Can they follow simple instructions? Do they know where they are? In some rehabilitation settings, we are supported by a clinical neuropsychologist who conducts a comprehensive evaluation of attention, perception, memory, and reasoning. We compile a great deal of information for making a diagnosis of language disorder with other cognitive systems *relatively* intact.

Multimodality Deficit

Sanjay Gupta kept referring to Gabrielle Giffords's verbal difficulties as a problem with *speech*. Speech is not language. It is important that SLPs know the difference between a language disorder and "the King's speech." On the surface, the difference is observed as an impairment affecting input and output modalities (language) as opposed to a disorder of a single output modality (speech).

When someone's name is on the tips of our tongues, it is also on the tips of our fingers. Finding the right word is the most common complaint with aphasia; and when a word is blocked, it can neither be written nor spoken. The person with aphasia has problems comprehending when reading as well as when listening. Moreover, the modalities are not impaired equally, and there is a typical pattern of comparative deficit. People with aphasia nearly always comprehend better than they talk or write, and reading–writing skills are usually more impaired than auditory–speech skills.

How do we measure language skill in each modality? Clinical tests tend to be structured like the one shown in Table 1.1. The clinician administers tasks at varying levels of difficulty. A client deals with words in some tasks, sentences in others, and paragraph-length material in the most difficult tasks. A common result is that the fewest errors are made at the word level and the most errors are made with paragraphs. The hypothetical results in Figure 1.1 represent the percentage of correct responses in each modality, and most people with aphasia display the pattern in this figure. A clinician uses such results to support a diagnosis of aphasia. Let us review some common modality-specific disorders to see how they contrast with aphasia.

Sensory disorders disrupt transmission of hearing, vision, touch, and so on to the brain. When someone has only aphasia, on the other hand, he or she hears speech and sees print as well as before the stroke. People with aphasia receive a hearing test anyway. When someone with aphasia does have a substantial hearing loss, the graph in Figure 1.1 is likely to look quite different. That is, the listening score, without a hearing aid, may be well below the reading score, an exception to the pattern for aphasia.

TABLE 1.1   **A model of assessment for aphasia consisting of tasks at different levels of language in each modality. The level of multiple sentences is represented by discourse (spoken) and text (written).**

	COMPREHENSION		PRODUCTION	
LEVEL	*Listening*	*Reading*	*Speaking*	*Writing*
Word	Listen to a word, then point to an object	Read a word, then point to an object	Name objects	Write names of objects
Sentence	Follow simple command	Follow simple instruction	Describe simple actions	Describe action
Discourse/ Text	Listen to a story, answer questions about it	Read a paragraph, then answer questions	Describe a complex picture	Write a letter

An enigmatic category of modality-specific disorders is **agnosia**, which is impaired recognition, even though sensory transmission is intact. It usually takes bilateral brain damage to cause this problem. With *visual agnosia*, an object can be seen but it cannot be identified. With *auditory agnosia*, a person hears a familiar sound, such as a hissing teapot, but does not recognize what the sound means. People with impaired word comprehension can recognize unusual sounds such as bird calls (Riege, Metter, & Hanson, 1980). *Tactile agnosia*, also called astereognosis, is the inability to identify an object by touch, even though the patient senses texture and temperature. Agnosias present the following challenges for clinical diagnosis:

- Whether a client has aphasia *or* an agnosia
- Whether a client has aphasia *and* an agnosia

FIGURE 1.1   General pattern of aphasia at two severity levels, when comparing performance among the language modalities.

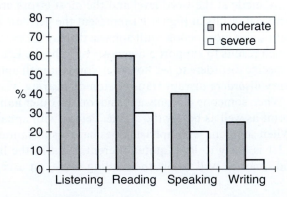

In either case of agnosia, the multimodality test pattern would differ from the one shown in Figure 1.1. The affected input modality would be distinctly depressed relative to other input modalities.

A person with aphasia often speaks with an easy flow. Speech articulation becomes difficult with **motor speech disorders** (Halpern & Goldfarb, 2013). The Mayo Clinic review discovered that these disorders accounted for 41 percent of Mayo's cases; aphasia accounted for 19 percent, although aphasia may constitute a larger proportion of the caseload in a long-term rehabilitation setting (Duffy, 2012). One type of motor speech disorder is *dysarthria*, which is a disruption of the execution of speech movements. The actor Kirk Douglas (2002) wrote of his struggle with this speech disorder following his stroke. Different types of dysarthria consist of muscle weakness, rigidity, or uncontrollable movement. Speech is often slowed or slurred, and the individual also finds it hard to chew and swallow food (i.e., *dysphagia*).

At the age of 42, Robert McCrum, editor-in-chief of a prominent publishing firm in England, suffered a right hemisphere hemorrhage that left him with the slurred speech of dysarthria. His retained language abilities made it possible to keep a diary of his convalescence. McCrum's speech therapy was very different from what would be provided for aphasia. One activity was to recite tongue twisters like "Theophilus Thistle, the thrifty thistle sifter, thrust three thousand thistles through the thick of his thumb" (McCrum, 1998). This sentence, too complex for someone with aphasia, facilitated the practice of a particular speech movement.

A person can have no muscular weakness or rigidity and still have trouble hitting speech targets, such as the lips for a /p/ or the back of the mouth for a /k/. **Apraxia of speech** (AOS) is an impaired programming of movement for the purpose of speaking. AOS can seem strange because the person can produce sounds and can even count to 10 or sing a song. The client may have no difficulty chewing and swallowing. Because the site of brain damage causing this disorder is similar to one that is responsible for one type of aphasia, an individual can have both aphasia and AOS.

In an audiotape made many years ago at the Mayo Clinic, a client with AOS is asked to describe John Steuart Curry's painting of a family on a Kansas farm escaping an approaching tornado (Darley, Aronson, & Brown, 1975). After an effortful description, the client was asked to repeat some of the more troublesome words including *tornado*. His attempts were roughly as follows: *torn-nati . . . excuse me . . . tornatio . . . tor-natoir . . . tor-na-toi . . .* and so on. The client had retrieved the word easily but struggled to reach the sound targets accurately and consistently.

This client at the Mayo Clinic had a stroke in the left hemisphere, which would make us consider his language. Here is some of his description of the painting: *I am looking at a drawing or a picture of what is apparently a tornado brewing in the countryside. This is having an immediate and frightening effect on a farm family . . .* and so on. Despite the hard work that went into forming syllables and the patience required of a listener, this is not aphasia. The vocabulary is sharp, and the syntax is complete.

Like the diagnostic challenges for sensory deficits, one person can have aphasia, another person can have a motor speech disorder, and someone else can have aphasia *and* a motor speech disorder. A referring neurologist examines the patient for clues to the underlying pathology, and an SLP makes a diagnosis relative to speech and language. When we see a slight droop in the right side of the face, the patient could have aphasia and an accompanying mild dysarthria. Nearly all people with brain damage are evaluated for safety of food and liquid intake. If the person with aphasia has a swallowing problem, it usually does not last long.

As a multimodality disorder, aphasia is not simply the sum of auditory, visual, speaking, and writing disorders. The damage causing aphasia is in one location, not four locations. In this sense, aphasia has been called a "central disorder." It is so central that the same aphasias occur in deaf users of *American Sign Language* (Poizner, Klima, & Bellugi, 1987). Thus, language functions are largely independent of each of the transmissive or peripheral functions of the nervous system (Table 1.2). Centralized functions have been identified historically with respect to linguistic components because word-meaning relationships are the same whether we are listening or reading. We do not possess one grammar for talking and another one for writing.

Propositional Language

When meeting someone with severe aphasia, the SLP may ask the individual to count to ten. Can he speak? We may have to prod a little, but counting often flows better than talking or when there was no talking at all. Fluent counting illustrates one fundamental feature of aphasia. People with aphasia retain so-called *subpropositional* forms, which "come 'ready made' or preformulated for the speaker" (Eisenson, 1984, p. 6). In addition to counting, subpropositional speaking acts include singing a song or producing routine greetings like "How are you?" or "I'm fine." A sudden emotion may propel an outburst of shocking profanities.

On the other hand, aphasia is an assault on the *propositional* language that we use intentionally for conversation and other communicative acts. Eisenson (1984) defined it as "a creative formulation of words with specific and appropriate regard to the situation" (p. 6). Difficulty primarily with propositional expression distinguishes aphasia from dysarthria, which puts constraints on all levels of verbal expression. Greetings, counting, singing, and profanity are proof that the neuromuscular mechanism is intact.

TABLE 1.2 Differentiation of aphasia from modality-specific communicative impairments, similar to Wepman and Van Pelt's (1955) historic construct.

	INPUT TRANSMISSION		CENTRAL PROCESSES	OUTPUT TRANSMISSION	
Function	Sensation	Recognition	Language	Programming	Execution
Dysfunction	Hearing loss	Agnosia	Aphasia	Apraxia	Dysarthria

Acquired Disorder

The person with aphasia was not born this way. We say that aphasia is acquired because its onset follows a substantial or completed period of language development and, for our purposes, a lifetime of language use. This circumstance is helpful for diagnosis of impairment, enabling us to compare current language abilities with language use prior to onset.

The term *aphasia* is also applied to language-specific disorders in childhood, and this double usage can lead to some confusion. Consumers of speech-language services may wonder if the adult and child versions are the same disorder. *Developmental language disorders* of childhood are diagnosed at an early age, and the cause often appears to have germinated prior to birth. Specific language impairment (SLI) is a developmental disorder with a symptom pattern that is consistent with aphasia (Leonard, 1998; Schwartz, 2009).

Describing Aphasia

Although the disorder hides inside someone's head, we can observe the resultant behavior. We must rely on clues or symptoms to diagnose aphasia and infer its nature. Also, describing the behavior of aphasia is a useful skill for notation in medical records and report writing. Terminology for categories of symptoms enables us to communicate a great deal more efficiently about our clients. By introducing terminology for symptoms, this section reveals more about what it means to have aphasia.

Symptoms of disorder come in contrasting categories. In his best-selling book *The Man Who Mistook His Wife for a Hat and Other Clinical Tales*, Oliver Sacks (1985) organized chapters around "loss" of function (e.g., not talking enough) and "excess" of function (e.g., talking too much). Another broad contrast is indicated in the following:

- Symptoms of omission (missing units of language)
- Symptoms of commission (erroneous units of language)

Word Retrieval

It is worth repeating. Many individuals with aphasia say things like, "I know what I want to say, I just can't think of the words." Each of us has experienced having a word on the tip of our tongue. For someone with aphasia, saying any word at any time is like reaching for a distant fruit on a tree. **Anomia** (also, *dysnomia*) stands for the general problem of finding and retrieving words. It is the most consistent feature of aphasia, common among all individuals with this disorder. This term should not be confused with the syndrome called "anomic aphasia." A syndrome is a unique pattern of symptoms (Chapter 2), and other syndromes of aphasia exhibit anomia.

Anomia appears as omissions and commissions. A person with aphasia may be unusually slow coming up with an intended word. When unable to find a word, he or she might talk around it saying, "I wear it right here, and I tell time with it. Mine goes tick, tick." "After I shower, I dry myself with it." This symptom of commission is called **circumlocution**, which tells us that an individual indeed knows precisely what he wants to say but could not find the word for it.

Someone with anomia may say "clock" when thinking of a watch. We use the term **paraphasia** when referring to a word substitution error. Often it appears accidentally and with surprise. Paraphasias differ according to the relationship between the intended word and the error (Table 1.3). Without a clear context, a client's intention can be difficult to identify. We identify paraphasias most confidently when we already know the targeted word, which is why we so often ask people to name objects, repeat words, or read words aloud.

A month after her brain injury, Gabby Giffords produced a variety of paraphasias (Giffords & Kelly, 2011). Shown a picture of a chair, she said, "spoon." For flowers, she said, "chicken." After some hints, such as "It's your favorite flower" and "They aren't roses," she called them "tulicks." What do we call these paraphasias? The first and second examples are real words but not very close to the target, and we would call them unrelated paraphasias. The third was close to the lexical form *tulips*, possibly a phonemic paraphasia.

Sentence Production

People with aphasia differ according to two styles of verbal production. One style is **nonfluent**, spoken with effort and with fewer words than normal. Sometimes we seem to be waiting forever for the next word to come. A listener has to be patient. The other general style is **fluent**, in which individuals talk with an easy flow of complete sentences. Aphasias are placed into two broad syndrome categories of nonfluent aphasia and fluent aphasia.

TABLE 1.3   A basic classification of paraphasias, including examples in Spanish. Neologisms are also known as nonword errors.

	ENGLISH		SPANISH	
Paraphasia	*Target*	*Error*	*Target*	*Error*
Phonemic	tiger	kiger	tigre	trigo
Semantic	tiger	lion	tigre	leon
Mixed semantic and phonemic	telephone	telegraph	cuchillo	cuchara
Unrelated	tiger	flag	tigre	bandera
Neologistic	tiger	floosis	tigre	banera

Labored nonfluent aphasia is usually limited with respect to grammar. In English, the symptom is one of omission called **agrammatism**, in which certain types of linguistic units drop out of utterances. When asked to tell what happened to cause him to come to the hospital, a patient might say one of the following:

- "Bathroom . . . shave."
- "Sleeping . . . get up . . . bathroom . . . fall down . . . um . . . Louise . . . um . . . ambulance."
- "I was standing mirror . . . shave . . . the . . . uh . . . fall on floor . . . and I did, too . . . no speech."

Knowing the situation, these fragments make sense and represent degrees of grammatical deficit. The omitted units are *grammatical morphemes,* including inflectional word endings such as *-ing* and closed-class or function words (e.g., *the, is, on*). The agrammatic individual produces mainly open-class or content words. In severe form, only one or two nouns are produced at a time.

With a fluent aphasia, the main problem is with producing content words such as nouns, verbs, and adjectives. Although sentences flow with correct structure, a person may have trouble finding a word she wants to use, or she may make word-finding errors. With a mild anomia, a person communicates fairly well. When a word does not come, he often resorts to general wording or circumlocution. In the following example, an auto mechanic explains how to drive a car:

When you get into the car, close your door. Put your feet on those two things on the floor. So, all I have to do is pull . . . I have to put my . . . You just put your thing which I know of which I cannot say right now, but I can make a picture of it . . . you put it in . . . on your . . . inside the thing that turns the car on. You put your foot on the thing that makes the stuff come on. It's called the, uh . . .

Other fluent aphasias can be "abstruse" (i.e., difficult to comprehend), a term that is used to characterize a type of production that clinicians call **jargon** (Marshall, 2006). This talk has the melody of normal utterance, but it is peppered with paraphasias of unclear origin. A listener is likely to be amazed and sometimes a bit amused at what is informally called word salad or gibberish. It is nearly the opposite of agrammatism (Table 1.4).

Howard Gardner (1974) asked one of his patients to talk about what brought him to the hospital:

Oh sure, go ahead, any old think you want. If I could I would. Oh, I'm taking the word the wrong way to say, all of the barbers here whenever they stop you it's going around and around, if you know what I mean, that is tying and tying for repucer, repuceration, well, we were trying the best that we could while another time it was with the beds over there the same thing . . . (p. 68)

The reply is mainly semantic jargon with one ambiguous paraphasia tossed in. What is *repuceration*? It could be a phonemic paraphasia for *recuperation* (i.e., phonological

TABLE 1.4   Traditional contrasting features of agrammatism (nonfluent) and jargon (fluent).

	AGRAMMATISM	JARGON
Utterance length	Reduced	Normal or increased
Content words	On target	Paraphasic substitutions
Grammatical morphemes	Omissions or errors	Occasional substitutions
Initiation and flow	Hesitant, slow	Smooth
Prosody	Reduced	Seemingly normal

reversal). Or, ignoring Gardner's question, it could be a neologism. This illustrates that individual paraphasias can be ambiguous. For diagnostic purposes, we are most interested in trends across a larger sampling.

Recurring or Stereotypic Utterance

Some people with severe aphasia are unable to say anything except involuntary and seemingly subpropositional utterances. Sometimes called formulaic expressions (Van Lancker Sidtis & Postman, 2006), these **stereotypic utterances** occur at the onset of aphasia and may persist for months. They may appear in any response, as if they were the only language forms available. Someone with severe aphasia may produce a repeated syllable such as "mem, mem, mem" uttered by poet Paul West soon after his stroke (Ackerman, 2011). A neologistic version was heard by Hughlings Jackson, a nineteenth-century neurologist, during a boyhood seaside holiday:

> . . . he lodged at a house where the landlady—as he discovered to his wonderment and awe—could say nothing but "watty." This unlikely disyllable was articulated with such a range of cadence that it could express a variety of emotions. Her laugh was merry and ringing, and when anything amused her she would say: "Watty, watty, watty." (Critchley, 1960, p. 8)

Sometimes this stereotypy consists of dictionary words. A common example is *yes* and *no* as the only verbalization. Another example is a phrase, such as "down the hatch." Ask the individual how he is doing, and he will say, "Down the hatch."

Explaining Aphasia

Why does someone have aphasia? We are sometimes amazed and often curious. How do we explain that one person speaks in fragmented sentences and another produces fluent jargon? Why do clients have trouble understanding some sentences but not others? We can look in a person's mouth and see muscle weakness, but we cannot see aphasia. Two types of explanation originate in an ancient philosophical conundrum called the "mind–body problem."

The Mind–Body Problem

Clinical investigators differ in their orientation to the internal processes of communication. Many focus on the concrete wiring of the brain, speaking of *neural* processes that encode and decode messages. Others are more "psychological," which is to say that they speak of *mental* processes that encode and decode messages. To be psychological is to speak of ideas and memories instead of convolutions and neurons. Aphasiology was born with a neurological orientation over a hundred years ago, whereas a convincingly scientific approach to the mind emerged only in the early 1970s.

The brain and the mind are not alternative versions of hidden processes. The mind is a brain function or "the brain creates the mind" (Damasio, 2007). For centuries, however, philosophers debated the nature of the mind, arguing over whether it exists or where it lives. In medieval Europe, laws were based on religious beliefs, namely, the Earth is the center of the universe, and material and spiritual worlds are completely separate. Drawings by Leonardo da Vinci show a belief that the mind or soul inhabits spaces inside the brain. During the 1600s, René Descartes was one of the first to speculate that memory and thought are managed in a material part of the brain. This was about as upsetting as Copernicus having the nerve to claim, with evidence, that the sun is the center of the universe.

Now, experimental psychologists speak of the mind as cognition. *Cognition* is "the collection of mental processes and activities used in perceiving, remembering, thinking, and understanding" (Ashcraft & Radvansky, 2010, p. 9). Cognitive science was born when these processes could be measured in the fractions of a second in which they occur. Just as archaeologists build models of Pompeii based on tiny fragments of its remains, cognitive scientists construct the most likely "functional architecture" of the mind from bits and pieces of behavior (e.g., Anderson, 1983).

Although most psychologists believe that cognition represents the jobs performed by the brain, they approach their work as if "the mind can be studied independently from the brain" (Johnson-Laird, 1983). Johnson-Laird added: "Once you know the way in which a computer program works, your understanding of it is in no way improved by learning about the particular machine on which it runs" (p. 9). At one time, texts on cognitive psychology contained almost nothing about the brain (e.g., Ashcraft, 1989; Solso, 1988), but the 1990s and beyond saw inclusions of cognitive neuroscience that began to address real-time neural operations (e.g., Ashcraft & Radvansky, 2010; Matlin, 2009).

The following treats neurological and cognitive orientations independently. This separation is not entirely artificial. A neuroscientist learns important things from studying pathologic brain tissue under a microscope without knowing the person's cognitive or communicative dysfunction. An SLP can make decisions about someone's language abilities without knowing what went wrong in the brain.

Neurological Explanation

Because many clinical features of neurogenic communication disorders depend on location and size of brain damage, Brookshire (2007) wrote that clinicians "must have at least rudimentary knowledge of the human nervous system and what can go wrong with it" (p. 2). Considering the previously cited symptoms of loss/omission and excess/commission, we may conclude that some symptoms result from the damage, and others are products of brain tissue that remains intact.

A distribution of faculties in the brain was contemplated while materialistic explanation of the human spirit was being rejected by church-guided authorities. Early in the 1800s, Franz Gall traveled to a tolerant Paris to escape the Austrian Kaiser's wrath because Gall was relating traits such as pugnacity and love of wine to areas of the brain. Relying on a pseudoscience called phrenology, Gall would detect wine lovers or those with strong "alimentariness" by feeling bumps on their skulls. Physicians, however, were looking forward to serious proof that human faculties could be localized in cerebral matter.

At the time the Civil War was beginning in the United States, Paul Broca performed an autopsy on a patient with a speech disorder and discovered a spot of damage in a frontal region of the left cerebral cortex. This discovery was received enthusiastically by the medical community. In 1874, Carl Wernicke published a doctoral dissertation about a severe comprehension deficit and damage in the left temporal cortex. He "proposed the first theory of language" that linked basic functions to centers in the brain (Amunts & Zilles, 2006). Diagrams of these centers proliferated in medical journals, and certain syndromes of aphasia came to be identified with Broca and Wernicke.

Doctors refer to the damage of any body tissue as a *lesion*. A lesion in the cerebral cortex causes aphasia. A few neuropathologies can destroy a small part of the brain, and such localized damage is called a **focal lesion**. Focal lesion in the brain is typically the consequence of disrupted blood flow or *stroke*. Yet stroke is not the only cause of focal lesions. A region of the cortex can gradually wither or shrink for mysterious reasons. Also, small parts of the brain can be scraped during lifesaving surgery, and surgeons try to avoid touching the areas for speech and language. A person may also accumulate several little strokes through the years, called a **multifocal lesion** pattern.

The role of location in explaining aphasia is based on the functional organization of the healthy brain. We can begin to think of this organization quite generally with respect to **posterior cortex**, which perceives, recognizes, and integrates sensory information, and **anterior cortex**, which is the platform for initiating volitional action. Four main lobes are a frame of reference for identifying sites of more specific functions. The frontal lobe, coinciding with anterior cortex, contains Broca's speech area. Posteriorly, auditory input lands in the temporal lobe, visual input, in the occipital lobe, and tactile input, in the parietal lobe. The laterally positioned Sylvian fissure divides the temporal lobe from the lobes above. Language functions reside on either side so that the anatomical area for language is often referred to as the **perisylvian region**.

The cerebrum has two halves, and the anterior and posterior regions of the cortex serve the same sensory and motor functions in each of these hemispheres. However, the left and right hemispheres have different cognitive responsibilities. When one hemisphere is damaged, its specialty is impaired, and the other hemisphere's expertise is relatively preserved. For most people, the left hemisphere is specialized for language, and the right hemisphere is specialized for high-level nonverbal functions. Most of this text is dedicated to left hemisphere lesions. One chapter deals with the specialties of the right.

The objective of neurological diagnosis is to figure out what happened to the brain. For example, fluent aphasia indicates that the posterior left hemisphere is damaged. However, it is still hard to tell in neurological terms why a person produces more neologisms than semantic paraphasias, or why someone simply omits grammatical morphemes. Why does a client not understand passive sentences? Scientists are currently engaged in using modern technology to explain specific linguistic behaviors in neurological terms. Contributing to this endeavor is the science of cognition, which provides a characterization of the hidden purposes of the brain.

Cognitive Explanation

What are those "central processes" in Table 1.2? Let us start with two basic features of cognition. One is the storage of information, or our fund of **knowledge**. It includes knowledge of the world and knowledge of the language we speak. The other feature of cognition is **process**, or the fleeting activity of the mind. A cognitive process is not just a plodding act of problem solving. It is also a quick mental response to a stimulus. Connecting a word to an idea is a type of mental process. Processes are temporal, and in principle, their duration can be measured. Studies of processing measure time.

A fundamental question pertains to how information is represented in our heads. What form does it take? This inner form is usually called a mental **representation**. Representation of a word, for example, may depend on whether it is in permanent storage or in a transient state. A neural representation can refer concretely to tissues and chemicals. Characterizing a representation in functional terms is more problematic. Cognitive scientists rely on analogies or metaphors. For example, a mental image may be like a photograph.

Cognitive functions are carried on the shoulders of **memory**. A psychologist explained that cognition is "the coordinated operation of active mental processes within a multicomponent memory system" (Ashcraft, 1989, p. 39). A memory begins with holding onto a representation beyond the life of a stimulus. This grip for a small fraction of a second allows the mind to do something in response to stimulation, such as recognizing the input.

What are the components of memory that Ashcraft mentioned? This information management system is like a library. A library stores books, acquires new ones, and has procedures for accessing its collection. In the mind, bits of knowledge are shelved in **long-term memory** (LTM). LTM contains different types of information. Representations are verbal, like novels, and visual, like picture books. Aphasia demonstrates that words and world knowledge are stored separately. Someone with aphasia knows what he wants to convey but cannot find the words. As shown in Chapters 12 and 13, different pathologies can single out one type of memory. Back to the library, organization of storage facilitates access so that we do not have to wander around all day looking for a book. Organization and access become a basis for investigations of aphasia in Chapter 3.

Now, let us turn to language processing. Our cognitive processing system has a limited capacity. The mind can do only so much multitasking (Eysenck, 2006). This limited work space is called **working memory** (WM): "a system that not only temporarily stores information but also manipulates it so as to allow people to perform such complex activities as reasoning, learning, and comprehension" (Baddeley, Eysenck, & Anderson, 2009, p. 19). Clinical investigators wonder if brain damage constrains working memory in a way that aggravates or even causes symptoms of aphasia.

Researchers have acknowledged that cognition operates at subconscious as well as conscious levels of awareness, which revolutionized the study of aphasia in the 1980s. Subconscious processing is said to be automatic. Scientists use so-called *fast tasks* and millisecond timers to measure automatic activity, as when the meaning of a word snaps to mind effortlessly. **Automatic processing** has the following characteristics:

- It is subconscious or beneath our awareness.
- It is obligatory (i.e., mandatory).
- It takes up little or no room in working memory.

In the presence of a stimulus, the brain does not just sit there waiting for our instructions. It activates on its own. Everyday comprehension and word retrieval, disrupted in aphasia, are automatic and obligatory.

In the clinic, we are more experienced with assessment and treatment of **controlled processing**, which has the following features:

- It can be conscious or in our awareness.
- It can be intentional and, therefore, optional.
- It is effortful and takes up room in working memory.

Also known as strategic or attentional processing, controlled processing is studied with *slow tasks* that allow enough time for decision making to occur. Unlike automatic processes, strategic processes clog working memory. When a client scans picture choices in a typical comprehension task, there is time for all sorts of thinking to occur.

The constructs of cognition have helped us to formulate explanations. For example, Schuell's (1969) clinical experience led her to believe that the "language storage system" is at least relatively intact. Most people who study aphasia think of it as an impairment of processing rather than a loss of linguistic knowledge. In this way, cognitive constructs provide a framework for locating a disorder functionally in the human information processing system.

Studying Aphasia

Clinicians support their beliefs about disorders and rehabilitation with personal experience, expert opinion, and research. Research extends our viewpoint beyond personal experience and sometimes runs counter to teaching. Some results surprise the experts. Fundamentally, science substitutes belief with fact (Lilienfeld, Lynn, & Lohr, 2003; Stanovich, 2007). One goal of this text is to encourage students to think briefly about how research is done and how it contributes to clinical thinking and method.

Approaches to Research

To say that something "drives" a study is to state the primary motivation and background that "informs" the design of an experiment. There are two approaches to observing the effects of stimulus manipulations on responses, namely, data-driven (i.e., descriptive) and theory-driven (i.e., explanatory) approaches. Historically, the former has tended to precede the latter in building our base of information.

   The data-driven, or empirical, approach focuses on the effects of independent stimulus variables on dependent response variables. For example, what is the effect of the length of instructions on the manipulation of objects? Empirical methods may expose unexpected deficits such as misnaming only musical instruments. An explanation may be added, called *post hoc analysis*. Post hoc analysis can be risky because the method may not have been designed for testing the chosen theory and an investigator ends up with an explanation jerry-built onto the data.

   A theory is a set of principles for explaining an observation or set of observations. A theory is especially necessary for representing something too big, too small, too old, or too obscure to be observed in everyday experience. For us, it consists of what could happen inside someone's head neurologically or cognitively to cause a behavior. We may overhear someone snipe that "it's only a theory," as if to say a theory is just a guess or is unhelpful. A sturdy theory, however, stands on *appropriate* evidence. A sturdy theory of aphasia could open a window to a sensible therapy.

   A rough example of a theory-driven study would be one intended to discover a client's ability to engage in mental activation of meanings when reading a word. In this case, a vast literature tells how mental activation can be studied (McNamara, 2005). Let us say our hypothesis is that people with aphasia are slower to activate concepts than neurologically intact people. This hypothesis obligates us to use methods that detect meaning activation and that measure its speed (Chapter 3).

   Empirically speaking, we question if a response is tied to a stimulus. Theoretically speaking, we ask if a response can be attributed to a hidden condition or process. Both approaches utilize predictions or hypotheses. Empirical hypotheses are based on previous findings. Theoretical hypotheses are based on assumptions about how hidden conditions might cause a behavior. Many studies contain a little bit of both approaches. Both data-driven and theory-driven methods may be said to be *quantitative* approaches to be contrasted with a *qualitative* approach, which emphasizes description of natural behavior in real-life situations (Chapter 4).

Research Designs

A study is planned around an independent variable, for example, a characteristic of people (e.g., brain damaged or not) or an ability of interest (e.g., naming objects). Manipulating a variable consists of at least one comparison. Sometimes a comparison is implied, such as "comparing" a client's progress two years after a stroke to an assumed plateau in natural recovery. Most comparisons, however, are explicit, such as comparing two participants (or groups) or comparing two tasks.

Deficient skills are identified with a between-group design where one group is neurologically intact (Table 1.5). The logic is similar to clinical diagnosis, in which we compare a patient's performance to a normal frame of reference. Comparisons of a brain-damaged group and a "control" group are less straightforward than comparisons of two healthy groups. Two healthy groups from the same population (e.g., college sophomores) should, in principle, be alike in every respect except for the variable being studied. This assumption underlies use of the traditional t-test for comparing the average scores. This assumption does not usually apply, however, when one group has brain damage (Clark & Ryan, 1993; Duffy & Myers, 1991).

A within-group design helps us learn as much as we can about a population or an individual. A single case is often examined when an investigator wants to answer a very specific question with a large number of tasks. Fastidious examination of an individual is useful when we are dealing with a widely variable population. We learn about rare disorders when it is difficult to assemble them in a group. Case studies generate hypotheses that can be tested later with a group and under more control. A group is preferred to maximize the applicability of results to a population.

Interdisciplinary Influences

Like other specialties in speech-language pathology, clinical aphasiology borrows concepts and methods from basic sciences. Aphasiologists have varying experience with these sciences, depending partly on their training. An SLP may have been mentored in

TABLE 1.5 Basic experimental designs and the empirical questions they answer.

DESIGN	COMPARISON	BASIC QUESTIONS	EXAMPLES
Between-group	Brain-damaged vs. neurologically intact	What deficits are caused by brain damage?	Trauma patients vs. normal participants
	Brain-damaged A vs. brain-damaged B	What is the result of damage to a particular area of the brain?	Left anterior damage vs. left posterior damage
Within-group	Task A vs. task B	Is there a pattern of retained and impaired language abilities?	Comprehending words vs. naming objects
	Item A vs. item B	Can a person have problems finding some words but not others?	Abstact vs. concrete words

speech science, neurology, linguistics, or cognitive psychology (Table 1.6). Scholars are drawn to aphasia because of the intersection of so many disciplines that are central to understanding human nature.

One could argue that **psycholinguistics**, the cognitive science of language processing, hits the nail on the head for representing the substance of language processing impairments. It is a field that claims an eclectic history consisting of philosophy, acoustics, and anthropology (Blumenthal, 1970; Osgood & Sebeok, 1965; Saporta, 1961). Psycholinguistics is more apparently a unification of *linguistics*, which is the study of language structure, and *cognitive psychology*, the study of mental processes. The data of linguistics is words and sentences per se, and the data of psycholinguistics comes from people processing words and sentences (Traxler & Gernsbacher, 2006).

Cognitive neuropsychology (CN) is a mainstay of European aphasiology. Its goal is to develop theories of cognition by studying the effects of brain damage. Regarding language, CN relies on single cases to test models of simple functions at the single-word level (e.g., Rapp, 2001; Whitworth, Webster, & Howard, 2005). It encourages a strategy for diagnosis and treatment. Psycholinguistic studies of aphasia may also be put forth under this heading to the extent that researchers also seek implications for normal language processes (e.g., Schwartz, Dell, Martin, et al., 2006; Zurif, Gardner, & Brownell, 1989). CN's place in cognitive psychology and psycholinguistics has been scrutinized and debated (e.g., Laine & Martin, 2012; Peach, 2012).

TABLE 1.6   **Disciplines that provide clinical investigators with paradigms for the study of language impairments.**

DISCIPLINE	ORIGIN	DOMAIN	PRINCIPAL METHOD
Linguistics	Philosophy, philology	Form and structure of language	Logical analysis of sounds, words, and sentences
Behavioral psychology	Experimental psychology	Stimulus-response relationships	Learning experiments; empirical research
Cognitive psychology	Experimental psychology	Mental representations and processes in cognition	Group studies of task accuracy and response time
Psycholinguistics	Cognitive psychology	Mental representation and processes in language functions	Group studies of task accuracy and response time
Clinical neuropsychology	Clinical psychology	Cognitive dysfunctions caused by brain damage	Group studies of standardized test performance
Cognitive neuropsychology	Cognitive psychology	Mental representation and processes in cognition (including language)	Case studies of brain-damaged persons; many tasks presented

Treating Aphasia

In 1925 in the United States, the field of speech-language pathology was established mainly to provide "speech correction" in public schools. Yet the great wars left many young adults to struggle with long-lasting language disorders. Physicians, psychologists, and speech pathologists responded with rehabilitation programs in military hospitals throughout the world. Therapies were pieced together from education, speech correction, and psychotherapy. Since then, clinical aphasiology has evolved into a full-fledged specialty with its own conference, the Clinical Aphasiology Conference, and its own journal, *Aphasiology*.

People with aphasia receive their rehabilitation initially in a medical environment and eventually just about anywhere with the help of family members. An SLP follows broad guidelines for health care and specific guidelines for aphasia developed by professional organizations. This section provides an introduction to the health care environment and clinical practice, including concepts that bolster discussions throughout this text.

Health Care Delivery

Between World War II and the mid-1970s, physicians and SLPs in the United States provided services without much guidance from the government. In the 1980s, health care costs skyrocketed along with double-digit inflation. **Managed care** became the collective term for approaches to the delivery of medical care that are intended to improve quality as well as contain costs.

The delivery of health care is determined partly by payment method. In theory, payment can be provided by the first party (patient) or by the second party (service provider). Yet, because the expense is usually too great for either party, health care is supported by **third-party payers**, who cover the cost on behalf of patients. A third party can be public (i.e., a government) or private (i.e., insurance). In many countries, the third party is exclusively the government, which results in some variation in rehabilitation around the world.

The first party receives services in different settings, depending partly on the stage of recovery. **Acute care** commences on admission to a hospital, and these hospital stays are as brief as medically reasonable. **Subacute care** (or postacute care) is a category established by the managed care industry to focus on rehabilitation as soon as possible. It is thought to provide a bridge between acute hospitalization and independence at home. **Chronic care** applies to long-term residual impairments such as aphasia (Table 1.7). An *inpatient* resides in the facility providing medical service, whereas an *outpatient* comes to the facility during the day and returns home after treatment. Currently, stroke survivors leave the hospital as soon as possible and receive therapies at a rehabilitation center or at home.

Health care delivery is different in countries where professional direct treatment is possible for months. This is not to say that comprehensive treatment programs are

TABLE 1.7   General categories of health care and typical settings in the United States.

CATEGORY	DEFINITION	SETTING
Acute	Immediate and short-term (e.g., stroke unit)	Acute care hospital
Subacute	Transition between acute hospitalization and independence at home	Rehabilitation hospital (inpatient or outpatient)
Chronic	Long-term for persistent diseases or conditions; living with permanent residual impairment	Home health care University clinic Nursing home

easily funded outside the United States. The Pat Arato Aphasia Centre in Canada provides group therapies and activities with a great deal of help from volunteers. After an initial seven years of relying on donations and bake sales, the center began to receive partial support from the Ontario Ministry of Health. Client fees and fundraising are still necessary to keep such programs going (Kagan, Cohen-Schneider, Sherman, et al., 2007).

WHO Framework

Since 1980, the World Health Organization (WHO) has provided a framework for evaluation and treatment of all medical conditions. The framework also contributes to conceptualization of rehabilitation for aphasia. In particular, it widens our perspective regarding what rehabilitation should entail. In regard for its common sense as well as its ubiquity, the WHO classification provides a foundation for clinical topics throughout this text.

Multiple versions of the WHO classification appear in the literature because there have been two major revisions. Originally, it parsed medical conditions into levels of "impairment, disability, and handicap." After complaints about this terminology, a revision expanded definitions with the more neutral terminology of "impairment, activity limitation, and participation limitation" (World Health Organization, 1997). A third and more complex classification emerged a few years later, now called the *International Classification of Functioning, Disability and Health* with the short moniker *WHO ICF* (World Health Organization, 2001; see Ross & Wertz, 2005; Table 1.8).

The intent of the 1997 classification is retained in the current version, but many authors prefer the middle one for its straightforward simplicity. For example, Worrall and others (2011) interviewed people with aphasia several months poststroke. Their rehabilitation objectives at this point were characterized as emphasizing the areas of activities and participation over attending to impairment. Similarly, this text leans on the terminology of the first revision.

TABLE 1.8   The first two frameworks from the World Health Organization, known as the *International Classification of Impairment, Disabilities, and Handicaps* (ICIDH-1 and ICIDH-2).

1980 ICIDH-1	ORIGINAL DEFINITIONS	1997 ICIDH-2	FURTHER DEFINITIONS	APHASIA
Impairment	Disordered system			
Disability	Functional consequences of impairment	Activity limitation	Reduction of personal activities	Communicative difficulties
Handicap	Social consequences of disability	Participation limitation	Reduced involvement in life situations	Loss of employment; social isolation

Aphasia Treatment

With respect to the WHO classification, aphasia rehabilitation has historically emphasized evaluation and treatment of language impairment. In the past couple of decades, we have progressed to an expanded view that recognizes consequences of impairment in activity limitations and participation limitations. Improving linguistic and communicative abilities are brought to bear on improving functional independence and quality of life.

Two varied contributions point to two fundamental approaches to treatment that absorb the WHO categories. One contribution is a collection of hypothetical case studies conjured in meetings of several aphasiologists in Italy (Martin, Thompson, & Worrall, 2008). The other is a large study of treatment effects in the Netherlands (de Jong-Hagelstein, van de Sandt-Koenderman, Prins, et al., 2011). Both groups divided aphasia rehabilitation similarly. One approach is **impairment-based**, focusing on linguistic or cognitive deficits (Chapters 5, 8, 9). The other approach is **communication-based** or *consequence-based* and addresses activity and participation limitations (Chapters 6, 10). Much of the information in this text will be identified with either of these two general approaches to rehabilitation.

What is new? We learn about "cutting-edge" treatment options at conferences and by sharing information as members of special interest groups (SIGs) in the American Speech-Language-Hearing Association (ASHA). One exploratory treatment is the modification of brain activity with a magnetic wand (end of Chapter 9). More down to earth is the rapidly expanding creation of applications for tablets and smartphones. **Apps** are employed for therapy and independent communication (Chapters 8, 10, 12). We can apply general-use apps such as calendars to aid memory and disorder-dedicated apps that have been mostly for children. More for adults are coming.

"Aphasia" Awareness

> If you'd been able to tell me unequivocally that Daddy had no more brain wattage than an eggplant, it would have been easier. Instead, I tended to feel around his aphasia for signs of the old self.
>
> "That was Lecia on the phone," I said.
>
> "Purty goo," Daddy came back.

In her memoir of her childhood in eastern Texas, Mary Karr (1995) was not afraid of the term *aphasia* when writing about her father.

Data proclaim, however, that the general public is ill prepared for this disorder. In 2002, questionnaires were given to nearly 1,000 people in shopping malls in Australia, England, and the United States. Only 14 percent had heard of "aphasia," and only 5.4 percent had knowledge of aphasia. A few thought that it is similar to dementia or Alzheimer's disease (Simmons-Mackie, Code, Armstrong, et al., 2002). A smaller study a few years later indicated that there is less knowledge of aphasia than of Parkinson's disease (Flynn, Cumberland, & Marshall, 2009). Researchers concluded that ignorance of aphasia diminishes an affected person's psychosocial adjustment and community reintegration, as well as funds for services.

Misconceptions about aphasia may have contributed in the case of Ruby McDonough, a resident of a nursing home in Massachusetts, where she was assaulted by a nurse's aide. In an initial district court proceeding, Ruby, who had expressive aphasia, was denied the right to accommodations so that she could give testimony against her attacker. It took a while, but the state Supreme Judicial Court, recognizing her intact intelligence, eventually ruled that she would be asked yes–no questions and would be allowed more than the usual time to respond (Miller, 2010).

The **National Aphasia Association** (aphasia.org) is a nonprofit organization in the United States dedicated to informing the public about this disorder (see Chapter 10, Table 10.5 for others). One of its programs educates emergency responders who are likely to be the first to come to the aid of someone with a stroke. In an independent effort, the actor Carl McIntyre has been traveling the United States, educating the public with a short film of his experience with aphasia (aphasiathemovie.com).

Besides public unfamiliarity, SLPs have wrestled with the term professionally. Clinicians in Europe and elsewhere have used the term *dysphasia*, whereas in the United States, we have used the term *aphasia*. Although the prefixes reflect a medically valid distinction between degree of loss (*dys-*) and total loss (*a-*), prevailing clinical usage has the terms meaning the same thing.

Referring to our clients has been more problematic. For a long time, we used the lazy phrase "the aphasic" (short for "aphasic person"). The adjective as a noun has been criticized for being linguistically clumsy. Then, "aphasic person" was felt to be insensitive to personhood, as people do not want to be defined by their impairment. A widespread accommodation in the clinical literature currently is to use the phrase "person with aphasia" (PWA) or "individual with aphasia" (IWA). The message may not have resonated in some circles. In Switzerland, for example, neuroscientists still use "aphasics" (Tschirren, Laganaro, Michel, et al., 2011).

One other thing. At a certain point in recovery, people do not want to be viewed as dependent "patients." Holland (2007) recommended that, once survival from a stroke is ensured, "people should now lose their 'patient' (i.e., helpless) designation" (p. 170).

Summary and Conclusions

This introductory chapter had a singular goal and a subtext. The goal was to help the reader acquire a general idea of what aphasia is in preparation for the details to follow. Aphasia is an acquired disruption of the cognitive system responsible for language comprehension and production. It is usually caused by a stroke, which leaves other cognitive functions relatively intact. Like Ruby McDonough in the Massachusetts courtroom, a person with aphasia knows what she wants to say. It is a problem with words, not ideas.

The subtext was to establish a foundation of thought for studying aphasia. Poststroke behavior is symptomatic of an internal dysfunction, one that we cannot observe directly. For clinical purposes, we measure and manipulate symptoms, but dysfunction is characterized in cognitive terms. Speech-language pathologists think about general processes involved in attaching meaning to sounds and putting thoughts into words. Clarity about knowing what we can observe and what we cannot observe contributes to the validity and strength of claims about cause and effect (e.g., Did our therapy remodel someone's brain?).

Many people with aphasia have other problems, such as a motor speech disorder or a problem with attention. Therefore, clinical management has multiple targets. Also, there are different aphasias. With some, finding nouns is harder than producing sentences. With others, producing sentences is harder than retrieving nouns. Such observations lead to decisions about targeting treatment of impairment for an individual and, thus, making the best use of time.

We can approach the language disorder from so many directions such as its psychology, its linguistics, its cognition, its neurology. We can reach back into philosophy and the history of medicine. We do evaluations, behavior modification, counseling, and report writing. We interact with hospital patients, their families, doctors, nurses, psychologists, and social workers. We can study this knotty problem. For now, at least, we know its name.

2 Neurological and Medical Considerations

Aphasia was introduced as being caused by focal lesions, usually, in the left cerebral hemisphere. This chapter explores these causes, with additional information that a speech-language pathologist (SLP) is likely to confront in a medical setting. This information includes medical treatments and technology for viewing the brain. The location of damage produces patterns of symptoms known as the syndromes of aphasia, which conclude the chapter. Colorful illustrations of most details are available online.

The main cause of focal damage is stroke or cerebrovascular accident (CVA). A stroke disrupts the distribution of life-giving nutrients to the brain. In the United States, it is the third most common cause of death over age 45, affecting nearly 800,000 people per year. Strokes occur more in women than men and more in Hispanic and African-American people than Caucasians (stroke.org; strokecenter.org).

Neuroanatomy, Neurophysiology

To understand what happens to the brain with a stroke, we should have some knowledge of the cerebral circulatory system. Like other tissues in the body, neurons thrive on the process of **metabolism**, or the exchange of nutrients and waste products between the circulatory system and nerve tissue. Arteries transport the nutrients oxygen and glucose from the heart to the brain. The brain's large appetite is reflected in its use of 15 to 20 percent of the body's blood while taking up only 2 percent of body weight (Sokoloff, 1989). The nutrients pass through the capillary membrane at the end of arteries, cross a space, and then pass through a neuron's membrane. The nerve cell transforms the nutrients into waste products that are carried away through veins. This process generates energy that is detected in brain imaging techniques presented later, and disruption of metabolism results in death of brain tissue.

Location of circulatory disruption contributes to the nature of deficit and recovery. Blood flow to the brain has three structural levels. First, arteries in the neck transport blood from the heart to the base of the cerebrum. These include the left and right common carotid arteries, each dividing near the larynx. The **internal carotid arteries** continue to the base of the brain. Behind the carotids, the vertebral arteries come together to nourish the brain stem and cerebellum. The second level consists of a horizontal polygon of interconnecting arteries at the base of the cerebrum called the circle of Willis.

The third structural level originates in the circle of Willis and consists of three cerebral arteries on each side, grasping the surface of the cortex. The trunk of the **middle cerebral artery** (MCA) emerges through the sylvian fissure between the temporal and parietal lobes. The MCA's anterior and posterior branches cover most of the lateral cortical convexity (i.e., the *perisylvian region*). In the left hemisphere (for most), it supplies the key language areas. A patient's medical report is likely to locate a stroke in the left middle cerebral artery (or **LMCA**), in its trunk, or in one of its branches. At its origin, the MCA is continuous with the internal carotid artery below and, thus, can suffer effects of blockage in the neck. The other cerebral arteries are rarely associated with aphasia.

Two mechanisms can disrupt metabolism. One is an ischemic stroke (or ischemia), which is an occlusion of an arterial vessel. The blockage keeps blood from getting to an area of the brain. The other mechanism is a hemorrhage, which is a bursting artery causing blood to accumulate around nearby brain tissue. In *Stroke for Dummies*, ischemia is referred to as a "white stroke" and hemorrhage, a "red stroke" (Marler, 2005). Ischemic stroke is much more common than hemorrhage.

Ischemic Stroke

Ackerman (2011) described her husband's stroke: "Paul shuffled out of the bathroom and stood at the foot of the bed, eyes glazed, his face like fallen mud. His mouth drooped to the right, and he looked asleep with open eyes that gaped at me in alarm" (p. 5). The most common cause is *atherosclerosis*, which is a proliferation of cells (i.e., blood platelets) along arterial walls and an accumulation of fatty substances (i.e., lipid) within the arteries. Another factor that could lead to ischemic stroke is high cholesterol. Atherosclerosis and high cholesterol are controllable risk factors (treatable) along with lifestyle factors such as smoking (changeable). Uncontrollable risk factors include age and a family history of stroke.

Types of Ischemia

Two types of occlusive or ischemic stroke produce similar clinical characteristics but result from different processes. Most ischemias are a **thrombosis**, which occurs from accumulation of atherosclerotic platelets and fatty plaque on the vessel wall, narrowing the passage (stenosis). It may take minutes or weeks for a thrombus to clog an artery. Dysfunction arises suddenly and worsens over minutes, hours, or even days during the final stages of accumulation. This *stroke-in-evolution* (or "progressing stroke") may proceed in a stepwise fashion, and maximum deficit is referred to as *completed stroke*. There is higher incidence of thrombosis among people with diabetes and high blood pressure than in the general population.

One signal of impending thrombosis is the **transient ischemic attack** (TIA), or "little stroke." TIAs are temporary disruptions of blood flow. They produce neurological signs indicating that platelet formation is underway, generally in the internal carotid artery. The signs stem from anything that the brain does and often consist of blurred vision, numbness or weakness on one side, aphasia, imbalance, or a combination of these signs. The event frequently lasts a few minutes and usually less than three hours. There is about a 20 percent chance of suffering a stroke during the first year after TIAs begin and a 30 to 60 percent chance in five years (Mlcoch & Metter, 2008).

TV viewers witnessed an apparent TIA when reporter Serene Branson garbled her words while broadcasting from the Grammy Awards in 2011. She started, "Well, a very heavy burtation tonight," and then she became incomprehensible. Neurologists speculated that she may have suffered a "ministroke" or, as Ms. Branson confirmed later, a migraine headache (cbsnews.com/8301-504763_162-20031790-10391704.html). She described her fear and confusion. "I knew what I wanted to say but I didn't have the words to say it" (hollywoodreporter.com/news/serene-branson-opens-up-terrifying-101504).

When a confirmed TIA's warning is heeded, the person usually receives medication to prevent a full stroke. The most common preventive treatment is *antiplatelets*, which inhibit platelet adhesion (e.g., aspirin, clopidigrel, or Plavix). *Anticoagulants*, such as heparin, improve blood flow and prevent clotting. High blood pressure (hypertension) is treated with *diuretics* that improve kidney function and *beta-blockers* that reduce pulse rate. *Vasodilators* relax the muscles of arterial walls.

Surgery is another preventive measure. *Carotid endarterectomy* entails inserting a shunt (small catheter) to keep blood flowing while the surgeon removes the thrombotic material. This procedure is usually performed in the fleshy neck, where the accessibly large common carotid divides. Also, the field of interventional radiology has been exploring *angioplasty* for clearing these arteries. The physician threads a balloon-tipped catheter into the blocked artery and inflates the tube to widen the vessel.

Unlike thrombosis, the origin and site of occlusion differ with an **embolism**. Platelets and fatty plaque break off a vessel wall, often near the heart, and then proceed until the cerebral artery becomes too small for the material to travel further. Medical history is likely to include cardiac disease. Clinical onset is more abrupt than thrombosis, and there are usually no warnings. Physicians often cannot determine an ischemia's origin and may refer to "thromboembolic CVA" in a medical report.

When metabolism is prohibited for about two minutes, the result is death (or necrosis) of neural tissue, called an **infarction**. The area of infarction varies in size depending on location of occlusion. A blockage in a main cerebral vessel starves a wide area. A blockage further along in a small branch starves a small area. Over time the necrotic tissue softens and liquefies, and then the waste is removed. The removal process is called *gliosis* because of the assistance of astroglial cells (astrocytes) that also hold cerebral neurons in place. Gliosis leaves a cavity on the surface of the cortex so that on autopsy an infarct looks like a crater on the moon.

In sum, ischemia refers to the occlusion of an artery, starving brain tissue of oxygen. Infarction is the resultant necrosis of brain tissue. We can say that ischemia causes infarction. However, we may see the terms used interchangeably when the type of stroke is identified in medical reports. In the following section, let us consider what happens after the moment of infarction.

Acute Phase

The target of acute medical treatment is an area surrounding an infarction known as the ischemic **penumbra**, a term defined in the dictionary as the grayish margin of a sunspot (and also is the name of a theater in St. Paul, Minnesota). Blood flow to this margin is reduced (called **hypoperfusion**), but the tissue is intact. In a strategy generally known as **thrombolysis** (i.e., clot busting), an emergency physician hopes to preserve neurons in the penumbra by administering a *tissue plasminogen activator* (tPA). tPA must be given within six hours after an ischemic stroke to avoid a risk of hemorrhage. Candidacy for thrombolysis is stringent, and the patient must be monitored very closely.

Scientists have discovered that an enzyme in vampire bat saliva serves the same neuroprotective function. For the bat, the enzyme thins a victim's blood so that it flows freely. Tested on mice, the enzyme may be less hazardous than tPA and could be administered up to nine hours after a stroke. Clinical trials on humans began in 2009.

The brain reacts to damage as if it is in shock. There is a suspension of functions that depend on structures remote from the infarct, called **diaschisis**. Two mechanisms contribute to diaschisis. One is a swelling of surrounding tissue, called *edema*, due to accumulation of fluid. It takes two or three days to peak and one or two more weeks to subside. Second, hypoperfusion extends widely in both hemispheres. Flow to the uninfarcted side improves spontaneously and dramatically within two or three weeks after onset (called spontaneous **reperfusion**). Diaschisis makes patients appear to be more impaired than they really are, and its temporary nature contributes to the appearance of early recovery.

In a hospital's stroke unit, a physician's main concern is patient survival. The patient is confined to bed with feet slightly elevated to avoid rapid lowering of blood pressure during stroke-in-evolution. Those with low levels of consciousness are nourished with intravenous fluids. Status of the penumbral region may be evaluated with magnetic resonance imaging or MRI, to be discussed later. Within two or three days after a completed stroke, physical exercises may begin to prevent muscle contractures. Self-care activities promote psychological and physical well-being.

Postacute Phases

Once survival is ensured, the physician initiates a plan for discharge knowing that infarction presents a relatively permanent condition. The plan includes postacute rehabilitation. When a patient is likely to have communication problems, the patient is referred to the SLP. A *consultation* or *referral* form contains the written request for services, which includes a provisional diagnosis, the patient's location in the hospital, and some medical history.

When postacute rehabilitation begins, diaschisis has not subsided. It usually takes the previously mentioned two or three weeks before the pattern of dysfunction mainly attributable to the infarct emerges. To obtain a reliable baseline, SLPs often delay full examination of language until medical stability is ensured and the lasting disorder is manifested. Meanwhile, medical treatment serves mainly to prevent another ischemia. Medication includes some of the drugs used for post-TIA prevention such as clot-dissolving antiplatelets (e.g., aspirin) and anticoagulants (e.g., heparin).

Research indicates that remote hypoperfusion lasts well beyond the early weeks of living with a stroke. However, Hillis (2007) advised that "functionally significant hypoperfusion beyond the infarct is probably uncommon beyond the first few days or weeks," although the issue "has not been adequately studied" (p. 170). In general, a chronic symptom pattern may be attributed to both infarction and some remote hypometabolism.

Hemorrhage

I have a terrific headache.

—*last words of Franklin Delano Roosevelt*

In a hotel lobby in Nicaragua, journalist Steve Fishman's (1988) vision suddenly became fuzzy, and then an arcing pain pounded in his head with each heartbeat. Eventually he wrote a book about his stroke, including neurological evaluations and neurosurgery (see also McCrum, 1998; Swet, 1998). A hemorrhage is a bursting artery causing blood to flood the brain's surface or invade brain tissue. The accumulation, called a **hematoma**, is a rapidly expanding mass that displaces and compresses adjacent structures. As reflected in FDR's last words, an excruciating headache, as well as nausea and vomiting, is a common initial sign of this sudden "space-occupying lesion." A hemorrhage can be caused by naturally weakened vessel walls or by tearing of arteries during traumatic brain injury.

Hemorrhages are labeled according to location. Mostly occurring in people with high blood pressure, an **intracerebral hemorrhage** (ICH) invades deep interior regions of the brain (e.g., thalamus, internal capsule, and basal ganglia). About half of these cases lose consciousness in minutes to hours after rupture, which may be precipitated by a sudden increase of blood pressure during physical activity or emotional stress. Medication reduces edema and blood pressure, and surgical evacuation is possible from some areas of the brain. However, for a spontaneous ICH, the death rate is 40 to 50 percent in the first 30 days, so that few of these individuals are likely to seek rehabilitation.

Subarachnoid hemorrhage occurs in a space within the meningeal membranes protecting the brain. It can be caused by a ruptured aneurysm near the circle of Willis. An **aneurysm** is a dilated blood vessel that could be the size of a pea to an orange, stretching and weakening the vessel wall. The rupture may be provoked by physical exertion but can be prevented by surgery when the aneurysm is accessible. Surgery includes trapping the reservoir by applying clips on both sides, clipping the neck of the bulge, or packing muscle around it. Plastics may be sprayed on the dilation and surrounding vessels.

Arterial walls also weaken in the condition of **arteriovenous malformation** (AVM), in which the capillary network between arteries and veins is absent. Vessels are twisted and tangled, occupying a tiny area or an entire hemisphere. Presumably a congenital condition, presence of AVM may not be signaled until hemorrhage or seizures occur in adulthood. A hemorrhaging AVM is usually less damaging than a bursting aneurysm. Jill Bolte Taylor's (2006) book and performances provide inspired testimony to the remarkable recovery than can occur with this uncommon type of stroke.

Tumor

A tumor (or neoplasm) is a nodule or mass of tissue that is caused by an abnormally increased rate in the growth of cells. Like a hemorrhage, it occupies space, pressing against nearby structures and obstructing circulation. Most hospitals use the World Health Organization's (WHO) classification. *Benign* growths do not spread to other parts of the body and are not recurrent. However, they can become large enough to be dangerous. *Malignant* tumors expand uncontrollably and are resistant to medical treatment. They may spread to other parts of the body via the bloodstream (called metastasis). They are graded from least malignant (Grade I) to most malignant (Grade IV). Doctors also distinguish *primary brain tumors*, which originate in the brain, from *secondary brain tumors*, which spread to the brain from elsewhere. An author may use the attention-seeking term "cancer-related aphasias."

Medical Diagnosis

General reductions of function are early signs of malignant neoplasms. Like hemorrhage, space-occupying pressure causes headache, nausea, and vomiting. Sensory impairments and dulled cognition may occur, and if the tumor is allowed to enlarge, impairment may evolve to stupor and coma. Specific dysfunctions depend on location and may include loss of vision or hearing when there is pressure on the optic or acoustic cranial nerves.

To determine whether a tumor is malignant, a pathologist performs a *biopsy* in which tissue or cells are removed from the body with a needle for examination under a microscope. Cells of a benign tumor are very much like their tissue origin. Cells of a malignant tumor are less recognizable. For areas that are difficult to reach, a biopsy can be guided by neuroimaging techniques that help the physician follow progress of the needle. Another advance is the use of very fine needles, called stereotactic biopsy.

Types of Tumors

Whereas hemorrhages are named for their location, neoplasms are named for their tissue origin. A common source is supportive cells throughout the central nervous system called glial cells. For example, an *astrocytoma* originates in the housekeeping astroglia cited earlier with respect to infarction and gliosis. The grades of malignancy can be determined based on rate of cell growth, differentiation of cell types, and number of abnormal cells.

Astrocytoma grade IV (*glioblastoma multiforme* or malignant glioma) is the most common primary brain tumor in adults. It is a rapidly growing mass likely to infiltrate both hemispheres through the commissures. Treatment consists of craniotomy (i.e., opening the skull) followed by *surgical resection*, which is the extraction of part or all of an organ or structure. Surgeons may report "gross total removal," but the tumor usually recurs in months. Survival averages about one year.

A couple of famous people were felled by this devastating glioma. George Gershwin, composer of "Porgy and Bess," suffered the earliest signs of a temporal lobe malignancy while conducting the Los Angeles Philharmonic Orchestra at age 38. He died two days after his surgery. Senator Edward M. Kennedy, at the age of 76, was diagnosed with a malignant glioma in the left parietal lobe. His doctors were unable to do a surgical resection safely, and they predicted survival of less than year. The senator battled longer than that and died 15 months after the diagnosis.

Astrocytoma grades I–II (low-grade astrocytoma) is much less common but has a more favorable prognosis. It expands slowly, and symptoms may appear years before the tumor is discovered. Complete removal is seldom accomplished, but repeated surgery can be beneficial when the neoplasm is accessible. Prognosis after surgery has been reported to be three to six years.

Meningioma is a benign tumor arising from the protective tissue covering the brain (*meninges*). After glioblastoma, it is the second-most-common primary brain tumor in adults. Unlike other tumors, it occurs more frequently in women than men. Meningiomas grow slowly and usually do not invade the cortex. Complete removal is possible, and prolonged survival is a frequent outcome.

Aphasia with Tumors

Several studies of left hemisphere tumors have shown that the resulting aphasia tends to be confined to a mild word-finding impairment (Davie, Hutcheson, Barringer, et al., 2009). In one of these studies, 17 pairs of participants were compared, one with tumor and one with stroke in similar locations. Regarding eight pairs with lesions in the left hemisphere, tumor caused less severe language impairment than stroke. When tumors intruded on Wernicke's language area, patients did not have aphasia at all (Anderson, Damasio, & Tranel, 1990).

Surgery for brain tumors may cause aphasia, and there have been only a few studies. Two of them found most of the aphasias to be mild and mainly with anomia regardless of lesion location. In one study, severity of aphasia was related to grade of tumor. Aphasia was worse with glioblastomas (Whittle, Pringle, & Taylor, 1998). More recently, researchers did not find this relationship in the acute period following surgery. Comprehension deficit was minimal and agrammatism was scarce following surgery (Davie et al., 2009). In general, because each tumor is unique, each surgery is unique and so are its consequences.

Investigators also wondered if guided stereotactic biopsy in the left hemisphere causes aphasia. Language was assessed with standard aphasia tests before and after a tissue sample was obtained. If the patient did not have aphasia preoperatively, the procedure carried a 9 percent risk of impairing language functions. If the patient already had aphasia, there was a high risk of aggravating the impairment (Thomson, Taylor, Fraser, et al., 1997a).

Focal Cortical Atrophy

For a long time most professionals in speech language pathology agreed that "aphasia in adults does not creep, it erupts" because strokes erupt, more or less (Rosenbek, LaPointe, & Wertz, 1989). Malignant glioma certainly has a progression of deterioration, but it is partially treatable and eventually ends in death in a relatively short amount of time. Progressive diseases, on the other hand, were associated with diffuse damage and generalized intellectual impairment. After extensive study, researchers have learned that progressive diseases can be more parochial than once thought.

At the risk of trespassing on Chapter 13, let us at least be introduced to pathologies suspected of underlying primary progressive aphasia (PPA). PPA is a gradual deterioration of language functions with relative preservation of other cognitive abilities. Marcel Mesulam's (1982) report of six cases led to widespread recognition of the syndrome but not widespread agreement over what to call it. PPA or something like it has been adorned with "aphasia without dementia," "semantic dementia," and other labels. Further complications arise in the literature because "there is no single agreed operational definition of the syndrome" (Croot, 2009, p. 311). More to the point of the current chapter, there is some variation in the proposed neuropathology of PPA, in part, because it is a relatively new area of research.

The pathologies may be referred to generally as *non-Alzheimer lobar degeneration*, in which degeneration shows up in brain images as **atrophy**, or shrinkage of part of the brain. Interior spaces or ventricles are enlarged because of the decreased mass of the surrounding brain matter. Also, in "pictures" of the brain or on autopsy, doctors see enlarged spaces (i.e., fissures) between thinning cerebral convolutions. With PPA, atrophy is concentrated in the language areas of the left hemisphere. The next question: What causes the atrophy?

Microscopic studies of diseased tissue in many patients have led to the conclusion that localized atrophy and the resultant PPA can be caused by different pathologies. Some of the causes are included in a spectrum under the heading of *frontotemporal lobar degeneration* (FTLD). The diseases in this spectrum overlap with etiologies of dementia (e.g., Pick's disease), and differentiations become quite technical with respect to the precise pathology. Researchers also suspect that a localized version of Alzheimer's disease may also be responsible for some cases of PPA (Croot, 2009).

Clinical Neurological Examination

A *neurologist* is the specialist responsible for evaluation and treatment of persons with brain damage. In a clinical examination, neurologists examine the basic status of sensory, motor, and cognitive systems in about 30 minutes. The physician wants to know the nature and site of neurological damage. Radiological tests confirm and elaborate a preliminary diagnosis. With the accuracy and availability of brain imaging technology, the neurologist no longer has to rely on clinical examination to localize a lesion. In addition to overseeing acute care, this specialist relates clinical findings to radiological findings and orders referrals to rehabilitative specialists so that impairments can be evaluated more thoroughly.

Clinical examination begins on first sight of a patient. Alertness indicates the status of deep cerebral regions and the brain stem. With a test called auscultation, the doctor presses a stethoscope lightly to the neck and each temple to listen for unusual rushing sounds in the bloodstream called *bruits*. Talking to the individual yields clues about cognition, including language. The doctor may administer a screening test such as the *Mini Mental State Examination* (Folstein, Folstein, & McHugh, 1975).

From head to toe (or vice versa) and alternating left and right sides, the neurologist examines motor and sensory functions to assess peripheral and central nervous systems. Tapping muscles for simple reflexes exposes either hypoactivity indicating peripheral damage or hyperactivity indicating central damage. Failure to react to stimulation on one side is called *hemianesthesia*, and paralysis on one side is called *hemiplegia*. In these instances, the normal side becomes a standard for estimating severity of unilateral impairment, which is common in the person with aphasia.

The visual system is unique because there is not a directly contralateral connection between the eyes and the cerebral hemispheres (occipital lobes). Instead, contralaterality exists between *fields of vision* and the hemispheres. When we look straight ahead, we see objects to the left and right of the center. The right occipital lobe receives what we see in the left visual field, and the left occipital lobe receives vision in the right visual field. The left and right optic nerves make these connections by crossing only partially at the base of the brain. At this crossing (optic chiasm), each optic nerve sends tracts to both hemispheres (diagrams can be found online).

Specific visual deficits are indicative of location of a tumor or other pathology, especially relative to the optic chiasm. If there is blindness of one eye, then the damage is between the one eye and the optic chiasm. If, on the other hand, a person does not see objects to the left or right of center with either or both eyes, the damage lies between the optic chiasm and an occipital lobe (or in the occipital lobe per se). The loss of one field of vision is called *homonomous hemianopia*. A "right field cut" can occur with aphasia because the optic nerve radiates through the parietal and temporal lobes on its way to the occipital lobe. The SLP should ask a client to look straight ahead and then should present objects to the left or right to determine if visual field affects responding to visual stimuli.

Clinical Brain Imaging

Chapter 1 addressed the reliance on theory to characterize phenomena hidden from everyday view. The brain can now be observed indirectly with special technology. Scientists and physicians view "images" of the brain. Neurologists request these images to help identify the pathology and locate the lesion. Research with this technology tells us about recovery and effects of language treatment. One of two types of imaging is spatial, or structural, imaging, producing a stationary picture of anatomy. The other is temporal, or functional, imaging, which is sensitive to neural activity in the cerebral cortex. Either structural or functional imaging can be used for clinical purposes.

Structural Neuroimaging

Cerebral **angiography**, or *arteriography*, is an X-ray procedure that exposes arteries in the head and neck. An opaque fluid is injected usually in a carotid artery to expose cerebral arteries to view. With ischemia, vessels seem to have disappeared beyond the occlusion. Tumors or other space-occupying lesions are inferred from distortion of the arterial pattern. *Digital-subtraction angiography* introduces a computer computation that improves image quality and reduces the amount of contrast medium injected into the bloodstream. *Magnetic resonance angiography* (MRA) displays cerebral arteries as bright white on a gray background. It exposes a variety of defects such as stenosis, occlusion, and aneurysm.

Computerized tomography (CT scan) relies on thin beams of X-rays from a scanner rotating around the head to provide a representation of cerebral structures. Varied intensities of the X-rays are sent to a computer that transforms the data into tissue densities. Results are displayed as tiny blocks of tissue, which is a "reconstruction" of structures in a particular plane of the cerebrum. Images of several planes are obtained in about 30 minutes.

CT scanning has been in use for a few decades (e.g., Mazzochi & Vignolo, 1979; Naeser & Hayward, 1978). Its advantages lie in its power of resolution of a lesion and detection of longstanding infarcts. Pathology is indicated by alterations in the expected densities of brain structures. Infarction is revealed as decreased tissue density, and hemorrhage is shown as increased density so that a CT is good at distinguishing between the two. Identifying an infarction can be improved with injection of a contrast agent. The main concern with this procedure is exposure to radiation.

A much sharper image *without radiation exposure* is achieved with **magnetic resonance imaging** (MRI). It is "widely used in acute stroke" or in *hyperacute stroke*, which is the first 24 hours after the onset of symptoms (Hillis, 2007). The body is placed in an area surrounded by a large electromagnet (people with metallic implants cannot be assessed). The magnet manipulates the "spin" of molecules within the nucleus of an atom. Then, a computer creates a picture of the brain from the electromagnetic signals generated by this manipulation.

MRIs provide sharp contrasts of gray and white matter. They are superior to CT scans in their sensitivity to subtle pathologies and early detection of diseases. Because the procedure does not require injection of a contrast medium (noninvasive), it can be used repeatedly and, thus, is suitable for longitudinal studies. Brookshire (2007) noted that "MRI scans take a long time, and the patient must remain motionless in a noisy, confining space, sometimes leading to claustrophobia and blurring of the MRI image because of patient movement" (p. 82).

MRI yields different types of information. *Diffusion-weighted imaging (DWI)* is sensitive to the extent of the acute infarction. *Perfusion-weighted imaging (PWI)* detects hypoperfusion indicative of brain tissue that is dysfunctional but salvageable by the return of blood flow. To reiterate, DWI locates the infarction, and PWI locates areas of blood flow reduction beyond the infarct. Combining the procedures can contribute to prognosis for the recovery of functions related to the region of penumbra.

Another MRI application is perhaps the first imaging technique to single out white fiber tracts that connect areas within the cerebrum. It is called **magnetic resonance tractography** (MRT) and may also be called diffusion tensor imaging (DTI) in case we want to look up more information about it. It has been used to study the arcuate fasciculus, a tract well known to aphasiologists because it links the temporal lobe to the frontal lobe in areas important for language and speech (Glasser & Rilling, 2008).

Functional Neuroimaging

Basic brain research involves detecting and measuring cortical process, especially in relation to the concept of "activation" in cognition (Sidtis, 2007). In one approach, electrical activity of neurons is measured in *electrophysiological neuroimaging*. The other method is *metabolic neuroimaging*, which measures blood flow or metabolism as reflections of neural electrical activity.

Attaching electrodes to neurons would be the most direct measurement, but implanting electrodes is impractical. Instead, scientists place electrodes safely on the scalp for **electroencephalography** (EEG). For a long time EEG was used for detecting pathology in a living person. It records activity at different locations on the scalp. A lesion is indicated by electrical activity in one location that differs from regular patterns detected at other regions. Although this method of localization is crude, EEG is still useful for identifying subcortical lesions and for estimating severity of damage when a patient is in a coma.

Because EEG is safe, it has been used extensively for studying the healthy brain. A refinement, called the *evoked potential* (EP) or event-related potential (ERP) detects neural response to a stimulus. A computer teases specific neural responses out of the complexity of EEG activity. The neural or evoked response appears as a positive or negative spike in the computed wave, and it is a neural correlate to response time in psycholinguistic research (Ward, 2010).

Metabolic imaging is used to infer the electrical activity of the cortex while a person is performing a task. Measuring **regional cerebral blood flow** (rCBF) is an indirect indication of metabolism, which increases where neural activation increases. Blood flow rate increases to support regions of heightened metabolism. A scanner detects variations in flow rate.

Positron emission tomography (PET) is a direct measure of metabolism and is more responsive than rCBF to rapid variations of activity. Radioactive tracers are combined either with oxygen or glucose and injected into arteries. A rotating scanner detects the rate at which tissue utilizes the radioactive nutrients. PET is considered the best method ("gold standard") for identifying dysfunctional brain tissue, but it is not the most feasible method in the first 24 hours after stroke (Hillis, 2007). It is expensive because a cyclotron must be available for producing the radioisotope. It takes a long 50 minutes for the scanner to rotate, and there is some exposure to radiation.

Less costly than PET, **single-photon emission computed tomography** (SPECT) employs a radioactive tracer nicknamed "Tc-99m." Investigators can "lock in" brain activity at the time of injection and view the localized activity later. This is advantageous for detecting neural activity that occurred while a person was performing a task. Although not requiring an on-site cyclotron, visualization is less precise and not particularly valuable for diagnosing lesions. rCBF, PET, and SPECT have been used to measure blood flow remote from a lesion.

Functional magnetic resonance imaging (fMRI) also detects brain activity by measuring blood flow (Song, Huettel, & McCarthy, 2006). First employed with humans in 1992, it is now widely used for research. It detects oxygen levels in the brain because magnetic properties of oxygenated blood are different from deoxygenated blood. This unique basis for fMRI is called **BOLD** for "blood oxygen-level-dependent contrast," and we are likely to see the label "BOLD fMRI" at conferences and in articles. Rich technicalities are buried in the "hemodynamic response function," which, in simple terms, is indicative of neural activity (Drake & Iadecola, 2007).

By taking a series of scans, a researcher identifies regions of the cortex that were activated while someone was performing a task. Like evoked potentials, fMRI has been used to study neural processing of language (e.g., Mason, Just, Keller, et al., 2003). Its emphasis on location is unlike EP, which provides an indicator of cortical events over time at one location. fMRI does not require a contrast medium and, thus, takes less time than PET and can be repeated on an individual. Also, it has better spatial resolution and is less expensive than PET. Disadvantages of fMRI include difficulty reaching certain areas of the brain and sensitivity to small movements prompting investigators to avoid overt speech during the procedure (Ward, 2010). Clinical use is restricted to assessing the risk of surgery.

Transcranial Doppler ultrasound (TDU) is a modification of ultrasound scanning that detects blood flow in a cerebral artery. In ultrasound scanning, high-frequency sound waves are transmitted into the head, and reflected echoes are detected and analyzed with a computer. With TDU, gel is applied to an area of the head where the bone is thin enough to allow the Doppler signal to enter and be detected (called the transcranial window). A technician directs the signal toward the artery being studied. High flow rates indicate arterial stenosis or arteriovenous malformation. The procedure may also determine if a secondary route of blood flow exists prior to surgery for diseased vessels.

Syndromes of Aphasia

Many people with aphasia exhibit what researchers call a **dissociation**, which is a clear deficit in one skill while other abilities remain relatively intact. It is as if a stroke has dislodged one function from the others. Some clients have more difficulty finding words (i.e., anomia) than forming sentences (i.e., agrammatism), whereas others have the opposite dissociation, namely, more difficulty with sentences than with words. This observation has a long history that includes Jakobson's (1955) "paradigmatic" and "syntagmatic" disorders. Researchers have interpreted such "double dissociations" to mean that one part of the brain deals with words and another part deals with sentence structure. For our purposes here, we are not worrying so much about the implications of aphasia for the healthy brain. Instead, let us turn our attention to the implications of lesion location for our clients' language difficulties.

A *syndrome* is a recurring pattern of symptoms. Multidisciplinary and international investigation has cluttered aphasiology with systems for labeling syndromes (e.g., Ardila, 2010; Kertesz, 2010). Chapter 1 introduced a broad and fairly consistent distinction between nonfluent and fluent aphasias. Nonfluent aphasias tend to be caused by damage in the anterior region, whereas fluent aphasias tend to be caused by damage to posterior regions.

In the system that is most familiar to clinical professionals, the main syndromes are differentiated according to three key areas:

- Severity of *comprehension* deficit
- Linguistic features of *spontaneous verbal expression*
- *Repetition* ability compared to spontaneous expression

We may focus on these functions when evaluating our clients, following the lead of some of the aphasia test batteries in Chapter 5. Although repetition is not a particularly functional skill, it can be a good test of speech articulation and short-term memory as well as providing a clue to syndrome diagnosis.

Broca's Aphasia

Let us start with nonfluent aphasias, Broca's aphasia in particular, partly because this syndrome is the main attraction in the research presented in the next chapter. It is named for a 19th-century French physician, Paul Broca, who helped to put localization of function on a scientific footing. It has been associated with "expressive aphasia" (Grodzinksy & Amunts, 2006).

Agrammatism, defined in Chapter 1, is the dominant feature of Broca's aphasia. Word finding is preserved better than sentence formulation. Auditory comprehension is slightly or moderately impaired. The clumsiness of apraxia of speech is likely to show up, especially with words that are difficult to articulate. The person with this aphasia is often a good communicator because the few words produced represent some of the message accurately. Also, our guesses as listeners are within the patient's comprehension ability.

"Broca's area" is located in the lower posterior region of the frontal lobe, in front of the motor area that distributes neural impulses to speech muscles. It is identified as areas 44 and 45 according to the Brodmann system used to identify cortical regions objectively or without attribution of functional significance. Broca's area "was the first brain region to which a circumscribed function, overt speech, had been related" (Amunts & Zilles, 2006, p. 17). Although not something we need to worry about too much, there appears to be widespread inconsistency with respect to the precise constitution of Broca's area (Lindenberg, Fangerau, & Seitz, 2007). With proximity to the motor region in the frontal lobe, Broca's aphasia is usually accompanied by a mild right facial weakness and right hemiplegia.

Chronic Broca's or agrammatic aphasia is caused by ischemic occlusion in anterior branches of the middle cerebral artery. The resulting infarction extends from Broca's area to neighboring areas in the temporal and parietal lobes. A lesion may extend into underlying white matter (Damasio, 2008). Lesions restricted to Broca's area can cause an acute Broca's aphasia that can resolve quickly (Kertesz, Harlock, & Coates, 1979). Such smaller lesions produce apraxia of speech or "Broca's area infarction syndrome" (Mohr, Pessin, Finkelstein, et al., 1978). Kertesz (1979) stated "there is a spectrum of syndromes produced by Broca's area infarct . . . the larger lesions produce the full-blown symptom complex of Broca's aphasia" (p. 187).

Hospitalized patients sometimes provide unique opportunities to study the relation between language functions and the brain. One day after surgery at Johns Hopkins Hospital, a 67-year-old man suffered a stroke and immediate (hyperacute) symptoms of Broca's aphasia. With an MRI given 4 hours postonset, the PWI component showed reduced blood flow to an intact Broca's area. Doctors wondered if this hypoperfusion caused the agrammatic symptoms. So, they administered language tests 5 and 32 hours poststroke. In between the patient was treated with intravenous saline to increase blood pressure and improve flow. PWI repeated at 36 hours poststroke revealed complete reperfusion of Broca's area. Moreover, the aphasia had disappeared, indicating that Broca's area was probably responsible for this temporary agrammatic aphasia (Davis, Kleinman, Newhart, et al., 2008).

Global Aphasia

As the label implies, global aphasia is a severe depression of language ability in all modalities. Some patients may not talk initially, and some produce noncommunicative verbal stereotypes. Yet these individuals are still alert and aware of their surroundings, and they express feelings and thoughts through facial, vocal, and manual gestures.

The following problems may mask language abilities and give the appearance of a comprehensive aphasia:

- Motor impairments that make it difficult to determine comprehension
- Extremely low level of arousal

- Extreme disorientation or confusion
- Depression or lack of motivation to communicate

The presence of these conditions may prohibit a clinician from having a clear view of the aphasia and lead to a conclusion that severity of aphasia is unknowable. A gloomy diagnosis of global aphasia may be honestly but carefully contemplated, especially soon postonset, because it can reduce support for speech-language treatment. It is generally best to wait a couple of weeks to see if spontaneous reperfusion improves the situation.

As might be expected with a broadly severe aphasia, CT scans identified lesions covering the entire language region (i.e., perisylvian) including Broca's and Wernicke's areas (Kertesz, Lesk, & McCabe, 1977; Mazzocchi & Vignolo, 1979; Naeser & Hayward, 1978). Lesions may also reach deep into white matter beneath the cortex. An exception to pervasive perisylvian damage is an occasional sparing of Wernicke's area in the temporal lobe (Basso, Lecours, Maraschini, et al., 1985; Vignolo, Boccardi, & Caverni, 1986). Also, global aphasia can arise from two separate strokes, in anterior and posterior branches of the left middle cerebral artery, instead of a single ischemic blockage in the main trunk of the LMCA (Damasio, 2008).

Wernicke's Aphasia

The most severe fluent aphasia is known by other names such as sensory aphasia, receptive aphasia, and *jargonaphasia*. A person with Wernicke's aphasia has poor language comprehension, produces jargon, and often lacks self-conscious awareness of this unusual speech. According to Mitchum and others (1990), neologisms are so characteristic that this aphasia is one of the few syndromes that can be identified by object-naming errors alone. The fluent jargon possesses sentence structure, indicative of a dissociation of word finding from syntactic construction. A patient may continue talking when it is his turn to listen, known as *press for speech*. People with Wernicke's aphasia may enter therapy with a poor "therapeutic set" because they do not realize why they are there (Sparks, 1978).

The syndrome pairing severe comprehension deficit and fluent jargon can be found with damage to Wernicke's area in the superior temporal lobe and neighboring regions (Kirshner, Casey, Henson, et al., 1989). In a small percentage of cases, some frontal lobe damage made the perisylvian landscape look like it should have caused global aphasia (Basso et al., 1985; Kirshner et al., 1989). However, there has been little controversy regarding the site of damage causing Wernicke's aphasia (Damasio, 2008).

Conduction Aphasia

Conversation with someone who has conduction aphasia goes smoothly. The key feature of this disorder is a disruption of *repetition* that is surprisingly severe relative to good comprehension and fluent spontaneous speech. When a client repeats phrases of increasing length and decreasing familiarity, verbalization deteriorates precipitously. The client may start with scattered phonemic paraphasias and end up producing bewildering jargon. Conduction aphasia is unique in that most conversational word-finding errors are phonemic paraphasias. Clients are usually aware of their errors and "produce repetitive self-corrections, known as *conduite d'approche*" (Bartha & Benke, 2003, p. 93).

Conduction aphasia is a relatively uncommon syndrome. It took Bartha and Benke (2003) five years to accumulate 20 cases for their research. To participate in their study in the category of conduction aphasia, a person had to have "a profound deficit in repetition displaying phonemic paraphasias and self-corrections . . . in the absence of a severe language comprehension disorder" (p. 95).

This aphasia has been thought to be an example of a "disconnection syndrome," meaning that a dysfunction is caused by a disrupted connection between structurally intact centers (Geschwind, 1965). The connections, called association tracts, are white axonal fibers beneath the cortex linking one cortical region to another within a hemisphere. The **arcuate fasciculus**, which can now be viewed with magnetic resonance tractography, is an association tract that carries impulses from Wernicke's area for listening to Broca's area for speaking. This connection enables us to repeat. For a long time, it was logical to think that the arcuate fasciculus is damaged in conduction aphasia.

CT scans of people with conduction aphasia showed anticipated damage to the posterior superior temporal cortex and inferior parietal cortex along with infarction of deep white matter below (Damasio & Damasio, 1980). Predicted by disconnection theory and a patient's good comprehension, posterior temporal damage spared Wernicke's area (Naeser & Hayward, 1978). However, the arcuate fasciculus need not be damaged (Anderson, Gilmore, Roper, et al., 1999). Damasio (2008) centered the typical lesion in the aforementioned temporal-parietal region but added that "conduction aphasia can result from somewhat different lesion patterns" (p. 29).

Contemporary structural and functional neuroimaging are highlighting lesions associated with symptoms of conduction aphasia. Fridriksson led a team of investigators using MRI to locate damage linked to acute repetition impairment. PWI (perfusion-weighted imaging) detected hypoperfusion in the left inferior parietal lobe and in the posterior arcuate fasciculus (Fridriksson, Kjartansson, Morgan, et al., 2010). In cases of explicit conduction aphasia, fMRI pinpointed damage in a similar posterior temporal area, thought to be required for phonological working memory (Buchsbaum, Baldo, Okada, et al., 2011).

Anomic Aphasia

Anomic aphasia (or "amnesic aphasia") is generally the mildest form of aphasia. It consists of slightly impaired comprehension and fluent coherent utterances that are weakened communicatively by failed word retrieval. Expressively, it is the word-finding dissociation mentioned earlier, the opposite of agrammatism. It should not be confused with the term "anomia," which stands for the general symptom of word-retrieval difficulty found in all syndromes. Anomic aphasia, the syndrome, has been reported to characterize most aphasias caused by tumors and closed head injuries.

Utterances can be vacuous, populated with generic terms (indefinite nouns and pronouns) filling the void of concept-loaded content words. An example is the description of how to drive a car in Chapter 1. Ambiguities, such as "that thing" or "somebody," can be resolved with situational context and knowledge of the topic. Clients retrieve some words quickly or engage in elaborate circumlocution while trying to think of names for objects. Although comprehension is quite good, word recognition difficulties can be detected when the client is pressed (e.g., *Did you mean clock?*). The individual may retrieve a word and then momentarily fail to recognize that the word is correct.

A site of damage responsible for anomic aphasia has been elusive. The syndrome is associated with damage to the posterior parieto-temporal juncture (i.e., angular gyrus). A fairly comprehensive structural and metabolic study of 12 patients with mild "anomic aphasia" was conducted by Illes, Metter, Dennings, and colleagues (1989). All participants had damage in the posterior superior temporal gyrus, but there were two subgroups. The most fluent group had good metabolism in both frontal lobes, but a slightly less fluent group had left prefrontal hypometabolism as well as deep damage in addition to the temporal damage.

Transcortical Aphasias

Repetition is again a key signifier, only this time for the opposite reason. In the rare transcortical aphasias, repetition is much better than would be expected from comprehension and spontaneous speech. **Transcortical motor aphasia** (TMA) is similar to Broca's aphasia. Someone with TMA struggles, sometimes agrammatically, to answer a question but repeats a long sentence without missing a beat. Lesions are generally located in the frontal lobe, superior and anterior to Broca's area (Berthier, 1999).

Similarly, **transcortical sensory aphasia** (TSA) seems like Wernicke's aphasia except for a remarkable ability to repeat. Echolalia, in which a person repeats a question instead of answering it, is a prominent feature. At the University of Manchester, United Kingdom, researchers selected four people with TSA to be samples of "semantic aphasia," which was defined as "a failure of control processes rather than damage to central semantic representations" (Soni, Lambon Ralph, & Woollams, 2012). According to CT scans, lesions causing TSA are usually posterior to and above the perisylvian language area.

A **mixed transcortical aphasia** (MTA) is sort of a combination of TMA and TSA. Language disorder is severe with poor comprehension and meaningless stereotypic utterances. Yet repetition can be compulsive. In other words, MTA is global aphasia with ability to repeat. It is as if intact mechanisms of speech recognition and production are "isolated" from intentions and meanings generated in the rest of the brain. The literature is inconsistent on the site of damage. Diffuse or multifocal pathologies produce MTA with frontal and parietal damage while sparing the language area. Cimino-Knight, Hollingsworth, & Gonzalez Rothi (2005) reviewed

TABLE 2.1   Summary of the contemporary clinical syndromes of aphasia.

GENERAL CATEGORY	SYNDROME	KEY SYMPTOMS	SITE OF LESION
Nonfluent/anterior	Broca's	Agrammatic production	Around and including Broca's area
	Transcorical motor	Like Broca's aphasia but with preserved repetition	Varied frontal lobe locations
Fluent/posterior	Wernicke's	Poor comprehension, jargon, press for speech	Wernicke's area (posterior portion of superior temporal gyrus)
	Conduction	Surprisingly impaired repetition	Temporo-parietal boundary (supramarginal gyrus)
	Anomic	Word-finding deficit, empty speech	Posterior temporo-parietal boundary (angular gyrus)
	Transcorical sensory	Like Wernicke's aphasia but with preserved repetition	Inferior temporo-occipital area
Mixed	Global	Poor comprehension; minimal production	Anterior & posterior perisylvian region
	Transcortical mixed	Like global aphasia but with preserved repetition	Diffuse or multifocal damage in frontal and parietal lobes

evidence indicating that the spared right hemisphere contributes to the preserved repetition ability.

Syndromes Summary with Commentary

The syndromes are important, at least, for reading this text. A great deal of research involves putting participants into these categories, mainly so that readers can identify a particular aphasia that is being studied. Researchers who are uncomfortable with acknowledging syndromes categorize individuals according to a key symptom (e.g., "agrammatic aphasia"). Many clinicians prefer to home in on specific symptoms and are not concerned with labeling per se, perhaps because many people with aphasia do not fit snugly into one of these categories. Yet the syndromes, at least the ones that are widely agreed on, provide us with a convenient shorthand for communicating a client's characteristics to other professionals (Table 2.1).

Exceptional Aphasias

Traditional diagnosis linked aphasia to pathologies that erupt and to damage of the left perisylvian region of the cortex. Removing neurologic causation from definition of dysfunction (Chapter 1) opens up the logical possibility of finding aphasias that creep.

Also, individual investigators may have an original take on what they observe and may come up with aphasias, such as "semantic aphasia," that are unfamiliar to many of us. "Exceptional aphasias" are those that are simply unusual and those that could, in some instances, be questionable because of inconsistent definition of dysfunction.

Crossed Aphasia

A referral of crossed aphasia is signaled when a patient has an infarct in the right hemisphere. Not everyone has language function located in the left hemisphere. Maybe 2 percent of right-handers have a reversed or "atypical" asymmetry with language functions in the right hemisphere and nonverbal functions in the left. Less than 4 percent of people with aphasia have crossed aphasia, in which *right-handed* individuals suffered a stroke in the right hemisphere (Coppens, Hungerford, Yamaguchi, et al., 2002).

There are two patterns of atypical language lateralization underlying crossed aphasia (Alexander, Fischette, & Fischer, 1989; Bhatnagar, Buckingham, Puglisi-Creegan, et al., 2011). Seventy percent of crossed aphasias are a **mirror image** of typical left hemisphere profiles. Most classical syndromes are possible (e.g., Sheehy & Haines, 2004). **Anomalous** profiles occur in the remaining 30 percent in which language seems to be managed outside the perisylvian right side. The anomalous cases tend to have large right perisylvian lesions but minimal aphasia.

Subcortical Aphasias

A cortical infarction can have depth, extending into subcortical regions. "Subcortical aphasias," however, are diagnosed when damage is primarily beneath the cortex in the left hemisphere. Reports of these disorders have raised eyebrows with respect to their implications for neural mechanisms of language as well as for the nature of aphasia.

Kirk and Kertesz (1994) compared cortical and subcortical aphasias and found similarities with respect to scores on a standard aphasia test. All subcortical patients were classifiable into aphasia syndromes, but subcortical damage caused more motor and sensory impairments. In general, there is some disagreement over whether forms of subcortical language disturbance are genuine aphasias or are merely similar to these syndromes. Kennedy and Murdoch (1994) argued that subcortical damage can produce the same classical syndromes, but they had reservations in using clinical tests to establish the true nature of a language disorder. Kirk and Kertesz also noted that subcortical language deficits "change dramatically over time," so that diagnosis may be quite different even three months after a stroke.

Researchers divided subcortical language disorders as to whether there is damage to the thalamus. Someone with a **thalamic lesion** is likely to have good comprehension and fluent word retrieval deficits (Raymer, Moberg, Crosson, et al., 1997). **Nonthalamic lesions** include the basal ganglia. Investigators have diagnosed anterior, posterior, and global aphasias. The anterior aphasias were like Broca's aphasia but without agrammatism. The posterior syndrome was similar to Wernicke's aphasia (Helm-Estabrooks & Albert, 2004; Naeser, 1988).

Early excitement has subsided over a possible discovery of subcortical language functions because "studies using perfusion-weighted imaging (PWI) have confirmed that aphasia only occurs after subcortical infarcts when there is concomitant hypoperfusion" (Davis et al., 2008, p. 51). The flow of nutrients to structurally intact regions is reduced, dampening the operation of Broca's and Wernicke's areas. Spontaneous reperfusion may be responsible for the dramatic recoveries observed by Kirk and Kertesz. Induced reperfusion may also have remarkable effects (Hillis, 2007; Hillis, Barker, Wityk, et al., 2004; Radanovic & Scaff, 2003).

Summary and Conclusions

Aphasia occurs because of neuropathologies that can single out the part of the brain responsible for language functions. For most people, the language areas nestle in the perisylvian region of the left cerebral hemisphere. Localized neuropathologies include ischemic and hemorrhagic stroke, tumors, and progressive focal atrophies. Regarding ischemic stroke, acute language impairments are caused by a region of dysfunction that includes the infarction and surrounding hypoperfused tissue. Early recovery is due in part to spontaneous reperfusion of structurally intact regions.

Family members, who were likely in a state of shock when the doctor explained what happened, may question the SLP about why a particular severity or pattern of language deficit occurred. Armed with knowledge of anatomy and neuropathology, we can help family members and patients understand the effects of size and location of lesion. We may anticipate residual capacities based on our knowledge of intact regions. Help can be obtained from the National Stroke Association (stroke.org). Books are available for patients and families, such as Stein's (2004) *Stroke and the Family*, Hutton's (2005) *After a Stroke: 300 Tips for Making Life Easier*, and Senelick's (2010) *Living with Stroke: A Guide for Families*.

Advances in neuroimaging have minimized dependence on clinical evaluation for diagnosing neuropathology. Although the technological developments are glorious, the indirectness of imaging techniques puts a perspective on what they do not tell us. They do not picture exactly what the brain is doing. They are pictures of blood flow and metabolism, not neurons at work. This perspective will be sobering as we ponder recovery in Chapter 7 and effects of therapy in Chapter 8. To complement brain images, the next chapter delves into cognitive theory of what the brain does.

In the clinic, we notice that each client is unique. The organization of language functions in the brain and lesions of diverse size and location are together responsible for some of this individuality. The result is a realization that "aphasia" stands for aphasias. At one time, the diagnosis of syndromes helped the neurologist identify site of lesion. Currently, the various syndromes alert us to the different kinds of acquired language disorders and, in all likelihood, the client-centered diversity of goals of treatment.

3 Investigating Language Impairments

What are the effects of damage in the perisylvian regions of the left hemisphere? At one level of research, investigators search for symptoms not usually exposed by clinical assessment. At a deeper level, investigators test cognitive explanations of familiar and freshly recognized symptoms. Research provides a foundation for improving language assessments and a platform for launching impairment-oriented therapies. It helps us understand the nature of our clients' difficulties, and this text provides an unapologetic look into the modern science of differentiating automatic and strategic processes.

This chapter is confined to auditory-oral language, beginning with comprehension and proceeding to production. Reading and writing are addressed elsewhere. Before forging ahead, it may be helpful to review introductions to cognition and research in Chapter 1. Studies are inserted to provide illustrations and evidence for claims.

Word Processing

Nearly all people with aphasia have difficulty comprehending language at some level, but many do not have problems understanding single words. The most common test of word comprehension is to present a word auditorily or visually and have a client point to a portrayal of meaning. About 50 percent make no errors or are within normal range in the picture-pointing task (e.g., Schuell & Jenkins, 1961). Difficulty comprehending individual words points to a severe aphasia.

If we are to understand comprehension disorder in contemporary terms, we should consider what happens mentally in a clinical word-comprehension task. Initially, the mind represents the stimulus, and the representation passes through levels of processing (Table 3.1). Accessing meaning can be thwarted because of a problem early in the process. An elderly individual with aphasia could have a preexisting hearing loss or a visual impairment. To prevent these problems from interfering with assessment of deeper levels, we should make sure that such clients are wearing hearing aids or glasses.

TABLE 3.1   Functional levels of word processing beginning with sensation and concluding with comprehension.

FUNCTIONAL LEVELS	SUBJECTIVE EXPERIENCE	PROCESS	ASSESSMENT
Sensation	*I hear something*	Initial detection of acoustic signal from the environment	Audiometric tests
Perception	*I hear the sounds "schadenfreude."*	Mental representation of a lexical stimulus, called a percept	Discrimination; identification
Recognition	*It sounds like a word. I've heard that word before.*	Activation of word in lexical memory (match percept to lexical representation)	Word naming; lexical decision
Comprehension	*I know what that word means.*	Activation of concept in semantic memory (match lexical representation to concept)	Point to picture

Speech Perception

Perception results in the mental representation of a stimulus, called a **percept**. Investigators once explored the possibility that a problem forming a percept might explain some comprehension deficits (Shewan, 1982). Speech perception with aphasia has been assessed in the following ways:

- *Discrimination* in which participants judge whether CV-syllable pairs are the same or different (e.g., /pa/, /ba/)
- *Identification*, or "labeling," in which an individual points to a letter for the phoneme
- *Discrimination-identification* in which a person hears a word (e.g., *pat*) and chooses between similar-sounding pictured options (e.g., a pat, a bat)

Most people with aphasia are within normal for discrimination (Fink, Churan, & Wittman, 2006). Labeling errors may be caused by a language deficit instead of a speech perception problem. Most with a deficit improve to normal perception within four months after a stroke (e.g., Franklin, 1989).

Wernicke's aphasia is of interest because of temporal lobe damage and severity of comprehension deficit. Someone with this aphasia may act as if he does not hear (Kirshner, Webb, & Duncan, 1981). Yet speech perception impairments are not specific to this syndrome and are often not sufficient to reduce language comprehension substantially (Blumstein, Cooper, Zurif, et al., 1977; Miceli, Gainotti, Caltagirone, et al., 1980). Lesion location may produce an "auditory-predominant" subgroup that has a modality-pattern differing from the common pattern (see Figure 1.1). In these cases, auditory processing is below reading ability (e.g., Kirshner, Casey, Henson, et al., 1989).

Word Recognition

Some readers may recognize *ashtanga pranam* but not know what it means. Recognition means that we have at least heard or seen a word before, and this experience has been stored in some way. Word recognition occurs when we match (or "map") a percept to the stored representation of the word. Let us put this operation into the memory system. If we heard a word seconds ago, then a representation may be active in working memory. However, we usually recognize words and other things with reference to a representation stored long ago in long-term memory. Entering the world of psycholinguistics, let us think about the study of simple word recognition and then comprehension.

A **lexical decision task** (LDT) is used to study word recognition. Remember this task because it is incorporated at all levels of language research. Usually a string of letters (e.g., BOOK or CHOT) is shown on a computer until a participant presses "Yes" or "No" indicating whether the string is a word. A nonword is a structurally possible foil. Researchers are mainly interested in response to the real word. It normally takes just over half a second (600 milliseconds) to respond to common words. In one study, participants with aphasia were as fast as normal controls and, also like the controls, responded faster to common words than rare words (Gerratt & Jones, 1987). The results indicated that people with aphasia are able to match the percept of a stimulus to the corresponding representation of a word in LTM, formally called a *lexeme*.

That 600 milliseconds (msec) is the time to press the button, and psycholinguists want to locate the moment of recognition occurring within this time frame. Experiments have supported an estimate that lexical access (i.e., recognition) normally occurs within 100 to 300 msec after the stimulus (McCrae, Jared, & Seidenberg, 1990).

Word Comprehension

To comprehend, we attach meaning to a lexeme, like attaching [pleasure in the misfortune of others] to *schadenfreude*. Meaning is stored in **semantic memory**. The core of semantic memory is universal in that most people have the same basic knowledge of living (animate) and nonliving (inanimate) things. Fringes of world knowledge vary according to locale, culture, and expertise. We store knowledge of objects as categories because we cannot remember everything we have seen or heard. A category, or **concept**, is the simplest unit of semantic memory. It is the mental representation of a class of objects or actions. Concepts are stored separately from lexemes. For example, a concept [hat] may be similar for everyone, but its lexeme varies from language to language and is stored in **lexical memory** (e.g., *chapeau, cappello, hoed*, or *hat*).

Concepts are organized, and this structure has an influence on processing (just as the organization of books in a library facilitates our search for a book). The prevailing view is that conceptual knowledge takes the form of a spatially characterized **semantic network**. A concept is represented as a **node** that is connected to other nodes, like those three-dimensional molecular structures in a physics class.

A network permits a general category like [vehicle] or a general attribute like [red] to be recorded once. A distance metaphor corresponds to the degree of relatedness among concepts, which is usually estimated from word association norms. Related concepts are close together, like "neighbors," and less-related concepts are more distant from each other.

When we hear or see a word like *nurse*, meaning flashes into the mind without cognitive effort. We have no control over it. It is said that word comprehension is an activation of a concept node in the semantic network. The challenge for researchers is to establish a method that addresses this fast process with minimal interference from irrelevant processes. Like the activity of neurons, activation of a node is imagined to spread automatically to related nodes nearby, called **spreading activation**. The notion of distances among concept nodes leads to predictions reflecting the time for activation to traverse from one node to the next.

Automatic activation of meaning is studied with a **semantic priming** task (McNamara, 2005). Word-pairs are presented, and a participant is asked to make a lexical decision about the second word (recall the LDT). The first word is called a **prime** (e.g., *nurse*) preceding a **target** for lexical decision (e.g., *doctor*). The method tests hypotheses about what happens in the mind when exposed to the prime.

Lexical decision is faster when a target is preceded by a semantically related prime (e.g., *nurse–doctor*) than by an unrelated prime (e.g., *flower–doctor*), and this difference is called the **semantic priming effect**. In explaining this effect, any prime (e.g., *nurse*) is presumed to activate nodes in its conceptual neighborhood (i.e., spreading activation), so that the related target concept [*doctor*] is likely to be active before the word is presented. With an unrelated prime (e.g., *flower*), a participant's mind is somewhere else when the target is presented (e.g., in an area about flowers).

The interval between visual prime–target pairs, when spreading activation occurs, is called the *stimulus onset asynchrony* (SOA). When words appear on a computer screen, SOA is the time between onset of a prime and onset of a target. Because timing of spoken stimuli is slightly different, terminology for the prime–target interval is different. In normal adults, speed of automatic activation is evident in semantic priming that occurs with less than 50 milliseconds of SOA (Simpson & Burgess, 1985).

It is important to note that lexical decision for the target is incidental to the process of interest, namely, what happens in the mind following the prime. The latter is inferred from the influence of the prime on the target in relation to characteristics of these words. Processing of the prime is more likely to be subconscious and automatic (i.e., implicit) when a person is not asked to do anything with the prime.

William Milberg and Sheila Blumstein conducted the first semantic priming experiments in aphasiology, and they had a surprising result. Participants with agrammatic aphasia (and presumably good semantics) did not have a semantic priming effect (Milberg & Blumstein, 1981; Milberg, Blumstein, & Dworetzky, 1987). The conclusion was that people with Broca's aphasia have a lexical–semantic deficit at the automatic level, which came to be known as the *automaticity hypothesis*. Later, however, Chenery and others (1990) found a range of people with aphasia capable of semantic priming, and Baum (1997) found semantic priming to be consistent in nonfluent (Broca's) participants but inconsistent in fluent participants. These apparently conflicting findings were worrisome.

Resolution of the conflicts arrived partly with adjustments to methodology. One problem was the complexity of Milberg and Blumstein's task because they used two-word primes. Katz (1988) simplified the task with one-word primes. Another problem with the early work was a reliance on a long prime–target interval of 500 milliseconds, which is enough time for controlled processing to overtake automatic processing. Shorter intervals became more common, and people with Broca's or Wernicke's aphasia displayed genuinely automatic semantic priming (Hagoort, 1997; Tyler, Ostrin, Cooke, & Moss, 1995).

A fundamental question concerns how the mind responds to ambiguity, which is a basic feature of linguistic processing. Semantically ambiguous primes, such as *bank*, facilitate response to targets such as *money* and *river* when the SOA is short. This type of result indicates that the mind activates multiple meanings automatically (a finding that we shall return to later). Katz (1988) discovered that people with Broca's aphasia activate multiple meanings in the same way. More recently, ambiguous primes like *fan* facilitated response to targets like *breeze* and *sport* with only a 100 millisecond prime–target interval for people with nonfluent aphasia (Klepousniotou & Baum, 2005). Therefore, Broca's aphasia does not necessarily include damage to spreading activation in semantic memory, casting doubt on the automaticity hypothesis for this type of aphasia (also, Grindrod & Baum, 2003; Janse, 2010).

Detecting Sentence Comprehension Deficits

When comprehending an isolated noun, a client does not have to deal with a functional role for that noun. Comprehending sentences, on the other hand, entails figuring out who is doing what to whom. In a sentence, a noun is an agent or recipient of an action, an instrument, or a location. In linguistic terms, this means figuring out the *thematic roles* of the nouns. Nearly all people with aphasia display a sentence comprehension deficit to some degree.

Aphasia Generally

Early study of sentence comprehension with aphasia was data-driven. There was scant interest in theoretical explanation. Investigators manipulated input to determine the attributes of sentences that contribute to comprehension difficulty and success. The results helped us determine severity of deficit and construct therapies that would be programmed to build complexity gradually.

Sentence comprehension is studied and assessed in several ways. Clients may match a sentence to a picture, follow instructions for manipulating toys or tokens, answer questions, or verify the truth of a sentence relative to a picture. Let us consider attributes of sentences that have been manipulated in each of these tasks.

One attribute is **complexity**, which was specified some time ago linguistically according to number of transformations applied to a simple active declarative statement such as *1a*:

(1a) The girl is reading a book.
(1b) A book is read by the girl.
(1c) A book is not read by the girl.

People with aphasia are challenged when the statement is turned into passive voice in *1b* and then by using two transformations, as in *1c*, for a negative-passive (e.g., Shewan & Canter, 1971). Complexity is also enhanced by embedding a clause within a statement, as in *2b*:

(2a) The man was greeted by his wife, and he was smoking his pipe.
(2b) The man greeted by his wife was smoking a pipe.

Sentence *2b* is shorter and says almost the same thing as *2a*, but the structure of *2b* is more difficult for people with aphasia to understand (Goodglass, Blumstein, Gleason, et al., 1979).

Another problematic attribute of sentences is thematic role **reversibility**. Let us consider the following example:

(3) The nurse kissed the girl.

Unlike the agent and recipient in *1a*, the agent and recipient in *3* can be reversed, and the sentence still makes sense. Thematically reversible statements can be difficult for people with aphasia (Heeschen, 1980). If we were to add complexity to reversibility (e.g., *The girl is kissed by the nurse*), we can make a sentence even harder for someone with aphasia to understand (Pierce & Wagner, 1985).

A related attribute known as the **canonicity** of a structure has a cultural implication. The active declarative of *1a* corresponds to the simplest and most common structure in English and in many other languages (e.g., agent–action–recipient), known as the canonical structure of a language. The canonical form in any language is the easiest structure to comprehend. Caplan and his colleagues studied canonicity in the context of center-embedded complexity:

(4a) The elephant that hit the monkey hugged the rabbit.
(4b) The elephant that the monkey hit hugged the rabbit.

Using an *enactment procedure* in which manipulating toy animals indicated comprehension, Caplan found that people with aphasia had more difficulty with *4b*, even though it is the same structure as *4a* (Caplan, Baker, & Dehaut, 1985). In *4b*, the recipient of *hit* appears before the agent, not after, as in *4a*. This canonicity effect also occurred with a picture-choice task (Caplan, Waters, & Hildebrandt, 1997).

One concern for diagnosing sentence comprehension problems is whether a deficit for a type of sentence is general across tasks (task-independent) or is unique to one task (task-dependent). A general problem points to the sentence structure as the culprit, whereas a task-specific problem points to the task and, perhaps, to a unique process in the task. Caplan and others (2006) explored this issue with 42 cases who were given sentence–picture matching and enactment tasks. They found only two cases of a general or task-independent deficit, mainly with passive sentences. For a large number of cases, difficulty with a particular type of sentence depended on the task used to assess it. Caplan called them "task-specific construction specific deficits." What this means clinically is that we should assess sentence-types with more than one task before a diagnosis targets a particular syntactic structure.

Asyntactic Comprehension

Broca's or agrammatic aphasia has been targeted in most studies. Grodzinsky (1991) called it "the flagship of the neuropsychology of language." Broca's aphasia gets so much attention for a few reasons. Deficits are substantive enough and participants are cooperative enough so that experiments run smoothly and produce reliable results. Also, the impairment appears to center on syntax, which gets many linguists excited about studying aphasia.

The manual for the *Auditory Comprehension Test for Sentences* (Shewan, 1979) shows that Broca's aphasia ranks in the midrange for major syndromes of aphasia (maximum score of 21):

- Anomic aphasia   14.8
- Broca's aphasia   12.5
- Wernicke's aphasia   9.7

Nevertheless, manuals for two major aphasia test batteries show a fairly wide range of deficit around the average score for Broca's aphasia (Goodglass, Kaplan, & Barresi, 2001; Kertesz, 2007). However, these numbers say nothing about whether this type of aphasia includes a particular kind of comprehension deficit cued by problems with a particular kind of sentence.

Explicit agrammatic production led early investigators to wonder if comprehension is damaged in a similar manner. They began by comparing lexical and syntactic factors in dealing with the attribute of reversibility. The most frequently cited early study is by Alfonso Caramazza and Edgar Zurif (1976). They compared reversible (*5a*) and nonreversible (*5b*) statements presented to participants who had either Broca's or conduction aphasias.

(5a) The girl that the boy is chasing is tall.
(5b) The apple that the boy is eating is red.

Because comprehension was thought to be relatively good with these syndromes, structurally complex sentences were used to heighten the challenge. Participants chose interpretations from two pictures. The foil differed either according to a lexical element or according to thematic role structure (i.e., reversal of agent and recipient).

Two findings have had a tenacious influence in the research community. First, participants with Broca's aphasia had particular difficulty with reversible statements (5a). Second, they made more thematic role order errors than lexical errors. Caramazza and Zurif concluded that people with Broca's aphasia are specially impaired when they must rely on word order to comprehend. Moreover, they retain access to semantic and pragmatic knowledge for comprehending thematic roles (e.g., apples do not eat). Suspicion of a unique syntactic problem grew with other studies showing mostly order errors when errors were made, even with reversible active sentences (e.g., Gallaher & Canter, 1982).

People with Broca's aphasia also had difficulty understanding passive sentences. Researchers started to identify this syndrome according to an "inability to interpret other than simple active structures" (Rosenberg, Zurif, Brownell, et al., 1985; see also Shapiro & Levine, 1990). Asyntactic comprehension has come to be diagnosed with the following:

- Deficit with thematically reversible sentences
- Deficit with noncanonical sentences (e.g., passives)
- Significantly more order errors than lexical errors

These criteria for identifying asyntactic (or agrammatic) comprehension can vary slightly, such as requiring a deficit only with reversible sentences. Some investigators may add a qualifier that clients additionally do well on word comprehension and grammaticality judgment tasks (Saffran, Schwartz, & Linebarger, 1998).

People with fluent aphasia and generally mild comprehension deficit appear to fare only slightly better with thematic role reversibility. Groups with conduction aphasia performed like those with Broca's aphasia (Caramazza & Zurif, 1976; Heilman & Scholes, 1976). Peach, Canter, and Gallaher (1988) compared anomic and conduction aphasia in comprehending thematic roles in active sentences. Both fluent groups were similar to people with Broca's aphasia, making significantly more subject–object order errors than lexical errors. Such findings are problematic for any claim that this comprehension pattern is unique to those with agrammatic aphasia.

Explaining Sentence Comprehension Deficits

Why do people with aphasia have difficulties with sentence structure? What happens in the mind to cause reversibility effects or canonicity effects? In explanatory research, the manner of obtaining the data is designed in a way that is appropriate for testing a particular theoretical account for what is observed. Following an introduction to explanation, let us consider attempts to identify internal language disorders in either lexical or syntactic systems. These system-specific proposals will be followed by more general cognitive territory such as attention and working memory.

Working Assumptions

Designing an appropriate theory-driven study requires giving some thought to the nature of language comprehension. According to Tyler (1987), core processes operate on a *principle of optimal efficiency* by assigning "an analysis to the speech input at the theoretically earliest point at which the type of analysis in question can be assigned" (p. 146). That is, the brain activates with the first syllable and proceeds from there.

Sentence comprehension is assumed to rely on three subsystems: a lexical processor, a syntactic processor, and an interpretive processor. Some psycholinguists focus on the lexical, and others specialize in syntactic structure. Others are more interested in the ultimate interpretation of sentences, especially in a narrative context (see Chapter 4). One hypothesis is that each processor operates as an autonomous subsystem and in a particular order (i.e., serially). A competitive hypothesis is that these components are interdependent and operate interactively or in parallel (i.e., simultaneously). Some investigators enter a study of aphasia believing in one of these assumptions, which may influence predictions about the effect of damage to one of the processors.

Researchers rely on two general types of procedure. The clinical tests noted previously are known as **off-line procedures**. That is, clients respond after a sentence is presented. This approach detects the cumulative result of all core processes or the *final interpretation* of a sentence. Conscious strategies contribute to the task's response (e.g., scanning pictures, decision making, pointing). These complications may account for results that depend on the task. **On-line procedures**, on the other hand, detect processes as they occur. Participants respond to a point within a sentence, before it is completed. The time to respond is indicative of relative processing load at the point of measurement. Consistent with the principle of optimum efficiency, the on-line approach is said to detect *intermediate interpretations* between the first syllable and the end of a sentence (Shapiro, Swinney, & Borsky, 1998; also, Poirier & Shapiro, 2012).

This definition of "on-line" (nothing to do with surfing the Web) is consistent with many areas of psycholinguistics. The term is deployed more broadly in the clinical literature, referring to any study of automaticity (e.g., semantic priming). Yet *on-line* has a temporal connotation and is restricted here to studies tapping into automatic processes in "real time." In aphasiology, for example, Caplan and Waters (2003) use a procedure called *self-paced listening*. Participants hear a sentence one segment at a time. They press a button signaling comprehension of each segment until the whole sentence is presented. The response time for each segment is the measure of cognitive effort at those points.

Lexical System

To study word comprehension in sentences, we might think that an appropriate method would be to put the semantic priming task into the middle of a sentence. This was done with neurologically intact adults, and it was discovered that an ambiguous word in a sentence instantaneously activates multiple meanings, even when prior context is biased to one interpretation (Seidenberg, Tanenhaus, Leiman, et al., 1982; Swinney, 1979). Thus, lexical-semantics can operate as an autonomous or "encapsulated" system, at least, immediately on hearing a word. On-line research also indicates that, a few syllables later, the context-sensitive meaning is the only meaning active.

Swinney, Zurif, and Nicol (1989) borrowed the method that places semantic priming within a sentence. Here is how it goes. A person with aphasia wears headphones for hearing the sentence, while sitting in front of a computer for viewing a target letter-string for lexical decision. Because of the two modalities, it is called **cross-modal priming**. An ambiguous word such as *plant* is placed in the spoken sentence such as 6:

> (6) The gardener was responsible for watering every *plant* * on the enormous estate.

While listening, participants made a lexical decision about a letter string (e.g., *tree, factory*) shown immediately after the ambiguous word (*). The word *plant* should act like a prime and activate multiple meanings. Unlike normal adults who were primed equally for multiple meanings, participants with Broca's aphasia were primed only for the dominant or most associated meanings (i.e., *tree*). Therefore, people with Broca's aphasia are, at least, slow to activate secondary meanings at more distant nodes.

If they are just slow, people with Broca's aphasia should activate multiple meanings eventually. To check this out, researchers placed the lexical decision five syllables later than the priming word. This allowed more time for activation to spread to other nodes, although by this time context narrows activated meaning in neurologically healthy people. Again, people with Broca's aphasia were primed only for the dominant meaning (Prather, Love, Finkel, et al., 1994). This could mean different things. One, participants were very slow to activate multiple meanings at this point. Two, participants were not slow but were unable to active multiple meanings. Three, multiple meanings were activated after a couple of syllables, and then context inhibited irrelevant meanings downstream from the ambiguous word (see also Swaab, Brown, & Hagoort, 1998). The results are frankly ambiguous.

Swinney's and Prather's studies included four participants with severe fluent aphasia. When the lexical decision was positioned five syllables after the prime, these participants maintained activation of multiple meanings. This is indicative of a different problem. Context failed to penetrate lexical access and inhibit irrelevant meanings. It is as if the lexical–semantic system was stuck in a modular mode. A failure to inhibit irrelevant information becomes pertinent later in this text.

In addition to meaning, the lexical processor activates information about syntax, which is carried by function words (i.e., free grammatical morphemes) and inflections (i.e., morphological structure of words). The lexicon also harbors knowledge of grammatical categories and the argument structure of verbs, called the *lemma*. One example reminds us that sentence comprehension entails figuring out who is doing what to whom. People with aphasia were asked to demonstrate comprehension of sentences in which position of *the* carried information about thematic roles. Researchers presented sentences in a picture-choice task with word-order and lexical foils:

(7a) She showed her baby the pictures.
(7b) She showed her the baby pictures.

Participants with Broca's aphasia had difficulty making word-order decisions (Heilman & Scholes, 1976). Elsewhere, participants with Broca's aphasia uniquely failed to distinguish definite and indefinite articles (Goodenough, Zurif, Weintraub, et al., 1977). Broca's aphasia developed a reputation for being insensitive to free-standing grammatical morphemes (e.g., Swinney, Zurif, & Cutler, 1980).

The notion of delayed lexical access was targeted at grammatical morphemes, similar to the locus of expressive deficits. Still, it is not clear how lexical deficits account for the asyntactic pattern. Lexical and/or semantic access for content words may not be as slow as once thought, but the possibility remains that word-meaning activation for sentences is a bit slow for some with Broca's aphasia. People with this aphasia also may have automatic processing capacities that break down in off-line tasks.

Syntactic System

A **syntactic parsing** mechanism assigns structure to a string of words (Carreiras & Clifton, 2004). To get a better idea of the nature of structure, let us consider Chomsky's (1957) famous sentence: *Colorless green ideas sleep furiously*. We can detect structure in this nonsense. The following *USA Today* headline, with its spacing, gives us another sense for assignment of structure:

(8) Cruise ship dumping poisons
seas, frustrates U.S. enforcers

As we read the first line with optimum efficiency, assigning structure at the earliest possible point, the headline reads, "the ship is dumping poisons." In the next line, we discover that this interpretation is incorrect, and we have to reanalyze the headline so that it reads, "the dumping poisons the seas." The word "poisons" is transformed from a noun to a verb. The difference in meaning is slight, but the structural ambiguity (called a *garden-path sentence*) makes us aware of syntactic structure. The study of structural assignment is challenging because we cannot literally see structure like we can see words. Linguists use "tree diagrams" to help us visualize these relations.

Theories of syntactic comprehension disorders have been divided into two categories (Choy & Thompson, 2010). *Representational theories* address the mind's encoding of structure and are proposed from a linguistic orientation. *Processing theories* refer to strategic and/or automatic mechanisms such as syntactic parsing and have a psycholinguistic orientation. Processing theories may also be identified with general cognitive systems such as working memory. Psycholinguistic and general cognitive theories may not be mutually exclusive, as language processes operate within the constraints of working memory.

A great deal of literature has been devoted to representational theories. Caplan and Futter (1986) proposed a **linearity hypothesis** stating that agrammatic individuals are fixated on assigning a canonical agent–action–recipient order to a string of words. This linear strategy works well for an aligned surface structure but causes trouble for sentences structured in a different thematic order. Evidence has come from Caplan's enactment procedure and picture-choice tasks.

Grodzinsky (1989) claimed that the impairment is an incomplete structural representation, rather than an assignment strategy. Normally, in passives, for example, a "trace" that designates thematic role is said to be left in the wake of *movement* of nouns from their canonical positions. Grodzinsky's **trace-deletion hypothesis** (TDH) has stated that people with Broca's aphasia delete traces and assign roles at random. The evidence has been below-chance off-line comprehension of sentences containing movement (Drai & Grodzinsky, 2006). There has been lots of debate (e.g., Caplan, DeDe, & Brownell, 2006; Caramazza, Capasso, Capitani, et al., 2005; De Bleser, Schwarz, & Burchert, 2006) and contrary on-line results (Hanne, Sekerina, Vasishth, et al., 2011). In a nutshell, Grodzinsky's TDH has favored a specific deficit in one aphasia, whereas others have detected more variability of deficit and not just in one aphasia.

Let us turn to process-oriented explanations. Proposals of an **impaired syntactic parser** began with the idea that syntactic information associated with inflection is not activated fast enough (Friederici, Wessels, Emmorey, et al., 1992). Evidence was provided with syntactic priming studies (Baum, 1988; Blumstein, et al., 1991; Haarmann & Kolk, 1991).

Verbs may have a direct influence on parsing because of the information that they carry about **predicate-argument structure**. Lemma knowledge includes the types of noun phrase that can be attached. For example, transitive verbs (e.g., *eat*) can take on recipients, but intransitive verbs cannot (e.g., *sleep*). Therefore, in an overlap between the lexicon and syntax, argument structure specifies the "frames" that can accompany a verb. Lewis Shapiro was interested in the influence of verb complexity according to the number of noun-phrase argument structures that can be attached. In particular, he looked for evidence of automatic activation of all possible argument structures, much like the multiple activation of word meanings.

To test the verb complexity idea, Shapiro looked into how this type of process had been studied before. He chose the cross-modal priming procedure and was interested in what happens at the site of the verb. People with Broca's aphasia activated multiple possibilities allowed by a verb, unlike restricted meaning activation. This effect dissipated downstream (Shapiro & Levine, 1990). Fluent participants, unlike Broca's aphasia, were impaired in activating verb-argument structures (Shapiro, Gordon, Hack, et al., 1993).

On-line studies have also addressed the linguistic phenomenon of movement and the processing of traces or "gaps." Edgar Zurif and David Swinney proposed a processing mechanism to handle gaps in sentences. The following types of sentences were presented over headphones for cross-modal priming (gaps are designated by the symbol for a trace [t]):

> (9a) The passenger smiled at *the baby* that the woman in the pink jacket fed [t] at the train station.
>
> (9b) The passenger smiled at *the baby* in the blue pajamas who [t] drank milk at the train station.

In *9b*, the "gap" is the pronoun. In *9a*, an empty space [t] implies movement of *the baby* from after *fed* to an earlier position. Antecedents (*the baby*) are thought to be *reactivated* at either of these gaps so that we can understand whom was fed and who drank the milk. If this is truly so, then the gaps should prime related visual targets (e.g., *diaper*) placed at the gaps.

Participants with Broca's aphasia failed to reactivate related targets at the gaps for both types of sentences, whereas normal controls evidenced antecedent reactivation or "gap filling" (Zurif, Swinney, Prather, et al., 1993). According to Zurif and Swinney, people with Broca's aphasia have a general deficit of concept reactivation rather than, according to Grodzinsky's TDH, a representational problem specific to movement (e.g., only *5a*). Further research indicated that the reactivation process is slow (Burkhardt, Piñango, & Wong, 2003; Love, Swinney, Walenski, et al., 2008).

Michael Dickey of the University of Pittsburgh and Cynthia Thompson of Northwestern University expanded the study of movement and filler-gap constructions. They developed two on-line techniques for their clinical research. They called one **auditory anomaly detection**, or a *stop-making-sense task*. Participants pressed a button as soon as a sentence "started to sound strange" (Dickey & Thompson, 2004). The other technique capitalized on an eye-tracking approach, used mainly to measure duration of eye fixations during reading. For studying aphasia, the investigators employed **eye-tracking while listening**. While participants listened to a story and answered questions about who was doing what to whom, Dickey and Thompson measured eye-fixations on a panel of objects, which included an agent and recipient of a sentence (Dickey & Thompson, 2009).

In one eye-tracking study, the investigators were interested in the processing of noncanonical questions containing wh- movement, as in *10*:

> (10) *Who* did the boy kiss [t] that day at school?

Participants with aphasia looked at the moved element as correctly and as quickly as control participants. This was surprising given the slowed-processing accounts of gap-filling, but it appeared that people with agrammatic aphasia comprehend wh-questions in real time (Dickey, Choy, & Thompson, 2007). However, on-line anomaly detection did expose some difficulty with other features of syntax (Faroqui-Shah & Dickey, 2009).

In conclusion, Caplan (1987) proposed the fundamental position that "syntactic comprehension impairments are often independent primary disorders of sentence processing" (p. 323). Moreover, the syntactic processor is not impaired in an all-or-none fashion but rather is impaired partially (Love & Brumm, 2012). Caplan (2002) advised that "caution must be observed in taking the pattern of performance . . . in sentence–picture matching or enactment (off-line tasks) as definitive evidence for a deficit in the unconscious, obligatory construction of syntactic structures" (p. 333).

General Theories of Comprehension Deficit

Some researchers have a different way of thinking about aphasia. Because language processing lives within cognition, it is logical that the underlying nature of aphasia includes a consideration of general systems. A common consideration is that some people with aphasia have accompanying cognitive limitations that exacerbate a language-specific impairment. For example, aphasia can be susceptible to breezes of **attention** difficulties. Distractions when multitasking may make some language processing with aphasia more brittle, even when the aphasia is mild (Murray, 2002; Murray, Holland, & Beeson, 1998). Attention is a complex component of cognition, discussed more in later chapters.

Short-term memory (STM) has been implicated because people with aphasia have difficulty with the immediate memory span task such as repeating a series of numbers or words of increasing length (e.g., Laures-Gore, Shisler Marshall, & Verner, 2011; Martin & Ayala, 2004). The deficit of repetition in conduction aphasia was purported to demonstrate a selective impairment of phonological STM (Shallice & Warrington, 1977). Short-term phonological encoding was reduced in most of Bartha and Benke's (2003) 20 clients with this aphasia.

Randi Martin at Rice University has been studying encoding in STM and has concluded that phonological STM has little to do with complex sentence comprehension in aphasia. However, she added that "some types of span deficits do cause sentence comprehension difficulties for patients" (Martin & Miller, 2002, p. 305). To examine such deficits, Martin used a **word padding** procedure in which several adjectives preceded a noun (e.g., *the rusty old red pail*). Some participants may not have retained *rusty* so that it could be connected to *pail*. Friedmann and Gvion (2003) put padding in complex sentences, and participants were unfazed by the amount of filler. These researchers concluded that STM does not explain comprehension deficits.

Working memory (WM) is where the cognitive workload is managed. Consciously strategic processing clogs WM, whereas automatic processing does not consume WM space. Another way of thinking about the capacity for mental manipulations is to speak of the **allocation of resources** when performing a task.

WM/resource allocation is tested in various ways. In *digit span backward*, digits are repeated in reverse order. The reversal requires that a mental manipulation be added to recall (Wright & Shisler, 2005). The *n-back test* consists of presenting lists of syllables or words and asking people to press a button when hearing an item heard 1-item back, 2-items back, and so on (Wright, Downey, Gravier, et al., 2007). Finally, the *dual-task paradigm* is like cognitive multitasking. A person performs two tasks at the same time, usually the main skill of interest and a distracter task. A deficit of resource allocation is indicated when performance on the main task is reduced with the distracter but is not reduced in a normal control group. The key ingredient is that the task demands something more than simple retention.

There are two general approaches in relating WM/resource allocation to comprehension deficits. In one, researchers show that people with aphasia are deficient in WM capacity or in managing dual tasks and then speculate that the deficit could be responsible for comprehension problems (e.g., Erickson, Goldinger, & LaPointe, 1996). Other investigators incorporate sentence comprehension into their studies. Caplan and Waters (1996) employed the dual-task paradigm. While taking a comprehension test, participants repeated a sequence of digits within their digit spans. The dual-task had no effect, indicating that WM capacity is not a factor for some people with aphasia. However, Wright and her colleagues (2007) found a correlation between the *n*-back test and off-line sentence comprehension. In general, the methods have been varied and the results have been mixed.

At the University of Pittsburgh, Malcolm McNeil took the strong position that a constrained WM accounts for most of what we know about aphasia. Initially, he argued that the variability of aphasic behavior cannot be explained solely with respect to impairment of language-specific mechanisms (Tseng, McNeil, & Milenkovic, 1993). Shuster (2004) took on this notion in *Aphasiology*'s Forum. Most of her concerns were essentially as follows:

- Resource allocation theory is too broad and flexible to be falsifiable (i.e., it can explain any result).
- Other theories can explain results used to support resource allocation (e.g., phonological coding deficit, slow processing speed).
- Some methodology has been inappropriate.

In reply to Shuster, there was some agreement regarding limitations of the methodology that had been used up to that point (McNeil, Hula, Matthews, et al., 2004). Later, McNeil, Hula, & Sung (2011) acknowledged that attentional resource explanations of aphasia have "a tendency toward vague usage of resource terminology" and that dual-tasks are "amenable to other interpretations."

Nevertheless, the Pittsburgh group went to work. Scores from a classic WM test predicted scores on a comprehension test and correlated with aphasia severity (Sung, McNeil, Pratt, et al., 2009). A word-by-word on-line version of the same comprehension test was presumed to tax WM capacity with adjective padding in simple instructions (e.g., *Put the black square by the red circle*, *Put the big red square before the big white circle*). Longer processing time for more adjectives was interpreted as evidence for a resource limitation (Sung, McNeil, Pratt, et al., 2011), although padding had not been a factor elsewhere (Friedmann & Gvion, 2003). In a dual-task paradigm, people with aphasia repeated stories while performing a visual tracking task. Absence of an effect of tracking difficulty was taken as evidence against a resource allocation problem (McNeil, Matthews, Hula, et al., 2006). In sum, evidence for an STM/WM/ resource allocation basis for aphasia has been mixed.

Word Finding and Retrieval

Turning to the more clinically accessible production of language, it has been observed that nearly all people with aphasia have some kind of difficulty with finding and retrieving words. Word retrieval is most often assessed with an object-naming task (or "confrontation naming"). Object-naming places word retrieval under a microscope in which we can examine difficulties with respect to an identified target.

There are many symptoms of word-finding deficit. People with aphasia may be unusually slow, may substitute generalities (e.g., *It's that thing you use for . . .*), may speak around the word (e.g., *You write and draw with it*), or make single-word errors that have different relationships to the target word (i.e., paraphasias, Chapter 1). Moreover, naming difficulty may not necessarily signify aphasia. Geschwind (1967) wrote of aphasic misnaming and nonaphasic misnaming, implying that errors in naming an object may be caused by an impaired language system (aphasic misnaming) or by another impairment such as visual agnosia (nonaphasic misnaming).

The CN Approach

Unlike the hidden result of comprehension, the outcome of word-finding can be heard or seen. Location of an underlying disorder may be hypothesized with respect to a theory of naming. Models begin with representing the stimulus as a percept and conclude with the motor response and then characterize mental events in between. The mental events may occur as follows: "The first step is the identification of the object as a member of a category whose stored representation provides a good match with the stimulus object. . . . Once a category representation has been activated, then the corresponding label is retrieved" (Brownell, Bihrle, & Michelow, 1986, p. 50).

The cognitive neuropsychological (CN) model in Figure 3.1 abbreviates the aforementioned mental events. It consists of independent processing components (in boxes) and routes between them. The model operates serially, that is, with each process informing the next process in a fixed order from the top down. Object recognition activates a concept in the semantic system (including the semantic network), which then points to the *phonological output lexicon* leading to speech production. For writing, lexical representation is called the *orthographic output lexicon.* Cognitive neuropsychologists tend to agree on the existence of semantic and lexical components, although terminology may vary (e.g., "conceptual system," "speech output lexicon"). Diagnosis is said to entail looking for the "functional lesion" in one of these components or in a route between them.

The most frequent question is whether an impairment lies in the semantic system or the lexical system (Nickels, 2001; Raymer, 2005). No one task leads to a diagnosis, because a single task like naming involves multiple processes. Similarly,

**FIGURE 3.1   A typical cognitive neuropsy-
chological (CN) model of object naming.
Diagnosis entails determining which component is impaired.**

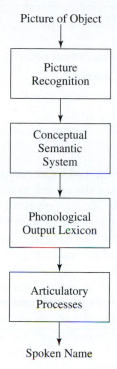

Picture of Object

Picture
Recognition

Conceptual
Semantic
System

Phonological
Output Lexicon

Articulatory
Processes

Spoken Name

a single error can have different interpretations (Mitchum, Ritgert, Sandson, et al.,
1990). Individual cases are presented with semantically and lexically oriented tasks
of sufficient variety to disclose a breakdown of one component and eliminate
breakdowns of other components. The strategy, called **componential analysis**, entails
comparing scores from a few tasks (Table 3.2) and then looking for common threads
among deficient and intact performances. Diagnostic criteria and task selection vary
among research teams (e.g., Antonucci, Beeson, Labiner, et al., 2008; Howard &
Gatehouse, 2006).

Let us start with the semantic component. A deficient semantic system would
send degraded conceptual information to the output lexicon. One type of evidence is
a comparison of naming errors to comprehension tasks that would reveal a common
semantic thread. Gainotti and his colleagues (1981) found an inconsistent relationship between type of naming error and type of word comprehension error. Another
research strategy is to compare naming to metalinguistic semantic tasks. Goodglass,
Wingfield, and Ward (1997) studied rapid decisions about categorical relationships

TABLE 3.2   Differential diagnosis of naming difficulties based on a process model of object naming similar to Figure 3.1.

PROCESS COMPONENT	DISORDER	RELATED TASKS
Object recognition	Visual agnosia	Match examples of an object; demonstrate use of object
Activation of semantic memory	Dementia or aphasia	Object classification; word–picture matching
Activation of lexical memory	Aphasia	Object naming; lexical decision task
Phonetic programming	Apraxia of speech	Complex word repetition
Motor execution	Dysarthias	Oral mechanism examination

between objects, but the tasks did not predict naming performance. At this point, semantics did not have a strong link to naming deficit.

Category-specific deficit points to semantic deficit (Warrington & Shallice, 1984). A client has a comprehension and naming problem in one conceptual domain (e.g., musical instruments). Category-specific deficits are seen mainly in dissociations between inanimate and animate things. In a comparison of cases, PS named 39 percent of animals and 90 percent of inanimate objects. Case JJ had the reverse dissociation, naming 91 percent of animals but only 20 percent of inanimate objects. JJ also favored animals in comprehension and written naming (Hillis & Caramazza, 1991). Scholars have entertained various explanations revolving around the idea that a semantic dissociation slices through a conceptual domain rather than attacking word forms (e.g., Capitani, Laiacona, Mahon, et al., 2003; Chialant, Costa, & Caramazza, 2002; Shelton & Caramazza, 2001).

Let us now turn to the output lexicon or words per se. Word familiarity is a lexical characteristic, perhaps, influencing how lexemes are stored (e.g., their threshold of activation). Early studies of aphasia established that familiar words are generally easier to find and retrieve than rare words. Although not typically assessed in CN case studies, one indication of partial lexical access is the **tip-of-the tongue (TOT) state**, in which properties of a word are conjured instead of the word itself. People with aphasia experiencing naming failure were instructed to point to the intended word's first letter, number of syllables, and *big* or *small* for size of the word. Participants guessed the word's properties over 60 percent of the time. It was as if an object activated parts of lexical form (Barton, 1971). In another study, some people with aphasia were less successful in reporting features of unspoken words, and a few others could not do it at all (Goodglass, Kaplan, Weintraub, et al., 1976).

Ellis, Kay, and Franklin (1992) provided a guide for distinguishing impairments at the semantic and lexical levels. Pervasive semantic deficits in comprehension and object classification are indicative of a problem at the semantic level. Another clue would be word-finding deficit in a particular semantic category. Then we use a process of elimination to diagnose a lexical impairment. We suspect that a disorder is confined to the lexical output system when word comprehension, object sorting, and other semantically based skills are relatively intact.

Psycholinguistic Study of Naming

CN models have been criticized for ignoring details, such as the differentiation of storage and process within the boxed components. Psycholinguists consider word-finding in the context of network structures and spreading activation processes. There are two fundamental positions. One, consistent with CN models, is that semantic and lexical processes operate in a **serial** fashion. Activation spreads sequentially from semantic memory to lexical memory (Schriefers, Meyer, & Levelt, 1990). The other position, more common in psycholinguistics, is that systems are **interactive**, meaning they operate simultaneously or "in parallel" (Dell & O'Seaghda, 1992).

When she was in London, Lyndsey Nickels (1995) conducted experiments comparing serial and interactive models to predict relationships between certain variables and paraphasias. Imageability of words was a semantic variable. Word length was a lexical variable. Word familiarity was related to both semantic and lexical modules. The interactive version predicts that all variables would affect both types of errors. A serial model is more selective, predicting that imageability would be related to semantic errors and length would be related to phonological errors. Results supported the serial model.

Gary Dell, a psycholinguist at the University of Illinois, suggested that word-form retrieval requires *two* steps after semantic activation, naturally called the "interactive two-step model" (Dell, Schwartz, Martin, et al., 1997). According to this theory, processing evolves as a series of "jolts" from semantics to grammatical information to sound. Dell performed sophisticated statistical analyses of naming errors. He also used computer simulations (i.e., computational modeling) of different versions of this theory, predicting naming patterns with aphasia (Schwartz, Dell, Martin, et al., 2006; Abel, Huber, & Dell, 2009).

There is an approach to picture-naming that is like priming methods called the **picture–word interference task**. It is employed "to track the activation of semantic and phonological processing during the course of naming" (Hashimoto & Thompson, 2010, p. 585). The experimenter simply measures time to name a picture, but a competitor word casually appears on the picture. This word is related semantically or phonologically to the picture's name. Like a prime, the printed competitor is incidental to the naming task. It is just there. It is presumed that the brain reacts to it, though, one way or another.

Tracking stages in the process is enabled by comparing effects of the overlaid competitors in interaction with brief intervals between appearance of the competitor and the picture. Hashimoto and Thompson (2010) presented this technique to eleven people with moderate-to-mild aphasias. Assuming that the semantic and phonological competitors tap into semantic and lexical processes separately, two normal effects emerged. An early semantic interference slowed naming, whereas a later phonological facilitation speeded naming. Without delving deeply into the logic of this paradigm, let us try to be content with the conclusion that semantics preceded the lexicon, indicating that people with mild aphasia have a conventional word-retrieval mechanism.

Action Naming (Verbs)

Twenty years ago, clinical researchers were mainly interested in the retrieval of nouns. Now, verbs are catching up in assessment and treatment. Verbs are more difficult to retrieve for some people with aphasia. Others have more difficulty with nouns, and others show no difference (Berndt, Mitchum, Haendiges, et al., 1997; Jonkers & Bastiannse, 1998). The dissociations between nouns and verbs have been classified as *grammatical category-specific deficits* in contrast to semantic category-specific deficits (e.g., Chialant, et al., 2002; Laiacona & Caramazza, 2004).

Researchers have suggested that greater difficulty with nouns tends to occur in posteriorly lesioned persons, whereas greater difficulty with verbs tends to occur in anteriorly lesioned individuals including those with Broca's aphasia (Bastiaanse & Jonkers, 1998; Kim & Thompson, 2000; Miceli, Silveri, Villa, et al., 1984; Williams & Canter, 1987; Zingeser & Berndt, 1990). Does this mean that noun retrieval is located in posterior regions and verb retrieval is located in the frontal lobe? Crepaldi and others (2011) investigated this *fronto-temporal dichotomy hypothesis* (FTDH) with a thorough review of the literature. They reported exceptions to this dichotomy, and neuroimaging experiments suffered from roadblocks to confident interpretation. Results possess "a great deal of inconsistency," and FTDH "is far from being even partially confirmed" (Crepaldi et al., 2011, p. 45).

To be confident that a dissociation is between grammatical categories, researchers control for *nuisance variables*, such as stimulus familiarity and complexity (Capitani et al., 2003). For example, a problem in naming actions may be caused by the way that actions are pictured. Kemmerer and Tranel (2000a) investigated a number of variables with brain-damaged people, some who were impaired and others who were unimpaired in action naming. They found that stimulus familiarity and complexity made little difference in the group data but that these variables did matter for a few individuals. Researchers still institute controls so that results can be interpreted with minimal ambiguity.

Word Retrieval with Fluent Syndromes

Therapy for fluent aphasias emphasizes word-finding over sentence-structuring, especially for people with **anomic aphasia**. Good comprehension enables these clients to perform about equally when naming verbal descriptions and naming objects (Goodglass & Stuss, 1979). Pashek and Tompkins (2002) found that word-finding can be better in the stream of narrative production than in picture-naming. We can conclude that confrontation naming is not necessarily predictive of word-finding in narrative production for mild aphasia, and therefore, we should assess word retrieval with naming, narration, and, probably, conversation.

Circumlocution is indicative of appropriate semantic activation (i.e., the concept to be conveyed) whereas the intended lexeme is elusive (Kohn & Goodglass, 1985). While the idea is active, could information about the word still be on the tip-of-the-tongue? In one study, when a participant could not name a famous person, he or she was asked questions about the person and the name. Participants with anomic aphasia differed from other syndromes. When they could not name, they produced semantic information 91 percent of the time but could identify the first letter only 7 percent of the time. The former was better and the latter worse than the other syndromes. People with anomic aphasia had a fairly intact semantic system but an occasional serious difficulty accessing an entire lexical form, or "access to phonology was more of an all-or-none phenomenon with the anomic group" (Beeson, Holland, & Murray, 1997, p. 333).

Sound-related errors (i.e., phonemic paraphasias) are a modification of an accurate lexical form and can be a distraction when listening to someone with **conduction aphasia**. Conduction aphasia does not seem to involve the all-or-none retrieval found in anomic aphasia. Most sound-related errors are nonwords (Wilshire, 2002; Schwartz, Wilshire, Gagnon, et al., 2004), but a few individuals produce a high rate of formal paraphasias such as *lazer* for *razor* (Gold & Kertesz, 2001).

Phonological problems of conduction aphasia are investigated with respect to either stage theory or interactive-activation theory (Caramazza, Papagno, & Ruml, 2000; Kohn & Smith, 1995; Wilshire & Fisher, 2004). A linguist at the University of Hamburg, Germany, compared published transcripts from a variety of syndromes to published records of normal slips of the tongue and slips of the pen. Phonemic paraphasia appeared to be comparable to slips of the pen but not slips of the tongue. Phonemic paraphasia was hypothesized to be a manifestation of an abnormally slow-moving structural activation system in the way that written production is more plodding than speech (Berg, 2006).

People with **Wernicke's aphasia** make more errors naming than those with other syndromes. The sample in Chapter 1 has complete sentences with grammatical morphemes in the right places. The sample is hard to interpret with one neologism (i.e., "repuceration") and words like *barbers* that have no connection to context. It is the number of neologisms or nonwords that set these clients apart (Mitchum et al., 1990). Moreover, they often ignore the strangeness of their own speech. In one recent study, severity of self-monitoring deficit was correlated with severity of naming and word repetition deficits but was not correlated with auditory comprehension deficit (Sampson & Faroqi-Shah, 2011). Also, people with Wernicke's aphasia appear less likely to exhibit the TOT state (Goodglass et al., 1976).

Word-finding in the flow of spontaneous speech is of greater concern for communication. Two kinds of jargon are recognized based on the type of paraphasias dominating utterances. Mostly semantic paraphasias is called *semantic jargon*, sounding like the speaker's language but with odd word choices. When neologisms dominate, *neologistic jargon* sounds like a strange language invented by the client. Semantic jargon is thought to be a less-severe form because it contains mostly real words.

Investigators have been interested in whether the word forms in jargon are related in any way to the user's language. Rinnert and Whitaker (1973) inventoried semantic paraphasias and found that 60 percent of error targets corresponded to association norms for the error and the target. Thirty-five years later, Bormann and others (2008) found that semantic paraphasias come from familiar options. Marshall (2006) concluded that "lexical access is rarely obliterated," at least, in milder semantic jargon.

Neologisms tend to consist of phonological sequences that are permissible in a client's language. Here is a brief example: "I appreciate that farshethe, because they have protocertive" (Buckingham & Kertesz, 1976, p. 66). Rare exceptions are forms like "chpicters." Investigators have distinguished two types. *Target-related neologisms* retain some phonological similarity to the target. Stenneken and colleagues (2008) examined *abstruse neologisms*, which have so little relationship to the target that, even in context, the lexical origin of the neologism cannot be identified. Even these neologisms had a strong phonological relationship to a client's language.

Hugh Buckingham, a linguist, speculated about a psycholinguistic basis for neologisms. One proposal was that a person with Wernicke's aphasia has a deep anomic aphasia but makes automatic or subconscious adjustments with a "random generator," somewhat wildly filling empty lexical slots with neologisms. This was called a *masking theory* (Buckingham, 1987). Neologisms become "strings of well-formed phonemes or syllables that fill in the gaps and compensate for words not retrievable from the lexicon" (Buckingham, 1981, p. 198). Thus, a lesion may produce an abnormal process in addition to damaging a normal process.

Sentence Production and Agrammatism

As soon as we train our sights on grammar, we think about Broca's aphasia or "agrammatic aphasia." Clinicians usually elicit sentences with picture description or an interview. More restrictive procedures include completing a sentence or short story and creating a sentence given a noun or verb. Faroqi-Shah and Thompson (2003) used pictures of simple actions to elicit active and passive sentences. In a picture, an arrow would point to either an agent or recipient, and clients were instructed to start a sentence with the target of the arrow. With the arrow pointing to a recipient of an action, a client would be steered to producing a passive sentence.

Symptoms of Agrammatism

A variety of grammatical phenomena can be heard in the speech of someone with Broca's aphasia. To encourage research, a vast archive of discourse from people with aphasia is available at a Web site called *AphasiaBank* (MacWhinney, Fromm, Holland, et al., 2010). Research has provided us with methods for identifying symptoms and for measuring deficits such as *Quantitative Production Analysis* (QPA; Berndt, Wayland, Rochon, et al., 2000; Gordon, 2006) and *Systematic Analysis of Language Transcripts*

(SALT; Armstrong, Ciccone, Godecke, et al., 2011; Miller & Iglesias, 2008). We attend to two broad features of grammar. One is grammatical morphology or lexical characteristics (e.g., Miceli, Silveri, Romani, et al., 1989). The other feature is syntax or phrase structure (e.g., Byng & Black, 1989). Awareness of the symptoms helps us to focus our diagnosis and, thus, our therapy.

Agrammatism, studied primarily in the English language (Bates & Wulfeck, 1989), has been portrayed as "telegramese" because of **grammatical morpheme omissions** (Gardner, 1974). These morphemes include *function words* (e.g., articles, conjunctions) and *inflectional attachments* marking pluralization, subject–verb agreement, and verb tense. Let us look at a couple of hypothetical descriptions of a woman in a kitchen:

- Function word omission: *Mother washing dishes . . . water flows sink.*
- Inflection omission: *The mother is wash dish . . . the water flow from the sink.*

Neat dissociations like this are rare, however. Usually agrammatism contains a mixture of function word and inflectional omissions.

Is telegramese a myth? Theories state that people with Broca's aphasia choose a "telegraphic register" as an adaptive strategy. Tesak and Niemi (1997) compared agrammatism in four languages to telegrams written by a large neurologically intact group. In normal telegrams, function word omissions ranged across languages from 61 percent (Dutch) to 77 percent (German). In agrammatism, however, there were only 7 percent omissions in Swedish and 66 percent in Dutch. Therefore, agrammatism and telegrams can be quite similar, but their similarity depends on the language.

Consistency of deficits has been debated vigorously. In one study, narratives were obtained from 29 people with Broca's aphasia. One subgroup produced more free-standing function words than bound morphemes, and another subgroup displayed the opposite pattern (Rochon, Saffran, Berndt, et al., 2000). The researchers distinguished between *morphological agrammatism*, which emphasizes problems with grammatical morphemes, and *constructional agrammatism*, which emphasizes short and simple phrase structure.

In addition to morpheme omissions, **grammatical morpheme substitution** is possible but is more likely in languages other than English (e.g., Swedish). Omission can no longer be considered a universal or definitive characteristic (Bates, Friederici, & Wulfeck, 1987b). Miceli redefined agrammatism as referring to "the omission of free-standing grammatical morphemes with or without the substitution of bound grammatical morphemes" (Miceli et al., 1989, p. 450). Focusing on verbs, studies showed that tense inflection (e.g., *the boy walked*) is harder to produce than agreement inflection (e.g., *the boy walks*) across a variety of languages (e.g., Kok, van Doorn, & Kolk, 2007).

Agrammatic individuals produce **structural simplifications** or what Rochon and others (2000) called constructional agrammatism. Simplifications may arise from a conscious strategy for coping with complexity (Chapter 10). Some structures are harder to produce than others. In the aforementioned study consisting of pictures with arrows, participants with Broca's aphasia produced 60 to 80 percent of cued active sentences but only 10 to 30 percent of the cued passives. On an optimistic note, providing a printed inflected cue (e.g., *was hugged*) improved production of passives dramatically to about 80 percent (Faroqi-Shah & Thompson, 2003).

Still keeping it simple, agrammatic individuals do not use subordinate clauses as much as neurologically intact adults (Bastiaanse, Edwards, & Kiss, 1996). Instead of embedding a phrase with modifiers, an agrammatic client may sequence ideas as a series of simple structures. For example, instead of constructing a noun phrase such as *a large white house*, a client may say "a large house, a white house." A client might say "girl tall and boy short" instead of "the girl is taller than the boy" (de Roo, Kolk, & Hofstede, 2003; Gleason, Goodglass, Green, et al., 1975).

Do people with agrammatism make **structural errors** such as an illegal word order? Or, do they maintain some integrity of their language like the phonology in Wernicke's aphasia? Syntactically speaking, English does not permit structures like *man the* or *ing-walk*, and such errors do not tend to occur with aphasia (Bates, Friederici, Wulfeck, et al., 1988). In Byng and Black's (1989) study, three element utterances were nearly always in the correct noun–verb–noun (NVN) order. Thus, linguistic difficulties are held together by fundamental linguistic rules.

Roelien Bastiaanse of the University of Groningen, the Netherlands, has directed students from several countries in the study of verbs in sentences. For example, she found that Italian agrammatic speakers tend to omit verbs and make inflectional errors (e.g., tense markers; Rossi & Bastiaanse, 2008). Those with a verb-finding problem often use vague verbs in narration (e.g., *get, do, have*) and tend to simplify sentence structure (Berndt et al., 1997). This difficulty with verbs could have implications for sentence production because of the grammatical information carried in a verb's lemma. As noted for comprehension, the lemma contains clues to predicate-argument structure, which specifies the "frames" that can accompany a verb (e.g., transitive vs. intransitive verbs). People with Broca's aphasia find transitive verbs to be easier to produce (Jonkers & Bastiaanse, 1998).

Predicate-argument complexity is manifested in whether a verb can take on one, two, or three arguments. Here are examples: one place: *The dog is barking.* two places: *The boy is catching the ball.* three places: *The woman is giving the money to the girl.* For people with agrammatism, Kim and Thompson (2000) found that action-naming accuracy was a function of this complexity. One-place verbs were retrieved around 80 percent of the time, and three-place verbs were retrieved a little over 40 percent of the time. In Italy, people with agrammatism prefer simple verb-argument structures (Rossi & Bastiaanse, 2008); and, in observation of Russian speakers, difficulty increases with a greater number of argument structures (Dragoy & Bastiaanse, 2010).

Debate over variability of symptoms is not confined to asyntactic comprehension. The quality of agrammatic syntax varies with the elicitation task. An unconstrained task like *Tell me about your illness* elicits worse structure than a more constrained task like *Tell me who is doing what to whom in this picture* (Sahraoui & Nespoulous, 2012). Yet this is just subtle variability of someone's agrammatism.

More seriously, some aphasiologists have questioned whether agrammatism is a legitimate entity. Miceli and others (1989) took the strong position that data "can no longer be ignored just for the obstinate protection of a fictional category of dubious theoretical value" (p. 475). Caplan (1991) countered that variability in agrammatism is indicative of the complexity of sentence formulation. In his opinion, agrammatism is an appropriate classification, and we just have to learn more about the intricacies of grammatical processes and, perhaps, be more flexible in defining agrammatism.

Speculation about grammatical oddities in the jargon of Wernicke's aphasia led to the term **paragrammatism** (not "agrammatism"). Paragrammatism consists of grammatical errors or symptoms of commission. Although a logical possibility, this term may not stand for a legitimate entity. For one thing, the errors do not appear or are hard to find. Phrase-level order errors that were absent in Broca's aphasia were also absent in Wernicke's aphasia (Bates et al., 1988). Also, jargon may contain fewer and simpler structures than normal, which is a feature of agrammatism (Gleason et al., 1980). "We conclude that the contrast between agrammatism (attributed to Broca's aphasia) and paragrammatism (attributed to Wernicke's aphasia) has been greatly exaggerated" (Bates & Wulfeck, 1989, p. 137).

Explanations of Agrammatism

What goes wrong in the linguistic mind to cause agrammatism? By now, the reader might anticipate that the list of answers is longer than desired. Initially, this multi-dimensional symptom was simply attributed to a dissociation of syntax from other components of language (Caramazza & Berndt, 1978). It was called the "no-syntax hypothesis" (Kolk & Van Grunsven, 1985). Problems with this hypothesis began with its ambiguity and its ambivalence on whether it refers to knowledge or processes.

Let us first consider grammatical knowledge in long-term memory. Is the disorder a "loss of grammar" that should be taken literally to be an erasure of linguistic competence? A common strategy for evaluating grammatical storage is to compare performance on a number of tasks. Schnitzer (1978) wrote that "a deficiency which affected all of the linguistic abilities would have to be either a remarkable coincidence or (more likely) a deficiency in the linguistic competence underlying all modalities" (p. 347). Caplan (1985) added that "disturbances found only in one language task have been considered to be disturbances in performance, sparing competence . . ." (p. 133).

For determining the status of linguistic competence, investigators often turn to a *metalinguistic task*. In such tasks we are thinking about language as in editing what someone has written. Some metalinguistic tasks involve "shallow processing" (Linebarger, Schwartz, & Saffran, 1983) and circumvent everyday comprehension and production (Baum, 1989). The most common task for grammar is *grammaticality judgment* or the detection of errors or violations of linguistic rules. The ability of agrammatic individuals to detect morphological and syntactic violations of all sorts has been demonstrated repeatedly in many languages (e.g., Devescovi, Bates, D'Amico, et al., 1997; Linebarger et al., 1983; Wulfeck, Bates, & Capasso, 1991).

These findings strongly support the view that people with Broca's aphasia retain grammatical knowledge.

Linguistic theories postulate a limitation on generation of a phrase structure or "syntactic tree." To fit into cognition, these theories could be referring to how the mind represents information during the formulation process. Caplan (1985) wrote of an "impoverished syntactic representation" that mirrors his linearity theory of comprehension. People with agrammatism activate a canonical form to convey any message (e.g., a simplification strategy). A different view is the *tree pruning hypothesis* (TPH) in which the highest nodes of a structural hierarchy are "impaired or inaccessible" or "do not exist" (Friedmann, 2006; Friedmann & Grodzinsky, 1997; Tissen, Weber, Grande, et al., 2007).

TPH has been evaluated in a number of ways. Studies have uncovered exceptions to the results supporting TPH (e.g., Burchert, Meisner, & De Bleser, 2008). For example, equal deficits of agreement and tense marking (and other results) led investigators at Northwestern University to conclude that agrammatic deficits "may result from disruption of differing underlying mechanisms and, therefore, they may require separate treatment strategies" (Lee, Milman, & Thompson, 2008, p. 893).

Schwartz, Lingebarger, and Saffran (1985) noted that "it is one thing to describe agrammatism in syntactic terms and quite another to locate the responsible deficit in a mechanism that constructs syntactic representations" (p. 86). In search of a mechanism, aphasiologists turned to Garrett's (1984) serial theory of production, which was originally intended to account for normal "slips of the tongue." In the model, formulation begins with an idea and concludes in two motor stages. In between, there are two levels of language formation. The first level, closest to the idea (or meaning), is a "deep" or abstract level of semantic–syntactic structure. The second level is closer to the surface where specific word forms are inserted into syntactically arranged slots.

Focusing on omission of function words, Garrett (1984) proposed that agrammatism is caused by damage in the surface level of the mechanism (formally called the positional-level) because this is where function words are selected. Also, evidence of intact deeper-level formulation is demonstrated by retention of basic canonical structure and logical location of agents and other thematic roles around a verb. Omission and substitution of grammatical morphemes as well as structural simplification have been interpreted as damage to the level closer to the surface (Caramazza & Berndt, 1985; Ostrin & Schwartz, 1986; Webster, Franklin, & Howard, 2001).

Thompson and her students introduced psycholinguistic methods. One procedure was *syntactic priming* in which participants with aphasia first repeated a sentence (an active or passive prime). Then, these participants, having been encouraged to use the same type of sentence, described a second picture (the target). An eye-tracker recorded eye-movements during sentence production. Errors included active sentences for passives and passively primed passives with role reversals. This combination of results and the eye-fixations were indicative of a structural impairment, not a morphological impairment (Cho & Thompson, 2010; also, Lee & Thompson, 2011).

Summary and Conclusions

This chapter covered what people with aphasia have in common and what makes some people with aphasia unique. Nearly everyone with aphasia has a problem with comprehension and some kind of difficulty retrieving words. Thus, general objectives of treatment are related to improving comprehension and improving access to words (Chapter 8). More specific language therapies are prompted, in principle, by an increase of precision in the observation of behavior and the diagnosis of impairments (Chapter 9).

Broca's aphasia received a lot of attention, but it is a swaggering flagship in a contentious sea. Clinical scientists tend to agree that people with this and other types of aphasia have not lost their knowledge of grammar and that impairments should be identified with processing. Yet experts differ regarding the characterization of processing and processing impairments. Adventurous researchers explore on-line procedures such as cross-modal priming, self-paced listening, and eye-tracking. We will have to wait to see what this work brings for separating automatic and strategic processing.

What does the research on attention and working memory say about our traditional definition of aphasia as a language-specific disorder? Researchers have approached the relationship between cognition and language impairment in two ways. Some boldly attribute language deficits to a general cognitive impairment, which indicates a modification of definition is in order. Others suggest that some people with aphasia have additional cognitive difficulties that accompany and may exacerbate the traditionally defined language impairment. This discussion will continue to be covered in journal articles and in conference presentations.

The robust conclusion that aphasia is an impairment of processing has had implications for how we approach therapy. The lack of agreement about a specific impairment is important for the clinical consumer of research to realize in case someone claims to have the answer. The lack of definite answers excites scientists and annoys clinicians. It is annoying for students when studying for an exam, but it also excites students who want to become the next great explorers. Rather than looking for simple answers, it may be good for now to understand methodologies and the thinking that goes into them.

CHAPTER

4 Investigating Communication and Participation

Functional or pragmatic aspects of aphasia coincide with the World Health Organization's (WHO's) former classifications of activity limitation and participation limitation (Chapter 1). The logic is that the language impairment (Chapter 3) puts a strain on communicative activities and participation for life. This chapter begins with the cognitive basis for pragmatic language use and then proceeds to more descriptive studies of functional verbal and nonverbal behavior. This sets a foundation for later chapters on functional therapies and other cognitive disorders. In conclusion, the chapter introduces participation by communicative partners and implications for quality of life, which become bigger topics for rehabilitation.

Cognitive Pragmatics

Relating words to meanings is not the whole story regarding language processing. People use language in various contexts for various purposes, and cognitive processes rise to these occasions. The study of natural language use is called **pragmatics**. For explanatory constructs, Tirassa (1999) drew attention to *cognitive pragmatics,* which is the study of mental processes responsible for the functional or natural use of language (see also Bara, 2005). We do not have to stray to recognize these processes, because the pragmatic mind is the same mind activated for basic language functions (Davis, 2007b).

Manipulations of contextual variables set the science of cognitive pragmatics apart from basic psycholinguistics. Contexts for the language system are **external**, such as a communicative situation, and **internal**, such as world knowledge and emotional states. Communication relies on these contexts in different ways. Conversation is more *situation dependent* because many referents exist in surroundings. Reading is more *knowledge dependent* because interpretation depends heavily on the reader's knowledge and imagination. "Rarely can we look around the room to make sense of what we have just read in a book" (Smith, 1982, p. 82).

The Problem: Speaker Meaning

In the messages exchanged in real-world language use, there is "a gap between the semantic representations of sentences and the thoughts actually communicated by utterances" (Sperber & Wilson, 1986, p. 9). A *speaker's meaning* can differ from the literal representation of a sentence or *sentence meaning*. In a notorious murder trial in England, a teenager's life hinged on his intent when he said "Let him have it, Chris" to a friend pointing a gun at a policeman. In this case, meaning lies in the speaker's intent and a listener's interpretation. Did the teenager mean "give him the gun" or "shoot him"? Interpretation probably depended on the situation and the listener's knowledge of the speaker.

How do we study or evaluate the exchange of hidden intentions? A solution to this problem includes finding some clear differences between sentence meanings and speaker meanings that can be presented in experiments. One approach to distinguishing these meanings was Searle's (1969) contention that the basic unit of communication is the *speech act*. Speech acts include asserting, greeting, warning, and requesting. When we ask politely "Can you open the door?" we are requesting rather than literally asking about someone's ability to open the door. The act of requesting is part of speaker meaning, and someone with aphasia can produce speech acts mainly because it does not take much verbalization to greet, warn, request, and so on.

People with aphasia understand the point of indirect requests. In one study, video vignettes contained a situation followed by a request (e.g., "Can you open the door?"). Another actor made either a pragmatically appropriate response to speaker meaning or an inappropriate literal response (i.e., "Yes"). A mixed group of participants with aphasia usually responded to speaker meaning, indicating their ability to relate the situation to the utterance (Wilcox, Davis, & Leonard, 1978). This ability was unrelated to clinical measures of literal comprehension. Other evidence supports the conclusion that aphasia does not impair the capacity to make nonliteral interpretations (e.g., Foldi, 1987).

Context (e.g., situation, topic) may determine whether a statement should be understood literally (e.g., *fan the flame* of the campfire) or figuratively (e.g., *fan the flame* of the relationship). Metaphors vary from those that stand alone (e.g., *he kicked the bucket*) to the novel metaphors of a creative writer, requiring external or internal context to be understood. A metaphor that stands alone, called an idiom, is readily interpreted figuratively rather than literally and is said to be "conventionalized" or "frozen" in meaning. It was thought that comprehending a metaphor involves more effort than literal interpretation, but Gibbs (2006), who has studied figurative language extensively, doubts that this is necessarily the case. He concluded that there is no single theory of metaphor comprehension and that figurative meanings can be activated very much like literal meanings.

The clinical study of metaphor comprehension began with presentation of phrases like *heavy heart* and *colorful music*. People with aphasia chose nonliteral meanings more often than literal meanings and scoffed at absurd literal options (Winner & Gardner, 1977). Similarly, idioms were easier than novel sentences for people with left-hemisphere dysfunction (LHD) to understand (Van Lanker & Kempler, 1987). People with aphasia are sensitive to indirectness, contrasting with the literalness of people with right-hemisphere dysfunction (RHD).

It has become common to follow traditional studies of strategic processing with a look at the same problem at the automatic level. Metaphoric interpretation is no different. Tompkins (1990) employed a semantic priming task in which a lexical target (e.g., *sharp*) was preceded by a metaphoric prime (e.g., *smart*), literal prime (e.g., *dull*), or an unrelated prime (e.g., *warm*). Both related primes facilitated target recognition for people with aphasia, indicating a built-in semantic connectivity for metaphor and literalness. Tompkins' study was also a rudimentary beginning for her investigations of RHD (Chapter 11).

The Mechanism: Inference

Inference is the general cognitive mechanism for deriving nonliteral, speaker meanings. A simple version is an elaborative inference in which literal meaning is supplemented, often automatically, with additional information. An example is to hear "The woman stirred the coffee" and think of [spoon]. "Inferencing" may be referred to as *inference generation,* not to be confused with production.

Do people with aphasia generate inferences without being asked to do so explicitly? A cross-modal priming task is suited for answering this question. In one study, pairs of sentences were presented such that the first sentence should leave one impression, but the second sentence should change that impression, called *inference revision* (Harris Wright & Newhoff, 2004). The impressions were detected with a lexical decision target presented after each sentence. An example follows:

(1a) Bill bumped the car in front of him while going around the curve. *accident*
(1b) At the end of the ride, Bill got out of the bumper car. *fair* or *accident*

The first sentence, *1a,* is likely to activate the concept of a traffic accident, but *1b* shifts the scenario to a ride at a fair. In the task, a spoken sentence (prime) preceded a visual word target such as those following the examples. After hearing each sentence, participants with aphasia made lexical decisions about word and nonword targets. Priming of *fair* would be indicative of inference revision. If *accident* continued to be primed after the second sentence, then participants would be presumed to have failed to revise their inference about the depicted scenario. So, how did the aphasic participants do?

Groups with nonfluent and fluent aphasia had moderate-to-mild language deficits. Participants with nonfluent aphasia activated the intended meanings for each sentence in a pair as did neurologically intact participants. Although most of the fluent group was mildly impaired, this group included several participants who generated the first inferences (e.g., *accident*) but not the revisions (e.g., *fair*). Therefore, with mild fluent aphasia, a person can have a subtle deficit of inhibiting an inference that is no longer appropriate and, thus, may have trouble arriving at a full interpretation of a speaker's intended meaning.

Prosody

Prosody has been considered to be a kind of context for linguistic processing. Researchers have spoken of *intonation* and *prosody* interchangeably, but intonation is actually a component of prosody (Seddoh, 2002). To be technical, prosody encompasses the timing, rhythm, and intonation of utterance, and intonation is the use of pitch to convey meaning (Fasold & Connor-Linton, 2006). There is a distinction between **linguistic** and **affective** prosody, whereby the former serves functions of meaning resolution, and the latter conveys emotions.

People with aphasia were expected to have difficulties with linguistic prosody. However, word stress for distinguishing meanings was shown to be intact, as participants with aphasia could tell the difference between *con*vict and con*vict, sore*head and sore *head, white*cap and white *cap* (Blumstein & Goodglass, 1972). At the sentence level, people with severe comprehension deficits, including Wernicke's aphasia, could recognize the difference between a statement and a question through prosodic contours (Green & Boller, 1974). People with Broca's aphasia had difficulty resolving global ambiguities such as *they fed her dog biscuits* (i.e., *dog* as a recipient or adjective) with stress and juncture cues (Baum, Daniloff, Daniloff, et al., 1982).

Years later, Walker and her colleagues (2002) looked at lexical stress, sentence-type contours, and pauses for clarifying ambiguous sentence meaning. An example of syntactic ambiguity follows:

(2) The boy said the girl is fat.

    (a) The boy said, the girl is fat.
    (b) The boy, said the girl, is fat.

The two possible interpretations are indicated by the commas in *2a* and *2b*. The task was to point to the picture that goes with the sentence (e.g., a fat girl, a fat boy). LHDs were worse than RHDs for all three types of prosody.

Baum and Dwivedi (2003) felt that Walker's off-line tasks provided an incomplete picture, especially because structural assignment probably occurs long before a person points to a picture. Baum and Dwivedi used garden-path sentences like those used in psycholinguistic studies of syntactic parsing. One example follows (keep in mind real-time structural assignment, reading left to right):

(3) The workers considered the last offer from the management was a real insult.

Inserting *that* after the first verb disambiguates the sentence, and so does subtle prosodic pause. A cross-modal priming task was used to determine if prosody facilitates the assignment of structure. Unlike Walker's results, both LHDs and RHDs showed deficits relative to controls.

Investigators have looked for a logical double dissociation, namely that LHD involves a deficit of linguistic but not emotional prosody and that, conversely, RHD involves a deficit of emotional but not linguistic prosody. To do so, researchers compared linguistic and affective prosody with both LHDs and RHDs. Although Walker and others (2002) found the double dissociation, Pell and Baum (1997) found that neither group had a deficit for emotional prosody. LHDs had the expected linguistic deficit.

Geigenberger and Ziegler (2001) used three receptive prosody tasks to compare relatively large LHD and RHD groups. For emotional prosody, participants were asked to identify a general positive or negative feeling in utterances. For pragmatic prosody, they reacted to appropriateness of prosodic cues for conversational turn-taking. For linguistic prosody, they comprehended sentences containing emphatic stress. Consistent with the predicted dissociation, LHDs with aphasia were impaired in the linguistic task and unimpaired in the more pragmatic tasks. RHDs are discussed in Chapter 11.

Regarding production of prosody, two studies by Baum and her colleagues in Montreal address syntactic phrasing and figurative expression. These investigators compared small mildly impaired LHD and RHD groups. First, participants were presented contexts to encourage production of either *The family that likes to eat, the Bergers, left hungry* or *The family that likes to eat the burgers left hungry* (see Shah, Baum, & Dwivedi, 2006). People with aphasia did well but were somewhat inconsistent. In the second study, word duration disambiguated possibly literal utterances such as *He hit the books* (Bélanger, Baum, & Titone, 2009). Participants produced such statements following different contexts, such as *Mike's exam was the next day, and he hadn't studied all semester* and *Frank was walking through the library when he tripped and fell*. This was not too hard. Both clinical groups performed like control participants.

Based on studies conducted through the 1990s, Baum and Pell (1999) had concluded that LH-stroke, not RH-stroke, causes an impairment in the comprehension and production of prosodic linguistic cues. Yet both LHD and RHD include a deficit in processing affective prosody, probably for different reasons (Pell, 2006). Partly because methods have been inconsistent, a stable double dissociation has not been established.

Nonverbal Modalities

Most people communicate more than what they say through the sound of their voices and body language. Audrey Holland (1975) helped to kick-start functional rehabilitation in the United States by pointing out that people with aphasia communicate better than they talk. They do so partly with retained unintentional emotion or reaction such as a frown or clenched fist (Buck & Duffy, 1980; Gardner, Ling, Flamm, et al., 1975). This section focuses on "nonverbal resources" (Hengst, 2003), which is a more complicated matter than we might think (Scharp, Tompkins, & Iverson, 2007).

The Question of Asymbolia

We shall turn to gesturing for rehabilitation, but for now let us consider a story regarding a particular kind of gesturing. Whereas we expect people with aphasia to be able to lean on gesture fairly easily, some have an accompanying difficulty with a type of gesture called pantomime. For a while, researchers entertained a mystery of why a gesturing deficit would accompany a language disorder, and some thought that language and gesture deficits might be symptoms of a deeper and broader disorder called "asymbolia."

To deconstruct this question, we need to consider the symbolic qualities of gestures. A truly symbolic gesture, like a word, has an arbitrary relationship to its referent. A salute or OK sign, for example, do not possess physical properties of their meaning, and yet they are understood by a community.

Curiously, inquiries into asymbolia targeted pantomime, which replicates a referent like in the game of charades. Duffy and Duffy (1981) found that pantomiming the use of objects was correlated with severity of aphasia and that motor impairment contributed little to pantomime performance. In another study, individuals with aphasia but without limb apraxia were impaired for imitating American Indian Sign Language (Amer-Ind) and American Sign Language (ASL; Daniloff, Fritelli, Buckingham, et al., 1986). ASL contains many arbitrary symbols, but Amer-Ind is loaded with pantomimic portrayals of referents. Thus, there was evidence that symbolic and nearly symbolic gesturing is related in some way to aphasia.

Because of the possibility of a motor confound, investigators decided to use pantomime recognition as an opportunity to determine whether a central disorder, like aphasia, could be inferred from coexisting receptive and expressive deficits. To assess recognition, a researcher produces a pantomime, and a participant identifies the referent in a set of pictures. Supporting the idea of asymbolia, there was an average of deficit in a group with aphasia (Duffy, Duffy, & Pearson, 1975), a correlation with overall language ability (Duffy & Duffy, 1981), and a correlation with receptive language ability (Ferro, Santos, Castro-Caldas, & Mariano, 1980). People with aphasia also had more difficulty recognizing pantomime than facial emotion (Walker-Batson, Barton, Wendt, et al., 1987).

However, not everyone with aphasia had a pantomime recognition deficit. The proportion of individuals with recognition deficits varied from 41 to 74 percent (Gainotti & Lemmo, 1976; Seron, Van Der Kaa, Remitz, et al., 1979; Varney, 1982). The range of recognition scores with aphasia in Duffy and Duffy's study overlapped considerably with the normal range. Other studies showed no relationship between pantomime recognition deficit and severity of aphasia (Daniloff, Noll, Fristoe, et al., 1982; Feyereisen & Seron, 1982). Despite the averages and correlations, many people with aphasia do not have pantomime recognition deficit, indicating that this problem is not a necessary component of aphasia.

Meanwhile, others claimed that pantomime deficit in people with aphasia is a movement disorder or a manifestation of limb apraxia (e.g., Kertesz, Ferro, & Shewan, 1984). Like Duffy and Duffy (1981), Wang and Goodglass (1992) found pantomime recognition and production to be correlated with each other and with auditory comprehension, but unlike the Duffy findings, pantomime abilities were not correlated with severity of aphasia. Wang and Goodglass also found a strong correlation between miming and a measure of motor praxis. Using a sophisticated analysis of their previous data, Duffy, Watt, and Duffy (1994) concluded that pantomime impairment has both a symbolic and a motoric basis.

Because pantomime may not be truly symbolic (Peterson & Kirshner, 1981), the issue of whether aphasia is subsumed in a more widely sweeping asymbolia may not have been resolved by this research. Investigators should probably add more symbolic gestures, such as a salute and OK sign, to the ageing body of research. Moreover, a clinician is more concerned about the communicative avenues available to a client with aphasia. For many individuals, pantomime can be one option with little training.

Drawing

If you cannot think of the word, can you draw it? Although many of us would say we are not artistic, most of us can draw to some degree. Because the right hemisphere is thought to be responsible for such visuospatial skills, we might expect people with aphasia to have retained whatever drawing skill they had. However, right hemiplegia accompanying nonfluent aphasia can restrict the usually preferred side for writing and drawing. This may be one reason why 30 to 40 percent of clients with left or right hemisphere strokes have some degree of drawing deficit when tested with copying tasks (e.g., Arena & Gainotti, 1978; Carlesimo, Fadda, & Caltagirone, 1993).

Chapter 11 has a discussion of drawing from the perspective of constructional skills with RHD. One point in that chapter is that drawing difficulties with LHD are different. People with LHD generally include accurate details and preserve the overall structure of an object, but they draw slowly and simply (e.g., Gainotti & Tiacci, 1970; Swindell, Holland, Fromm, et al., 1988). What is important for the present discussion is whether drawing with aphasia is recognizable or can convey meaning.

In one study, clinicians examined copying and sketching ability of three individuals with severe aphasia, right hemiparesis, and little drawing experience. The participants were right-handed and drew with the left hand. All three produced intelligible copies and sketches of objects. The wives of two of the patients were surprised with their husbands' newly discovered artistic skills. The study indicated that drawing can be a communicative option (Kashiwagi, Kashiwagi, Kunimori, et al., 1994).

More recently, Sacchett and Black (2011) suspected that drawing can be a window to thought processes of people with aphasia. Two individuals with severe nonfluent aphasia were instructed to draw the main event in short scenes "as if you were trying to get it across to somebody else." One participant sketched representations equivalent to controls, containing all elements and arrows showing direction of action. Pictures by the other person with aphasia were ambiguous about the main event, with missing elements and arrows. The investigators attributed these different performances to different abilities in conceptualizing events.

Discourse and Text

Let us return to verbal behavior. *Discourse* is a term that has been used to refer to numerous things. Broadly it refers to "the use of language above and beyond the sentence" (Schiffrin, 2006, p. 169). Monologue and dialogue are examples of discourse and share features of processing simply because each entails dealing with strings of sentences in a functional context. Dialogue is the same as *conversational discourse,* a special topic to be covered later. For reading and writing, this level of language is known as *text.* We are still in the realm of pragmatics because language is normally used as discourse, which provides a context in which single words and sentences are understood and produced.

We study discourse production with aphasia for different purposes. One aim is to determine the nature of impaired word finding and syntax in a somewhat natural productive circumstance (i.e., spontaneous speech). The other purpose is to determine a person's more pragmatic abilities with respect to discourse-specific levels and functions. We should consider the method for *elicitation* and the method for *analysis* somewhat independently. For example, we may elicit discourse but analyze word-finding, which is beneath the discourse level (e.g., Herbert, Hickin, Howard, et al., 2008).

Discourse Elicitation

Stimuli and instructions steer a client toward producing a particular type of discourse (Table 4.1). The types of discourse in the table are produced as monologue, that is, with the client talking and the clinician listening. Description, narration, or exposition also arise in dialogue such as an interview (e.g., *I'd like to ask some questions about your job*) or a conversation (e.g., *Let's discuss what we like about our jobs*). In some studies, an interview can be an awkward means of eliciting conversation, and it may be "semistructured" to loosen it up a little.

Clinical researchers have been interested in whether the condition for eliciting discourse matters when we are attempting to measure language production. One concern is whether standardized test conditions are valid for assessing the way people normally talk. In one study, a test of describing object functions was compared to

TABLE 4.1 Methods for eliciting different kinds of monologue. Description has been the most commonly elicited form in clinical evaluation.

DISCOURSE TYPE	VISUAL STIMULUS	INSTRUCTION
Description	Complex picture	Tell me everything you see in this picture.
Procedure	None	Tell me how you make a sandwich.
Narration	Complex picture	Tell me a story about this picture.
	Picture sequence	Tell me the story being told in these pictures.
	None	Tell me the story of Cinderella.

conversation (Roberts & Wertz, 1989). There were some differences favoring conversation (i.e., longer utterances, better word finding) and others favoring the object-functions test (i.e., better syntax). For description, content of pictures may make a difference. Pictures of the Kennedy assassination elicited more words than a drawing used in an aphasia battery (Bottenberg, Lemme, & Hedberg, 1987). Thus, a full picture of sentence-level capacities may require observation in formal and natural conditions and with different topics.

When we show someone a picture and ask for discourse, instructions are likely to determine the type of discourse that will be produced. In a study of healthy older adults, Harris Wright and Capilouto (2009) presented complex pictures used in two prominent aphasia test batteries. They asked one group to describe the picture in a fashion typical for clinical assessment (i.e., "Talk about what is going on in the pictures") and asked another group atypically to tell a story (i.e., "I want you to look at the picture and tell me a story"). Not surprisingly, the latter instructions were more likely to elicit narrative. Olness (2006) found a similar result for people with aphasia.

Doyle and others modified a story-retelling procedure for computer presentation to determine how many stories is enough. Twelve stories were each represented by six-frame drawings. An audio version was synchronized with the pictures. The investigators were particularly interested in whether four subsets of three stories each would produce comparable results. It turns out that there was no significant difference among the four subsets, indicating that three stories should be as informative diagnostically as 12 (Doyle, McNeil, Park, et al., 2000). The retell procedure, touted for its uniqueness, was shown to be valid relative to more familiar discourse elicitation tasks (McNeil, Sung, Yang, et al., 2007).

Within-Sentence Analysis

Although software for syntactic and semantic analysis has been used for aphasia (Armstrong, et al., 2011), the main story regarding within-sentence analysis has been the measurement of **informativeness**. Investigators look for the presence of predefined content units without regard to their relationships to each other. The main objective has been to have a reliable measure that discriminates aphasia from normal performance in discourse production.

Initially, Yorkston and Beukelman (1980) divided descriptions of a test picture (i.e., *Cookie Theft*, see Chapter 5) into content units the size of a word or short phrase. A **content unit** was considered to be "a grouping of information that was always expressed as a unit by normal speakers" (p. 30), such as *cookies, from the jar, mother,* and *in the kitchen*. A group with mild aphasia did not differ from normal elderly participants in amount of information, but the people with aphasia were much less efficient with fewer units per minute (also Craig, Hinckley, Winkelseth, et al., 1993).

At the Veterans Administration Medical Center in Minneapolis, Linda Nicholas and Robert Brookshire worked on improving content analysis so that it is independent of a particular picture. They started by counting the most informative words in a narrative, which they called a **correct information unit** (CIU; Nicholas & Brookshire,

1993). The percentage of words that are CIUs and the number of CIUs per minute separated people with aphasia from the controls. Obtaining 300 to 400 words from four or five stimuli led to the most reliable score (Brookshire & Nicholas, 1994). However, the consistency of this measure when repeated on individuals is questionable (Cameron, Wambaugh, & Mauszycki, 2010; Oelschlaeger & Thorne, 1999).

Nicholas and Brookshire turned their attention to a more elaborate system for identifying **main concepts**, still wanting to establish a reliable measure that is sensitive to deficit (Nicholas & Brookshire, 1995b). Main concepts are statements that form a "skeletal outline" of the essential information in pictured stories. One study showed that people with aphasia produce fewer complete and accurate main concepts than neurologically intact individuals. To determine validity of these measures, Doyle and others (1996) asked volunteers to rate the informativeness of several narratives produced by people with aphasia. Both the CIU and main concept measures were strongly related to the subjective judgments. This method continues to be used for people with aphasia (e.g., Harris Wright & Capilouto, 2009).

McNeil and Doyle and their colleagues (2001) created their own information unit (IU) analysis for the story retelling procedure mentioned earlier. An IU was a "word, phrase, or acceptable alternative from the story stimulus that is intelligible and informative and that conveys accurate and relevant information about the story" (p. 994). This procedure was reliable, and rate (i.e., percentage of IUs per minute) identified deficit better than the percentage of IUs per se (McNeil, Doyle, Park, et al., 2002).

Between-Sentence Analysis

The special qualities of discourse come from interrelationships among statements establishing **coherence**. A conversation of alternating single sentences makes sense because the statements are about a topic holding them together. Coherence is studied at two levels. A local or *microstructural level* pertains narrowly to the overlap of meaning between sentences. This overlap is known as **cohesion**. As the minimum level of discourse, it needs only pairs of statements for targeted study. A global or *macrostructural level* pertains to broad themes and structural schemes. It is the "upper limit of structural organization" where an entire discourse or text is held together (Stubbs, 1983). This level is necessarily invoked for research and assessment with three or more statements.

Quantifying coherence begins with parsing a transcript of discourse for various purposes. One purpose is to have a frame of reference for computing density of different forms, such as number of words per sentence or number of sentences per episode in a story. Also, investigators like to have a basis for examining meaningful relationships among the parts of a discourse. The most common units include the following:

- **Sentence**, a standard syntactic unit containing a subject and predicate
- **T-unit**, a more complex syntactic unit containing a main clause and attached subordinate clauses
- **Proposition (p-unit)**, an informational unit consisting of a predicate and its arguments

A sentence may be the most ambiguous of the three. Mentis and Prutting (1987) divided spoken narratives into sentences according to pauses and intonation, which may not correspond to punctuation in text or a transcript. A T-unit could be the following: *The heroic policeman who apprehended the thief turned over his weapon before the investigation began.* This could be classified as a sentence or a T-unit containing the equivalent of two or three sentences and three propositions (e.g, *the policeman apprehended the thief; the investigation began*).

One team of clinical researchers combined the notions of main concept and proposition to form a unit called the "main event" (Harris Wright, Capilouto, Wagovitch, et al., 2005). Identified beforehand by the investigators for stories to be presented to participants, a main event was defined as being an independent event and important to the story. Some of the main events included two related propositions. Sequentially pictured stories produced more of these events than single pictures, and people with aphasia produced fewer main events than intact adults (Capilouto, Harris Wright, & Wagovich, 2006).

One cohesive device is *anaphora*, which is a lexical unit referring to previous information. One type of anaphora is the pronoun. In a cohesion analysis, the first thing to look for is the presence of such elements. Then, we search for a **cohesive tie** between an anaphor and an antecedent. Incomplete ties are noted when an antecedent cannot be found. In interviews, participants with fluent aphasia produced the usual number of cohesive elements but also produced more incomplete cohesive ties than controls, indicating that pronouns and other anaphors were difficult to interpret (Glosser & Deser, 1991).

The **theme** of a discourse contributes to overall coherence, as we expect every statement to be related to a topic in some way. Moreover, types of discourse possess a macrostructure. Storytelling is the most frequently studied form of discourse, perhaps because its macrostructure is more apparent than the other forms. **Story grammars** are theories of what we know about narrative structure. It has a beginning, middle, and end. Thorndyke's (1977) linguistic-like hierarchy contains functional categories of *setting, theme, plot,* and *resolution.* Then *plot* branches into multiple *episodes,* and so on. We may recognize the setting category (i.e., place, characters) such as "Once there was a wily fox who lived in a forest." Stein and Glenn's (1979) grammar has a plot starter called the *initiating event* from which all follows: "One day the fox left the forest to explore a henhouse in a nearby village."

Using story grammar as a frame of reference, researchers initially counted narrative categories. People with aphasia were deficient in number of thematic statements (Gleason, Goodglass, Obler, et al., 1980). They tended to repeat major themes and omit details. In another study, participants conformed to narrative structure and produced sufficient events, but they were deficient in certain story categories such as setting, resolution, and evaluation (Ulatowska, et al., 1983). Bloom and others (1995) resorted to rating stories according to key characteristics and also found overall story structure to be preserved.

Coelho developed measures of narration for studying traumatic brain injury. Originally, analysis addressed cohesion (i.e., number of complete cohesive ties) and story content (i.e., number of episodes, T-units within an episode; Coelho, 2002; Coelho, Youse, Lê, et al., 2003). Later he got closer to story grammar with **goodness of narratives**, which retained the episode counts and added *story completeness* by counting the number of critical story components out of five (e.g., characters, events, resolution; Lê, Coelho, Mozeiko, et al., 2011). Results are in Chapter 12.

Christiansen (1995b) compared syndromes by rating the relevance of propositions in stories told from cartoons. Participants with Wernicke's aphasia were distinctive in producing more irrelevant statements than the other participants. Those with Broca's and conduction aphasia were more coherent. Then Christiansen (1995a) focused on mildly fluent aphasias, and they displayed storytelling problems consistent with their syndromes. Those with anomic aphasia produced mostly information gaps and fewer propositions than the other groups. Those with conduction aphasia produced more repetitions than other violations. Those with mild Wernicke's aphasia continued to produce more irrelevant propositions than other violations.

More recently, Olness and her colleagues (2010) found that narrative structure and prominence of information were fairly intact for all but severely impaired people with aphasia. In general, it has been concluded that left-hemisphere stroke impairs microlinguistic parameters (e.g., content units) and preserves macrolinguistic characteristics of discourse (i.e., cohesion and coherence).

Discourse Comprehension

Like a theory of any cognitive function, a full account of discourse comprehension contains both a knowledge structure and a processing system. The network of semantic memory is broadened to account for knowledge of complex situations generally known as **schemas**. For example, we have a schema for weddings. Our schema for narrative structure (i.e., story grammar) lets us know when someone is telling us a story about a wedding. Processing is constrained by what is called the **bottleneck problem**. That is, only small chunks of a discourse can squeeze into working memory as we listen or read. Theories of comprehension propose different levels of representation for holding previous input temporarily and for accumulating a representation of the entire discourse (Kintsch, 1998).

Clinical tests of discourse comprehension have been used mainly for finding subtle language comprehension deficits. The usual method is to read a paragraph to a client and then ask questions about what was just heard, thereby testing recall as well as general comprehension. In some aphasia batteries, many questions can be answered without having heard or read the paragraphs (Nicholas, et al., 1986). Familiarity of content improves performance using this method (Jones, Pierce, Mahoney, et al., 2007). Nicholas and Brookshire developed a test of discourse comprehension that is presented in Chapter 6.

Few studies of aphasia have targeted comprehension at the microstructural level (e.g., cohesive devices). We could put the aforementioned study of inference by Harris Wright and Newhoff (2004) in this category. Chapman and Ulatowska (1989) presented short vignettes in which two characters were introduced in the first sentence, and a subsequent sentence referred back to one of the characters, as in the sentence-pairs of *4*.

> (4) The customer shouted angrily at the waitress that the meal was awful.
> The waitress was new at the job and did not know how to respond.
> or
> She was new at the job and did not know how to respond.

Participants were given response cards showing the two characters and were asked questions such as "Who was new at the job and did not know how to respond?" People with aphasia responded less accurately with the pronominal anaphor than the lexical anaphor (see also Kahn, Joanette, Ska, et al., 1990). Studies of comprehension hinging on macrostructure are even harder to find.

Conversation

The dynamic interaction of conversation differs from formal clinical interactions. For example, tests and treatments tend to have someone practice comprehending repeatedly or producing utterances repeatedly; whereas people take turns talking in the give-and-take of conversation. This section covers two distinctive aspects of conversation, namely exchange of new information and management of turn-taking. These features are ingredients of treatments such as PACE therapy and "language-action" in constraint-induced therapies (Chapter 10). Closing this discussion is an introduction to the ethnographic study of aphasia and conversation analysis.

New Information

Conversation is conducted as if there were a tacit agreement or "social contract" between participants. Grice (1975) called it the *principle of cooperation*. According to Grice's "maxims," a speaker tries to be informative, truthful, relevant, and concise, and a listener assumes that this is what the speaker is trying to do. Let us focus on the informativeness maxim as we turn our attention to the *shared responsibilities* of participants in a conversation. More specifically, we shall pay more attention to a clinician or others engaged in conversation with someone who has aphasia.

The informativeness maxim gives us another way of examining speaker meaning. It states that a speaker tries to convey new information in addition to rehashing information a listener already knows. Comprehension is said to be a process of relating new information to information already known, called given or old information. A speaker uses linguistic devices to help a listener identify what is new and what is old. For example, a pronoun signals that we are referring to information that a listener should already know from a previous utterance, the situation, or knowledge of the world. When a speaker estimates what a listener already knows, a speaker is said to be assuming the point of view of the listener or what some call "theory of mind" (see Chapter 11).

Conditions can be devised to observe someone conveying new information. A blunt procedure is to put a **barrier** between a client and a listener so the listener does not see the client's stimuli. Each participant may be provided with a set of pictures of slightly differing events. People with aphasia can be quite good at verbalizing information that is distinctive enough so that listeners can choose the picture being described (Busch, Brookshire, & Nicholas, 1988).

The notion of a word attached to a concept (e.g., naming) now becomes a collaborative act in which partners work together to convey reference to an object in mind or in the situation, known as *referential communication*. Julie Hengst (2003) employed a barrier to study referencing by young adults with aphasia. In one task, a partner directed the other person to place a picture in a location on a board, but the partners were unable to see each others' workspaces. All participants, including family members, were successful in exchanging information. The individuals with aphasia communicated occasionally with partial words, spellings, and paraphasias.

Another manipulation of new information is the **familiarity of a listener**. A client may talk to one who is already familiar with a message or another who is unfamiliar with the message. Clinicians, spouses, and strangers contribute differently with respect to common knowledge and communicative strategies. Stimley and Noll (1994) had familiar and unfamiliar examiners administer verbal subtests of an aphasia battery to people with aphasia. Familiarity mattered for the more difficult subtests, as the clients scored significantly better with the unfamiliar examiner. The authors guessed that familiarity breeds reduced effort. Familiarity of a listener may not matter for storytelling (Bottenberg & Lemme, 1991; Brenneise-Sarshad, Nicholas, & Brookshire, 1991). In a study of people with Broca's aphasia, Doyle and others (1994) found that familiarity of the communicative partner had little effect on the use of statements, requests, answers, and ambiguities.

Conversational Management

Clinical investigators have borrowed methods from sociolinguistics and anthropology or have invented their own approaches to studying the interactive characteristics of conversation. Attention is likely to be given to the local management system of turn-taking or the global structure of conversation, whether it be face-to-face or over the telephone. Like trying to tame a wild horse, clinicians are working on reliable methods of observation directed by frameworks specifying structural features of conversation.

Unlike some TV news interviewers, people with mild to moderate aphasia tend to follow conversational rules. In the typical conversation, speaker turns rarely overlap (i.e., simultaneous talking), and gaps between speakers often span less than a second. This precision stems from an inherent predictability of a speaker turn, which enables a partner to anticipate when a switch from speaking to listening will occur. We may be concerned about the comprehension deficit and press for speech of Wernicke's aphasia. However, these individuals also appear to be sensitive to turn-taking conventions (Schienberg & Holland, 1980).

There are different types of turn sequences. One is the **adjacency pair**, in which a speaker turn (first part) is followed by a predictable response from the other speaker (second part). For example, a greeting follows a greeting; an answer follows a question. Other types of turn sequences may encompass three or four turns. One of these is the **repair sequence**, in which a speaker modifies a turn because it failed to convey a message. Repairs are likely to be frequent in conversation with someone who has aphasia because either participant may not get a point across.

The study of repair behavior now considers two variables. In addition to listener familiarity, the other variable pertains to whether a partner's repair is self-initiated (without prompting) or other-initiated (with prompting; e.g., Dressler, Buder, & Cannito, 2009). Lubinski, Duchan, and Weitzner-Lin (1980) found that neurologically healthy adults prefer self-initiated repairs. Other-initiated repairs are rare, and when they occur, they are usually modulated with prefaces such as "You mean . . .?" or addendums such as ". . . , I think."

Ferguson (1994) studied precursors of repairs in conversations between people with aphasia and either familiar or less-familiar individuals. In particular, she looked for trouble-indicating behavior by either participant, such as commenting about a word-finding problem or halting the conversation. Not surprisingly, normal participants indicated more trouble and used more repairs when interacting with someone with aphasia compared to interacting with intact partners. Visiting participants made more other-repairs than the familiar participants who lived with the person with aphasia, indicating that unfamiliar partners are more likely to seek a "speedy remedy" for trouble.

Ethnography and Conversation Analysis

Ethnographic research (also known as "qualitative research") extends the previous section on conversation. The ethnographic approach originated in anthropology and sociology with the main goal of studying human behavior in its natural state (Mey, 2001). In aphasiology, this research has been cultivated internationally. In the United States, Nina Simmons-Mackie and Jack Damico collaborated in Louisiana, and Julie Hengst directed studies in Illinois. Qualitative research has been pursued in Canada by Guylaine Le Dorze and Claire Croteau and in the United Kingdom by Ruth Lesser, Lisa Perkins, and Anne Whitworth, as well as by Ray Wilkinson and Suzanne Beeke. Alison Ferguson has been developing this approach in Australia. This research appears most frequently in the journal *Aphasiology*.

There are special methods for observation. Researchers aspire to obtain data that is "authentic," avoiding a contrived stimulus or task (e.g., Ferguson & Harper, 2010). For obtaining authentic conversations in the home, researchers train participants to use recording equipment so that naturalness is not compromised by the presence of an investigator. In one study, a couple received no instructions on the conditions or frequency of recording (Oelschlaeger & Thorne, 1999). Hengst and others (2005) videotaped conversations at restaurants, stores, and a high school football game. A researcher was present but functioned as an observer. Hengst (2006) also set up a gamelike situation to observe playful interactions between individuals with aphasia and their routine partners. Luck and Rose (2007) did a naturalistic study of an interviewing technique that would elicit the best information.

Ethnomethodology consists of many observations of a single participant, but unlike cognitive neuropsychology, research is mainly empirical with questions such as "Is repetition a naturally occurring behaviour in the conversation of a person with aphasia?" (Oelschlaeger & Damico, 1998, p. 972). Observations are recorded as field notes, and data are likely to be reported as transcripts and descriptions rather than as numbers (Beeke, Wilkinson, & Maxim, 2007; Davidson, Worrall, & Hickson, 2003; Le Dorze & Brassard, 1995). In exploring methodological variations, Armstrong and colleagues (2007) concluded that "transcription-less" analysis (i.e., directly from audio and video recordings) provides the same information as transcription-based analysis for three types of discourse, including conversation.

A formalized analysis of natural conversation is naturally called **conversation analysis** (CA). For the study of brain-damaged individuals, guidelines began with Perkins, Whitworth, and Lesser's (1997) *Conversation Analysis Profile for People with Cognitive Impairment* (CAPPCI; see also Lesser & Perkins, 1999). From this foundation they developed a similar *Conversation Analysis Profile for People with Aphasia* (CAPPA; Booth & Perkins, 1999; Booth & Swabey, 1999). An investigator may focus on a feature of conversational management and present a transcript of dyadic turns that exemplifies a participant's realization of that feature.

Interpretation begins with comparing the descriptions of behavior to what is known about normal conversation. In this vein, CA "is informed by two domains of data: prior aphasiological knowledge and the experience and expertise of conversation analysts with talk and conduct in interaction among language-unimpaired speakers" (Heeschen & Schegloff, 1999, p. 365). Interpretation consists of "explaining the essence of the social phenomenon and its meaning in the participants' lives" (Damico & Simmons-Mackie, 2003, p. 133), including inference of motivation (Oelschlaeger & Damico, 1998).

Investigators in London applied ethnomethodology to the study of a father's agrammatism in conversations with his daughter at their home (Beeke et al., 2007). The researchers advocated extending assessment beyond "sentence-level testing" to include natural interactions, in which they found the father's grammar to be reflective of turn-taking strategies. He compensated for verb-retrieval difficulty by gesturing to convey events. The investigators detected a greater variety of intentions in conversation (i.e., speech acts), including commenting, assessing, and reasoning despite the absence of sentences.

Frankel, Penn, and Ormond-Brown (2007) attempted a "merging of two distinct and historically separate paradigms" to relate cognitive abilities to conversational behavior. They compared performance on an executive functioning battery with performance in conversation. The battery consisted of an assortment of neuropsychological tests ranging from digit span to card sorting. Relationships were established via logical analysis rather than with an experimental design and statistics. For example, it was decided that good performance in a test of forward planning was reflected in a conversational sample that the researchers interpreted to be an example of verbalized forward planning.

Conversational Gesturing

Gesturing serves at least two functions during conversation. One is communicative with either the automatic gestures that show emotion or the volitional gestures that express ideas. Gestures also signal conversational moves, thereby regulating an interaction. Clinical researchers are especially interested in severely nonfluent or global aphasias for whom gesturing may be a necessary compensatory behavior (Simmons-Mackie & Damico, 1997).

Simmons-Mackie and Damico (1996) identified **discourse markers** that people with nonfluent aphasia employ in managing conversational interaction. They observed the following markers in two individuals:

- Initiation or alerting (e.g., raised finger indicating desire to begin or maintain a speaking turn)
- Termination or reorientation (e.g., hand clasp to end a failed communicative attempt)
- Participant role request (e.g., eye gaze and body movements to relinquish speaking turn)
- Affiliation or politeness (e.g., "Is good" as a response to an offer)
- Truth level (e.g., "I don't know" amid trying to convey something)

Also, severely nonfluent people with aphasia indicate when they are not comprehending, and they signal for help (Herrmann, Koch, Johannsen-Horbach, et al., 1989).

Researchers have also studied whether communicative gestures arise naturally. People with severe aphasia displayed better gestural ability in a new information condition than in a formal test of limb apraxia (Feyereisen, Barter, Goossens, et al., 1988). Yet communicative use of gesture decreased when a barrier was placed between clients and partners, indicating that people with aphasia are sensitive to the viability of gesture as a communicative option (Glosser, Wiener, & Kaplan, 1986). Gesturing style in Broca's and Wernicke's aphasia corresponded to the nature of their verbal expression (Duffy, Duffy, & Mercaitis, 1984). In Hengst's (2003) study with a barrier task, participants tapped into several nonverbal resources, including displaying cards over the barrier, full body postures, and drawing in the air.

People with aphasia were videotaped while describing a complex picture to someone who had not seen it. Then they were asked questions to create a more interactive condition (Hadar, Wenkert-Olenik, Krauss, et al., 1998). The researchers tracked gestures that supplemented language. Participants with conceptual deficits beyond aphasia gestured differently from normal controls. This result anticipated the aforementioned problem with drawing that was related to event conceptualization (Sacchett & Black, 2011). Participants with deficits restricted to word-finding gestured more like controls.

Communication Partners

At this point, we shall consider two general areas of research concentrating on significant others in the life of someone with aphasia. One area is conversation, turning our
attention to the partner's role in the exchange of meanings. The other area of research
focuses on relationships between husband and wife, parent and child, and so on, as
the person with aphasia progresses following the occurrence of a stroke. Student clinicians worry about becoming involved with the second area, but the speech-language
pathologist (SLP) can help a family member provide positive support. This section
provides the background that supports our family counseling.

The contributions of others in conversations may help or hinder communication by a participant with aphasia. Support groups and organizations such as the
National Aphasia Association (aphasia.org) provide lists of "do's and don'ts" such as
the following:

- Don't exclude the person with aphasia from conversation.
- Wait. Give them time to speak.
- Allow the person time to understand your message.

Drawn mainly from everyday experience, these suggestions became targets of ethnographic studies.

Simmons-Mackie and Kagan (1999) used conversation analysis (CA) to identify
strategies that characterize conversational partners who had been judged previously
as "good" or "poor." During repair sequences, the good partners used strategies that
were "face-saving" for the person with aphasia. For example, these partners would
adopt communicative behaviors, such as gestures, that were used by the person with
aphasia. The poor partners preferred talking, such as asking the person with aphasia
to talk instead of gesturing. These partners emphasized getting information, rather
than fostering a relationship.

One communicative partner action is called *speaking for* behavior, which "don't"
lists tend to discourage. In multiparty interactions, this seemingly overprotective
behavior may squelch participation by the person with aphasia. In a series of studies building to 26 couples in interviews, severity of aphasia was a factor. The spouse
spoke for the most severely impaired partner most often, whereas the spouse offered
repairs of speaking turns for the moderately impaired and little help for the mildly
impaired (Croteau & Le Dorze, 2006; Croteau, Le Dorze, & Morin, 2008).

In refining these observations, investigators identified three slightly different
speaking roles. When *speaking on behalf of another,* the partner speaks as if he or
she were the person with aphasia, coauthoring a message. This role is similar to the
"speaking for" behavior just discussed. *Speaking support* consists of cueing or prompting to help the person with aphasia convey a message. It seems consistent with repairs.
The third role, *speaking instead of another,* has a participant speaking to others about

the person with aphasia. Calling the first two roles "interactive co-construction," Ferguson and Harper (2010) suggested that these roles can reinforce the collaborative nature of conversation in which each participant, leaning on shared knowledge, helps another in the exchange of messages. Each role occurred in multiparty interactions, with speaking support directed only to the person with aphasia (see also Purves, 2009; Simmons-Mackie, Kingston, & Schultz, 2004).

Also, aphasia distorts family dynamics. Immediately after a stroke, the family is likely to be overwhelmed with the sense that they nearly lost a husband, wife, father, or mother. Suddenly a partner appears to be vulnerable to the slightest encroachment, and a skittish spouse wants to protect him or her 24 hours a day. The devoted spouse may return home from the hospital only overnight, sleeping partly dressed in case there is an emergency. Spousal adjustment hopefully follows a path from selflessness to a renewed sense of self, a path that may parallel the progress of the individual with aphasia. These stories have been told by accomplished authors whose husbands had been accomplished wordsmiths (Ackerman, 2011; Hale, 2003).

Family members assume unaccustomed roles. A traditional male client may no longer be able to provide income, sign the checks, and park the car. Dalhberg noted the following: "Since I'd grown up in middle-class America, I was used to taking care of 'masculine' details. I signed into hotels, picked up the bags, gave taxi directions, and ordered in restaurants." His wife added: "I looked forward to the time Clay would be able to do the managing again. It wasn't the physical exertion I minded as much as the loss of my female enjoyment of being 'taken care of'" (Dahlberg & Jaffe, 1977, p. 52). With heightened responsibilities, a spouse becomes increasingly fatigued and drops some favorite activities to attend to the afflicted partner (Labourel & Martin, 1993; Le Dorze & Brassard, 1995; Ponzio & Degiovani, 1993).

Zraick and Boone (1991) found that spouses developed attitudes toward their spouse with aphasia that diverged from "control spouses." With an attitude assessment called Q-methodology, spouses sorted and ranked 70 attributes according to what was most and least representative of the person with aphasia. In general, spouses had more negative attitudes than poststroke controls, indicating that spouses' attitudes had changed after onset. The most prevalent perceived characteristics of the impaired spouse were *demanding* and *temperamental* in contrast to *mature* and *kind* for controls. Least prevalent for the clinical group included *sexy, mature,* and *intelligent.* Spouses of nonfluent individuals had more negative attitudes than spouses of fluent individuals, which in part could have been due to the more frequent presence of hemiplegia in the nonfluent group.

The same themes show up in contemporary research. Twenty couples were examined along dimensions of agreement/disagreement and understanding/misunderstanding (Gillespie, Murphy, & Place, 2010). Primary family caregivers were conflicted by a "desire to support independence . . . but feeling compelled to be protective" (p. 1559). Conversely, the partners with aphasia were conflicted about receiving help and not wanting to appear dependent. Couples agreed regarding the scale of communication deficit, but they disagreed regarding "speaking for" behavior as spouses thought that the individuals with aphasia were more in favor of it than they were. The partners with aphasia mistakenly thought that their caregivers knew they did not like being corrected. Caregivers would be "protective in their actions but encouraging in their words." Also, they tried to conceal their burden of care with respect to household matters, paying bills, and so on.

Children of people with aphasia have not received much attention in family research. Le Dorze, Tremblay, and Croteau (2009) followed a 31-year-old daughter's adaptation to her father's aphasia. The investigators conducted three interviews, namely when the father started outpatient treatment, at end of this treatment, and three months after the treatment. The daughter was evolving. Negative consequences subsided, and positive adjustments emerged. Obtaining information about aphasia and services relieved some of the stress. Because she was living with her parents, the daughter's experiences were similar to those of a spouse. Such studies identify problem areas for comprehensive rehabilitation, and we shall return to the process of family adaptation in Chapter 10 where the SLP's role as a facilitator is discussed.

Life Participation

A family's adjustments facilitate participation by the person with aphasia. Life participation pertains to reentry into family, work, and society. Enhancing this involvement has become the primary objective of *social and life-participation approaches* to rehabilitation (Elman, 2005; Hilari & Cruice, 2013; Simmons-Mackie, 2008). Clinical specialists have focused on the notion of **quality of life** (QoL) for defining the outcome of rehabilitation. This "intuitively appealing" phrase has been formalized "not only as an aggregate of broad domains but as the product of personally weighted life domains filtered through the individual's own perspective" (Hirsch & Holland, 2000, p. 37). In other words, QoL varies among individuals, and perhaps the most potent indicator of someone's progress is whether he or she believes that life is getting better.

As a general concept, the study of quality of life with aphasia has a long history (e.g., Backus, 1947). This history may not be recognized by Google searches because the issues were identified in other terms such as "emotional and psychosocial adjustment," "role changes," and so on (Davis, 1983). In today's terms, health care professionals are interested in the impact of all medical conditions, known as *health-related quality of life* (HRQoL, HRQOL, HR-QOL; Bowling, 2004). The literature until 2007 suggested that, in addition to the interpersonal changes cited previously, return to work is often at a less-demanding level (Dalemans, De Witte, Wade, et al., 2008). Thirty people with mild to moderate aphasia cited several factors contributing to QoL, such as indoor and outdoor activities, verbal communication, company of people, body functioning, fear of another stroke, mobility, and independence (Cruice, Hill, Worrall, et al., 2010).

Leaders in life participation studies include Linda Worrall and Louise Hickson in Australia and Madeline Cruice in the United Kingdom, as well as the aforementioned pioneers of ethnographic research. In attempting to quantify the impact of aphasia on participation, an activities checklist demonstrated that people with aphasia have reduced social contacts and activities relative to controls (Cruice, Worrall, & Hickson, 2006). In California, Candace Vickers (2010) used social network and participation questionnaires to demonstrate the shrinkage of social networks once a person had aphasia.

In a series of studies examining accessibility to society and media, Worrall's research team found that people without aphasia respond positively or negatively depending on their familiarity with aphasia or the person with aphasia. Media are challenging, with one culprit being Web sites that are too complex to read and navigate (Worrall, Rose, Howe, et al., 2007).

Worrall and Hickson have been particularly interested in identifying environmental barriers and facilitators that influence community participation. One clinical implication is that if we can anticipate and identify important factors for an individual client, then we can manipulate these factors so that they become facilitators instead of barriers. Interviews of 25 persons with aphasia revealed barriers related to other people (e.g., knowledge, attitudes), the physical environment (e.g., ticketing machines, background noise), and society (e.g., absence of services, complexity of institutional procedures). Facilitators included plain speaking, patience, color-coded signs, and access to others with aphasia. Generally, people with aphasia desired more awareness of their disorder and more opportunities for social interaction (Howe, Worrall, & Hickson, 2008). Ethnographic methods, instead of interviews, were necessary for studying those with severe aphasia; and not surprisingly, social exclusion was a common observation (Parr, 2007).

Summary and Conclusions

This chapter concludes an introduction to basic research regarding the language and communication problems of aphasia. The chapter put the impaired language system into the contexts of its use. It began with cognitive pragmatics (i.e., inference), made a stop with nonverbal supplements to language, and then proceeded to consequences for activities (e.g., discourse, conversation, communication partners) and for life participation (e.g., quality of life).

These summaries of research are essential for understanding the nature of aphasia and for asserting an expertise in aphasiology. Furthermore, there is the well-worn axiom that research begets clinical method. Research foreshadowed clinical practice when studies by Harold Goodglass and his colleagues went into creating a commonly used assessment battery (Chapter 5). This information may inspire clinicians to develop heretofore unheard of assessments and therapies.

The opening topic of cognitive pragmatics provided a construct that extends into the study of pragmatic language impairments characteristic of right-hemisphere dysfunction (Chapter 11) and closed head injury (Chapter 12). Prosody, affective prosody in particular, is an issue with RHD. Discourse becomes twisted for different reasons with these cognitive disorders. All these matters point to the contexts in which people with aphasia reach for compensatory communicative strategies.

Evaluation of people with aphasia includes attention to consequences of language impairment. Basic research has guided SLPs in development of assessments for identifying communicative abilities and measuring functional outcome (Chapter 6) and development of therapies capitalizing on narrative and conversational competencies, as well as nonverbal expressive abilities (Chapter 10). Family members can be part of the rehabilitation team, and their assistance is facilitated by our understanding of their role in communication and their own adjustment needs. Finally, quality of life is a longstanding concern dressed in new clothing with fresh energy for defining practical goals and providing meaningful documentation.

5 Clinical Assessment and Diagnosis

Rehabilitation begins with diagnosis and assessment. An accurate diagnosis points to the correct treatment. The purpose and extent of assessment depends on the time postonset and the setting. Acute assessment in the hospital is likely to be brief. Much later, let us say at a university clinic, it may be more extensive partly to provide experience for a supervised graduate student. In between, at a rehabilitation center, initial testing may consist of picking the most essential parts of a comprehensive aphasia battery, given the time available.

A complete evaluation addresses each of the World Health Organization's (WHO's) levels of deficit (Chapter 1). This chapter emphasizes the assessment of *impairment*, featuring large batteries and brief screenings. In the past, evaluation of consequence-based limitations was relegated to interviews and notation of vocational and social information on a page of an impairment test booklet. A surge in assessment of communication and life participation comprises the second half of Chapter 6.

The First Visit

During initial hospitalization, the speech-language pathologist's (SLP's) goals are tied to a patient's survival. What is the status of swallowing? What are communicative abilities? Differentiating language from speech disorders is helpful for consulting with family and planning for discharge. A quick bedside screening exposes specific linguistic deficits, some temporary. A more detailed analysis of language impairments can be done once the individual arrives at a rehabilitation unit or center.

After receiving a referral, the SLP reviews the **medical history** maintained at the nurse's station. The chart contains an admission summary with the neurologist's initial diagnosis and possibly some early radiologic findings. A social worker may also have obtained some family and vocational history. For her first visit with the patient, the SLP is likely to possess the following information:

- Date of the cerebral incident
- Medical history, including possible complicating conditions

- Current medications
- Family or potential caregivers

The first meeting takes 5 to 15 minutes, depending on the patient's medical condition. The SLP explains who she is and why she is there. She asks the individual's full name and if the patient knows where he is and why he is there. Knowing that aphasia is a problem with words, not ideas, the SLP empathizes: "I know. You know what you want to say, but just have trouble finding the words." The person with aphasia discovers someone in the hospital who understands the problem and thinks that this visitor is likely to be helpful. The SLP explains what the individual can expect, especially with respect to rehabilitation. She is reassuring.

The SLP returns later to do a more complete bedside evaluation following the framework for aphasia assessment introduced in Table 1.1. All that is needed is common objects in a hospital room, a pen, and some paper (Table 5.1). The patient answers some yes/no questions, points to things, and names and describes some other things. If the patient cannot verbalize spontaneously, the SLP wants to see if he or she can count or recite the days of the week. Counting may uplift a severely impaired individual by showing that he or she has a capacity for speech production (e.g., Crary, Haak, & Malinsky, 1989).

Standardized Testing

The inconsistency of informal assessment makes it difficult to measure progress reliably. Henry Head, a British physician early in the 20th century, was one of the first to standardize aphasia assessment. He was particularly vexed by inconsistent response as "one of the most striking results produced by a lesion of the cerebral cortex"

TABLE 5.1   A bedside examination illustrating the minimal ingredients of an initial evaluation.

COMPREHENSION		PRODUCTION	
Listening	*Reading*	*Speaking*	*Writing*
Is your name [Fred]? (No)	*Point to the object on this card.*	*Count to ten.*	*Write your name.*
Point to the [window] (lamp, etc.).	*Do what it says on this card (e.g., point to your nose).*	*Say Methodist Episcopal.*	*Write down some things you see in this room.*
Point to the table and ceiling.		*What do you call this (e.g., clock, pillow)?*	
Is Washington, D.C., the capital of France?		*Tell me what happened to you.*	

(Head, 1920, p. 89). A person with aphasia names an object one moment and fails to name it the next. If we tested naming just once, we might misdiagnose a patient as having severe impairment or no impairment. Head decided that a response had to be observed at least three or four times in what he called "serial tests." He would place common objects (e.g., knife, key, matches) on a table and would ask a patient to point to them by name and then try to name them. He used the same objects for each task. He did the same thing for each patient and recorded exactly what was said.

Testing for aphasia began with the harnessing of Head's ideas as test batteries, short ones and long ones. A test **battery** provides comprehensive assessment of language functions. Corresponding to the content introduced in Table 1.1, a battery covers the four language functions (i.e., listening, reading, speaking, and writing) at all levels of language (i.e., word, sentence, discourse/paragraph). Each battery featured in this chapter contains this content, although it is organized differently among the batteries.

Validity of an aphasia test is derived from our knowledge of aphasia or, more simply, from the definition of aphasia as a specialized cognitive disorder. The test minimizes influences of intelligence and education so that we have as pure an assessment of language as possible. For example, we do not ask questions about world history or science. Also, the test minimizes the influence of extralinguistic context that could provide clues to comprehending input.

In the 1930s, physicians developed the *Halstead-Wepman-Reitan Aphasia Screening Test* as a quick evaluation at bedside (Halstead & Wepman, 1949). Two hundred were distributed to military neurologists and neurosurgeons during World War II. One version fit into a shirt pocket, and another version was absorbed into the larger Halstead-Reitan neuropsychological battery (Reitan & Wolfson, 1993). Longer batteries in our history include Eisenson's (1954) *Examining for Aphasia*, Wepman and Jones's (1961) *Language Modalities Test for Aphasia* (*LMTA*), and Schuell's (1965) *Minnesota Test for Differential Diagnosis of Aphasia* (*MTDDA*).

The *MTDDA* was the most widely administered test in the United States and Great Britain in the 1960s and 1970s. It evolved methodically through seven revisions over 17 years, beginning with the first version in 1948 (Brown & Schuell, 1950). The sixth form was made available to clinics in 1955 on a limited basis for experimental use. The marketed form did not appear until 1965 (Freed, 2009). After Schuell's death in 1970, Sefer revised the test slightly (Schuell, 1973).

The full "Minnesota test" is lengthy, taking from 2 to 6 hours. It covers the four language modalities with 46 subtests. To shorten test time, Schuell (1966) suggested establishing a baseline and ceiling within each section of the full *MTDDA*. For each modality, a clinician establishes a **baseline** by starting with a subtest on which the client should make a maximum of one error (i.e., avoiding absence of impairment). To establish a **ceiling**, the clinician should stop testing on the task producing 90 percent failure (i.e., avoiding obvious maximum difficulty). Thompson and Enderby (1979) created a short form of the *MTDDA* by eliminating the subtests and items that are too easy or too difficult. Their version had only 5 items per subtest, contrasting with the original 20 to 32 items.

Over the past 50 years, aphasia test batteries have arisen out of different viewpoints regarding aphasia and the way to approach measurement of behavior. This chapter presents a modest variety of current batteries. Why is it useful to be familiar with different batteries? First, we may have a protocol at a rehabilitation facility that consists of a collection of subtests from different batteries. Second, we may be referred a client from a rehabilitation center that employs another test. Third, our broad knowledge helps us to follow conference presentations and literature that depend on a variety of tests.

Administering the Formal Test

Administering an initial test is shaped by keeping in mind the goals of this assessment. We want to confirm a diagnosis that has probably already been made. We want to obtain a baseline from which to measure progress, anticipating that we shall give the test, or part of it, the same way in the future. Mainly we want to plan treatment for the next few days. For example, we want to discover the type of stimulation that will produce a challenge at a high level of success (Chapter 8). In the assessment, we learn what is so difficult that practice would be impossible and what is so easy that the activity would seem like a waste of time.

Middle-aged and elderly adults are not accustomed to being tested, and so the mere idea of "a test" may provoke anxiety. The SLP should spend some time getting to know the person with aphasia before formal testing, giving the individual time to adjust to the setting. Adults may associate a test more with "getting a grade" than with planning treatment or documenting progress. The purpose and general characteristics of testing should be explained. Most adults are very understanding.

The initial assessment may provide a client with a first impression of the clinician, and we can be more aware of the client's point-of-view by considering the extremes. Based on a survey of 50 people with aphasia, Skelly (1975) found that several were offended by testers who were either "bellicose or indifferent." Skelly elaborated:

> One patient said that a questioner "barked at me as if I were a dog. I thought he might hit me if I answered." The reverse effect obtained with another aphasic person: "I felt he couldn't care less and probably wouldn't listen even if I did say something" (p. 1141).

Skelly figured that we would not want our performance to influence a client's performance.

An affable test administrator is relaxed and positive. The tester provides general encouragement rather than feedback about success or failure on particular items. We want to obtain information about current level of function. Clients look for clues about how they are doing by watching us score responses. The score sheet should be hidden and notation made for each response. If only errors are recorded, the client may become distracted and believe that performance is worse than it actually is. Consider when we just made a few errors on a midterm exam and then leave the room fearing that we failed the test.

We want to obtain the maximum amount of information in the shortest time. With most tests, we may have a sympathetic urge to see if a frustrating error can be forgotten with a little help. Through the kindness of providing a hint, we may learn something about responsiveness to intervention. However, assessment is not supposed to be therapeutic. We can avoid veering off track by scoring only what came before the hint and moving quickly to the next item. Consistent with strategies for abbreviating a battery, tasks that become obvious failures or successes can be aborted.

Results should be reported to the client and family as soon as possible. Not being informative during the test enhances validity and reliability. Being informative afterward contributes to a realistic perception of the impairment, especially regarding a client's ability to comprehend language. Selected results can be encouraging. Also, the client has a right to know. The results should be explained in a way that the client and family can comprehend.

There are some considerations when we repeat a test to measure progress. Now the client has some experience with being tested, which may result in greater tolerance as well as more frustration with failures that have been avoided in therapy. Because the measure should be reliable, administration should not be changed to make the test easier. General encouragement continues. Frustration is allowed and acknowledged as being natural.

Documenting Syndromes: The Boston Exam

Confirming a syndrome is a secondary objective in most rehabilitation settings, but a battery with this objective addresses aspects of language that can expose the uniqueness of someone's aphasia. The "Boston Exam" started the syndrome orientation in assessment. Harold Goodglass and Edith Kaplan first published the *Boston Diagnostic Aphasia Examination* (*BDAE*) in 1972. Nearly 30 years later, a third edition provided extensive revisions and additions (Goodglass, Kaplan, & Barresi, 2001). In addition to confirming syndrome, its features are as follows:

- Analysis of spontaneous verbalization
- A Short Form
- Extended testing

The *BDAE-3* is accompanied by a DVD of demonstrations. The test has been translated throughout the world, such as in Finnish (Laine, Goodglass, Niemi, et al., 1993) and Portuguese (Radanovic & Mansur, 2002). There are also Spanish and French versions (Roberts, 2008).

Content and Scoring

Initially, the *BDAE* was distinctive with its analysis of conversational and expository utterance prior to systematic testing. Conversation is elicited with an interview. Then a client describes the **Cookie Theft** picture: a kitchen setting in which a child, perched precariously on a tilting stool, is reaching for a cookie jar while a woman, appearing unaware of the crime, is washing dishes with water overflowing. This picture has been ubiquitous in research, including an elicitation of discourse from 225 healthy adults in the United Kingdom (Mackenzie, Brady, Norrie, et al., 2007). Google "cookie theft" and examples pop up online. In the test, Cookie Theft description is supplemented with cartoons for eliciting narratives.

The bulk of the *BDAE-3* contains four sections, each focusing on a language modality. Auditory and spoken modalities are presented before reading and writing (Table 5.2). Each major section contains standard subtests used since the first edition and optional *extended tests*. Auditory comprehension starts with words and then shifts to commands and short stories. Oral expression begins with tests for apraxia of speech (i.e., "agility") and then tests of automatic or subpropositional production such as counting and singing. Repetition, which is important for identifying conduction and transcortical aphasias, comes next. The complete test, including reading and writing, can take up to 3 hours to administer. However, clinicians tend to give it in parts, sometimes according to the aforementioned baseline-ceiling strategy used by Schuell with the *MTDDA*.

For those of us familiar with earlier editions, some of the changes were merely cosmetic, such as revising the clunky section title *Understanding Written Language* to the simpler and more direct title *Reading*. The body-part identification subtest was eliminated, and a few of these items were inserted into the word comprehension section. Goodglass removed the "animal naming" test (i.e., word fluency) and inserted

TABLE 5.2　Most of the sections and subtests of the *Boston Diagnostic Aphasia Examination*. Examples of extended testing are noted in boldface.

AUDITORY-ORAL			WRITTEN LANGUAGE	
I. Conversational and Expository Speech	*II. Auditory Comprehension*	*III. Oral Expression*	*IV. Reading*	*V. Writing*
Interview	Point to body parts, objects, actions, letters, numbers	Oral and verbal agility	Identify letters and numbers	Mechanics
Conversation		Automized sequences and melodies	Word–picture matching	Alphabet and numbers
Cookie Theft description	**Word categories**		**Grammatical morphemes**	Write to dictation
Cartoon narratives	Commands	Repeat words and sentences		Written naming
	Complex material (short stories)	Answer questions	Oral word and sentence reading	Cookie Theft description
		Boston Naming Test	Sentence–paragraph comprehension	
	Syntactic processing	**Naming in categories**		

the *Boston Naming Test* (Chapter 6). He transferred oral reading subtests from *Oral Expression* to *Reading*, which is consistent with cognitive neuropsychology's use of such tests. Clinicians, however, do not forget the important role of speech in determining performance on these tasks.

The **Short Form** is "a brief, no frills assessment, but one that still documents the performances that are essential for diagnostic classification and quantitative assessment" (Goodglass, et al., 2001, p. vi). It consists of most of the original subtests but only a few of the items from each subtest. The selected items are in boldface in the complete scoring booklet, but the Short Form has its own record booklet and set of stimulus cards extracted from the full test. Most correlations between subtests of the Short Form and the Standard Form were in the 1990s. The Short Form was used successfully in the remote delivery of assessment via two linked computers (Hill, Theodoros, Russell, et al., 2009).

Standardization and Interpretation

A revised normative sample of people with aphasia was assessed between 1976 and 1982. This sample was used to relate raw scores to percentiles. Then standardization samples of 85 people with aphasia and 15 elderly normal volunteers were obtained to support the third edition. The data mainly consist of internal agreements among items in each subtest.

For establishing validity, the lack of summary scores has made it difficult to compare the *BDAE* to other tests statistically. Comparisons to another test with a similar purpose will be reviewed shortly. There has been some study of the relationship between test patterns and site of lesion. Naeser and Hayward (1978) found agreement between independent classification with the test and predicted site of damage determined with CT scans for 19 patients.

Diagnosis of syndrome is supported with a rating of speech characteristics and a subtest summary profile. The manual provides examples and ranges of performance that are typically seen in cases of Broca's, Wernicke's, anomic, and conduction aphasias. In particular, the *profile of speech characteristics* is a convenient guide for classification. We analyze the transcripts of discourse according to a profile consisting of six scales characterizing dimensions of extended utterance. The scales address motor agility, phrase length, grammar, prosody, paraphasias, and a judgment of word-finding relative to fluency. These dimensions distinguish clients who, for example, have good grammar but lots of paraphasias from those that have poor grammar with few paraphasias. We complete the profile by comparing utterance characteristics to auditory comprehension and repetition as they were determined during formal testing.

Extended Testing

Noting that "aphasia assessment has been under pressure to change from a number of directions" (Goodglass et al., 2001, p. vi), the authors modified the Boston approach in two opposite directions. One direction, already discussed, provides for shortened testing. The other direction extends testing beyond the original battery with the application of neurolinguistic or cognitive neuropsychological research.

Let us see what the Boston team considered to be important new developments. The assessment begins with eliciting discourse, and type of discourse is expanded with cartoon-based narratives (Chapter 4). The word comprehension section is extended partly with tests of words by categories such as living and nonliving things. This is for detecting seldom-seen category-specific deficits (Chapter 3, 13). In another extension, a client grapples with syntax by responding to reversible possessives (e.g., *the ship's captain*) and sentences with embedded clauses (e.g., *The child calling her mother has dark hair*). As a nod to cognitive neuropsychology, word reading is supplemented with a number tasks involving phonologically and morphologically based decisions (Chapter 6).

Syndromes Quantified: The *WAB-R*

At the University of Western Ontario, Andrew Kertesz introduced the *Western Aphasia Battery* (*WAB*) as a modification of the *BDAE* (Kertesz & Poole, 1974). The test was first published in 1982 following earlier appearances in studies of aphasia (Kertesz, 1979; Kertesz & McCabe, 1977; Kertesz & Phipps, 1977). Roberts, Code, and McNeil (2003) reviewed 100 studies published in 2001 and 2002 and found that researchers documented participant selection most often with the *WAB* (i.e., 23 studies). The Boston Exam followed with 14 studies, also indicating that many tests are used for this purpose. A revised edition, the *WAB-R*, appeared 25 years after the first edition (Kertesz, 2007).

Kertesz perceived a problem with inconsistent definitions of syndromes. Consistency is possible "only if aphasia types are objectively defined, and classification criteria used in different centers are objectively compared" (Ferro & Kertesz, 1987, p. 374). To this end, the *WAB-R* has the following salient features:

- Content similar to the Boston Exam
- Summary scores including an overall score
- Syndromes identified by score patterns
- A bedside version

One difference from the *BDAE* is that subtests within main sections do not have a particular order of difficulty. Another difference from the *BDAE* and the original *WAB* is that objects, instead of pictures, are used for word-level subtests.

Content and Scoring

Like the *BDAE*, administration begins with obtaining a sample of spontaneous speech through interview and picture description. For the *WAB*, the picture is a scene of a picnic and outdoor activities. The test battery examines the auditory-oral language

TABLE 5.3 **Sections and subtests for the language portions of the *Western Aphasia Battery*.**

	AUDITORY-ORAL (AQ)			GRAPHEMIC	
Spontaneous Speech	*Auditory Verbal Comprehension*	*Repetition*	*Naming and Word Finding*	*Reading*	*Writing*
Interview	Yes/No questions	*window*	Object naming	Sentences	Name and address
Description of picnic scenario	Word recognition	*The telephone is ringing.*	Word fluency	Commands	Write a story about a picture
	Commands	*Pack my box with five dozen jugs of liquid detergent.*	Sentence completion	Words	Write to dictation
			Answer questions	Spelling recognition	

abilities of auditory comprehension, repetition, and word-finding, leading to the most well-known summary score called the **Aphasia Quotient** (AQ). Visual language and other subtests are bundled as a "supplemental" section for reading, writing, apraxia, and additional constructional (e.g., drawing), visuospatial, and calculation tasks (Table 5.3). Reading has a distinctly cognitive neuropsychological flavor with a variety of quick word-level tasks.

The entire test could take a couple of hours, and Kertesz recommended dividing it into segments across sessions. The manual indicates that the AQ can be obtained in 30 to 45 minutes (i.e., spontaneous speech, auditory comprehension, repetition, naming). Another 45 to 60 minutes is needed for the remainder of the test.

Summary scores set this test apart from the Boston Exam. Scores are obtained for the four sections of the oral language test. The spontaneous speech section is rated with two 10-point scales, one for information content and another for fluency. The fluency scale is used in classification. For example, 0 to 4 represents levels of nonfluency, and 5 to 10 depicts levels of fluency. The following scores have been calculated in various studies (see also Figure 5.1):

- *Aphasia Quotient* (AQ): Used with the test since 1974, the AQ is the summary score for auditory-spoken language. Forty percent of the score is derived from the spontaneous speech rating scales. Possible score is 100.
- *Language Quotient* (LQ): The LQ is a composite of all language sections, including reading and writing (Shewan & Kertesz, 1984).
- *Cortical Quotient* (CQ): This is the only score besides the AQ that was mentioned in the original test manual. The CQ represents performance on all subtests, verbal and nonverbal.

FIGURE 5.1   The tiered structure of summary scores for the Western Aphasia Battery. A Performance Quotient (PQ) for Part 2 appeared in early investigations (Kertesz, 1979; Appell, Kertesz, & Fisman, 1982).

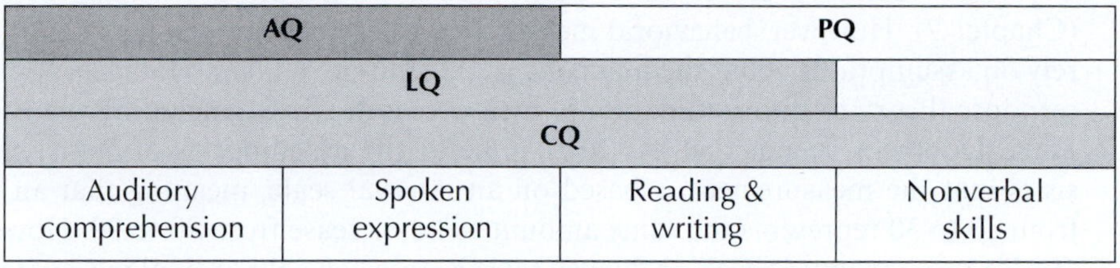

AQ		PQ	
LQ			
CQ			
Auditory comprehension	Spoken expression	Reading & writing	Nonverbal skills

Standardization and Interpretation

Originally, typical scores were reported for 215 people with aphasia, 63 neurologically intact individuals, and 53 brain-damaged people without aphasia (Kertesz, 1979). For a sense of what the AQ means, we can start with healthy people whose mean AQ was 99.6. The tendency for anomic and conduction aphasias to be mild and moderate impairments is indicated in mean AQs of 83.3 and 60.5, respectively. Broca's and Wernicke's aphasias scored means of 31.7 and 39.0, respectively. Broca's aphasia had the widest variation of all the aphasias. Persons with global aphasia had a mean AQ of 10.5.

Criterion-related validity was supported by comparisons to the *Porch Index of Communicative Ability* (Ross & Wertz, 1999; Sanders & Davis, 1978), and the *Lisbon Aphasia Examination Battery*'s "quociente de afasia" or quotient of aphasia (Ferro & Kertesz, 1987). The studies indicated that the *WAB* assesses aphasia like other batteries. For reliability see Shewan and Kertesz (1980).

A diagnosis of aphasia is supported with an AQ cutoff score of 93.8 (Kertesz & Poole, 1974). In one study, people with aphasia who surpassed the 93.8 score were considered to be "recovered" (Holland, Greenhouse, Fromm, et al., 1989). Ross and Wertz (2003) suggested that "the use of cut-off scores for differentiating normal from aphasic performance is problematic" (p. 313). These investigators compared 18 people with aphasia and 18 healthy adult controls. Four of the participants with aphasia had an AQ above the cutoff of 93.8. Therefore, blind use of such scores for diagnosis can lead to identifying a mild aphasia as normal and vice versa. Test scores should be supplemented with medical history, history of symptoms, communicative interactions, and other sources of evidence. For example, if someone has an AQ of 95.8 but also had a stroke a week ago, we might investigate for mild aphasia.

The *WAB-R* specifies ranges of test scores for key language functions as the basis for syndrome diagnosis. These key functions are the fluency scale and scores from auditory comprehension, repetition, and naming subtests. Conduction aphasia, for example, is recognized by scores that are low in repetition relative to higher scores in spontaneous speech fluency and auditory comprehension (Figure 5.2). For informal diagnosis, we pay special attention to these four areas (i.e., fluency, listening comprehension, naming, and repetition).

The summary scores have been used for measuring progress or recovery (Chapter 7). However, behavioral measures can be tricky for statistical analyses that rely on assumptions about the numbers. In Pittsburgh, William Hula has applied item response theory to the examination of measures for aphasia, including the *WAB* (e.g., Hula, Donovan, Kendall, et al., 2010). One of the assumptions of statistical analysis is that the measurement is based on an interval scale, meaning that an increase from 20 to 30 represents the same amount as an increase from 80 to 90. However, the *WAB*'s spontaneous speech or fluency scale is an ostensibly ordinal measure in which an increase from 2 to 5 is not an amount that is equivalent to an increase from 7 to 10. Even the ranking implied by the scale points is not self-evident.

FIGURE 5.2 Decision tree illustrating the manner in which the *WAB* classifies aphasias according to fluency, auditory comprehension, and repetition.

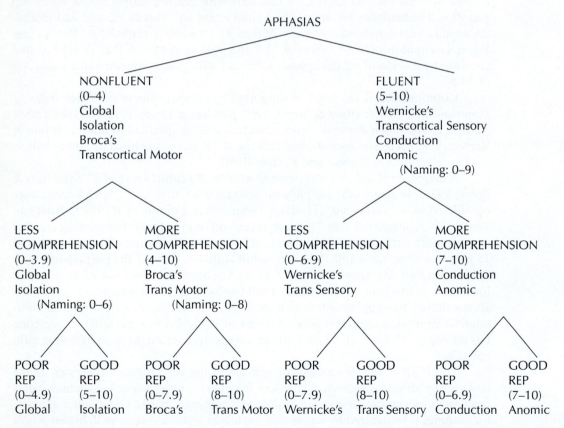

Analysis of Syndrome Diagnosis

Wertz (1983) had questioned the validity of the *BDAE* with respect to its classification of aphasias, and this concern spread to the *WAB*. Wertz, Deal, and Robinson (1984) compared the two tests given to the same 45 people with stroke-based aphasia. There was only 27 percent agreement as to classification. In a follow-up study, Crary, Wertz, and Deal (1992) performed cluster analyses with each test. They found 38 percent agreement between *BDAE* diagnosis and cluster membership and 30 percent agreement with the *WAB*, leading to the conclusion that the tests classify aphasias differently.

In Ferro and Kertesz's (1987) comparison of the *WAB* to the similar Lisbon aphasia test, they found only a partial overlap of aphasia types derived from the tests. A major discrepancy was between global and Broca's classifications. The main issue was the amount of comprehension deficit that would turn a nonfluent patient into someone with global aphasia. Another problematic discrepancy was in diagnosing conduction aphasia. To examine the goal of classification, Swindell, Holland, and Fromm (1984) compared *WAB*-derived syndromes to clinical impressions. They found that the test agreed with clinical experience for only 54 percent of the people with aphasia that were studied. Agreement was greater for nonfluent aphasias than fluent aphasias. Swindell recommended that, when we document diagnosis of a syndrome, we supplement scores with descriptive notes.

Psychometric Constraints: The *PICA*

Bruce Porch was disturbed by flexible administration and vague scoring when he embarked on his doctoral dissertation in the late 1950s at the VA Medical Center in Albuquerque, New Mexico. He wanted to achieve *reliability* for measuring progress and comparing clients. So, he applied psychometric principles to construction of the *Porch Index of Communicative Ability* (*PICA*), first published in 1967. It has the following salient features:

- Relatively small number of subtests
- Restrictive rules for administration
- Multidimensional scoring

Initially, many SLPs were wary of the rigidity of administration and cool reliance on numbers for describing clients. It just seemed too calculating for what had been the art of assessment. Furthermore, it was startling that a 40-hour workshop was needed to learn the scoring system. Now the *PICA* does not seem to be used as much as other current batteries (Roberts et al., 2003), but it has had a prominent place in clinical research and provides psychometric perspective on aphasia assessment.

Content and Scoring

The *PICA* contains 18 subtests of the four language modalities and other functions. The other functions include pantomime and basic object matching and copying. Reminiscent of Henry Head's serial method of the 1920s, each subtest utilizes a constant set of 10 common objects arranged neatly (i.e., cigarette, comb, fork, key, knife, matches, pen, pencil, quarter, and toothbrush). The objects are the same throughout the assessment so that functions can be compared without content variation. Also, the order of subtests is unusual. Auditory, reading, and verbal tasks are mixed together in subtests I through XII. Writing and copying are together at the end in subtests A through F.

The main sections of most aphasia batteries start easy and become gradually more difficult. The *PICA,* on the other hand, appears to proceed from difficult to easy. For example, describing the function of an object comes before naming the object. The organization was established to discourage a learning effect from repeated use of the objects across subtests. That is, if word comprehension were to come before naming, as in other batteries, a client would have heard the word before the naming test. The general principle is that minimal linguistic information is provided early. As a result, the sequence does not follow a strict hierarchy of difficulty. Actually, some earlier subtests are likely to be easier than later subtests for many people with aphasia.

Explicit prescriptions for administration apply to the physical conditions of testing as well as what a clinician is to say and do for each subtest. It can take 1 hour for a well-trained clinician to give the *PICA*, but it often takes about 90 minutes.

Having learned the scoring system at a "*PICA* workshop," an SLP assigns a score of 16 to 1 to each of the 180 responses (18 subtests, 10 items each). The definition of points in this **multidimensional scoring scale** begins with the basic concept of correctness (or traditional +/− scoring). The scale's sensitivity to nuance recognizes degrees of correctness and degrees of incorrectness. Incorrectness can garner scores of 1 to 7 (e.g., 4 is unintelligible, 7 is related). Correctness spans scores of 8 to 16 (e.g., 10 is a self-correction, 13 is correct but slow). The manual defines each scale point for each subtest, with subtle variations among subtests. The skill of assigning these scores quickly is learned in the workshops and then practiced over a professional lifetime.

Standardization and Interpretation

Did Porch achieve his goal of reliability? A convincing answer contains some details. Test-retest reliability, important for measuring progress, was examined for 40 participants who were retested in 2 weeks or less. Correlations were 0.90 or less for the subtests. Stability of summary scores was between 0.96 and 0.99. Thus, reliability is stronger for scores representing more subtests. Similarly, agreement among three scorers was 0.93 or better for subtests and 0.97 or better for summary scores. Of course, this strong reliability holds for workshop-trained examiners (Porch, 1967).

Reliability is not worth much if a test is not valid. The *PICA* has strong criterion-related validity with respect to other standardized tests but falls short of reflecting natural communicative abilities in daily life (Holland, Frattali, & Fromm, 1999; Keenan & Brassell, 1975; Sanders & Davis, 1978).

Mean scores are used for documenting and interpreting performance. The most specific summary score is the individual subtest mean. An average such as 12.25 is called a *response level*. The average for all 180 scores is the **overall score**. At one time, subtests were grouped according to the output functions in Table 5.4. Now, there are summary scores for both input and output functions (e.g., auditory, reading, verbal, and writing). To enhance communication of results, response level scores can be translated into **percentiles** relative to a large sample of people with aphasia. As implied in the discussion of reliability, the overall score is more reliable than subtest scores.

Data summary forms are provided to help a clinician identify patterns of performance and to facilitate meaningful documentation. Modality-specific conditions, such as motor speech deficits or illiteracy, are revealed by depressions of speech or reading modalities beyond what would be expected with respect to the typical pattern among modalities for aphasia.

The studies of reliability produced a basis for detecting real progress. Shifts between first and second testing showed a mean improvement of around 0.38 points. This indicates that a subtest shift of 0.40 or more is needed to represent real change as opposed to normal between-test variation. Reliable change scores (i.e., differences between a test and retest) can be determined for general and specific abilities. A 10 percent increase in the overall score is considered to be a reasonable treatment goal, whereas a 5 percent change "has a limited effect on communicative ability" (Porch, 1981, p. 105).

Shortened *PICA*

Changing the structure of the *PICA* voids use of the interpretive devices provided with the test. Yet, if we were to shorten the test, would an overall score from the shortened *PICA* be equivalent to an overall score obtained from the complete test? A regression analysis determined that 10 subtests and five objects per subtest produce an equivalent overall score (DiSimoni, Keith, Holt, et al., 1975).

TABLE 5.4 **Healthy adults (Duffy, Keith, Shane, et al., 1976) and people with aphasia (Porch, 1981) are compared according to original categories based on type of response. "Gestural" includes comprehension subtests.**

	OVERALL	GESTURAL	VERBAL	GRAPHIC
Normal Adults				
Range	13.40–14.99	13.73–15.00	13.48–15.03	11.18–15.03
Average	14.46	14.66	14.55	14.12
Left-Hemisphere Damage				
95th percentile	14.44	14.74	14.62	13.91
50th percentile	10.89	12.96	10.77	8.22

Another short *PICA*, called the SPICA, had similar results (Holtzapple, Pohlman, LaPointe, et al., 1989). This version was even shorter, consisting of four subtests but with the 10 objects (instead of the earlier five). The overall score from the SPICA was significantly different from the overall obtained with the *PICA*. Another SPICA with five objects was reliable but had less sensitivity to recovery over 4 weeks than the complete test (Lincoln & Ells, 1980; Phillips & Halpin, 1978). A shortened *PICA* may be good for a single assessment but may not be the best means of measuring change.

United Kingdom: CAT

The most influential aphasia batteries for English-speaking communities were created from the 1960s to the 1980s. Research since then (e.g., on-line experiments) might have, in principle, stimulated the creation of something significantly different. So, what is new? The *Comprehensive Aphasia Test* (*CAT*) was created in the United Kingdom (Swinburn, Porter, & Howard, 2005) and was promoted as being "the first new aphasia battery in English for 20 years" (Howard, Swinburn, & Porter, 2010). Its unique features are listed here:

- Cognition pretest
- Linguistic variables incorporated in the test
- Quality of life post-test
- Outcome prediction

The test incorporates variables, such as sentence structure, that became important in research. Goodglass and others (2001) had advanced the *BDAE* similarly through its "extended testing." The *CAT* is different because the new variables are contained in the main battery.

The *CAT* takes 90 minutes to 2 hours to administer, a little more than the *PICA* and less than the *BDAE*. The battery consists of three main parts. The first, called the *Cognitive Screen*, searches for visual, memory, and math deficits that may accompany aphasia or undermine obtaining a clear view of language abilities. A word fluency subtest in this section is usually found in the language component of other batteries.

The main part of the test is the *Language Battery* with sections for language comprehension, repetition, spoken output, reading aloud, and writing. In addition to alternating between listening and reading, the language comprehension section proceeds from words to sentences. Linguistic variables for sentences reflect some of the variables covered in Chapter 3 and include subject-object reversibility and actives versus passives. The dedicated reading aloud subtest reflects the emphasis on word-level cognitive neuropsychology in the United Kingdom.

More recent concerns regarding life participation or quality of life prompted inclusion of the final part of the battery, the *Disability Questionnaire*. The client marks rating scales assessing degree of disability in the four language modalities as well as self-image and emotional impact of aphasia.

Interpretation with the *CAT* includes prognosis. The last time prediction was based on test scores soon after onset was with the *PICA*'s various mathematical computations. With the *PICA*, we started with a "high-low gap" in which highest scores were thought to be indicative of a person's potential overall (e.g., Porch, Collins, Wertz, et al., 1980). There was some critical analysis of this method (e.g., Aten & Lyon, 1978; Wertz, Deal, & Deal, 1980, 1981), and the goal of test-based prediction of quantified language outcomes faded from the clinical imagination.

A modest version of statistical prediction was resurrected with the *CAT*. In a study of recovery, early scores (i.e., 1 and 3 months postonset) were related to scores at 1 year postonset. That is, early scores, with the help of graphs and considerable caution, were thought to predict later scores. However, the manual states that prediction "is not particularly accurate for individual subjects" (Swinburn et al., 2005, p. 134; also, Bruce & Edmundson, 2010).

Revival: Eisenson's *Examining for Aphasia*

Following his death in 2001, Jon Eisenson's *Examining for Aphasia* of 1954 was rejuvenated by LaPointe as *Examining for Aphasia*-4 (*EFA-4*; LaPointe & Eisenson, 2008). The current version retains the original overall structure and most of the subtests. It is supplemented with a "revised context" of test forms, normative data, and guidelines for analysis. Areas of modernization are listed here:

- Relabeling and reorganization
- Subtest additions and omissions
- New norms and interpretive scoring

One advantage of the *EFA-4* is that it takes less time than other batteries. The complete test, called the *Diagnostic Form*, takes 60 minutes. A *Short Form* takes about 30 minutes.

Without changing too much of the content, LaPointe replaced diagnosis-oriented labeling (e.g., subsections for "aphasia") with less-judgmental function-oriented labeling (e.g., subsections for "language"). Tests for agnosia are now called tests for recognition. Tests for apraxia are called tests for volitional movements (Table 5.5). The changes give the appearance of broadening the test's applicability to scores not necessarily attributable to aphasia or other disorders. The clinician has to decide on the disorder that produces the test performance.

There is a difference between the preliminary or prelinguistic section of this test, focused on transmission, and the preliminary section of the *CAT*, which aims at cognition. Where recognition is involved, the *EFA-4* presumes an examination of modalities, whereas the *CAT* adds a memory component and points to recognition as a cognitive function. The *CAT* is indicative of current interest in cognitive problems accompanying aphasia. The *EFA-4* maintains a traditional distinction between central and peripheral communication disorders (Table 1.2).

TABLE 5.5   Organization of *Examining for Aphasia*-4 (EFA-4; LaPointe & Eisenson, 2008).

PART I. RECEPTIVE AND EVALUATIVE TASKS		PART II. EXPRESSIVE AND PRODUCTIVE TASKS	
A. Recognition	1. Visual, 2. Auditory, 3. Tactile	**C. Volitional movements**	6. Nonverbal, 7. Verbal tasks
B. Language comprehension	**4. Auditory verbal comprehension**	**D. Language production**	**8. Meaningful speech**
	4a. Word identification: Body parts		8a. Automatic or serial speech
	4b, c. Comprehension of oral & multiple-choice sentences		8b–f. Naming, word-retrieval
	4d. Auditory discourse comprehension		8g, h. Arithmetic processes
	5. Silent reading comprehension		**9. Meaningful writing**
			9a, b. Write numbers and letters to dictation
	5a. Sentences		9c. Spelling (write words to dictation)
	5b. Paragraphs		9d. Writing from dictation (sentences)
			10. Tell a story (optional)

EFA-4 is certainly not a copy of the original battery. Reorganization and additions characterize the expressive section. Word-finding is tested earlier, so that the time-consuming writing subtests are delayed according to current custom. Word-finding is assessed more broadly. Object-naming continues to focus on body parts, and both versions of the *EFA* contain a test that consists of answering questions with a word (e.g., *Where do you buy coffee?*). There is the more current interest in divergence or "generative naming" of word fluency tasks (Chapter 6). A unique "category-naming" subtest asks clients to recognize the commonality among three items such as *Paris*, *Tokyo*, and *San Francisco*. "Oral reading comprehension," which entails reading a story aloud, is at the end of the meaningful speech section.

Subtest scoring is a fairly simple 3-point scale. With respect to the category naming example, we assign 2 points for correct (e.g., *cities*), 1 point for a related response (e.g., *country*), and 0 points for incorrect or no response. To facilitate interpretation in a manner similar to the *PICA*, subtest raw scores can be converted to percentiles relative to a sample of 58 people with aphasia. This answers the question of how a client ranks relative to a general population of people with aphasia. Validity of the test for basic diagnosis is indicated by an accurate prediction of 48 of 57 participants as having aphasia and 41 of 51 participants as not having aphasia.

Bedside Screening and Brief Batteries

The informal bedside screening described at the beginning of this chapter strains validity and reliability with respect to repeated testing, different examiners, and comparison to other clients with aphasia. Standard protocols ensure that everyone in the clinic does the screening the same way.

In many rehabilitation settings, SLPs select subtests from a comprehensive battery (except with the *PICA*). They may use the baseline and ceiling strategy described previously for the Minnesota Test. For a severe aphasia, they may select the easiest subtests in each modality to discover language abilities. For a mild aphasia, they may select only a few of the most difficult ones to discover deficits. They may postpone the slower tests of reading and writing. Also, abbreviated or "short forms" of batteries are available (e.g., *BDAE*, *WAB*, *EFA-4*).

Another approach is to employ a published screening test. In screening tests, each modality may be examined with a series of items sampling subtest areas, rather than with whole subtests. Brief tests emerged in the 1970s, such as the *Aphasia Language Performance Scales* (*ALPS*; Keenan & Brassell, 1975). Later, the *Frenchay Aphasia Screening Test* (*FAST*) was developed in the United Kingdom for nonspecialists, such as nurses and occupational therapists, to assist in identifying people with linguistic disturbances (Enderby, Wood, & Wade, 2006).

With a typical test time of 40 to 50 minutes, the **Aphasia Diagnostic Profiles** (ADP) is indicative of what clinical aphasiologists consider to be essential for exposing aphasia in its different forms (Helm-Estabrooks, 1992). The ADP contains just nine subtests and yields profiles for word retrieval, severity of aphasia, and alternative communication. It also yields a syndrome classification profile based on the four regions of assessment employed by the *WAB*, namely verbal fluency, auditory comprehension, naming, and repetition (Figure 5.2). The test was standardized at 42 sites in the United States and Canada on 290 adults with neurological impairments (222 with aphasia) and 40 adults without brain damage.

The ADP contains several unique features. For assessing verbal fluency, two questions and a grocery store picture elicit samples of spontaneous connected language. The picture arouses interest with a butcher's cut finger and a stack of cans about to fall. Writing is tested quickly by filling in a form with personal information. Along with reading and writing, an "elicited gestures" subtest contributes to the alternative communication profile (e.g., blow out a candle, wave goodbye). Conduction aphasia may be exposed with repetition that starts easy (e.g., *I love you*) and becomes more difficult (e.g., *If they come, he will go*). Someone with apraxia of speech may trip over tongue twisters such as *happy hippopotamus* or *Chuck challenged Chick to a game of quoits*.

The **Bedside Evaluation Screening Test** (BEST-2) is a portable test that can be given in 20 minutes or less (Fitch West, Sands, & Ross-Swain, 1998). Absence of a section for writing speeds up testing. Seven subtests are constructed for conversation, spoken production, auditory comprehension, and reading. The second edition was standardized on nearly 200 adults with aphasia. Norms are separated for those younger or older than 75 years. Confidence in the test was indicated by its use for measuring acute aphasia severity in a study of early cerebral hypoperfusion (Fridriksson, Holland, Coull, et al., 2002).

Diagnostic Decisions

The details of an aphasia test can distract us from our fundamental objectives. In the acute care setting, we are mainly involved in discharge planning. Will the individual continue as an inpatient for rehabilitation? Can she return home safely and participate in rehabilitation as an outpatient? Did we learn anything that might contribute to rehabilitation?

Here are the questions we are likely to answer in acute and subacute settings. Does the patient have a speech or language disorder? If it is a language disorder, is it aphasia? If it is aphasia, does the patient have a focused language impairment of word-finding or sentence construction? Does the patient have additional transmission problems such as an agnosia or dysarthria, or additional cognitive issues such as a low level of arousal or memory difficulties? Does the medical diagnosis present a favorable prognosis? No matter what test we use, our questions are the same.

"Too often examiners base their diagnoses on test results. They forget that tests do not diagnose problems; people do" (Fitch West et al., 1998, p. 20; see also Ross & Wertz, 2003). We interpret our observations according to what we understand aphasia to be, namely a disorder of language processing as opposed to hearing loss or a low level of consciousness. An inexperienced clinician may have a tendency to "overdiagnose" a patient who is not talking, especially in the first couple of weeks after onset. The clinician may have the urge to say that someone has one or more of the main communicative disorders studied in graduate school, while forgetting that a patient may be silent for reasons that are unrelated to aphasia (see Chapter 2 on global aphasia). Sometimes it is more accurate to say that we cannot be sure of language abilities (or speech abilities) until a lethargic patient becomes more alert and has more energy.

Another source of error is the potential for **cultural bias** in standardized tests. The mistake would be to consider a low score as indicative of aphasia in individuals who may be at a cultural or linguistic disadvantage when taking a particular test (see next section on bilingualism). In one study, socioeconomically matched healthy African Americans and caucasian Americans submitted to the oral expressive subtests of the *BDAE* and the *WAB* (Molrine & Pierce, 2002). There were no differences between groups with tasks requiring convergence on a single response. Although African Americans performed worse with divergent tasks, they also performed within normal limits. Molrine and Pierce concluded that "these common standardized aphasia assessment instruments were not unduly biased" against African Americans (p. 147).

No matter which test we use, we want to determine just a few things, such as the status of the four primary language modalities to diagnose aphasia. We also want to determine the retained skills that can be useful communicatively. A test battery with 30 subtests does not mean that a client could have 30 disorders. The 18 subtests of the *PICA* and the 46 subtests of the MTDDA do not mean that Porch and Schuell

Clinical Assessment and Diagnosis   **111**

disagreed on the number of problems that could be diagnosed. We know that people with aphasia can have a few specific language disorders in word finding or sentence construction. In general, any test is harnessed to help us document fundamental deficits.

So, what do we do with the results? We conduct three levels of comparison, summarized in Table 5.6. We look for **common threads** such as problems with language in all modalities. Task comparison is essential because no single task is diagnostic of a disorder. For example, a low repetition score by itself could be indicative of a hearing loss, short-term memory deficit, or motor speech disorder. In task comparison, we look for common threads such as difficulties only in tasks requiring lengthy verbal input or only in tasks requiring speech output. Then, within a single task, comparing items may direct us to a focus for treatment. A client may make comprehension errors with particular sentence structures or may make particular types of errors in naming tasks (see Chapter 3).

As we identify specific language problems, we are starting to plan for treatment. We **prioritize** with respect to an individual's communicative needs as well as the time we have. What will a client be most motivated to work on? What is most likely to improve in the next month or so? What problems can the family help us with? For some clients, improving comprehension (e.g., yes/no response) goes a long way to improving communicative interaction. For some clients, reading or writing skills are relatively unimportant. We may be writing our initial report in the rehabilitation unit (Figure 5.3).

Assessment may also be conducted for specialized purposes beyond planning for treatment and measuring progress. For example, questions of **competency** consider whether individuals are able to function in their own best interest or in the best interests of those for whom they have been responsible. What is the person's capacity to stand trial, assume parental responsibilities, live independently, and conduct business and personal affairs? Ability to understand one's will, called testamentary capacity, is indicated by assessment of language comprehension (Ferguson, Worrall, McPhee, et al., 2003).

TABLE 5.6   Levels in analysis of aphasia tests.

COMPARISON	DEFINITION	DIAGNOSTIC ISSUES
Function	Comparing status of language modalities	Aphasia versus sensory loss, agnosias, or motor speech disorders
Task	Comparing task performances within a modality	Level of language impairment such as words, sentences, or discourse/text
Item	Comparing specific items within a task	Impairment of a linguistic feature such as verbs or passive sentences
		Impairment of a semantic category such as living things or vegetables

FIGURE 5.3   Summary of an initial speech and language evaluation in a rehabilitation unit.

Pocumtuck Medical Center Speech-Language Pathology		
Name: Maxwell Chipotle	Location: Rehabilitation Unit	Date: 4-17-07

INITIAL EVALUATION SUMMARY

   Dr. Chipotle is a 65-year-old male who suffered an ischemic stroke on April 10, 2007. He is a professor at the local university. After 5 days in acute care, he was referred to the Rehabilitation Unit by Dr. Irving Waxman.

History
   Medical diagnosis was a thrombotic stroke causing aphasia and moderate hemiparesis on the right side. There were no sensory deficits. A CT scan showed an area of infarction in the region of the left middle cerebral artery distribution, specifically in the inferior left frontal lobe sparing part of the 3rd frontal convolution but extending into the inferior parietal region and superior temporal region.   After 2 days, Dr. Chipotle became aware of his surroundings and was able to recognize hospital staff and family.
   While in acute care, he was evaluated briefly by Patricia Burns, speech-language pathologist, who determined that Dr. Chipotle has a severe aphasia, mild dysarthria, and no swallowing difficulties. He was in an acute confusional state at the time of initial evaluation. He was able to gesture most basic needs, and by the 4th day was able to produce a few words communicatively. It was recommended that he be transferred to the Rehabilitation Unit for further evaluation and determination of post-acute rehabilitation needs.

Subjective Observation
   During initial interview, Dr. Chipotle was attentive and cooperative. Normal conversation was overwhelming, but he understood simple instructions. He was still limited in verbal expression. He became somewhat agitated when he could not express himself.

Objective Language Evaluation
   Dr. Chipotle was given selected portions of the Boston Diagnostic Aphasia Examination to evaluate auditory-oral language abilities.
   In auditory comprehension, he scored 31/37 for word comprehension, 10/15 for following commands, and 5/12 for answering questions about short paragraphs. In general, he had difficulty with the most complex material.
   In verbal expression, he described the Cookie Theft picture producing six nouns, one verb, and one 2-word phrase that were appropriate. He scored 38/60 for picture naming and answered 5/10 simple questions with one word. He had only minor difficulty repeating "Methodist Episcopal" but repeated 4/10 sentences accurately.

Conclusions
   Dr. Chipotle has some functional comprehension and limited agrammatic verbal production. He can communicate most basic needs. His speech and test results conform to a pattern of severe but still evolving Broca's aphasia. Repetition showed that apraxia of speech is minimal. This diagnosis is consistent with site of lesion and hemiparesis. Individuals with this type of aphasia often make excellent progress. His rapidly improving comprehension, good health, and motivation are all positive signs that he can progress substantially.

Recommendations
(1) Dr. Chipotle should receive language treatment to improve auditory comprehension, word-finding efficiency, and phrase length.
(2) Reading and writing abilities should be evaluated, especially because these skills are important to him with respect to his professional interests.
(3) The speech-language pathologist should meet with family members to answer questions and introduce them to the rehabilitation process.

Aphasia in Bilingual Individuals

Michel Paradis (1998) of McGill University was a little uncomfortable contributing a chapter on bilingualism for a book about "aphasia in atypical populations." He wrote that "there is nothing atypical" about bilingual people with aphasia. Most of the world is bilingual, and "bilingual aphasia" is the most transparently relevant issue for aphasiology with respect to cultural diversity. Being bilingual could refer to possessing any knowledge of a second language (Roberts & Kiran, 2009) or to "those people who use two or more languages in their everyday lives" (Grosjean, 1989, p. 4; see also Centeno & Ansaldo, 2013; Weekes, 2010).

Assessing these individuals means testing in each language. Some aphasia batteries, such as the *BDAE*, are translated into other languages. The *Aachen Aphasia Test* (AAT) originated in German and then was converted to Dutch, Italian, and Portuguese (Huber, Poeck, & Willmes, 1984; Roberts, 2008). For a dedicated bilingual battery, Paradis and Libben's (1997) *Bilingual Aphasia Test* (BAT) is available in several languages and includes the following parts:

Part A: multilingual history
Part B: comparative assessment of impairment in each language
Part C: translation abilities and language interference detection

The BAT is "one of the few published tests in Russian" (Ivanova & Hallowell, 2009) and is commonly employed for research (e.g., Muñoz & Marquardt, 2008; Tschirren, Laganaro, Michel, et al., 2011).

Questions are mounting concerning the equivalence of difficulty between test translations for comparing severity of language deficits (Roberts & Kiran, 2009). Compounding what Roberts (2008) called "the test mess" is the wide variety of bilingual backgrounds that a client brings to rehabilitation. By interviewing a family member, we should delve into the following factors before assessment begins:

- Relative ability in each language (linguistic level, style, reading, writing)
- Situations and purposes for which each language has been used (home, work, recreation)
- Persons with whom each language has been used (family, friends, colleagues)
- Translation abilities

This information leads to assessment that is appropriate for a particular language. For example, we would not assess reading and writing in a language not used for these purposes. We would employ work-related content with the language used at work. The same considerations apply to planning treatment.

What are we likely to find when comparing languages? Paradis (1977) found that 41 percent of the cases he reviewed seemed to have aphasia equally between the two languages spoken. Paradis noted that other studies showed as high as 90 percent having similar deficit across two languages. Controlled studies, which began to appear in the 1980s, also identified comparable deficits between languages such as noun–verb dissociations (e.g., Miozzo, Costa, Hernández, et al., 2010; Vogel & Costello, 1986). Any comparison between languages can be complicated by a dissociation between comprehension and expression. Good comprehension can be retained in two languages, whereas verbal expression is more impaired in one language.

Bilingualism is difficult to study, and similarly, bilingual aphasia is difficult to assess (Solin, 1989). A client brings individual characteristics of bilingualism to assessment, and the SLP considers at least the age of learning the second language (L2) and proficiency in using L2. Thus, a client may already have a predisposition to perform worse in one language for reasons that have nothing to do with aphasia. A study of late L2 learners (later than age 6) with aphasia revealed no difference between their two languages in overall test scores. A closer look showed that syntactic judgment was more impaired in L2 (Tschirren et al., 2011).

The language behavior of a bilingual person also varies according to the situation, especially with regard to the other conversational participant. When conversing with monolingual people, bilinguals enter a **monolingual mode** in which they *may* suppress or deactivate the language not known by the listener. When conversing bilinguals share the same two languages, both participants enter a **bilingual mode** in which they activate both languages. A bilingual person with aphasia is likely to display different behaviors depending on a clinician's linguistic status.

One dilemma is to distinguish aphasia from normal bilingual behavior, and one distinction may be between code switching and language mixing (Perecman, 1984). **Code switching** is normal and is the alternating use of two or more languages in a conversation. While speaking in one language, a person inserts a word or phrase from another language, perhaps because the insertion conveys a meaning better. Someone with aphasia may exhibit *unintentional* code-switching called **language mixing**. It gets our attention because it is not appropriate for the situation, as when talking to a monolingual clinician. Mixing may be indicative of a difficulty in accessing languages independently or a deficit in the ability to suppress a language (Gianico & Altarriba, 2008; Kohnert, 2008).

Situational code-switching can be more subtle. Four Hispanic people with aphasia conversed with healthy Hispanic individuals in monolingual English, monolingual Spanish, and bilingual modes. Code-switching in the monolingual mode turned out to be appropriate in this community. Thus, appropriateness of bilingual behavior is relative, such that code-switching is diagnosed as language mixing when inappropriate for the particular community (Muñoz, Marquardt, & Copeland, 1999).

Ideally, each language would be examined in each interactional mode for brief formal testing and conversation. This means that the assessment would be conducted by a monolingual SLP and a bilingual SLP (or family member). Roberts (2008) suggested that hiring a translator is fraught with difficulties. In the monolingual mode, conditions should lead to a deactivation of the language not being used, which is most likely to occur when the examiner truly does not know the other language. Pretending not to know the other language is rarely foolproof (Grosjean, 1989).

A family member may be enlisted to translate and administer a second test in the language not known by the clinician. Regarding the amount of time between test administrations, Vogel and Costello (1986) placed 30 minutes to 2 days between tests of object naming. They claimed that 15 to 20 minutes seemed too brief to minimize interference (or maximize deactivation of one language). Thirty minutes to 1 hour was sufficient for most participants. Paradis and Libben (1997) recommended assessing languages on separate days.

For obtaining behavior samples in the bilingual mode, the client should feel comfortable code-switching. Grosjean (1989) recommended that we learn about how aphasia has affected the special skills used in this mode, such as whether the client uses the "wrong" language, mixes languages to the same extent as before, or mixes in the same way as before. Has the ability to translate languages changed? Naturally, translation abilities should be assessed by someone who knows both languages.

Summary and Conclusions

Communicative disorder is diagnosed with two comparisons. One is a comparison to what we think of as normal. As noted in Chapter 1's discussion of research and a control group, comparing a test score to normative standards helps us to identify a deficit. Informally, we compare an observation to our sense of healthy language. Also, we compare an individual's poststroke behavior with a determination of prestroke behavior. We may ask a family member, "What changed suddenly, after the stroke?" This comparison is especially helpful with respect to subtle language difficulties and functional skills beneath the radar of formal assessment.

Comprehensive batteries provide different examples of how aphasia is assessed generally. Five batteries were summarized in this chapter:

- *Boston Diagnostic Aphasia Examination* (*BDAE*)
- *Western Aphasia Battery-Revised* (*WAB-R*)
- *Porch Index of Communicative Ability* (*PICA*)
- *Comprehensive Aphasia Test* (*CAT*)
- *Examining for Aphasia-4* (*EFA-4*)

The first three of these appeared in a span of 15 years, between 1967 and 1982. They have been revised and their standardization updated. The motivation for developing new tests is likely to come from further changes in health care management and discoveries about the nature of aphasia that make a difference in rehabilitation.

To minimize costs, acute and subacute assessments are shorter than a complete battery. The clinician prioritizes the time for evaluation, given the number of sessions that will be reimbursed. Clinicians adjust according to what is minimally needed to classify a patient for reimbursement and get therapy started. A clinician in a rehabilitation hospital wrote in an ASHA blog, "Our current language evaluation includes a hodge-podge of tasks from a variety of standardized language assessments . . . and does not always paint a full picture."

Fundamental diagnoses can be accomplished in an informal evaluation. Tests provide documentation of a diagnosis, and subtests are useful for setting baselines from which to measure progress. Measurement of progress is generally based on specific tasks reflecting treatment objectives, a topic of much discussion in the treatment chapters.

CHAPTER

6

Supplemental and Functional Assessments

Tests are continually invented to help us deal with problems that the large batteries do not solve. Two of these problems are posed by each end of the aphasia severity continuum. A test battery may be so difficult for the most severe aphasia that it does not expose capabilities that we depend on for starting therapy. Conversely for the slightly impaired, a test may not be difficult enough to expose deficits that would point to goals of treatment. The following are the main uses of supplemental tests:

- Assess special populations such as the most mildly or severely impaired
- In-depth evaluation of a language skill, such as reading
- Assess skills not represented in traditional batteries, such as functional communication

This chapter starts by climbing the levels of impairment before dealing with its consequences. Special topics include the diagnosis of reading disorders according to cognitive neuropsychology (CN) and the differential diagnosis of phonological and motor speech impairments. Admittedly, the chapter is a hodgepodge, a mix of published tests and strategies culled from research, tied together by the concepts of supplemental or targeted evaluation.

Word Comprehension

We are concerned about word comprehension mainly with severe aphasia (i.e., Wernicke's aphasia, global aphasia). Clinical examination usually consists of a **picture-pointing** task. Responses may be influenced by the number of choices and the relationships between or among choices. Pictured foils may be for words that are either phonologically or semantically related to the correct choice. People with aphasia tend to make more semantic errors than phonological errors (Gainotti, Caltagirone, & Ibba, 1975; Rogalsky, Pitz, Hillis, et al., 2008).

Suppose we want to assess word comprehension with a different task. Breese and Hillis (2004) compared the picture choice task with a rarely used **word/picture verification** task in which a client decides whether a single picture is a match to a clinician's spoken word. Of the 50 percent of participants with a deficit on the tasks, nearly 80 percent performed worse with the verification task, demonstrating that this task is more likely to diagnose a word comprehension problem. Verification could be more about making true/false decisions than about activating a meaning on hearing a word.

Word comprehension can be detected more subtly with **word sorting**. Clients may group words on their own or according to conceptual categories designated by an examiner. Nonfluent and fluent groups have exhibited knowledge of categorical and functional organization (Germani & Pierce, 1995; McCleary, 1988). When deficits appear, they usually occur with posteriorly lesioned fluent aphasias (e.g., McCleary & Hirst, 1986). The ability to deal with semantic implications of words is utilized in therapies for word retrieval, such as semantic feature analysis (see Chapter 8).

There may be subtle changes in **semantic memory** for some persons with aphasia. One clinical evaluation of conceptual knowledge is to have clients match or sort *objects* (not words) according to common semantic categories. Some individuals with aphasia sort objects into these categories normally (Milton, Wertz, Katz, & Prutting, 1981), but many others exhibit deficits and do worse than persons with right-hemisphere damage (Gainotti, Carlomagno, Craca, et al., 1986; Grossman & Wilson, 1987).

Howard and Patterson's (1992) *Pyramids and Palm Trees* (PPT) assesses "a person's ability to access detailed semantic representations from words and from pictures" (p. 5). Routes to conceptual knowledge are addressed with triads of pictures or words for concrete objects. One item, called the given item (e.g., *ticket*), has to be related to one of the other two (e.g., *car, bus*). There are six main subtests beginning with matching within the object and word sets and then presenting the given item as printed for picture pairs, as pictured for word pairs, or as spoken for either the objects or the words. A clinician can choose subtests to administer and may wish to address pure semantics with only the picture triads.

In the manual for the PPT, the authors encourage clinicians to diagnose with reference to a comprehensive CN model containing input and output components and centralized semantic components. Nine impairments are proposed, but only two of these can be inferred from distinctive subtest patterns. Regarding the other impairments, three, for example, should cause the same pattern of performance. The manual concludes that "a particular pattern of performance on the Pyramids and Palm Trees Test cannot be unequivocally related to a specific underlying level of impairment" (p. 15).

Could a word comprehension deficit in aphasia be related to a deficit in semantic knowledge? Researchers have compared a word comprehension task and a semantic task mainly with objects. In one study, 8 of 16 people with aphasia were identified as having deficient word comprehension. Three of the 8 did well with the semantic task, whereas 5 were diagnosed as being "nonverbally impaired" (Chertkow, Bub, Deaudon, et al., 1997). People with Wernicke's aphasia have displayed a somewhat surprisingly intact semantic memory (Koemeda-Lutz, Cohen, & Meier, 1987), but others have displayed impairment (Cohen, et al., 1980; Kiran & Thompson, 2003a). Thus, a clinically measured conceptual deficit may or may not accompany word comprehension problems. The problem may be in the meaning activation process.

Model-Based Assessment of Reading

CN reading models locate impairments that could be responsible for a pattern of performance on a variety of tasks. When we can point to an impairment, a model indicates alternative routes to successful reading. Reading problems are especially important to individuals who want to use a computer and who are particularly fastidious about their spelling (Rapp, Folk, & Tainturier, 2001).

Figure 6.1 identifies components of a CN model for reading aloud, the pivotal task for this assessment strategy. Such models usually navigate two routes from visual input to spoken response. In the primary or **lexical-semantic route,** a percept of the stimulus activates the lexicon (i.e., input-related form), which activates semantic storage, which then activates the lexicon again (i.e., output-related form) to guide speaking. An alternate route, **grapheme-phoneme conversion** (GPC), bypasses

FIGURE 6.1 Typical cognitive neuropsychological model of stages in reading words aloud. Functional equivalents are noted in parentheses.

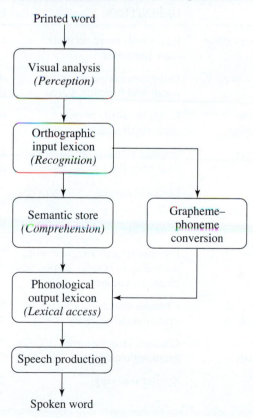

the semantic system, providing a capability for reading an unfamiliar word aloud. The ability to pronounce unfamiliar words or nonwords depends on a rule-based spelling-to-sound conversion mechanism (i.e., phonological reading). In principle, alternative routes are suggestive of compensatory therapy options when another route is damaged.

To find a culprit in producing an acquired dyslexia, clinical researchers use a "componential analysis." They manipulate stimulus variables and record spoken reading errors (i.e., paralexias). A daunting number of stimulus variables and types of errors are shown in Table 6.1. When we read through them, we can appreciate the intricacy of what seems to be a simple activity. Some variables relate strictly to word form, such as whether a string of letters is a real word, a nonword, or a pseudoword that comes close to being a real word. Other variables invoke the semantic system, such as a word's concreteness or imageability. Comprehensive assessment expands to other tasks, such as word repetition, to determine if a disorder is specific to an input modality.

TABLE 6.1   Symptoms observed in reading aloud as a function of word characteristics and paralexic error.

	SYMPTOM	DEFINITION	EXAMPLES
Stimulus factors	Word superiority effect	Real words more accurate than nonwords	*clean* better than *blean*
	Grammatical category effect	Difference between content words and function words	*tree* better than *the* *the* better than *tree*
	Concreteness or imageability effect	Concrete words more accurate than abstract words	*camera* better than *danger*
	Regularity effect	Regular words more accurate than irregular words	*mint* better than *pint* *cove* better than *love*
Paralexias	Visual	Looks like word	"plant" for *planet* "camping" for *campaign*
	Phonological	Sounds like word	"cambane" for *campaign*
	Regularization	Pronouncing an irregular word according to regular grapheme–phoneme conversion rules	"hayve" for *have* "sue" for *sew*
	Inflection (morphological)	Changes structure, not grammatical category	"plant" for *plants* "running" for *run*
	Derivational (morphological)	Changes structure and grammatic category	"strange" for *stranger* "territorial" for *territory*
	Semantic	Similar meaning	"coast" for *seashore* "tear" for *crying*

Investigators commonly relate core performance patterns to classification of dyslexias (e.g., McCarthy & Warrington, 1990). Research often entails finding cases with basic symptoms of a category and then doing further analysis to explain the symptom pattern. One case, DE, who had a traumatic brain injury followed by a stroke, was studied for over 30 years (Rastle, Tyler, & Marslen-Wilson, 2006).

Classification begins with a distinction between *peripheral dyslexias* and *central dyslexias,* roughly corresponding to sensory and cognitive levels of function, respectively (Table 6.2). Peripheral dyslexias are caused by impairments outside the reading system such as attentional deficits with a right-hemisphere stroke. Central dyslexias are disorders of the reading process per se. Most of these dyslexias tend to be part of a more pervasive disorder such as aphasia with a left-hemisphere stroke. The following are key characteristics of the central impairments:

- In **phonological dyslexia,** there is a severe difficulty pronouncing nonwords and unknown words, and word familiarity is a strong factor.
- In **surface dyslexia,** spelling-sound regularity is a strong factor. Nonwords and function words can be read aloud by the aforementioned conversion or GPC mechanism.

TABLE 6.2   Types of dyslexia. Central dyslexias consist of phonological, surface, and deep types.

CLASSIFICATION	SYMPTOMS	DIAGNOSIS
Visual (peripheral)	Visual paralexias Reading one letter at a time	Possibly "pure alexia"
Attentional (peripheral)	Visual errors with left or right side of words	Attentional neglect of the left or right side of a word
Phonological	Word superiority effect (real words much easier than nonwords) Good nonword repetition (auditory input)	Impaired conversion route
Surface	Strong regularity effect Regularization errors No semantic errors Nonwords and function words better than content words	Damage to lexical or semantic stages of the primary route
Deep	Mainly semantic errors Morphological errors Visual and derivational errors Strong word superiority effect Content words better than functors Concreteness effect	Impaired grapheme–phoneme conversion, or Damage to mapping input to semantics to output

■ **Deep dyslexia** is the reverse of surface dyslexia in the sense that nonwords and function words are harder to read than real content words. A client makes semantic errors and morphological errors (Rastle et al., 2006), and impairment may be linked to a semantic processing deficit (Riley & Thompson, 2010). Sometimes errors are visually mediated, such as reading *sympathy* as "orchestra." This error may have been accessed via the percept "symphony."

When a component process is impaired or a route is blocked, persons with acquired dyslexias appear to use compensatory strategies for reading aloud or for reading comprehension. One such strategy was suggested based on a large group study of 340 Italian-speaking people with aphasia, which provides a different perspective relative to the presentation of single cases (Ciaghi, Pancheri, & Miceli, 2010). Whereas picture-naming errors were common (i.e., semantic paraphasias), semantic paralexias in reading aloud, a key sign of deep dyslexia, were found in only nine cases, or 2.4 percent. Someone with aphasia avoids semantic paralexias by taking an unimpaired GPC route or, namely, by pronouncing familiar words. The analysis was that the few cases of semantic paralexia occur when the compensatory GPC route is damaged along with the lexical-semantic deficit of aphasia.

Another compensatory strategy is **letter-by-letter reading,** which is abnormally slow. There is a large increase in reading latency as the length of a word increases. It can take up to 3 or 4 seconds to read three-letter words and a 2- to 3-second increase for each additional letter. A letter-by-letter reader is often identified as someone with pure alexia or vice versa. However, reading one letter at a time is observed with various types of dyslexia. Other compensatory strategies include the following:

■ *Reading by sight* to compensate for the spelling–sound conversion problem in phonological dyslexia
■ *Reading by sound* to compensate for semantic route damage in surface dyslexia

Other investigators are wary of dyslexia classification. Hillis and Caramazza (1992) claimed that classification is arbitrary and is "not informative with respect to the nature of damage that underlies the reading disorder" (p. 250). They argued that classification-based studies are "empirically inadequate" mainly because of testing that is biased to a classification. Also, classified cases can have different explanations (e.g., Berndt, Haendiges, Mitchum, et al., 1996). Hillis and Caramazza (1992) advocated that "all theoretically relevant aspects of performance in language and other cognitive tasks should be considered in determining the level of impairment for every patient" (p. 251).

Can we relate this literature to familiar constructs for diagnosing aphasia? In the case studies, CN investigators often ignore syndrome and location of lesion. As a result, it can be difficult to relate the case to others. Also, there does not seem to be a fixed relationship between dyslexia classification and category of aphasia. Different syndromes can have the same reading impairment, and one type of aphasia can have different types of reading impairment. We cannot take a shortcut to diagnosing a dyslexia, such as by diagnosing Broca's aphasia and then assuming that the individual has a particular reading disorder.

Modular Impairment: *PALPA*

Researchers in Europe have been critical of aphasia batteries, claiming that they "were not designed primarily with the aim of elucidating the underlying nature of language disorder" (Byng, Kay, Edmundson, et al., 1990, p. 72). In 1992, the "much-longed-for PALPA" (Marshall, 1996, p. 197) was welcomed with open arms because it "beautifully fills this gap" (Basso, 1996, p. 191). ***Psycholinguistic Assessments of Language Processing in Aphasia PALPA*** was developed by Janice Kay, Ruth Lesser, and Max Coltheart in the United Kingdom and in the environment of cognitive neuropsychology (Kay, et al., 1992). Accordingly, the PALPA reflects a fascination with word reading disorders while promoting a fundamental and valuable diagnostic strategy consisting of the search for "common threads" noted near the end of Chapter 5. The previous section on reading prepares us for understanding this test.

The test manual's introduction was reproduced in the Clinical Forum of the journal *Aphasiology* (Kay, Lesser, & Coltheart, 1996a). Later, the test was examined in an entire issue of this journal, where the editor referred to an activity called "PALPAring" (Code, 2004, p. 75). PALPAring is a regional activity. In 217 citations of this test over 10 years, 139 originated in the United Kingdom. The United States followed with 34 (Kay & Terry, 2004). The test emphasizes word-level language and is flexible in subtest selection. It is sometimes used in the United States for description of research participants (e.g., Hashimoto & Thompson, 2010; Kiran & Roberts, 2010).

Description

The PALPA consists of 60 subtests with an organization shown in Table 6.3. The authors recommend, however, that the test not be given from subtest 1 to 60. Subtest

TABLE 6.3 A summary of most of the subtests for the *Psycholinguistic Assessments of Language Processing in Aphasia* (PALPA; Kay, Lesser, & Coltheart, 1992).

SECTIONS	SUBTESTS	FUNCTIONS INCLUDED (SUBTESTS)
Auditory processing	1–17	Auditory lexical decision (5–6) Repetition (7–12) Rhyme judgments (14–15)
Reading and spelling	18–46	Letter discrimination (18–21) Visual lexical decision (24–27) Oral word reading (29–37) Spelling to dictation (39–46)
Picture and word semantics	47–54	Word-picture matching (46–47) Synonym judgments (49–50) Picture naming (53–54)
Sentence comprehension	55–60	Sentence-picture matching (55–56) Locative relations (58–59) Pointing span for nonverb sequences (60)

selection should be flexible, and the test is "not designed to be given in its entirety to an individual" (Kay et al., 1996a, p. 160). Selecting a group of subtests may be based on a hypothesis of impairment, such as one that focuses on reading. Instructions for administering each subtest contain "suggestions for where to go next," especially when a client has difficulty with a subtest. Each subtest is scored for accuracy, and an examiner is also encouraged to pay attention to type of errors.

The auditory and reading sections through subtest 46 (three-fourths of the test) mainly deal with word form, such as phonology and syllable length, or grammatical variables, such as morphology and grammatical class. They are considered to be tests of input processing. Only a few of these subtests deal with the relation of a word to another cognitive representation, such as meaning. Five subtests manipulate image-ability as a variable (i.e., whether a word evokes a concrete visual image). There are nine subtests of oral word reading. As indicated in the previous section, an important aspect of reading assessment is performance with nonwords (e.g., *bem*). Deficient pronunciation of nonwords is indicative of an impaired GPC process (Figure 6.1). Some of these subtests infiltrated the Boston Exam (Chapter 5).

Testing the meaningful use of words begins in earnest with subtest 47, which is the classical test of word comprehension by pointing to pictured choices. Much has been made of this subtest, especially because the authors recommended that this is "a good place to start an initial assessment of auditory processing . . ." (Kay et al., 1996a, p. 177). Cole-Virtue and Nickels (2004) studied subtest 47 and concluded that the pictured choices have some confounds that might hamper interpretation, such as semantically similar distractors also being visually similar to the target word.

Standardization and Interpretation

The subtests were given to 25 people with aphasia and 32 individuals who were generally the partners of those with aphasia. Performance with aphasia is not reported in the manual. The norms for the non-brain-damaged controls appear at the beginning of most subtests. A diagnosis of deficit is judged to be two standard deviations below the controls' mean. The authors also recommend considering a score's relationship to chance when the response is a binary yes/no (i.e., 50 percent).

Interpretation "is based on the assumption that the mind's language system is organized in separate modules of processing, and that these can be impaired selectively by brain damage" (Kay et al., 1996a, p. 160). The modules are illustrated in models similar to Figure 6.1 for reading. Any one of the models in the manual "forces one to think hard, and with precision, about the patient's performance . . ." (p. 173). The idea is to infer a specific cognitive impairment from a pattern of subtest scores. The general lesson is that reliance on one subtest can be problematic. For example, when giving a definition for a homophone (e.g., *week, weak*), the process of interest can be masked by formulation problems. Once a decision on impairment is made, the isolated component becomes a target for treatment. Examples of how the PALPA is used for diagnosis appear in the journal *Cognitive Neuropsychology* (e.g., Tree, Kay, & Perfect, 2005).

The suggestions for where to go next are a useful guide to grouping subtests for the purpose of diagnosing impairments in particular components of the models. Dismissively, Marshall (1996) speculated that "the PALPA expects too much of the practicing clinician . . . It calls for an alternative way of thinking about aphasia" (p. 198). However, some strategies should be familiar to the most traditional clinical aphasiologists, such as comparing the same mode of output with different modalities of input to determine if a problem is output related (i.e., cannot produce the response in any condition) or input related (i.e., can produce the response to some input modalities but not others).

What worries some aphasiologists is the limited language processing theory behind PALPAring, when compared to the psycholinguistics presented here in Chapter 3. One response from the authors is that their "simple" model can be "a helpful way of *introducing* this way of assessing and thinking about language disorders, not because we believe it to be a particularly valid 'model' of language structure" (Kay, Lesser, & Coltheart, 1996b, pp. 203–204; see also Basso, 1996; Wertz, 1996).

Sentence Comprehension

Climbing the language ladder, there are a variety of methods for assessing sentence understanding, some available from test publishers, others suggested in experiments. A broad strategy minimizes the possibility of a test-dependent diagnosis. The view of a client's comprehension may differ depending on whether it is assessed with picture choice or verification (Mitchum, Haendiges, & Berndt, 2004).

Token Tests

This is an example of tackling the problem of batteries that are not difficult enough. The auditory sections of the PICA and BDAE were found to have low ceilings for people with aphasia, meaning that the challenging end of the tests does not have enough room for mildly impaired people to show deficit (Morley, Lundgren, & Haxby, 1979). Auditory language input is usually the least impaired modality, and mild comprehension deficits are found in anomic, conduction, and Broca's aphasias.

At the University of Milano in Italy, Ennio DeRenzi and Luigi Vignolo created the Token Test for the purpose of identifying and measuring subtle auditory comprehension deficits. Response would be based on processing language with minimal help from a situation, props, and topic. The test is a series of instructions to identify and manipulate bland shapes of different shape, color, and size. With contextual factors cleared away, it concentrates on the influence of linguistic length and complexity (DeRenzi & Vignolo, 1962). The Token Test, in its different incarnations, has been used widely in clinics and for research.

Boller and Vignolo (1966) published a complete list of commands, and so their version became the basis for most subsequent versions. The test has five parts. Parts I through IV contain 10 items each, and they differ according to information given about the tokens and length of command. Part V contains 22 commands of varying syntactic construction, and the commands are generally more complex than the items in previous sections. The complete test contains 62 items. The following illustrates each part of the 1966 version:

   I. Touch the yellow rectangle.
  II. Touch the large blue circle.
 III. Touch the red circle and the yellow rectangle.
  IV. Touch the small yellow circle and the large green rectangle.
   V. (1) Put the red circle on the green rectangle.
        (11) Touch the white circle without using your right hand.
        (20) After picking up the green rectangle, touch the white circle.

A variety of scoring systems have been used. Originally, errors were counted for each element of each command, with total possible errors being 250. Most clinicians followed Boller and Vignolo's recommendation of scoring each command as correct or incorrect and then having a best score of 62 (e.g., Swisher & Sarno, 1969; Gallaher, 1979).

Normative information must be pieced together from many studies (Table 6.4). For mild aphasia, comprehension difficulty may not show up until sentences are both long and complex, reflected in errors only on Parts IV and V (Morley et al., 1979; Noll & Randolph, 1978). The test can be difficult for others with aphasia (e.g., Hartje, Kerschensteiner, Poeck, et al., 1973). Problems with Part V in LHDs without aphasia led to a diagnosis of "latent aphasia" (Boller & Vignolo, 1966).

The first abbreviated Token Test was a subtest of the *Neurosensory Center Comprehensive Examination of Aphasia* (Spreen & Benton, 1977). There were 39 items instead of 62. A 16-item version was equally capable of deficit identification (Spellacy & Spreen, 1969). Norms were also developed for a 36-item Token Test with a cutoff of 29 for identifying aphasic deficit (DeRenzi & Faglioni, 1978). DeRenzi eliminated the color blue because of problems that elderly adults have in discriminating between blue and green.

McNeil and Prescott (1978) borrowed principles of the PICA to reduce inconsistencies in the family of Token Tests. Like the PICA, their ***Revised Token Test*** (RTT)

TABLE 6.4   As an indication of what to expect, here are some sample scores on the Token Test (Noll & Randolf, 1978; Swisher & Sarno, 1969).

POPULATION	RANGE	MEAN
Neurologically intact adults	48–62	59.7
Mild aphasia	18–59	43.5
Wide range of aphasia severity	0–58	23

has structural balance with 10 sections and 10 commands in each section. A 15-point multidimensional scoring system is applied diligently to each element of each command, and a clinician ends up with a score for each subtest and an overall score. The RTT takes around 30 minutes to administer. The test was employed frequently in research on auditory processing with aphasia (e.g., Hageman & Folkestad, 1986).

Testing time was cut nearly in half with the *Five-Item RTT*. It consists of the first five items of each subtest except for a complete subtest IX, totaling 55 commands. Arvedson and her colleagues (1985) wanted to determine if this version yields the same information as the full test. Results showed that the overall score predicted the overall score with the complete test. Arvedson suggested that the short version is substitutable for the overall score, but she was cautious about more specific analyses. Park, McNeil, and Tompkins (2000) found that reliability is nearly as high as the full RTT.

Not long ago a **computerized RTT** (CRTT) appeared in research on working memory (Sung et al., 2009; Sung et al., 2011). Validity and reliability studies were reported in unpublished presentations at the Clinical Aphasiology Conference in 2008. An experimental reading version (CRTT-R) was developed for one of the studies, and it was thought that the recording of response time for command elements would detect subtle reading deficits related to the padding of modifiers before the nouns.

Enactment Procedure

Caplan (1987) argued that traditional forms of testing do not permit examination of important syntactic and semantic features. He preferred a procedure in which people manipulate toy animals in response to instructions. More types of errors are possible, permitting more facile identification of difficulty. Caplan employed a ***Thematic Role Battery*** to assess the ability to assign thematic roles to noun phrases in a variety of simple and complex reversible sentences. In one study, 14 structures generated a battery of 168 items (Waters, Caplan, & Hildebrandt, 1991).

People with aphasia understand a variety of syntactic structures, but comprehension gets worse as syntactic complexity increases. In particular, sentences preserving the canonical order of English, as in *1a,* have been easier than deviations from canonical order, as in *1b* (Caplan, Baker, & Dehaut, 1985).

(1a) The elephant hit the monkey that hugged the rabbit.
(1b) The elephant that the monkey hit hugged the rabbit.

In *1b,* the recipient of *hit* (elephant) appears before the agent. Except for the most severely impaired, individuals with aphasia use word order to comprehend but still have difficulty when a sentence deviates from canonical order.

Complexity effects were replicated with a two-picture choice task, indicating that findings are robust across test procedures (Caplan, Waters, & Hildebrandt, 1997). These procedures were used to support arguments in debates over representational theories of syntactic impairment (Chapter 3). Love and Oster (2002) used similar sentence types for the *Subject-relative, Object-relative, Active, Passive Test of Syntactic Complexity* (S.O.A.P.), in which response was picture-choice instead of enactment.

Short-Term Memory (STM)

The belief that the short-term buffer of working memory is essential for sentence comprehension led to development of the **Temple Assessment of Language and Short-Term Memory in Aphasia** (TALSA; Martin, 2012). Its 14 subtests include basic language tasks (e.g., sentence comprehension) and STM components that compare phonological and semantic encoding and that stretch memory span. A sentence repetition task uses padding to challenge buffer capacity (see Chapter 3). The TALSA was used to evaluate a treatment of STM for people with aphasia (Kalinyak-Fliszar, Kohen, & Martin, 2011). It is not likely that a speech-language pathologist (SLP) will have time to give the test in its entirety, but individual subtests may be valuable, partly, as a source of ideas.

Reading Sentences and Paragraphs

For more thorough examination of reading capacities, clinical aphasiologists have created printed versions of auditory comprehension tests (e.g., McNeil's CRTT-R), borrowed reading batteries from the field of education, or created their own silent and oral reading tasks. These tests are considered when treatment objectives focus on reading needs, such as returning to jobs requiring reading skill.

Throughout several editions of his text, Brookshire (2007) suggested borrowing reading batteries. Nicholas and Brookshire (1987) used the *Nelson Reading Skills Test* (*NRST*) to evaluate the need to read paragraphs to answer test questions about them, called **passage dependency.** NRST paragraph tests were found to have better passage dependency than paragraph items in standard aphasia batteries (Nicholas, MacLennan, & Brookshire, 1986), which indicated that the NRST is a more valid assessment of text comprehension. Other favored reading batteries included the *Gates-MacGinitie Reading Tests* (MacGinitie, MacGinitie, Maria, et al., 2006) and the reading subtest of *Peabody Individual Achievement Test-Revised* (Markwardt, 1989).

The second edition of the *Reading Comprehension Battery for Aphasia* (*RCBA-2*) contains ten subtests from word to paragraph levels (LaPointe & Horner, 1998). Unique sections include a subtest for functional tasks such as reading common signs, a checkbook, and a phone directory. A supplement (*RCBA-S*) was added for the second edition. It contains seven subtests exploring word-level reading in a manner similar to the PALPA. Subtests include letter discrimination and recognition, word–nonword discrimination, and oral word and sentence reading.

People with aphasia are often meticulous readers. Van Demark, Lemmer, and Drake (1982) measured an average time of about 45 minutes to administer the main RCBA. They compared 19 nonfluent and 7 fluent people with aphasia. Both groups had PICA scores indicative of moderate impairment. With a maximum score of 100, the nonfluent group averaged 70.73, and the fluent group averaged 77.85. The mean and range for all participants were 71.34 and 31 to 97, respectively.

Word Retrieval

Some kind of problem with word retrieval is a fundamental component of aphasia. Naming tests are the most convenient means of measuring this deficit and, for some, aphasia in general. Differences between naming tests and conversational word-finding have been reported through case studies. However, group studies show that picture naming can be a valid indicator or predictor of anomia in natural conversation (Herbert, et al., 2008; Mayer & Murray, 2003), except occasionally for mild aphasia (Chapter 3; Pashek & Tompkins, 2002).

Naming Tests

The **Boston Naming Test** (Kaplan, Goodglass, & Weintraub, 1983), first intended to detect mild word-finding impairments, is incorporated into the BDAE-3. The *BNT* contains 60 drawings to elicit words of varied familiarity. It is graded in difficulty similar to the previously developed *Graded Naming Test* (*GNT*) by McKenna and Warrington (1980; Warrington, 1997). The *BNT* begins with common words such as *bed* and *tree,* and at the end it presents infrequently used words such as *trellis, palette,* and *abacus.* We provide cues when a patient is slow to respond, and we cease testing after six consecutive failures. The score is derived from the total correct with the maximum being 60. Cued and uncued versions of the test proved to be reliable (Huff, Collins, Corkin, et al., 1986). The *BNT* has been translated for several European and Asian languages (Patricaou, Psallida, Pring, et al., 2007).

Because of some of the unusual vocabulary (e.g., *protractor, tripod*), there have been several norming studies, focusing on older adults and helping us decide whether difficulty may be due to something other than aphasia (e.g., Henderson, Frank, Pigatt, et al., 1998; Tombaugh & Hubley, 1997). Investigators have found age and education to be influential, depending on how participant groups were selected (Patricacou, et al., 2007). Race has been an inconsistent cultural factor. After a comprehensive review, Hawkins and Bender (2002) concluded that few of the norming studies were representative of the general population. They suggested that norms be subdivided by level of education and that clinicians also consider premorbid vocabulary when using *BNT* scores to diagnose aphasia.

The **Philadelphia Naming Test** (*PNT*) arose out of Dell and Schwartz's studies of aphasia and was developed at the Moss Rehabilitation Research Institute (Roach, Schwartz, Martin, et al., 1996). The unique contribution of this test is its detailed error analysis leading to theoretical interpretation. The *PNT* consists of 175 nouns of different frequency and syllable lengths. Pictures are presented on a computer with PowerPoint, and naming latencies are measured. The goal is to analyze errors according to "what they reveal about the mental processes underlying normal and pathological word retrieval" (pp. 129–130). The *PNT* can be downloaded at the Web site for the Neuro-Cognitive Rehabilitation Research Network, which is a collaboration between the institute and the University of Pennsylvania (NCRRN.org).

Word Fluency

In expanding the range of word-finding test conditions, Chapey and her colleagues (1977) argued that "divergent thinking" should be considered in addition to the "convergent thinking" of object-naming tasks. Confrontation naming converges on one idea and one response. In a divergent mode, we freely generate a quantity and variety of responses. Once part of the Boston Exam, the word fluency task is divergent and entails producing a number of words to a single stimulus, which can be a concept or a letter.

In a **categorical or semantic word fluency** task, we ask someone to produce as many members of a category as possible, usually in 60 seconds. Speed maximizes the number of words produced within the time limit, and the speaker can be highly strategic by searching groups of words. The task has been adorned with a variety of names such as "category generation" (Hough, 1989), "category naming" (Grossman, 1981), "word-naming" (Joanette, Goulet, & Le Dorze, 1988), or "controlled association task" (Cappa, Papagno, & Vallar, 1990).

Some details from the research give us an idea of how this task provides a perspective on our clients. Grossman (1981) used 10 categories such as sports, birds, furniture, tools, clothes, and weapons. Normal adults produced around 14 words per category. People with nonfluent aphasia produced 5.3 words, and fluent individuals produced 6.7. These levels are fairly consistent (e.g., Adams, Reich, & Flowers, 1989). However, this skill fluctuates as normal adults displayed a wide range of 9 to 41 animal names (Borod, Goodglass, & Kaplan, 1980).

Productive strategies are identified as *clustering* (i.e., generation within semantic subcategories) and *switching* (shifting from one cluster to another; Hough & Givens, 2004). In his study of word fluency, Grossman (1981) examined the succession of words produced to a category such as "birds." Participants with Wernicke's aphasia started by producing examples of high typicality (e.g., *robin*) and proceeded to examples of low typicality (e.g., *pelican*). Yet they were also likely to produce words that do not belong in the category. Clustering and shifting are indicative of strategic processing.

Whereas categorical-fluency induces generation of words from a semantic base, **letter-fluency tasks** induce generation from a lexical base by having individuals fish for commonalities of word form. The letter-word fluency task was introduced by Borkowski, Benton, and Spreen (1967). Six letters were difficult for normal adults; for example, *J* elicited 4.83 associations, whereas moderate difficulty was observed with *N* (8.23). Easy letters (*F, A,* and *S*) went into the aptly named and commonly used FAS test, with these letters eliciting 10.22 to 11.50 words from persons without brain damage. Damage to either hemisphere caused a large drop in production (see also Collins, McNeil, Lentz, et al., 1984).

Because word fluency scores are likely to start on the low side for nearly anyone with aphasia, we may be tempted to consider this strategy for measuring progress. However, five administrations of the category test over a 2-week period showed that word fluency can be quite variable with acute and chronic aphasia (Boyle, Coelho, & Kimbarow, 1991). A sample of individual ranges for foods included 1 to 8 words for one person and 14 to 23 words for another. For some, performance varied depending on the category used, such as 8 to 10 for animals and 9 to 17 for foods. This lack of consistency suggests that a single word fluency test, certainly with just one category, is unreliable for measuring progress.

Verbs: Comprehension and Production

In Chapter 3, the importance of verbs for sentence comprehension and production was presented with research by Bastiaanse, Thompson, and others. Verb complexity, determined by argument structure, influences verb processing. Because aphasia batteries do not address verb complexity, there have been attempts to develop action naming and verb comprehension tests. These include *An Object and Action Naming Battery* (*OANB*; Druks & Masterson, 2000) and a *Verb and Sentence Test* (*VAST*) for naming and comprehension (Bastiaanse, Edwards, Maas, & Rispens, 2003; Bastiaanse, Edwards, & Rispens, 2002).

More recently, Cho-Reyes and Thompson introduced the **Northwestern Assessment of Verbs and Sentences** (*NAVS*). The *NAVS* consists of five subtests. Verb Naming entails naming actions with verbs that take on three levels of argument structure. Verb Comprehension involves pointing to pictures used for the naming test. Argument Structure Production entails producing a sentence from the same pictures with printed-word cues and arrows pointing to arguments for the verb. In the Sentence Production Priming test, like Sentactics® treatment (see Chapter 9), a priming action is modeled and then the target action is a reversal of the action. The Sentence Comprehension subtest presents the pictures used for the priming test. Initial data with the *NAVS* was obtained from people with agrammatic and anomic aphasias (Cho-Reyes & Thompson, 2012; see also Thompson, Lukic, King, et al., 2012).

Speech Disorders

This text has not had much to say about production of speech sounds or phonemes with aphasia. Blumstein (1973) compared the speech of people with Broca's, conduction, and Wernicke's aphasia. She concluded that the groups were identical in the kind of phonemic errors produced. Subsequent studies left a similar impression that any sound-level error by anyone with aphasia should be called a phonemic paraphasia. Yet are all sound-level errors the same disorder? This is a diagnostic problem, and several researchers contributed to solutions.

Because Blumstein's participants were fluent and nonfluent, researchers began to wonder if the widespread use of "phonemic paraphasia" was obscuring important differences in the speech of people with aphasia. This has been a particular concern regarding Broca's aphasia, which is caused by a lesion near the motor areas of the brain. Others recognized that this aphasia is often accompanied by apraxia of speech (AOS) and/or mild dysarthria, just as someone with aphasia can also have limb apraxia and right-side paralysis (Duffy, 2012; Halpern & Goldfarb, 2013).

The ability to differentiate levels of impairment is a function of **level of observation** (Canter, Trost, & Burns, 1985). *Internal analyses* depend on observing structures or events within the speech mechanism, such as evoked potentials in the brain stem, muscle contraction, or velar movement. *Acoustic analysis* records the speech signal with devices such as a spectrograph, which measures sound duration and voice onset time (VOT) for voiced sounds. Both of these analyses observe the external result of the mechanism. The common clinical strategy is *perceptual analysis* or classifying what we hear. As observation gets further from the neurological events, the chance of misdiagnosis increases. Thus, the opportunity for error is greatest in our clinical perceptual analysis. Sound-level errors across syndromes in Blumstein's perceptual analysis sounded alike but were not necessarily the same disorder internally.

Researchers set out to obtain telling observations of VOT, sound duration or timing, and velar movement. Fluent and nonfluent/Broca's aphasias were compared. Sometimes people with conduction aphasia were compared to people with AOS. This research indicated that nonfluent aphasia is accompanied by a disruption of the motor system, whereas motor function in fluent aphasias is normal (Itoh, Sasanuma, Hirose, Yoshioka, & Sawashima, 1983; Itoh, Sasanuma, Tatsumi, et al., 1982; Seddoh, Robin, Sim, et al., 1996; Williams & Seaver, 1986).

Clinicians do not usually have such laboratory support. So, can we hear differences in the speech of nonfluent and fluent aphasias? Table 6.5 is a summary of differences uncovered in research. Two research teams compared Broca's, conduction, and Wernicke's aphasias (Canter, 1988; Canter et al., 1985; Monoi, Fukusako, Itoh, et al., 1983). Conduction aphasia had more substitution errors taken from elsewhere in the same word, called transpositions. Buckingham (1989) called them "linear ordering derailments" that can be anticipatory (e.g., *papple*) or perseverative (e.g., *gingered*). Speech with Broca's aphasia contained more transitional disruptions from one sound or syllable to the next. Errors increased as a function of production complexity in Broca's speech but not in fluent aphasias.

In sum, phonemic errors in conduction aphasia are diagnosed as a disorder at a "prearticulatory" phonemic level in the language system, whereas AOS (accompanying Broca's aphasia) is a disorder in the articulatory or motor system. AOS contributes to the nonfluency of these cases. We can say that the person with AOS produces an accurate lexical representation with difficulty, whereas conduction aphasia involves an inaccurate lexical representation produced skillfully.

TABLE 6.5   Differential diagnosis of phonological disorders, including the terminology used to designate functional levels. For those familiar with Garrett's (1984) model of language production, his terminology is in boldface.

DISORDER	CNS LOCATION	FUNCTIONAL LEVEL	SPEECH SYMPTOMS
Conduction aphasia	Posterior cortex	**Phonological process (positional level)** Premotor stage	Fluency More errors in final position Sequence errors Transposition anticipatory preservative No distortions
Apraxia of speech	Anterior, premotor cortex	**Regular phonological processes (phonetic)** Prearticulatory or motor programming	Laborious More errors in initial position Transition errors Distortions and substitutions
Dysarthria	Motor cortex and below	**Motor coding process (articulatory)** Execution	Varied distortion and substitution Respiratory and phonatory deficit Impairment at all functional levels

Severe Aphasia

Whereas the original Token Test assesses one end of the severity continuum, the *Boston Assessment of Severe Aphasia* (*BASA*) aims at the other end (Helm-Estabrooks, Ramsberger, Morgan, et al., 1989). When impairment is severe, general batteries are too difficult or too language-oriented to expose communicative capabilities that can be reinforced in therapy. In the BASA, 61 items are distributed among sections for auditory comprehension, oral and limb apraxia, gesture recognition, oral and gestural expression, reading comprehension, and visuospatial functions. This test has detected significant improvements in communicative functions in severely impaired individuals up to 18 months post onset (Nicholas, Helm-Estabrooks, Ward-Lonergan, et al., 1993).

Functional Communication and Outcomes

Chapter 4 staked out the territory of functional communication as consisting of alternative modalities and contextual influences on language use, such as communicative purposes and situations. It is a short step to documenting the activities of living.

Functional assessment has been mandated by legislation and payment providers, and newer methods are influenced generally by constraints on time for assessment. These methods are important for measuring progress and determining outcome of rehabilitation.

Assessing Gesture

Whereas Chapter 4 introduced gesturing and drawing as nonverbal communicative options, this section turns to the present chapter's theme of assessment. Diagnosis comes into play when considering **limb apraxia,** which can interfere with communicative gestures. It is a disorder of skilled movement (or **praxis**) that, similar to apraxia of speech, is not attributable to paralysis. A movement, such as brushing teeth, can be performed in natural circumstances but not when invited to perform the action. Thus, limb apraxia may not be experienced explicitly until a clinician hunts for it (DeRenzi, Motti, & Nichelli, 1980). Because it occurs with damage to the left parieto-temporal lobe boundary, patients often do not have hemiplegia (DeRenzi & Lucchelli, 1988).

Evaluation is usually done with three tasks, namely imitation, movement on command, and natural or spontaneous movement. Movements are examined according to *transivity,* such as transitive actions on objects (e.g., dialing a phone) or intransitive actions without objects (e.g., an OK sign), and according to *complexity* such as a single movement (e.g., drinking) or a sequence of movements (e.g., making coffee). Clinical researchers often study transitive movements as pantomime, that is, pretended movement without the object in hand (i.e., "mime").

To facilitate diagnosis, researchers have categorized movement errors, especially for mimed transitive gestures such as combing, hammering, erasing, or smoking. Rothi and others (1988) looked for content errors (e.g., wrong pantomime), temporal errors (e.g., wrong sequence of movements), and spatial errors (e.g., unusual amplification of movement). One spatial error is what Raymer and others (1997) called body-part-as-tool (BPT) in which someone uses a body part as the tool. An example is the use of a straightened finger as a toothbrush when miming the appropriate action, as opposed to pretending to hold a toothbrush. Researchers have reached opposite conclusions regarding whether BPT responses are symptoms of a disorder (e.g., Duffy & Duffy, 1989; Haaland & Flaherty, 1984; McDonald, Tate, & Rigby, 1994). Intact adults do these things, too. Subsequent research showed that a truly pathological BPT error occurs only after someone is reinstructed to pretend to hold the tool (Raymer et al., 1997).

Duffy and Duffy's (1989) **Limb Apraxia Test** (*LAT*) is one device for assessing praxis. The *LAT* relies on the imitation task to specify response parameters precisely, minimize verbal instruction, and minimize the influence of cognitive problems that may appear when making movements on command. The test also avoids conventional intransitive gestures. Eight subtests are constructed according to the following factors:

- Movement with and without objects
- Simple (i.e., one to three components) and complex (i.e., four to six components)
- Sequenced (i.e., complete movement) and segmented (i.e., one component at a time)

A control group showed that there is no difference between left- and right-hand performance of the tasks. Sixty-eight percent of LHDs performed beneath the range for normal controls.

The Test of Oral and Limb Apraxia (*TOLA*) by Helm-Estabrooks (1991) evaluates movement a little differently. The section on oral apraxia instructs a client to perform nonrespiratory actions with the mouth such as "lick a lollipop" and respiratory actions such as "cough" and "blow out a candle." Oral and limb movements are observed first on command and then by imitation. Transitive and intransitive gestures are compared. Correlated with a rating of spontaneous gesture, the *TOLA* may be predictive of natural gestural use (Borod, Fitzpatrick, Helm-Estabrooks, et al., 1989).

A test of pantomime was developed to determine if miming is available. The ***Assessment of Nonverbal Communication*** (Duffy & Duffy, 1984) contains two tests of recognition and two tests of production. For recognition, a videotaped demonstration can be obtained for maximizing consistency of presentation. Response is made with a choice of four pictured objects. Like the naming task, the SLP shows a picture of an object, and the client demonstrates its use. Finally, in a "referential abilities" test, the client's gesture is evaluated by a third person, who must decide what was conveyed by choosing one of four pictures. One foil is an object that would be used in the same location in space as the correct object, thereby requiring a precise gesture.

Discourse Comprehension

Discourse is a string of sentences in narration or conversation. The ***Discourse Comprehension Test*** (*DTC*) consists of 10 stories played on a tape recorder. Each story is followed by eight yes/no questions. Some test questions address **main ideas** that are central to the theme of the story, and others address **details** peripheral to the story line. Inferencing is assumed to be assessed by presenting questions about information that is implied in a story (Brookshire & Nicholas, 1993). People with aphasia made more errors than neurologically intact individuals. Yet both groups displayed the same pattern with respect to main ideas and details (Nicholas & Brookshire, 1995a). Elsewhere, people with Broca's and conduction aphasias performed poorly in recalling main ideas (Christiansen, 1995b).

Nicholas and Brookshire (1995a) found both quantitative and qualitative similarities among aphasia, RHD, and traumatic brain injury. They noted that "this does not necessarily mean that the underlying reasons for their performance deficits are the same" (p. 78). They added that "evaluation of the underlying reasons . . . would appear to be a productive area for future research" (p. 78). Tompkins and others (2009) wondered if inferencing is really tested by asking questions about the recall of implied information. The DTC did not correlate with an inferencing task.

Conversational Discourse

Research methods such as ethnography and conversational analysis (discussed in Chapter 4) are valuable in determining the effect of aphasia on functional language use but are cumbersome for clinical assessment. The research has shown us what to look for. Regarding outcome documentation, Holland (1998) suggested that whereas "third-party intermediaries like to see numbers . . . they have never told us what to count" (p. 846). She added that, besides our "professional obsession with counting linguistic units," we can count "sociolinguistic units of conversation, such as ideas encoded, topics maintained . . . repairs completed, messages transmitted and so forth" (p. 846).

Conversational interaction has been employed as *social validation,* which is a generalization probe in single-participant experiments. It assesses whether progress reaches "the demands of the social community of which the client is a part" (Kazdin, 1982). What is a generalization probe? Unless a clinical procedure (e.g., using a phone) is identical to a functional objective (e.g., to improve using the phone), a functional outcome is documented with respect to something beyond the therapy. A barrier activity may be a treatment, but improving natural conversation is the goal. An SLP takes a moment before or after a treatment to determine whether a client is progressing with respect to the objective. Generalization is discussed further in Chapter 8.

Thompson and Byrne (1984) used a probe called a *novel social dyad* to observe production of trained social conventions. The dyad was a five-minute conversation with an unfamiliar person (i.e., undergraduate students). The clinicians also gave the probe to intact adults for interpreting peak levels reached by participants with aphasia. The range of scores exhibited by the controls exposed a problem with interpretation of natural progress: "We really don't know what patients are supposed to do when they go out into the real world because we don't always know what non-brain-damaged people do" (p. 142). In the United Kingdom, another rating of 10 minutes of conversation was offered as a "Therapy Outcome Measure" (Hesketh, Long, Patchick, et al., 2008).

Communication Activities of Daily Living

Communication Activities of Daily Living (*CADL-2*) is a test and an opportunity to observe a client trying to solve a few everyday communicative problems (Holland, Frattali, & Fromm, 1999). The following seven areas are evaluated.

- Reading, writing, and using numbers
- Social interaction
- Divergent communication
- Contextual communication
- Nonverbal communication
- Sequential relationships
- Humor/metaphor/absurdity

There are 50 items, and test time averages 30 minutes. The *CADL-2* provides a booklet for a client to mark a birthday party on a calendar, fill out an address form, and make a short shopping list while looking at a color photograph of the fruits and vegetables section of a supermarket. Scoring is done with a 3-point scale applied to each item, with the best score per item being a 2. Maximum score is 100.

Ross and Wertz (2002) included the *CADL-2* in a study of relationships among several tests of aphasia and a general estimate of quality of life. Eighteen participants with chronic aphasia averaged a score of 74.9. There were no significant correlations between Holland's test and quality of life. Thus, a measure of activity limitation may not necessarily correspond to feelings of life satisfaction.

Mahendra (2004) translated the *CADL-2* into Hindi and modified it for an illiterate population in India, providing an example of how a test needs to be modified to be used in a different culture. The *CADL-2*'s restaurant menu was changed to reflect Indian cuisine and included photographs of selections, which is common in India and helpful for illiterate individuals. Bus schedules are rare, and people in rural areas do not relate to the car speedometer that appears in *CADL-2*. Some could not state their home addresses, not because of aphasia, but because they tend to identify their houses by structural features and landmarks. In all, the investigator deleted 14 items to create a culturally appropriate *CADL-2* of 36 items with a maximum score of 72.

Another test that samples communicative problems in the clinic is the *Amsterdam-Nijmegen Everyday Language Test* (*ANELT*). The SLP presents scenarios of common situations and asks the client for what he or she would say. Verbal responses are evaluated according to scales for understandability and intelligibility (Blomert, Kean, Koster, et al., 1994). More recently, a new quantitative measure was introduced for the test (Ruiter, Kolk, Rietveld, et al., 2011).

A fairly straightforward approach to documenting participatory changes is to compare what a client does after therapy with what he did before therapy. Before therapy, a client is likely to have discontinued certain activities because of a stroke or other brain injury. For example, a client stopped working after a stroke but, after therapy, returned to work (Morris, Franklin, & Menger, 2011). Lyon recorded activities such as grocery shopping, maintaining a bank account, participating on a church committee, volunteering at a day-care center, and so on (Lyon et al., 1997; see also Caporali & Basso, 2003; Hinckley, 2002).

Communication Profiles and Scales

SLPs quickly estimate how clients function in their worlds by using rating scales. The first of these scales is the **Functional Communication Profile** (FCP), which rates mostly language functions of "everyday urban life" (Sarno, 1969). Based on interviews and testing, a clinician estimates abilities in five categories: movement, speaking (e.g., saying nouns, noun–verb combinations), understanding (e.g., for conversation, television, movies), reading, and other (e.g., writing, calculation). Functional performance is defined as the use of language "without assistance, cues, or artificial conditions." While the interview is freshly in mind, each item is rated on a 9-point scale. Wertz and others (1981) modified the FCP so that family or friends could rate a client's communication, and the researchers called this modification the *Rating of Functional Performance* (RFP).

In 1992, the American Speech-Language-Hearing Association sponsored development of a universal measure of functional communication. ASHA sought advice from an international panel. The developers especially wanted to assess the use of language and other communicative skills in activities of daily life. The result is the *ASHA Functional Assessment of Communication Skills* (*ASHA-FACS*), which covers four domains summarized in Table 6.6 (Frattali, Thompson, Holland, et al., 1995).

To obtain observations, the clinician becomes familiar with a client's communicative behavior and solicits judgments of family members and other caregivers. Each of the items is rated according to two scales. One is a 7-point scale of Communicative Independence. The other is a 5-point scale of Qualitative Dimensions of Communication, which is intended to assess the nature of functional deficit. As reported in 1995, a second pilot test produced data on 32 individuals with aphasia due to stroke and 26 individuals with traumatic brain injury. One study found that the *ASHA-FACS* and the *Western Aphasia Battery* (*WAB*) are strongly correlated (McIntosh, Ramsberger, & Prescott, 1996). Psychometric properties have also been examined (Donovan, Rosenbek, Ketterson, et al., 2006).

For the **Communicative Effectiveness Index** (CETI), a family member or friend is asked to rate communicative ability for 16 situations that were determined to be most important to family members. Situations include getting someone's attention, having coffee-time visits and conversations, conveying physical problems such as aches and pains, starting a conversation with people not close to the family, and conversing with strangers. Ratings are based on a scale with respect to "not at all able" at one end and "as able as before stroke" at the other end (Lomas, Pickard, Bester, et al., 1989).

Patrick Doyle and his colleagues translated the concept of "burden of stroke" into an assessment tool called the **Burden of Stroke Scale,** or BOSS (Doyle, McNeil, Hula, et al., 2003). An interviewer assists a client in reporting limitations in areas that include mobility, self-care, sleep, cognition, and social relations. Doyle was interested in obtaining a measure of the psychological distress associated with each of these areas. The BOSS contains a *Communication Difficulty* (CD) scale and a *Communication Associated with Psychological Distress* (CAPD) scale. Presented to

TABLE 6.6   Domains assessed with the *ASHA-FACS*. Only some of the 44 items are listed under the domains (Frattali et al., 1995).

SOCIAL COMMUNICATION	COMMUNICATION OF BASIC NEEDS	DIARY PLANNING	READING/WRITING/ NUMBER CONCEPTS
Uses of names of familiar people	Recognizes familiar faces or voices	Tells time	Understands signs
Explains how to do something	Expresses feelings	Dials the telephone	Follows written directions
Participates in telephone conversation	Requests help	Keeps appointments	Writes or types name
Understands nonliteral meaning and intent	Responds in an emergency	Follows a map	Completes forms
			Makes money transactions

281 stroke survivors in the Pittsburgh area, both scales distinguished communicatively impaired survivors from those not communicatively impaired, supporting validity of the scales (see also Doyle, Hula, McNeil, et al., 2005).

Clients may end up not doing much with an enhanced language process or communicative skill if they lack confidence in their abilities. Babbitt and others (2011) at the Rehabilitation Institute of Chicago have been developing an evaluation tool called the **Communication Confidence Rating Scale for Aphasia** (CCRSA). Clients rate themselves on 10 items such as abilities to talk with people, follow news and sports on TV, speak on the telephone, and discuss finances.

Minimally, reimbursement systems rely on pre- and post-treatment estimates of functional status. The American Speech-Language-Hearing Association (ASHA) has developed its own **National Outcomes Measurement System** (NOMS; Mullen, 2003). According to ASHA's Web site (asha.org), Centers for Medicare and Medicaid Services have classified NOMS as an approved reporting agency. Upon patient admission and discharge, SLPs may use the agency's Functional Communication Measures (FCMs) to document progress. The FCMs consist of eight 7-level rating scales that include four for the language modalities and similar scales for motor and cognitive functions.

Overall Functional Outcome

SLPs participate in general decision making regarding a client's welfare. Rehabilitation teams decide on whether a person will be discharged to home (a good outcome) or long-term institutionalized care (a poor outcome). In one study, 172 patients were examined initially during the first 2 weeks after onset (Henley, Pettit, Todd-Pokropek, et al., 1985). Researchers recorded information about medical history and obtained CT scans, measures of sensory and motor functions, a rating of activities of daily living, and a couple of measures of cognitive functions. CT scan data were not predictive of discharge outcome. Predictors of independent living included attentiveness, cooperation during testing, and high scores on motor-sensory and cognitive evaluations.

At rehabilitation centers, a client's functional independence is rated soon after admission and then at discharge. Professionals are likely to differentiate *instrumental activities of daily living* (IADLs) from traditional *activities of daily living* (ADLs), the former being more difficult than the latter (Cullum, Weiner, & Saine, 2009). ADLs are the daily essentials such as feeding ourselves, bathing, dressing, and grooming. IADLs include housework, managing money, shopping, and use of technology. Rating scales to assess ADLs encompass the domains of several professions (e.g., Mahoney & Barthel, 1965). Current scales are used to track progress, measure outcomes, and assist in determining costs of rehabilitation.

A national task force developed the ***Functional Independence Measure*** (*FIM*; State University of New York, 1990). It is a widely used multidisciplinary scale intended to measure overall severity of disability or "burden of care," and it is incorporated into Medicare and Medicaid's reimbursement system. Although an SLP does not complete an FIM, the clinician contributes to it. It consists of 18 items classified into the following six subscales:

- Self-care (eating, grooming, bathing, dressing, toileting)
- Sphincter control (bladder and bowel management)
- Mobility (bed, chair, toilet)
- Locomotion (walking or wheelchair, stairs)
- Communication (comprehension, expression)
- Social cognition (interaction, problem solving, memory)

These subscales are grouped into *motor* and *cognitive* domains with communication and social cognition included in the latter.

Each member of the rehabilitation team uses a fairly reliable 7-point scale for rating abilities in his or her domain (Cook, Smith, & Truman, 1994; Hamilton, Laughlin, Granger, et al., 1991). The SLP rates functional comprehension and expression, reserving lowest ratings for complete dependence on a helper and highest ratings for independence requiring no helper.

The *Functional Assessment Measure* (*FAM*) was incorporated into the *FIM,* resulting in an outcome assessment called the *FIM + FAM* (Hall, Hamilton, & Keith, 1993; Hawley, Taylor, Hellawell, et al., 1999). The *FAM* adds 12 items, producing the 30-item *FIM + FAM*. The developers had traumatic brain injury in mind and added more items for assessing language and cognition. For example, there are additional items for reading and writing. This measure has a rating scale for each item, rather than a single general scale.

Life Satisfaction

Chapter 4 indicated that life participation can be evaluated with respect to quality of life. The World Health Organization helped to make this territory explicit by developing a general health-related QoL measure. The brief *WHO Quality of Life* questionnaire (WHOQOL-BREF) poses 26 questions with each to be rated on a 5-point scale (WHOQOL Group, 1998). Some of the questions are listed as follows:

- How would you rate your quality of life?
- To what extent do you feel your life to be meaningful?
- How safe do you feel in your daily life?
- How satisfied are you with the support you get from your friends?

This questionnaire has been translated and standardized in countries around the world. The items distinguishing aphasia had to do with independence, social relationships, and the environment (Ross & Wertz, 2003). Also, with narrow exceptions, these QoL measures did not correlate with traditional language and communication tests, indicating that perception of QoL is unrelated to severity of aphasia (Ross & Wertz, 2002). There are several such measures (Table 6.7).

TABLE 6.7 **A sample of quality of life measures cited in the aphasia literature. There are many others (see Bowling, 2004).**

	ASSESSMENT	DESCRIPTION	REFERENCE
General	*Ryff Scales of Psychological Well-Being*	Measures agreement on 24 statements in 6 areas	Ryff (1989)
Health-related	*Sickness Impact Profile* (*SIP*)	136 items in 12 categories of daily life	Bergner et al. (1981)
	Dartmouth COOP Charts	Illustrations for nine questions about well-being	Nelson et al. (1987)
	WHOQOL-BREF	Short version, 26 items in 4 domains	WHOQOL Group (1998)
Stroke-related	*Stroke-Specific Quality of Life Scale* (*SS-QOL*)	49 items in 12 domains	Williams et al. (1999)
	Stroke-Impact Scale 2.0 (*SIS*)	64-item self-administered questionnaire; 8 domains	Duncan et al. (1999)
Aphasia-related	*Stroke and Aphasia Quality of Life Scale-39* (*SAQOL-39*)	39 questions in 4 domains	Hilari et al. (2003)
	Aachen Quality of Life Inventory (*ALQI*)	Pictorial version of a pared-down SIP	Engell et al. (2003)
	Quality of Communication Life Scale (*ASHA QCL*)	15 minute administration	Paul et al. (2004)

ASHA published the *Quality of Communication Life Scale* (*ASHA QCL*) for neurologically impaired populations. It takes around 15 minutes to administer and is recommended as a complement to the *ASHA-FACS* for assessing participation and documenting outcomes (Paul, Frattali, Holland, et al., 2004). Bose and her colleagues (2009) compared the *QCL* to the SAQOL-39 (Table 6.7) and showed that the two scales differed with respect to separating people with aphasia from control participants. With ASHA's *QCL,* people with aphasia were lower in the socialization/activities subdomain; whereas with the SAQOL-39, people with aphasia were lower in the communication subdomain. Therefore, the two scales have different sensitivities for living with aphasia. Another study relied on these two scales together as a measure of quality of life (Cranfill & Harris Wright, 2010).

In general, the source of information varies. For a client's **self-report,** questions or statements may be simplified (Hoen, Thelander, & Worsley, 1997). The *Dartmouth COOP Charts* may be good for people with aphasia because questions and response options are illustrated with aphasia-friendly drawings. The scales address nine areas including daily activities, physical fitness, and quality of life, and they take about 3 minutes to administer (Nelson, Wasson, Kirk, et al., 1987). An adaptation of the *Aachen Quality of Life*

Inventory (*ALQI*) consists of transforming items (e.g., *often alone*) into pictorial form (e.g., a person sitting alone). Ratings are depicted with a thumbs-up or thumbs-down and a neutral, frowning, or weeping face (Engell, Hütter, Willmes, et al., 2003).

Cruice and her colleagues (2003) gave a few QoL measures to moderately or mildly impaired people with aphasia. Impairment (*WAB*) and disability (*CADL*) were correlated to QoL measures, which indicated that language, communication, and life satisfaction are interrelated. Later, these investigators examined **proxy reports** using the same measures (Cruice, Worrall, Hickson, et al., 2005). The proxies were mainly spouses and children, and they were significantly more negative than people with aphasia in rating of quality of life, physical functioning, overall health, and vitality. They agreed with the people with aphasia for rating physical fitness, feelings, and daily activities. The investigators concluded that proxies do not reflect the life satisfaction of people with aphasia. Some clinicians advocate that outcome documentation come from the client rather than others (Worrall & Cruice, 2005).

In conclusion, health-related scales for a variety of medical conditions tend to be standardized, but the aphasia-related measures provided through the 1990s tend to be nonstandardized for validity and reliability (Hirsch & Holland, 2000). A decade ago, Ross and Wertz (2003) concluded that "no comprehensive, conceptually coherent, psychometrically sound assessment of QOL with aphasia exists" (p. 362; see also Ross & Wertz, 2005). A more recent study by Bose and others (2009) reinforces this view. Others argued that there are plenty of excellent assessments (Worrall & Cruice, 2005). It is likely that standards vary for evaluating these measures.

A summary of outcome assessment need only refer to *Living with Aphasia: Framework for Outcome Measurement* (*A-FROM*). Developed by Kagan, Simmons-Mackie, and several others (2008), it uses diagrams and charts to pull together all aspects of outcome measurement in the following four overlapping areas:

- Severity of aphasia
- Communication and language environment
- Personal identity, attitudes, and feelings
- Participation in life situations

A-FROM incorporates participation in work and play and satisfaction with quality of life. It makes sure that we think of everything that could be assessed as outcome.

Summary and Conclusions

This chapter introduced assessment strategies and tools that supplement the aphasia battery. These methods cover a range of linguistic and communicative functions dealing with impairments and consequences of impairments. The chapter began with comprehension of words, then sentences. Then it shifted to language and speech production. Functional assessment began with gestures as an alternative mode of communication, and it reached full bloom with measures of communication and ratings of life participation and satisfaction. These themes will not be forgotten in the following chapters on recovery and treatment.

7

Recovery and Prognosis

Will he talk again?

Will she get better?

How long before we have a normal conversation?

People with aphasia, their families, and payment providers have a stake in our ability to predict recovery. Because of the chronic limitation of brain injury, some prefer the term *progress* to the word *recovery*. Nevertheless, researchers still use the latter term. They have measured linguistic recovery and have explored factors that influence progress. However, this has become a sedentary area of clinical research. Most of the more recent endeavors continue the neurological story that was started in Chapter 2. At the end of the current chapter, the story becomes an explanation of progress, or what happens in the brain in the weeks and months after a stroke.

Stroke

Let us begin with a discussion of stroke in general. Chapter 2 noted that, during the acute period, intact regions far from the site of infarction are dysfunctional because of hypoperfusion of blood flow. As a result, most people with a stroke are perplexed and broadly impaired when entering a hospital. Rapid early improvements are the result of a subsiding of this disorienting diaschisis. Lifting the early cloud of global confusion reveals the structural *sparing* of regions of the brain rather than recovery from infarction per se. Progress later is understood with respect to how the brain deals with the chronic damage.

Most people with a stroke experience some degree of **spontaneous recovery**, regardless of whether they enter rehabilitation. In a longitudinal study of 92 persons with ischemic stroke, researchers followed functions of daily living for 2 to 3 years. They observed statistically significant progress during the first 3 months postonset. Between 3 and 6 months, there was slight improvement, and no change was detected on average after 6 months (Skilbeck, Wade, Hewer, & Wood, 1983). These results are indicative of a long-held view of recovery in general.

The *Functional Independence Measure* (*FIM*), introduced late in Chapter 6, was evaluated for its predictive value for anyone with a stroke. When given 6 days after admission to an acute care hospital, the scale predicted discharge to home, a rehabilitation center, or a nursing home (Mauthe, Haaf, Hayn, et al., 1996). When the *FIM* was given later during admission to a rehabilitation center, around 2 months after stroke, the severity level of the full scale was suggestive of outcome 60 days later (Oczkowski & Barreca, 1993). It was also predictive of "burden of care" at home, measured according to the minutes of assistance per day provided by a caregiver (Granger, Cotter, Hamilton, et al., 1993). Thus, the *FIM* contributes to decisions regarding discharge from rehabilitation.

Recovery of Language

Spontaneous recovery of language has been documented in a variety of circumstances, including studies in which untreated and treated individuals were compared. In one study, participants with aphasia "were prevented from attending therapy by extraneous factors, such as family or transportation problems, but were willing to come back once again to the unit after six months or more in order to take the second examination" (Basso, Capitani, & Vignolo, 1979, p. 191). For bolstering an evidence-based clinical practice, most of this section presents data that shows what we can expect for language behavior. In particular, this section explores different aspects of recovery, such as "how much" and "how fast."

Measuring Progress

Sarno and others (1971) stated that "improvement which is not reflected in the patient's daily life is not improvement in fact" (p. 74). Still, we respect reliably measured progress. We are vigilant in assessing both **clinical improvement** with valid tests of linguistic skills and **functional improvement** in solving communicative problems of daily living. With respect to clinical improvement, most investigators have measured clinical progress with the measurement-oriented *Porch Index of Communicative Ability* (*PICA*) or the *Western Aphasia Battery* (*WAB*). In the clinic, we probe generalization of goal-related skills as noted in the next chapter.

In directing large studies of recovery and treatment efficacy, Robert Wertz was interested in the performance of various clinical tests (e.g., Ross & Wertz, 1999). Covering intervals up to 1 year after stroke, he compared the impairment-related PICA and two functional measures. These assessments were not correlated with respect to measuring change at any point in the first year, indicating that impairment-related and functional (or pragmatic) tests measure different aspects of recovery (Irwin, Wertz, & Avent, 2002). Lyon and his colleagues (1997) found no progress over a 5-month period with respect to the Boston Exam and the *Communication Activities of Daily Living* (*CADL*). However, significant change was detected with more subjective questionnaires related to a client's (a) comfort, confidence, and skills when conversing with family members or strangers and (b) life satisfaction and general comfort with self and others. This research indicates that perceived progress can also be measured.

The following sections introduce the components of linguistic recovery, including amount, outcome, and rate. Most of the data is from clinical measures taken in rehabilitation programs, but studies of spontaneous recovery are given special mention. *Variability* is a central theme, and it will be shown that predictions differ depending on the component of recovery being considered (Connor, Obler, Tocco, et al., 2001; de Riesthal & Wertz, 2004). Before embarking on this adventure, it would be good to review the scores associated with the *PICA* and the *WAB* (Chapter 5).

Proportion of Clients That Improve

What is the likelihood that language improves after stroke? Long ago, it was reported that only about 50 percent of people with aphasia made recognizable improvement (Basso, et al., 1979; Godfrey & Douglass, 1959; Marks, Taylor, & Rusk, 1957). The percentage of clients that improve was used as the dependent measure in a large efficacy study in Italy (Chapter 8). Fifty-nine percent improved in the first 2 months without therapy. The proportion dropped after the first 2 months, and the treated group did much better (Basso et al., 1979).

Later, according to the more sensitive *PICA*, 90 percent of untreated individuals improved over the first 10 weeks postonset, an indication of the pervasiveness of spontaneous recovery. The proportion dropped to 79 percent between 10 and 22 weeks (Lendrem & Lincoln, 1985). Thus, these reports depend on the assessment method, and sensitive and reliable measurement paints a more hopeful picture than the earlier studies.

Amount of Improvement

Reliable measurement enables us to quantify progress without relying on subjective judgment. Of course, amount of improvement is determined by subtracting an earlier test score (i.e., pretest) from a later score (i.e., post-test). The result is called a "difference score" or "change score" in the literature. Change scores have been reported for a variety of intervals between the first and second test. For a moment, let us give the nature of these intervals a little scrutiny to sharpen our analytical skills.

In studies, *initial scores* have been obtained at different times postonset. Sarno and Levita (1971) obtained functional ratings for 28 patients at bedside within 2 days, when a few had "a total lack of responsiveness and, quite probably, total absence of consciousness" (p. 177). To avoid invalid and unreliable results, researchers and clinicians prefer to wait until the medical condition stabilizes and pattern of language deficit is apparent before giving the first comprehensive test (e.g., Wallesch, Bak, & Schulte-Mönting, 1992). The first score has often been obtained around 1 month after onset (e.g., Deal & Deal, 1978; Wertz, Collins, Weiss, et al., 1981), depending on the time of admission to a rehabilitation center (Pickersgill & Lincoln, 1983). One result of this strategy is that there is little data regarding recovery during the first month.

In studies of spontaneous recovery, the *final score* may not always be obtained at the point of maximum recovery. Investigators tend to give the final test at 3 or 4 months postonset, possibly missing the progress that might be made later. Lendrem and Lincoln (1985) retested at 6-week intervals beginning at 10 weeks postonset and concluding at around 8 months. When we are scrutinizing the literature, noting when initial and final scores were obtained helps to identify the boundaries of results.

In studies of people in rehabilitation, on the other hand, the final test has often been given around 1 year postonset rather than at 3 or 4 months (e.g., Wertz et al., 1981). Also, change scores have been based on either final scores at termination of treatment (Deal & Deal, 1978) or *peak scores* achieved before treatment was terminated (Bamber, 1980; Hanson & Cicciarelli, 1978). Thus, end points have been tied to different clinical circumstances, and later final scores usually are not indicative of spontaneous recovery.

The most consistent fact is that people with aphasia are widely variable in amount of recovery, making prediction seem to be quite daunting. In a study of mostly untreated individuals, the WAB's Aphasia Quotient (AQ) progressed an average of 16.64 percentage points (Kertesz & McCabe, 1977). Yet one subgroup improved 5.16 points and another 36.80 points (these groups will be identified later). The *PICA* also demonstrated wide ranges of spontaneous progress (e.g., Lendrem & Lincoln, 1985). Three small-sample studies of treated people with aphasia had remarkable agreement in average amount of change over the first year postonset (Table 7.1). We may be tempted to inform a client that he or she is likely to improve around 3.30 overall points in the first year. Unfortunately, we cannot promise this improvement, which may amount to 0.10 or 7.16 response level points.

How do we interpret a change score? Researchers speak of "significant progress" with respect to statistical analysis. In Lendrem and Lincoln's (1985) study, spontaneous progress did not become statistically significant until 5 months postonset. We may distinguish *statistical significance* and *clinical significance* of recovery data. With a large experimental group, a small change score may be statistically significant; but it may not represent a meaningful change in someone's life. For an individual, a small change may be clinically significant. For example, progress merely in answering yes/no questions may have a profound impact on communicative interaction.

TABLE 7.1 **Amount and variability of change in *PICA* overall scores in three studies of mixed aphasic groups.**

	N	INITIAL	FINAL	CHANGE	RANGE
Hanson and Cicciarelli (1978)	13	9.48	12.72	3.24	0.98–4.29
Deal and Deal (1978)	17	9.14	12.52	3.38	0.51–7.16
Bamber (1980)	13	8.40	11.65	3.25	0.10–6.18

Outcome

In Chapter 6, outcome was assumed to be the product of rehabilitation as well as some perceived or even mythical end-point of recovery. The aforementioned final or peak scores are a numerical indication of level of language ability around a year after stroke. Yet have outcomes actually been determined beyond this point? In research, the conclusion of recovery is demonstrated with a series of measures suggestive of a "plateau" of slightly variable scores. This set of scores indicates that the final linguistic outcome usually falls short of a return to normal function.

Kertesz (1985) categorized outcomes of mostly untreated individuals with AQs taken at an average of 2 years postonset. He found a balanced representation with 27 percent in the excellent category (75–100 AQ); 24 percent were good (50–75); 24 percent were fair (25–50); and 25 percent ended up in the poor category (0–25).

The final scores in Table 7.1 are indicative of average *PICA* overall outcomes for people with ischemic stroke who were in treatment until a year postonset. Outcomes ranged from 8.69 to 14.88 across the three studies. Thus, many were far from a neurologically intact group (Table 5.4). About one-third of the clients in the table reached into the "normal" range. Substantial progress was found in cases receiving therapy well beyond the first year (e.g., Broida, 1977; Hanson, Metter, & Riege, 1989; Sands, Sarno, & Shankweiler, 1969).

Saying that someone might end up with a 12.00 on the *PICA* does not say much about quality of life. Schuell and her colleagues (1964) documented the number of individuals that returned to school, entered vocational training, or reentered employment. In her youngest group with "simple aphasia," 14 percent entered school or vocational training, and 19 percent resumed employment. In a group with Broca's aphasia, 33 percent entered vocational training, and 27 percent found work. Schuell explained that the less-impaired people had difficulty accepting a downgrade from their previous employment. Among the most impaired groups, no one entered vocational training or became employed. Caporali and Basso (2003) followed 52 clients up to an average of 5 years after stroke. Nine were employed.

Rate of Improvement

Although final outcome varies, we may still wonder how long it takes to get there. It is one thing to say that a person with aphasia may improve 3.30 points, and it is another thing to say that it will take 4 months or 4 years. Our information comes from research that has regularly employed certain time frames, namely, from onset to 3 months, 3 to 6 months, 6 to 12 months, and beyond 12 months. Most data come from the first 12 months.

A "recovery curve" for aphasia is consistent with what was noted earlier for stroke in general (Skilbeck et al., 1983). Progress is more rapid in the first 3 months postonset than in any period thereafter. Lendrem and Lincoln (1985) found statistically significant progress between 4 and 22 weeks (1 to 5.5 months). A comparison of 10 weeks to 34 weeks yielded change that was not significant. The shape of this curve

FIGURE 7.1   **Hypothetical recovery curves drawn from studies of recovery, with variation according to initial severity of aphasia. Mild aphasia has a test ceiling effect.**

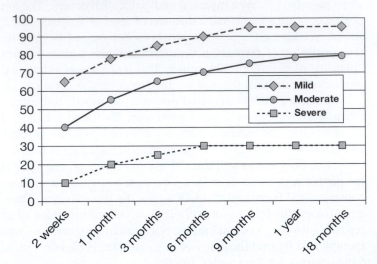

applies to both spontaneous recovery and progress during rehabilitation (Figure 7.1). For one group of people with aphasia receiving language treatment until 11 months postonset, 65 percent of their progress occurred within the first 4 months (Wertz et al., 1981).

Duration of spontaneous recovery has been an important factor in determining the efficacy of treatment. For individuals in a rehabilitation program, we are tempted to conclude that progress can be attributed to a treatment when the improvement is observed after spontaneous recovery is assumed to have run its course. Since a study by Butfield and Zangwill (1946), the belief has been that spontaneous recovery lasts around 6 months (or even less). Any progress afterward is thought to have been caused by therapeutic intervention (see discussion of efficacy in Chapters 8 and 9).

Like the other components of recovery, rate is highly variable. In studies of those receiving treatment, one took over 7 months to improve 4.01 points overall on the *PICA*, whereas another took about 8 months to improve only 0.98 points (Bamber, 1980; Hanson & Cicciarelli, 1978). Also, duration of recovery can be quite different between clients improving the same amount. Two people with aphasia improved almost 3.00 points but took about 4 and 19 months, respectively, to do so. Two others, who improved around 5.00 points, took 7.7 and 30.4 months, respectively.

Pattern of Improvement

An overall measure that absorbs all language functions can be misleading. It obscures progress in specific language abilities as well as communicative abilities. A person with aphasia may progress substantially in one function while regressing in another, canceling each other in an overall score. It can be more informative and optimistic to address specific communicative functions. Most comparisons in the research have been between auditory comprehension and oral expression.

Spontaneous recovery for 4 months postonset was differentiated according to eight subtests of the WAB (Lomas & Kertesz, 1978). The observations included two auditory comprehension tasks, one repetition test, and five expressive tasks mainly requiring word retrieval. Comprehension fared better than verbal expression. Auditory comprehension has had a better outlook for treated individuals, as well (Basso et al., 1979; Kenin & Swisher, 1972; Prins, Snow, & Wagenaar, 1978).

Following recovery to its peak, Hanson and Cicciarelli (1978) reported that the *PICA's* verbal functions improved more than auditory functions. However, auditory functions peaked sooner than expressive functions (i.e., 5.5 months vs. more than 8 months). Reported progress in auditory functions may be smaller because this initially less-impaired function reaches a test's ceiling. Standard tests keep us from measuring further progress, which was the main reason for creating the Token Test (Chapter 6). Also, when someone is followed long enough, verbal expression appears to overtake auditory functions in amount of progress (Figure 7.2). When discussing prospects with a client and the family, it can be hopeful to stress the outlook for comprehension and its importance for communication.

Considering the recent interest in relating general cognitive functions to language with aphasia (e.g., attention, working memory), we should consider a study of pattern of recovery in which language and cognitive functions were compared. Measures were obtained in the acute phase and 6 months later. For people with stroke-related

FIGURE 7.2 Hypothetical recovery curves drawn from studies of recovery, this time comparing the same overall curve with auditory comprehension and verbal expression. Note the ceiling effect for comprehension.

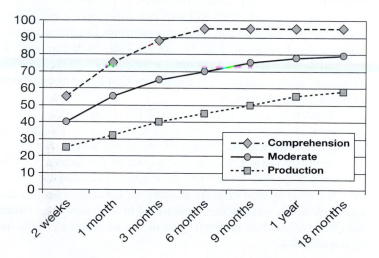

aphasia, correlation between language and cognitive functions was weaker than for people with traumatic brain injury (Vukovic, Vuksanovic, & Vukovic, 2008).

Approaches to Prognosis

The documentation of amount, rate, and outcome of recovery demonstrated that it is nearly impossible to predict the long-range future based on an early and general diagnosis of aphasia. We must identify more specific factors that are related to whether a person with aphasia does or does not get much better. Long ago, Porch, Collins, Wertz, and Friden (1980) identified three strategies of prediction, two of which are preserved here:

- **Statistical prediction**, or the use of early test scores to predict subsequent test scores, perhaps with a mathematical formula
- **Prognostic variable approach**, in which we compare "a patient's biographical, medical, and behavioral characteristics against how these variables are believed to influence change in aphasia" (p. 312)

The goal of statistical prediction was believed to have been achieved with the *PICA* and, more recently, with the *Comprehensive Aphasia Test* (*CAT*) (Chapter 5). The most common clinical strategy is the prognostic variable approach.

Rational use of prognostic variables relies on studies of factors that are thought to be predictive of recovery. A "real factor," such as size of lesion, influences the recovery process. A database called PLORAS, for "predicting language outcome and recovery after stroke," aims at enabling clinicians to compare a client's lesion with images of a large number of stroke patients and their language test scores (Price, Seghier, & Leff, 2010). Other factors, such as the timing of initial test, may be useful predictors (i.e., correlated) but do not influence recovery.

Prognostic indicators fall into two other broad categories. *Endogenous factors* are attributes that a person with aphasia brings to rehabilitation. The clinician can do nothing about many of these factors (e.g., size of lesion, age). *Exogenous factors* are external to our clients and are often a function of clinical decisions or circumstances. Timing of initial evaluation is a predictor that depends on when treatment is initiated or when a referral is made.

Speech-language pathologists (SLPs) try as soon as possible to predict whether prospects are favorable or unfavorable. We gather information regarding medical history, neurological diagnosis, and initial test results. We also attend to motivation and support system. The collective impact of the factors is estimated, and prediction is framed in general terms. The most striking development in the past 20 years has been the investigation of brain imaging for concrete clues to a client's future. What we know about the main factors is presented in the following sections dealing with several comparisons, such as between types of stroke, levels of initial impairment, and types of impairment.

Type of Stroke

The gradual recovery described so far is mainly characteristic of ischemic stroke. Hemorrhage is likely to have different outcomes because the hematoma "displaces the fibre bundles without completely destroying them" (Basso, 1992, p. 340). Hemorrhage can produce alternating periods of progress and plateau, and improvement may not begin for months following a small intracerebral hemorrhage (Rubens, 1977a). In Kertesz and McCabe's (1977) study of spontaneous recovery, some people with hemorrhage had large and rapid recovery, whereas others had little or no recovery. Two studies showed better recovery with hemorrhage than ischemic stroke (Basso, 1992; Holland, Greenhouse, Fromm, et al., 1989).

In another comparison between hemorrhage and infarct, Nagata and others (1986) measured cerebral blood flow during a period beginning at 2 to 4 weeks postonset and concluding at least 3 months after onset. In a group with infarction, blood flow gradually improved and was correlated with recovery. Among those with hemorrhage, blood flow was variable and was not related to recovery. Their explanation pointed to the instability of compression by a hematoma on adjacent brain tissue.

One case study followed a professional author's writing for over 3 months. He started out with semantic jargon in speech and writing. He was an example of unusual recovery after intracerebral hemorrhage. After admission to a rehabilitation program, his spontaneous writing samples lengthened and word-retrieval improved. He made a complete linguistic recovery in a relatively short time (Pickard, McAllister, & Horton, 2010).

Severity of Impairment

Recalling the mind-body conundrum (Chapter 1), we can address two sides of severity, namely brain damage and the resulting dysfunction. Let us start with **severity of brain damage**. The hope is that neuroimaging can provide a concrete aid in predicting linguistic outcome (e.g., PLORAS; Price et al., 2010). Not surprisingly, larger lesions are related to less recovery, which is most evident when comparing very large and very small lesions (Goldenberg & Spatt, 1994; Kertesz, Harlock, & Coates, 1979; Knopman, Selnes, Niccum, et al., 1984; Mazzoni, Vista, Pardossi, et al., 1992).

Naeser and her colleagues (1998) examined 12 people with aphasia one year and then 5 to 12 years poststroke. Lesion borders expanded over this period of time. The reason for this slight increase in lesion size is not understood. The possibilities include degeneration of adjacent cells, hypoperfusion creating the appearance of degeneration, or problems in other small arteries. Curiously, Naeser also found significant progress in naming and phrase length in those with nonfluent speech. Evidently the gradual expansion of lesion borders need not have a negative effect on language behavior.

Considering that a stroke affects neural activity, it is reasonable to think that a picture of early poststroke activation might predict language recovery. This possibility for the future was pursued in Germany for 21 patients by Saur and others (2010). fMRIs were given 2 weeks after stroke, and language was retested 6 months later. Activation patterns predicted these language scores with 76 percent accuracy. Accuracy increased somewhat when age and initial test scores were also considered. The investigators suggested that predictive early fMRIs could lead to targeting early intensive therapy.

Severity of lesion is related to **severity of dysfunction**, and we believe that our clinical measure of dysfunction can be predictive of recovery. We believe that "there is a negative correlation between severity of aphasia in the early recovery period and the amount of improvement which occurs during the recovery process whether or not speech therapy is given" (Sands et al., 1969, p. 204). That is, the more severe the impairment before 1 month postonset, the smaller the change score. However, there have been some technicalities in the research that should be acknowledged.

In a few studies, oddly, people with the most severe aphasias changed the most (Bamber, 1980; Hanson & Cicciarelli, 1978). Later, de Riesthal and Wertz (2004) pored over data from an earlier large treatment study and found that an initially more severe aphasia was predictive of a *larger* amount of progress. These counterintuitive results make some sense when considering that the studies did not appear to include the most severe aphasias. Also, these analyses were hampered by the ceiling effect because initially mild aphasias had little room to improve with common aphasia tests. Thus, some results may have been a function of assessment circumstances instead of a more likely reality.

The value of severity of deficit as a predictor may depend on when the first test is administered. Wallesch and others (1992) found the first 2 weeks to be an unstable platform from which to predict recovery. Severely impaired patients are unpredictable, which is one reason for delaying a prognosis until the end of the acute period. However, Mazzoni and others (1992) found that, at 15 days postonset, severe and moderate impairments were associated with small and moderate amounts of improvement, respectively, over the subsequent 6-month period. It is possible that the platform begins to become more stable at the end of the first 2 weeks (see Figure 7.1).

Lomas and Kertesz (1978) studied spontaneous recovery with four groups based on initial levels of comprehension and verbal fluency. The groups were tested initially within 1 month postonset and were retested up to 4 months later. The low-fluency/high-comprehending group (e.g., Broca's aphasia) made the most progress. The low-fluency/low-comprehending (i.e., "global aphasia") made the least progress. The two high-fluency groups (i.e., "posterior aphasias") made moderate amounts of progress. People with low comprehension improved mainly in receptive functions, whereas those with high comprehension improved both receptively and expressively. Separating comprehension and production produced results that were more consistent with clinical experience.

Initial severity of auditory comprehension deficit appears to be an indicator of how a client may proceed with *expressive language*. Gaddie and others (1989) found that high-comprehending people made more recovery of language production than low-comprehending individuals. In another study, good initial word comprehension was predictive of good recovery in naming (Knopman et al., 1984).

Type of Impairment

Site of lesion and type of aphasia are also interrelated sides of the brain–behavior coin because syndromes are born out of lesion locations. Type of aphasia has been studied according to the general distinction between nonfluent and fluent disorders or according to specific syndromes.

Site of Lesion

Location of lesion in the left hemisphere has a pronounced effect depending on whether it is in the primary language zone around the sylvian fissure or in the encircling borderline areas. The latter tends to cause transcortical aphasias. Recovery occurred more often in people with penetrating trauma in marginal zones than in those with perisylvian damage, and several with marginal damage made rapid and complete recovery (Luria, 1970). Rapid and near-total recovery of transcortical aphasias has been observed (Kertesz & McCabe, 1977; Rubens, 1977a).

Deficits caused by a **subcortical lesion** recover differently from those caused by a cortical stroke. Investigators tend to distinguish thalamic from nonthalamic sites. With thalamic hemorrhage, aphasic symptoms disappeared completely by the end of the second month (Rubens, 1977a). Participants in Kirk and Kertesz's (1994) study recovered dramatically by 3 months postonset. Kennedy and Murdoch (1991) assessed four cases with nonthalamic hemorrhage. Each case had some aphasic symptoms at 3 months, but two of these cases had AQs above the 93.8 cutoff for language deficit in most of their assessments over time. Subcortical language deficits generally resolved dramatically over time, which was explained later as reperfusion of blood flow to cortical language areas, not as any restored language function of the subcortical structures (Hillis, 2007).

Broad Classification of Dysfunction

Site of cortical damage is related to syndrome. The easiest classification is anterior/nonfluent and posterior/fluent aphasias. Early comparisons of these categories produced mixed results (e.g., Butfield & Zangwill, 1946; Godfrey & Douglass, 1959; Prins et al., 1978; Sarno & Levita, 1979). In the study by Mazzoni and others (1992), nonfluent aphasias had less progress in verbal expression and reading than fluent aphasias. Yet the two groups were quite alike in recovery of listening and writing. As a group, these studies are inconsistent. The dichotomy may be too broad for meaningful study of recovery, especially when a variety of aphasias is encapsulated in the fluent category (e.g., anomic, Wernicke's).

Research focuses increasingly on the specific syndromes. However, there have been few direct comparisons. Pashek and Holland (1988) followed syndromes with the *WAB*. Lendrem and Lincoln (1985) compared four syndromes according to the *PICA* overall score, failing to capture the quirks of each syndrome. Reporting some of their results, the following sections focus on individual syndromes.

Global or Severe Aphasia

We are especially concerned about people with chronically global or severe aphasia. In Kertesz and McCabe's study of spontaneous recovery, global aphasias changed by an average AQ of 5.16 in contrast to a nearly 37-point improvement by those with Broca's aphasia.

Holland, Swindell, and Forbes (1985) followed individuals who presented with global aphasia when admitted to the hospital. The researchers recorded conversations daily during acute care and then administered the *WAB* regularly for about a year. Some people evolved to other forms of aphasia by the time of hospital discharge, whereas others remained in a severe state for months. A good sign was when verbal expression changed rapidly in the early conversations. Those without early progress continued to have chronic global aphasia. In another study of people with global aphasia diagnosed within the first 30 days, four remained global and seven evolved to Broca's aphasia within the next 2 or 3 months (McDermott, Horner, & DeLong, 1996).

For people with severely global aphasia, it may be a disservice to report progress in terms of overall or general scores. During early spontaneous recovery, low-comprehending individuals improve in comprehension but not expression (Lomas & Kertesz, 1978). Within 1 year postonset, seven severely impaired individuals receiving treatment made significant gains in auditory language comprehension and gesturing, and most of this progress occurred between 6 and 12 months postonset (Sarno & Levita, 1981). Also, severe aphasia has better prognosis for word comprehension when Wernicke's area is spared (Naeser, 1994).

Brookshire (2007) concluded that "the presence of global aphasia in a neurologically recovered patient is an ominous prognostic sign for recovery of functional language" (p. 335). Preliminary research indicates that progress is possible in some cases. The problem lies in identifying the cases that are most likely to improve. Positive indicators are lesions that are mainly subcortical, an intact Wernicke's area, and signs of progress during the acute period.

Wernicke's Aphasia

Wernicke's aphasia is also a severe impairment, but with fluent verbal production sometimes in excess. Comprehension is also depressed. Lendrem and Lincoln (1985) found that people with this aphasia had poorer outcomes at 8 months than other syndromes. Elsewhere this group displayed a bimodal distribution of recovery (Kertesz & McCabe, 1977). Some improved little. Others improved by at least 20 *WAB*-AQ points. Four of 13 ended up in the anomic category. Those with higher initial test scores and less jargon did better than others.

Kertesz and others (1993) wanted to determine if lesion size and location would be predictive of recovery in 22 cases of Wernicke's aphasia diagnosed between 14 and 45 days poststroke. Patients were grouped according to whether they had good, moderate, or poor recovery after 1 year. Poor recovery was related to damage extending beyond Wernicke's area to the supramarginal and angular gyri bordering the parietal lobe. Good recovery was associated with small lesions sparing much of the superior and middle temporal gyri.

Naeser (1994) reported results of a similar strategy in which people with Wernicke's aphasia were classified at 6 months as having good or poor recovery. There was a distinct relationship to the amount of damage to Wernicke's area. All of those with good recovery had damage in half or less than half of Wernicke's area, whereas all poorly recovered cases had larger lesions. Eaton, Marshall, and Pring (2011) described a case that improved over a 21-month period in word production tasks and in self-monitoring. Connected speech showed little change.

Broca's Aphasia

Broca's aphasia is like Lomas and Kertesz's low-fluency/high-comprehending group. In Kertesz and McCabe's study, four people with this aphasia improved an average of 36.8 AQ points. Compared to the others, this syndrome had the greatest amount of recovery and had varied outcomes of fair, good, and excellent (see also Lendrem & Lincoln, 1985). With respect to early evolution, people with Broca's aphasia either remain in the same category or progress to a milder, more fluent form (McDermott et al., 1996).

More recently, Dickey and Thompson (2007) described the progress of an agrammatic individual who had undergone 2 months of a therapy called Treatment of Underlying Forms (see Chapter 9). An interesting aspect of recovery was a dissociation between morphology and syntax. The client improved in producing sentence structures but not in producing grammatical word endings. Others may exhibit the opposite dissociation. The problem is that we do not know which it will be. When studying recovery, investigators have seldom delved into specific linguistic characteristics, preferring to report general test scores.

Conduction Aphasia

Conduction aphasia has been judged to be between Broca's and anomic aphasias in overall severity of language impairment. People with conduction aphasia seem to remain in a milder form of this syndrome or follow the fluent path to anomic aphasia, sometimes within the first 3 months (McDermott et al., 1996; Pashek & Holland, 1988). In Kertesz and McCabe's (1977) study, conduction aphasia had an amount of recovery comparable to Broca's aphasia and reached nearly maximum AQs in some cases. Most anomic, conduction, and transcortical aphasias had excellent outcomes, and many rose above the "normal" standard of 93.8 for the AQ.

Gandour and others (1991) followed one case for 6 months after onset. Initially, this individual followed simple commands and produced fluent utterances with occasional paraphasias. However, when asked to repeat "No ifs, ands, or buts," he said "sucklent incadiblems." He evolved from a "reproduction" form of conduction aphasia (i.e., reading aloud as impaired as repetition) to a "repetition" form (i.e., reading aloud resolved). Chronic short-term memory impairment was indicated by progress in Part V of the Token Test (varied structures) but no progress in Parts III and IV (longer commands). Phonemic paraphasias disappeared by 6 months postonset.

Other Factors

Several other factors have been studied extensively or have been suspected to be prognostic based on common sense or theories of functional organization of the brain.

Age at Onset

Chronological age may be more of a predictor than a real factor. Kimmel (1974) reminded us that "when we find age changes or age differences, it is important to keep in mind that these findings only point to changes that occur with age but do not indicate the possible causes of these changes" (p. 33; see Tompkins, Jackson, & Schulz, 1990). Growing older is accompanied by changes in biological function, susceptibility to disease, and cognitive and social changes.

The experimental support for age as predictor has been mixed. Correlations between age and recovery were not significant in several studies (e.g., Basso et al., 1979; de Riesthal & Wertz, 2004; Keenan & Brassell, 1974; Kertesz & McCabe, 1977). Sands and others (1969) had been impressed with age because five people making the most change averaged 47 years of age, and five making the least change averaged 61 years. Holland and others (1989) found age to be a strong predictor over 2 or 3 months postonset. McDermott and others (1996) found clients younger than 65 making more progress than those above 65. A similar result occurred with respect to age 70 (Pashek & Holland, 1988).

Pashek and Holland warned that age by itself is a precarious predictor, and older individuals may differ according to whether they have dementia and other pathologies. Basso (1992) concluded that age is not a very important factor in recovery. We may contemplate age as a predictor with respect to extremes, especially whether youthful middle age or older adulthood is accompanied by environmental or medical conditions that create a positive or negative climate for therapeutic success.

Gender

Gender has been considered because of the possibility that men and women differ in distribution of cognitive functions between the cerebral hemispheres. Evidence indicates that verbal and nonverbal abilities are more evenly distributed in women, whereas men have a more familiar asymmetric division of labor. Some of the evidence is indirect such as comparisons between verbal and nonverbal tasks. More direct evidence has included PET and fMRI readings with some support for the difference, especially when language tasks are used (Clements, Rimrodt, Abel, et al., 2006).

If functions are more evenly distributed in women, then women should have a more favorable prognosis because their right hemisphere has more linguistic capability.

Gender was found not to be a factor in a few studies (e.g., Kertesz & McCabe, 1977; Lendrem & Lincoln, 1985; Sarno & Levita, 1971). However, it was a factor in the predicted direction in a few other studies. In a study of nearly 400 people with aphasia in Italy, females improved more than males in spoken language but not in comprehension (Basso, Capitani, & Moraschini, 1982). In cases of severe aphasia, women had more improvement than men in auditory comprehension (Pizzamiglio, Mammucari, & Razzano, 1985). Mustering enough participants with aphasia for gender comparison has been hampered by the male-dominance of veterans' research hospitals.

Handedness

Handedness, or *laterality* of motor skills, is commonly assessed by clinical neuropsychologists. Similar to gender, handedness could be a clue to recovery because of evidence that left-handed people have more bilateral representation of language in the brain than right-handers (Springer & Deutsch, 1998). However, these differences apply to half of left-handers at the most. This factor is of particular interest with respect to right- and left-handed people with aphasia and a left-hemisphere stroke.

Data on this question are scarce, partly because left-handers are relatively rare and because of the tendency to study only right-handers. In a study of traumatic injuries, Luria (1970) found an effect of familial left-handedness. That is, pure right-handers without family history of left-handedness did not recover as quickly as those with this family history. Basso and her colleagues (1990) found that non-right-handed people with stroke-related aphasias did not differ from right-handed people with aphasias. Borod, Carper, and Naeser (1990) followed the progress of left-handed individuals and found patterns of change that were similar to right-handers. Thus, handedness cannot be counted on for enhancing a prognosis based on a predisposed capacity for language in the undamaged hemisphere.

Race

Race was considered in Holland and others' (1989) multivariate analysis of spontaneous recovery, and they found that it did not matter. Wertz, Auther, and Ross (1997) compared African Americans and Caucasians across the course of a 44-week treatment study that began a month poststroke. Progress was measured with the *PICA*, Token Test, and a word fluency task. The two clinical groups did not differ in initial severity nor in amount and rate of improvement of auditory and oral language skills over 10 months. Thus, there is no scientific support for considering race to be a prognostic factor.

Time of Initial Test

The recovery curves of Figure 7.1 tell us many things, depending on how we look at them. One of those things is that the amount of recovery depends on when we initially test a client after stroke. We can expect a smaller amount of improvement the later someone is referred. For example, Pickersgill and Lincoln (1983) measured overall progress of 1.01 points with the *PICA* over an 8-week period, much less than the change scores in Table 7.1. Their participants were tested initially at an average of 5 months postonset at the time of admission to a rehabilitation program.

Yet timing of the first test within the first 2 months is probably unrelated to change measured over a year, as indicated in Bamber's (1980) study and in an analysis of data reported by Hanson and Cicciarelli (1978). Thus, starting time within 2 months is not likely to be predictive of subsequent progress, but a program started much later is likely to be accompanied by less improvement.

Premorbid Brain Structure

A person with aphasia could bring a favorable brain structure to the recovery process. One characteristic is *morphological asymmetry*. Burke and others (1993) reviewed previous work indicating that people with global aphasia and a *right* hemisphere larger than the left recovered better than those without this asymmetry of brain size. Others found no relationship between structural asymmetries and recovery. Burke's team decided to do their own study and reviewed medical charts at the Albuquerque VA Medical Center from 1976 to 1986. They came up with a different result.

Burke's team compared the size of each hemisphere to *PICA* overall scores recorded initially at 1 month poststroke and at 1-month intervals until a year after the stroke. Posterior width asymmetry favoring the left was associated with faster recovery and higher outcome at 1 year than right posterior asymmetry or equal hemisphere size. This posterior asymmetry included portions of Wernicke's area and the temporoparietal boundary. The research team concluded that a larger *posterior left* hemisphere is a more efficient language processor and provides more intact brain for facilitating recovery.

Years later, another retrospective study honed in on the arcuate fasciculus of the left hemisphere (i.e., fibers connecting Wernicke's area to Broca's area). Using a recently developed imaging technique for exposing fiber tracts (Chapter 2), Hosomi and others (2009) found that those with aphasia persisting for 30 days had smaller left arcuate fasciculus tracts than those without persistent aphasia. The observation falls short of long-term recovery, but it offers a tantalizing prospect for further investigation.

Additional Considerations

Other factors make sense but have not been studied much. Some, such as motivation, are difficult to measure for research purposes. *Length of hospital stay* was a moderate predictor, as 20 days or less was more favorable than 21 or more days. Like age, this is one of those indicators tied to more direct or "real" influences, such as the reasons for a short stay (e.g., smaller infarct, less-severe deficit, good medical condition).

Other contemplated factors are *education* and *estimated premorbid intelligence*. de Riesthal and Wertz (2004) found that neither correlated with language outcome

1 year after stroke. A retrospective review of hospital records indicated that neither education nor *occupation* relates to rate of recovery, although these indicators of "socioeconomic status" were related to early severity of aphasia and severity years later (Conner et al., 2001). If we want to predict a return to work, Hinckley's (2002) review of pertinent studies indicated that severity of aphasia is not a factor and that there are several stronger factors including workplace flexibility, social support, motivation, motor impairment, and cognitive abilities.

Bilingual Recovery

Do the languages of a bilingual person recover differently? Long ago, exceptions to equivalent recovery of two languages were associated with the so-called rules of Ribot and Pitres. The rules indicated that any difference would have something to do with which language is the native tongue and/or which is the most familiar language.

- *Rule of Ribot* ("primacy rule"): the first learned or native language recovers first
- *Rule of Pitres*: the most frequently used language recovers first

Obler and Albert's (1977) review of the literature indicated that Pitres's rule describes recovery more often. That is, the most recently used language recovers faster more often than the other languages. The reliability of this characterization is confounded by definition of most frequent/familiar language, partly because functional bilinguals use two languages depending on the situation.

Paradis (1977) had a different impression from 138 cases of bilingual aphasia that were reported in the literature. He found many possibilities (Table 7.2). Contrary to the previous conclusion, nearly half the cases improved according to a **synergistic** pattern (often called *parallel* recovery) in which progress in one language is accompanied by comparable progress in the other language. Subsequently, Paradis and others (1982) described *alternate antagonism* (or "seesaw recovery"); "for given periods of time, the patients could speak only one language, and the available language would alternate for consecutive periods" (p. 56). A critical suspicion regarding the literature is that clinicians may be more inclined to report differences between languages or journals may be more inclined to publish them.

On a smaller scale, Fabbro (2001) reported on the severity and recovery of aphasia by Friulian-Italian bilinguals who live in the Friuli, in northeast Italy bordering Slovenia. Code-switching rarely occurs. Of the 20 individuals studied, 65 percent exhibited the synergistic parallel pattern of recovery in which Friulian and Italian were impaired equally and recovered at the same rate. This percentage is in line with Table 7.2. The other bilinguals with aphasia had a version of the synergistic differential pattern, depending on which language was more severely impaired at the beginning.

More recently, Green and his colleagues (2010) decided to dig into processes that might be related to bilingual recovery. They studied two people with very different sites of lesion (subcortical and posterior) but both with parallel recovery of languages.

TABLE 7.2   Patterns of recovery between languages in bilinguals (Paradis, 1977)

PATTERN	DEFINITION	PERCENTAGE
Synergistic (parallel)	Two languages progress at the same rate and were similarly impaired at the beginning; nearly identical recovery curves	41
Synergistic (differential)	Two languages improve at the same rate but were impaired to different degrees at the start; curves separate but parallel	8
Selective	One language improves but the other does not	27
Successive	One language recovers after another; one seems dormant while another is progressing, and the dormant language starts improving weeks or months later	6
Antagonistic	One language progresses but the other regresses	4
Mixed	Two systematically intermingled languages	?

Each participant had a European native language and English as a second language. The investigators drew on a previous hypothesis that inability to control language selection contributes to selective recovery, and then they simply wondered about the status of this ability for those with equal recovery of languages.

Let us consider two of the three tasks used to examine the basic cognitive capacity to manage or suppress conflicting information. One was a lexical decision task, introduced in Chapter 3. The feature of interest was the ability to inhibit activation of a real word while rejecting a nonword. The other verbal test was a Stroop task in which participants named the ink color of a color name. Conflict suppression comes into play when the ink color differs from the color name. One participant had a deficit of conflict suppression on both tasks, whereas the other participant was deficient mainly with lexical decision. Thus, despite their parallel language recovery, both bilingual individuals showed some impairment in verbal control. The investigators decided that more research of this type is needed.

The Targeted Prognosis

The variability of recovery indicates that prediction is elusive. What do we say to a client and the family regarding the client's prospects? What do we say in a discharge staffing? As indicated before, we generally follow the *prognostic variable approach* for these scenarios, and much depends on the time postonset of the decision and the period of recovery being considered. That is, acute phase prognosis is likely to be expressed differently than postacute phase prognosis, and predicting the next 2 weeks (short-term goals) is a little easier than predicting the next year and beyond (long-term goals).

Our overarching desire is to be as positive as possible, especially for encouraging a client and family members to do the work of rehabilitation. The data, as well as the nature of injury, tell us that people with a stroke do not return to the way they were before. The data also tell us that we can be more positive when predicting progress than when predicting recovery. We can be more positive when we target comprehension and other retained abilities that can be used for communication.

Shortly after a stroke, the doctor is likely to advise the family to "wait and see." Because of diaschisis (or remote effects), it is difficult to know the pattern of dysfunction and how serious the permanent impairments will be. The doctor can be vaguely positive if the lesion is small, the patient is middle-aged and otherwise healthy, and the family is supportive. If the lesion is large and the patient is elderly and weak, it is still best to wait a few days to see if the patient shows signs of gaining physical strength and psychological vigor.

SLPs may be comfortable making a general prognosis during the subacute (or postacute) phase, soon after admission to a rehabilitation unit. At this time, we can obtain a better picture of the fundamental impairment. *We see signs of progress. Auditory comprehension is improving. We are hopeful that speech will get better, but we cannot predict how much.* Outlook is related to (a) severity of language impairment and (b) amount of progress in the first few days since the stroke. We also know that therapy makes a difference in recovery (Chapters 8–10). We do not promise more than the wounded brain will allow. We want to be realistic.

Clients will want to tie prognosis to specific life goals. Returning to work is one example. Paul Berger had to adjust his sights as he attempted to return to a real estate development department. He had some difficulties, and at some point, an attempt was made to adjust his responsibilities to fit his strengths (Berger & Mensh, 2002). How positive we can be depends on the skills required for each activity. Predicting a return to work may require evaluation by a state department of vocational rehabilitation. Prognoses can be targeted toward realistic possibilities, and all the factors should be considered at a staffing and with the client and family.

Explaining Recovery

We know that people with aphasia progress in language abilities. The question now is *why* does language function return to some degree? What happens in the damaged brain? Do undamaged areas learn to perform language functions? Popular media and some of the literature extend the promise of a brain that rewires itself (e.g., Doidge, 2007). Is this true? It sounds good, but what does it mean?

Acute and Early Recovery

There is not much to say about the first week or two after a stroke that has not already been said. It is a dramatic period of adjustment. One study showed that the right hemisphere increased activation within the first 2 weeks after a stroke and then settled down to normal activity over the rest of the first year. It is notable that left-hemisphere activity also increased gradually within the first two weeks (Saur, Lange, Baumgaertner, et al., 2006).

Soon after a stroke, the brain does not appear to grow new neurons or shift connections. This chapter began by noting early recovery caused by a subsiding of disorienting diaschisis. The mechanism of this sometimes dramatic recovery is most likely to be *reperfusion* to structurally sound regions. Hillis and Heidler (2002) found that recovery of auditory word comprehension in the first 3 days following stroke is associated with restoration of blood ipsilaterally to Wernicke's area. This restoration occurred spontaneously in some individuals and with medical treatment in others.

Recovery with Chronic Aphasia

Now, let us consider adjustments in the brain occurring long after the acute stage. Two types of change are considered. One is the structural repair of damaged regions through the birth of new neurons (i.e., neurogenesis), and the other is a compensatory contribution from structurally intact regions. It has been hypothesized that both processes could occur spontaneously (without intervention) or therapeutically (with medical or behavioral intervention). Both contribute to widely acknowledged **neuroplasticity** or the brain's capacity to change (Meinzer, Harnish, Conway, et al., 2011; Papathanasiou, Coppens, & Ansaldo, 2013).

Regarding neurogenesis, does the brain eventually grow new neurons, especially in the region of damage? *Spontaneous regeneration* of damaged nerves was demonstrated in animals in the 1930s and 1940s by Weiss and Sperry (i.e., without infusion of an experimental drug). Sperry cut the optic nerve of salamanders. The nerve returned, and sight was restored. After damage to the motor cortex on one side in adult rats, dendritic arborization or "sprouting" occurred nearby and in the opposite hemisphere (Keefe, 1995; Rose, 1989).

From zebrafish to humans, neurogenesis (also called rewiring) has been detected. In the late 1990s, nerve cell regeneration was observed in the hippocampus and in some cortical regions of mammals (i.e., rats, monkeys) by Elizabeth Gould at Princeton (Gould & Gross, 2002; Gould, Reeve, Graziano, et al., 1999). Fred Gage at the Salk Institute in La Jolla, California, with the help of Peter Eriksson of Götenborg, Sweden, detected regeneration in the human hippocampus (Eriksson, Perfilieva, Björk-Eriksson, et al., 1998; Kemperman, Kuhn, & Gage, 1997).

Some are now inclined to gloat over the demise of a "dogma" that brain cells do not regenerate. However, we may be sobered by that fact that most of the contrary findings come from artificially infarcted rats and monkeys. When researchers refer to neurogenesis in the "aged brain" or "adult brain," they are often referring to elderly mice and regions away from language (e.g., Lee, Clemenson, & Gage, 2012). Yet animal modeling is where hope begins in medical research. Restorative therapies tested in rats have excited the imagination for some day inducing human brain cell regeneration (see Chapter 9).

Other theories are based on the notion of functional flexibility in the established brain. According to *functional substitution*, a structurally intact area assists in or even takes over an impaired function. More specifically, the idea that the right hemisphere (RH) takes over language functions used to be called the "spare tire" theory. However, the process is likely to be more complex than one that simply occurs in one side or the other (Sebastian & Kiran, 2011).

Substitution is facilitated if the RH (or any intact region) had a capacity for the impaired language function before the stroke. This might apply to individuals, such as females and left-handers, with an unusual functional organization in the brain. A *spontaneous* substitution (i.e., without therapy) may indicate that language skills already existed in the substituting region. A demonstration of this in normal adults would contribute to this theory of recovery.

One group of studies relied on indirect "observation" of brain function with techniques for studying functional asymmetry. Dichotic listening, for example, has demonstrated a left-ear advantage in people with aphasia, which is indicative of a preference for using the RH (Moore, 1989). Other indirect evidence for a shift of language function came from presentation of words to the visual fields. Ansaldo, Arguin, and Lecours (2002) studied someone who responded faster with words in the left field (RH) than with words in the right field (LH) at 2 and 6 months postonset. At 10 months, the fields were equivalent. It was presumed that the LH (right field) caught up with the compensating hemisphere.

Neuroimaging techniques address the questions more directly. Investigators measure cerebral metabolism with PET or blood oxygen levels with fMRI while an individual performs a simple language task (Chapter 2). Some studies entail comparing a participant to normal controls, whereas other studies consist of repeating tests after a stroke so that a participant serves as his own control. Repeated testing is considered to be stronger evidence for changes in the brain (Thompson, 2005).

Cappa and his colleagues (1997) obtained PET scans from eight people with aphasia 6 months after stroke. Improvements in Token Test comprehension and spoken naming were correlated more with changes in the RH than in the left. Other studies indicated that the RH assumes an increased role in language functions during the chronic phase (Blasi, Young, Tansy, et al., 2002; Thurlborn, Carpenter, & Just, 1999). Compared to healthy controls, people with aphasia had greater activation in the RH during simple lexical tasks (Cao, Vikingstad, George, et al., 1999; Gold & Kertesz, 2000; Weiller, Isensee, Rijntjes, et al., 1995). Without repeated measurement, however, we do not know if these findings represent change.

With modern brain imaging, compensatory changes have been identified in the ipsilateral hemisphere (i.e., same side as the lesion) as well as in the contralateral hemisphere. Karbe and colleagues (1998) concluded that "left hemispheric structural reorganization is significantly more effective than the right hemispheric compensation" (p. 227; see also Fernandez et al., 2004). More recently, Fridriksson and others (2010) compared 15 people with aphasia to healthy controls using fMRI to detect cortical activity during a naming task. There was a linear relationship between naming ability and degree of cortical activation in intact regions of the left hemisphere. In addition to ipsilateral compensation, some recovery has been associated with perilesional regions (i.e., surrounding the infarction).

After comparing eight people with aphasia to eight matched healthy controls, using fMRI during semantic judgment and naming tasks, Sebastian and Kiran (2011) concluded that recruitment of intact areas of the brain is related to the task. Multiple regions of the brain are brought to bear in an individual's recovery.

Repetitive transcranial magnetic stimulation (rTMS) is presented in Chapter 9 as an experimental therapy for modifying cortical activation. Heiss and Thiel (2006) explained how rTMS is used to develop hypotheses of neural mechanisms for recovery. These mechanisms include recruitment of undamaged regions of the damaged hemisphere and disinhibition of homologous regions in the opposite hemisphere. In one study in Germany, RH compensation did not occur in patients with rapidly progressing tumors but did occur in those with slow progression, indicating that reorganization involving the RH takes some time (e.g., Thiel, Habedank, Herholz, et al., 2006).

The data so far indicate that changes in the LH near the infarct may be more impressive than changes in the RH. This finding has been reinforced in studies of people receiving therapy (Chapter 8).

Differing from spontaneous substitution, *therapeutic substitution* is indicated if a region's increased involvement is linked to language therapy. In any case, the prospects of a rewired brain viewed through brain imaging technology have captivated authors such as Bob Guns (2008), a stroke survivor, for his self-published book called *Rewire Your Brain, Rewire Your Life*.

Summary and Conclusions

Important decisions about services are based on notions of recovery. This chapter encourages an analytical approach to viewing the literature and, hopefully, contributes to thinking about individual clients. Recovery is greatest and swiftest during the first 2 or 3 months postonset and slows down afterward. Some believe that language does not improve after 6 months or a year, and the notion of an impending "plateau" is anathema to those who do make progress years later. Fortunately, research has demonstrated progress beyond 1 year.

A physician wants an SLP's opinion about prospects for recovering language, especially if the patient is to be recommended for language treatment. The targeted prognosis becomes important as a substitute for focusing on the obvious such as speech. We want the physician and family to be thinking about recovery of specific skills and of an ability to interact in some fashion. We make a point of documenting recovery of language comprehension, verbal expression, and other communicative skills. A person with aphasia may never have a "normal conversation" as we know it, but many come close.

Like physicians, SLPs shy away from prediction during the first week after onset. We are more willing to make a general prediction later in the first month. Prognosis pertains to the likelihood that a person with aphasia can benefit from treatment. This is close to a binary decision, namely either the person can benefit from treatment or treatment is not likely to help. Our job is to document initial severity of deficit and follow early spontaneous progress. Of course, the physician's opinion regarding type, size, and site of lesion is important. An infarction that preserves the comprehension area, along with some early spontaneous progress, are all fairly positive signs.

8 Treatment of Language Impairment

Three chapters are dedicated to treatment. Chapters 8 and 9 emphasize the impairment-based orientation introduced early in the book. Chapter 10 follows with the communication-based orientation. This chapter begins with therapy settings and some notes on getting started. It then proceeds to principles of stimulation that apply to any type of aphasia and setting. Hildred Schuell, who coauthored our first clinical text for aphasia (Schuell, Jenkins, & Jimenez-Pabon, 1964), believed that "what you do about aphasia depends on what you think aphasia is" (Sies, 1974, p. 138). Her vision was advanced by Robert Brookshire, her successor at the Minneapolis VA Medical Center.

Following the introduction to principles, stimulation method is illustrated later with a review of naming therapies. Although basic research contributes ideas for procedure, clinical research furnishes evidence for effectiveness. Naming is followed by topics touching on more general aspects of treatment. For example, computers have become another form of treatment delivery. Then, evidence for the efficacy of language stimulation is surveyed. Reasons for treatment effects have been sought in neurological studies (see Chapter 7). Finally, there is more information about the health care system in which this therapy is provided.

Rehabilitation Team and Settings

Poststroke care is the responsibility of a rehabilitation team operating in a variety of settings (Table 8.1). Besides a speech-language pathologist (SLP), the team minimally includes a physical therapist, occupational therapist, and social worker.

- *Physical therapy:* To improve strength and range of motion of large muscle groups. The therapist's concerns include ambulation and transfers between bed and wheelchair.
- *Occupational therapy:* To improve fine motor skills. The therapist is particularly concerned with manipulation of utensils for grooming, eating, and other self-care tasks.
- *Social services:* For psychological, residential, and vocational needs; discharge planning.

TABLE 8.1   **Rehabilitation settings in the United States, including common estimates of length of stay or length of therapy.**

SETTING	TYPE OF CARE	NOTES	LENGTH OF THERAPY
Acute care hospital	Inpatient Acute	Ensure survival; discharge when medically stable	Less than 7 days
Rehabilitation hospital	Inpatient Postacute or Subacute	Often in acute care facility; full rehabilitation services	Less than 4 weeks
Rehabilitation center	Outpatient Chronic	Independent facility; long-term rehabilitation	Weeks or months
Home health care	Residential Chronic	Client's home; home health agency (HHA)	Weeks or months
Nursing home	Residential Chronic	Skilled nursing facility (SNF)	Weeks or months
University clinic	Outpatient Chronic	Supervised student practicum; experimental treatments	Months to years

Reasons for more integrated teamwork in recent years include the sharing of reimbursement resources. In rehabilitation centers, team members meet regularly so that, for example, language treatment can be coordinated with occupational therapy.

Getting Started

For an ischemic stroke, the acute hospital stay revolves around survival and averages around 4 days. The SLP can do little more than evaluate the patient for swallowing and explain the availability of rehabilitation. If the patient remains in the Stroke Unit for a longer period, the SLP may conduct a bedside evaluation and note suggestions for future therapy. Once the patient is admitted to a subacute rehabilitation unit or hospital, an SLP is likely to be required to evaluate swallowing within 24 hours of the doctor's order and evaluate speech and language within 72 hours.

Opinions on when to begin formal therapy depend partly on the approach being considered. Wepman (1972) worried that there could be an adverse reaction to "direct therapy" during the acute and subacute periods. According to Wepman, such treatment should be delayed beyond diaschisis and until chronic aphasia becomes apparent. We should provide only "a supportive psychological role" during a potentially delicate time.

On the other hand, Eisenson (1984) insisted that direct therapy begin "as soon as the patient is able to take notice of what is going on and is able to cooperate in the effort" (p. 180). A neurologist believed "that the therapy should be as intensive as the general medical situation will allow" (Rubens, 1977b, p. 1). Usually the medical situation allows relatively intensive therapy when the person with aphasia enters the rehabilitation facility, where a complete therapy plan is instituted.

Starting therapy may also be based on presumptions about recovery. One belief is that therapy is only effective during the period of spontaneous recovery. Robey (1998) analyzed 55 studies and found that treatment can be effective when started sooner than 3 months postonset, between 3 to 12 months postonset, and 12 months or later. Yet the magnitude of effect decreased over time, so Robey concluded that people with aphasia "should receive treatment as early in their recoveries as possible" (p. 181) because it was most effective in the first 3 months.

Holland and Fridriksson (2001) had some suggestions for management through the 4-week period immediately following stroke. Like Wepman, they recommended informal conversational therapy (i.e., encouraging patients to talk) and counseling the client and family regarding communication. This counseling includes providing information about aphasia and the rehabilitation process. Patients and families need to know that their perceptions and feelings are understandable and common.

We choose impairment-oriented therapy based on the diagnosis of *language* disorder. In writing about her husband's aphasia, Ackerman (2011) observed a therapist instruct as follows: "I want you to listen carefully and repeat after me. Let's start with the consonant M." The therapist "continued through ME and MO and back to MA again, over and over . . ." (p. 189). Unless the person has severe apraxia of speech, most clients with aphasia can start with whole words. Our main goals are aimed at a deeper level of formulation.

When we train our sights on language impairment, we translate assessment results into initial goals. When assessment shows an impairment of word-retrieval, one goal is to improve word-retrieval. The goal, however, is usually expressed in behavioral terms, following a strategy summarized by the acronym SMART, which stands for specific, measurable, achievable, realistic, and time-bound objectives (Wade, 2009). Such a goal might be as follows:

- Increase spoken picture naming from 30 percent to 60 percent in 2 weeks

Wording may vary, but the goal specifies a stimulus and a response that can be counted. Assessment scores and early therapy may have provided the evidence that the goal is realistically achievable.

A group in Australia concluded that some applications of SMART may not have worked out too well. From interviews with 50 people with aphasia, 48 family members, and 34 clinicians, the researchers found that clients "often feel confused or excluded by the goal-setting process" (Hersh, Worrall, Howe, et al., 2012, p. 231). A client's goals and clinician's goals may differ (Rohde, Townley-O'Neill, Trandall, et al., 2012). Setting goals should be collaborative between the client and clinician. The supplemental acronym SMARTER suggests goals that clinicians and clients establish together (Table 8.2).

TABLE 8.2   **Comparison of SMART and SMARTER approaches to treatment goal setting.**

SMART Nature of goals	Specific	Measurable	Achievable	Realistic	Time-bound		
SMARTER Process of goal setting	Shared	Monitored	Accessible	Relevant	Transparent	Evolving	Relationship-centered

Cognitive Stimulation

Impairment-based direct therapy originated with Schuell's "stimulation-facilitation." She would stimulate to facilitate. Her colleagues Frederick Darley (1982) and Jon Eisenson (1984) were on the same wavelength. Schuell's lasting influence has been preserved in Duffy and Coelho's chapters (e.g., Coelho, Sinotte, & Duffy, 2008). To be modern, the term *cognitive* is added to the idea of stimulation. For language, in particular, we could say that we do *psycholinguistic stimulation* as we try to influence the inner worlds of comprehension and formulation. The following sections highlight key overlapping principles, beginning with process-oriented goals.

Psycholinguistic Objectives

According to Brookshire (2007), "most clinicians and investigators agree that aphasia is not a loss of vocabulary or linguistic rules, but is caused by impairments in processes necessary for comprehending, formulating, and producing spoken and written language" (p. 338). He wrote of "reactivating" these processes. Although some still speak of learning words as a goal, we do not have to spend our limited time restoring a lost vocabulary or teaching a whole language.

Brookshire recommended a *treat-underlying-processes approach*, pointing us to the targeting of mental abilities that underlie a response pattern. We are not concerned with a particular word-set or a particular structure as long as a client is exercising the targeted process. Schuell said it a long time ago, "I do not teach aphasic patients words. I stimulate language processes and they begin to function. Words come out that I never used" (Sies, 1974, p. 138).

The processing target is reflective of a common thread underlying a variety of communicative circumstances or tasks. For example, "to improve word-retrieval" has implications for speaking and writing activities. Brookshire (2007) believed that "improving a process also improves the abilities that depend on the process" (p. 255). Activities may begin with picture naming as the core but are expanded to divergent or word fluency tasks and sentence production.

Some process-oriented targets should be familiar by now, such as comprehension and word-retrieval, and others are more specific derivatives of research in

Chapter 3. For right-hemisphere dysfunctions (Chapter 11), treatment has been aimed at coarse coding and suppression of alternative meanings. Cognitive goals (e.g., to expand working memory) may go into a clinician's thinking but are not a preferred approach to objective documentation, for which SMART behavioral goals are chosen (e.g., to increase number of digits to be repeated).

The Task

The procedures of language treatment are similar to the procedures of research and assessment. In research and assessment, tasks are designed for observing both failures and successes. In treatment, the same tasks are constructed for eliciting an individual's best performances. Brookshire, Nicholas, and others (1978) studied 40 videotaped treatment sessions conducted in various regions of the United States (see also Horton, 2006). The clinicians carried out basically the same interaction structure. Therapy tasks contained the following components:

- Clinician's stimulus (antecedent event)
- Client's response
- Clinician's feedback (consequent event)

Although these components should not be a revelation, our recognition of them heightens our sensitivity to variables in all of our treatment procedures.

The clinician's stimulus and response are specified in instructions to the client (e.g., "When I show you a picture, you say its name"). When we want a client to focus on comprehension, the stimulus is a word or sentence and the response is simple (e.g., pointing to a picture). We do not want language production difficulties to distract from comprehending. For focusing on production, the stimulus is nonverbal, such as a picture of an object, and the client is asked to make a verbal response. Working memory should not be cluttered with distracting linguistic demands. Table 8.3 shows core tasks for general objectives.

One decision pertains to the composition of items in the stimulation task. Do we present 10 words five times each or 50 different words? In their Language Oriented

TABLE 8.3 Some basic tasks in treatment.

AREA TO IMPROVE	CLINICIAN'S STIMULUS	PATIENT'S RESPONSE
Auditory comprehension	Says a sentence while showing three pictures	Points to one of the pictures
Reading comprehension	Shows a sentence while showing three pictures	Points to one of the pictures
Spoken word finding	Shows a picture of a common object	Says name of the object
Written word finding	Shows a picture of a common object	Writes name of the object

Treatment (LOT), Shewan and Bandur (1986) stated that "the same stimuli are not used over and over again . . . different stimuli at a comparable level of difficulty are presented to elicit responses" (p. 13). For example, a client could say "car" in response to "You buy a _____," "You wreck a _____," and "You fix a _____." Conversely, more than one response is acceptable for one stimulus (e.g., You drive a *car, Ford, tractor, golf cart,* and so on). There can be a wide range of acceptability in the latter task as long as the response can be appropriate and, for process-oriented treatment, as long as the client is finding words.

In general, there are two positions regarding item variety, namely that stimulating a process permits great variety and that teaching words is consistent with limited variety. When a wide net is cast for item content, it has been argued that progress is more likely to carry over to untreated content, especially when unanticipated content depends on the same process.

The Success Principle

We start therapy with what a client can already do, which is determined directly or indirectly in initial testing. We rely on tasks that produce a high frequency of accurate responses. Let us call it "the success principle." Brookshire (2007) wrote that "I try to keep patient performance between 60% and 80% immediate and correct responses during the beginning of a given task . . . it is a good idea to limit most brain-damaged patients' percentage of uncorrected error responses to no more than 10% to 15% of all responses . . ." (p. 260). In a day filled with communicative frustrations, the therapy session becomes an island of uplifting linguistic achievement.

By following the success principle, we ensure that a client is processing somewhat normally. Repeated failure, in effect, is the practice of an ineffective or aberrant process. Empirically speaking, errors beget errors. Brookshire (1972) discovered that a naming error on one trial increased the likelihood of an error on the next trial. Brookshire and Nicholas (1978) found that three or four consecutive errors reduced the chance of subsequent correct response to almost nil, possibly due to mounting frustration. When a client starts making 30 percent or more errors, we adjust the task to make it easier, or we switch to a different task in which normal processing is resumed. Success with a task apprises us of processing adequacy, and we are always ready to make adjustments when a task becomes difficult.

In the United Kingdom, a similar approach is called "errorless learning" (e.g., Conroy, Sage, & Lambon Ralph, 2009b). In a comparison of naming therapies, a participant was given the correct response in *errorless therapy* and was provided with hints to the target in *errorful therapy*. The difference between Lambon Ralph's and Brookshire's approaches is subtle. Following the latter's success principle, a client is not necessarily given the correct response at the start. Success is based on how a client performs no matter what the stimulus is, and a few errors are permissible so that the task is challenging. A client may feel that time is being wasted by activities that are completely errorless.

The Antecedent Event

How do we enhance the prospects for successful responding? We begin with Schuell's belief in bombarding a client with stimulation and that each stimulus should elicit a response. Again, she stated, "I stimulate language processes and they begin to function" (Sies, 1974, p. 138). Called the antecedent event in behavioral therapy, the stimulus is the impetus for improving responses. In behavioral therapy, the consequent event manipulates responses. Coelho and colleagues (2008) added that "responses should be elicited, not forced . . . If a stimulus is adequate, there will be a response" (p. 408).

Darley (1982) suggested that we maximize the "arousal power" of a stimulus. We adjust input variables for comprehension according to familiarity, length, semantic redundancy, and syntactic structure. For a verbal production, a pictured stimulus may be supplemented with linguistic cues to the response. Rosenbek and his colleagues (1989) wrote that "our feeling that good clinicians can—by their stimulus selection, ordering, and presentation—elicit responses from all but the most severe or sullen patients, causes us to emphasize antecedent over consequent events" (p. 137).

Schuell added more specifically that "I am going to depend largely on auditory stimulation, because I think language is most dependent on this perceptual system" (Sies, 1974, p. 139). Another reason for relying on listening is that it is usually the least impaired of the modalities. Antecedent power is then increased with *multimodal stimulation*, supplementing an auditory stimulus with a written word or sentence. For unplanned enhancement, a clinician keeps blank cards handy.

Feedback, Especially for Errors

In operant conditioning, "consequences of the behavior serve to control the frequency of its occurrence" (Mowrer, 1982, p. 204). Reinforcement should increase the frequency of a behavior, and negative feedback (or "punishment") should decrease the frequency of a behavior. In therapy for aphasia after a good response, clinicians usually use adult verbal praise such as "good" or "nice job." After errors, Tonkovich and Loverso (1982) administered a "verbal reproof" such as *No, that wasn't right*. Thompson and Byrne (1984) said simply *No, not quite*. Scott and Byng (1989) programmed a computer to emit a "cheerful sound" after a correct response and a "negative tune" after an error.

Schuell and others (1964) stated that "the objective is to get the language processes working, not to teach the patient that whatever he says is wrong" (p. 342). Based on his study of clinical interactions, Brookshire (2007) concluded that "many clinicians tend to avoid negative feedback, perhaps because they do not wish to discourage their patients" (p. 271). Instead of correcting errors we *stimulate the client again*, calling it **restimulation**. We first say "Let's try it again," and then reinstate the initial stimulus. If simple repetition does not work, we supplement the reinstated stimulus with cues such as the first sound in a naming task. We are still trying to elicit, not force, responses.

When stimulation is powerful enough to elicit a good response most of the time, there should be little need for restimulation. If a client exhibits frustration, making errors at a frequency of more than 30 percent, then we modify the task so that the stimulus is more powerful. Often the restimulation becomes the initial stimulus (i.e., antecedent event) in the modified task. It can be like returning to a previous level of the task or a previous task.

Many clients are aware of the difference between their response and their target. Yet we may be tempted to supply informative feedback such as explaining the difference (e.g., "It's not a complete sentence" or "Close, but you should have put *was* in front of the verb"). The client tries to understand the suggestion and respond, leading to an extension of a task's trial. Before we realize it, we are swerving away from the task, possibly confusing the client, and taking time away from the planned stimulation. We can short-circuit such temptations by proceeding immediately to the next item or by changing the task. The point is to stimulate processing success, not teach grammar.

Most clients are self-motivated. Tasks do not have to be tricked up, and a client will practice the way a basketball player repeats shots. For feedback, many clinicians prefer to provide general encouragement (e.g., "You're doing fine," "You're doing much better today").

Programmed Stimulation

Therapy changes as a client changes. Programmed learning is part of our heritage, and we heed the principles in the backs of our minds to keep stimulation on a track specified by a goal. LaPointe (1985) called it programmed stimulation. The long view is that therapy starts with maximum dependence on the clinician for eliciting a response (e.g., imitation) and then proceeds in the direction of the client becoming independent of the clinician.

Treatment of aphasia is a series of little victories. Principles of programming state that moving from an initial task to meeting a short-term goal requires small steps. If the next step is similar to the current step, then capacities employed successfully in the current step should transfer readily to the next step. Mostly the same processes are being used in each step, and the next step should present an easily surmountable new obstacle.

In principle, a small step is created by changing one variable in the current task to make a slightly different task. We may make a stimulus sentence slightly more complex, or we may increase the length of an expected response. An approach to stimulus adjustment is called **fading**, in which we gradually remove supportive cues so that the stimulus becomes more like real life. Fading is like arousal power in reverse and is what Conroy and others (2009a) called "decreasing cue therapy." Another technique is called **shaping**, whereby we reinforce imperfect responses in a way that closes in on the best response.

Formal programs usually include a somewhat flexible response criterion as the basis for moving to the next step. In Shewan and Bandur's (1986) LOT, a 70 percent criterion is frequently recommended. A client has to achieve this level of accuracy on consecutive blocks of 10 trials before processing is considered sufficient for handling the next level of difficulty. Others may consider a 90 to 95 percent criterion, especially because a task should start at a 70 to 80 percent level (e.g., Brookshire, 2007).

In the United States, however, fussy programming has become more of an ideal than a reality. With managed care, the traditional principles of programming might be modified in at least two ways. A short-term goal is likely to be functional, such as requesting an item at a grocery rather than producing a particular linguistic form. Second, a unit of progression is likely to leap multiple steps rather than just one at a time. With bursts of improvement, clients skip steps. For example, once a client starts producing verbs, other elements of a sentence may naturally follow without having been targeted in treatment. As Schuell stated, "Words come out that I never used" (Sies, 1974, p. 138).

Measurement and Generalization

The health care system demands that clinicians document progress. Informally, we can note the return of an activity that had been suppressed since onset. We can take three approaches to measurement:

- Charting performance of treatment tasks
- Repeating a standardized test (e.g., "pre–post-test")
- Regular probing with tasks that are independent of treatment

Probably the least time-consuming approach is to measure performance in the task(s) used as treatment, indicated by the practice of setting criteria for changing tasks (e.g., LaPointe, 1985). A change of 70 to 95 percent accuracy would indicate that a client is improving (as well as becoming successful with increasingly difficult tasks). Graduate students are often required to measure treatment in clinical training.

Measuring the treatment, however, presents conflicts between principles of treatment and principles of measurement. One conflict is between conducting therapy at a high rate of accuracy (e.g., 80 percent) and starting measurement at a low base-line to show change. Another conflict is between maintaining a flexible responsiveness to clients in therapy and maintaining the consistency required for reliability of measurement. Both conflicts can be resolved by separating the tasks for therapy and measurement. Treatment can be flexible and at a high rate of success, and an independent measurement device can begin at a relatively low level and can be consistent.

The difference between treatment and measurement tasks coincides with the desire to measure generalization. It has become common practice for clinical researchers to measure both acquisition and generalization. *Acquisition* refers to a new behavior appearing consistently during a training activity. *Generalization* is progress beyond the treatment, either in other conditions or with untrained responses. In single-case experiments, investigators look for generalization that is related to a treatment activity, such as word-finding treatment with naming and generalization to words used in conversation. The common ground between the therapy and the measure is the process being treated (i.e., word retrieval).

Clinicians can measure three types of generalization (Table 8.4). The importance of **stimulus generalization** has been known for a long time. Starting with the naming of objects, Taylor and Marks (1959) moved clients to using their treated vocabulary in "everyday life without the help of a picture, a word card, or a therapist" (p. 16). Stimulus generalization consists of the absence of clinical assistance and the presence of "everyday life." In a more recent example, action naming therapy relied on pictures as stimuli, but generalization was detected with videos for eliciting the same verbs (Conroy et al., 2009a).

The second type is **response generalization**, which is a logical consequence of the process approach. An improved word-finding process, for example, should show up beyond the words of a therapy. As Schuell stated, words started coming out that she never used. Third, **maintenance** refers to generalization across time. Is an improvement maintained, let us say, 6 months after discharge?

A **generalization probe** takes a few minutes to administer and is usually given at the end of a session. These postsession probes may be given daily, on alternate days, or once per week. However, there can be a learning effect when repeating items, which is minimized by spacing probes a few days apart. Reliability is maximized by using at least 10 items and, of course, by administering the task the same way each time.

A generalization probe is linked to a treatment activity by a goal as well as a process. Sometimes the goal is long-term, such as improving natural conversation while the therapy is still focused and simple. The treatment is the means to achieving the goal, and the generalization probe tells us whether we are meeting the goal. Because a treatment is a means to an end, goals should point to behaviors that differ from the treatment. For example, a treatment may consist of repetition, but our goal is *not* to make a client a better imitator. Instead, our goal may be to improve spontaneous verbalization (Table 8.5). Some theory-based therapies, intended to improve production, do not contain a production task.

The degree of difference between a treatment task and a generalization probe varies as a function of whether a goal is short-term or long-term. We can think of the

TABLE 8.4   The three types of generalization.

TYPE	DEFINITION	TREATMENT	TRANSFER
Stimulus	Trained response to stimuli that differ from treatment	Yes/no to a list of questions	Yes/no to other questions at home
Response	Untrained response to the stimuli used in treatment	Says "car" to picture of a Toyota	Says "Toyota" to same picture
Maintenance	Trained stimulus-response pairs after completion of treatment	Says 10 food names in 60 seconds	Same outcome 6 months later

TABLE 8.5   Relationships among a goal, a therapy, and a generalization probe.

BEHAVIOR GOAL	TREATMENT PROCEDURE	GENERALIZATION PROBE
Improve naming from baseline of 40% to 80%	Sentence completion	Simple naming using words not practiced in treatment
Increase sentence length in conversation	Repeat phrases of increasing length	Conversation at the end of a therapy session

differences as the distance between the treatment and the probe. A clinician may be more interested in naturalistic changes in everyday activities (i.e., more distant) than improvement with untreated words or sentences with the same clinical task (i.e., less distant).

Word-Finding and Retrieval

Everyone with aphasia struggles with finding words and activating them for production. Therapy often begins with the object-naming task but proceeds quickly to more functional activities. Looking ahead, we move up the linguistic ladder to sentence structure in the next chapter. Naming therapies are presented here, alone, because they elegantly illustrate earlier principles such as reliance on stimulation and the search for generalization. Furthermore, neurologically based studies of treatment, presented later, so far depend on naming to represent the impairment-based component of therapy.

Cue Responsiveness

Cues elicit words automatically, without our having to provide the word being practiced. We proceed from automatic to volitional production, which coincides with the ideas of programming steps and fading supportive stimuli. The current section is about the arousal power of cues. Later we shall consider their use as therapies across multiple sessions.

Cues for naming fit into two broad categories (Table 8.6). Semantic cues provide information about meaning with respect to associations that are superordinate, functional, or locational (e.g., "It's a sport," "It is played on a diamond"). These cues are said to activate an area in semantic memory. A lexical cue provides information about the word itself. A phonological cue is usually the first sound or syllable (e.g., "It starts with /b/"). It gives no information about meaning. These cues point to a form in the mental lexicon. Either type of cue is more effective in eliciting names than a picture alone (Stimley & Noll, 1991).

In the research, cues have been presented either prior to showing an object, called *prestimulation* (Pease & Goodglass, 1978; Stimley & Noll, 1991), or they have

TABLE 8.6   Common cues used to facilitate spoken object naming. They are employed in the semantic and lexical therapies to be discussed shortly.

SEMANTIC CUES	EXAMPLE	LEXICAL CUES	EXAMPLE
Definition	"It uses ink and you write with it."	Phoneme (first sound/syllable)	"puh"
Function	"You use it for writing."	Rhyming word	"It's not ten; it's a _____."
Semantic associates	"Pencil," "ink," "It's like a pencil."	Spelling	"pen"
Sentence completion	"A ball-point _____." "You write with it. It's a _____."	Modeling	PEN
Location	"You find it on a desk."		

been presented as restimulation after naming difficulty or an error (Li & Williams, 1990; Kohn & Goodglass, 1985; Love & Webb, 1977). Generally, cues are more effective as the severity of naming deficit decreases. The first sound is more effective than semantic cues and other lexical cues such as a printed or rhyming word. In one study, phonemic cues elicited names about 50 percent of the time, and semantic cues were effective around 30 percent of the time (Li & Williams, 1989), although some exceptions have been observed.

Phonemic cue superiority has been slightly more pronounced for Broca's aphasia relative to aphasia in general. Some investigators left the impression that phonemic cues are especially useful for cases of Broca's aphasia that have the most difficulty in naming (Bruce & Howard, 1988; Love & Webb, 1977). Regarding fluent aphasias, cueing has been more effective for conduction aphasia than the other fluent syndromes. Cues have been least productive for Wernicke's aphasia.

A more recent study compared phonologic cues with purely visual cues consisting of the initial mouth shape in articulating a word (Wunderlich & Ziegler, 2011). The mouth shapes are of interest because there are apps for smartphones that provide this visual information. In the study, both auditory and purely visual cueing improved picture naming for 16 participants (10 with Broca's aphasia). However, auditory cues alone had a pronounced effect for only five participants, and mouth shape by itself had a pronounced effect for only three.

Theory-Driven Naming Therapy

The serial-stage naming model of cognitive neuropsychology (Chapter 3) mediated a transition from empirically based cueing to theory-driven cueing. Process-oriented goals became more specific, as we began speaking of targeting semantic and lexical stages of word-retrieval. The United Kingdom has been a hub for cognitive neuro-psychological (CN) oriented case studies, beginning with the work of David Howard and continuing with Julie Hickin, Wendy Best, and Ruth Herbert. Anastasia Raymer has pursued this approach in the United States. The interactive-activation theory of psycholinguistics has been championed by Kati Renvall and Matti Laine in Finland and by Mary Boyle and Nadine Martin in the United States (for reviews, see Nickels, 2002; Raymer & Gonzalez Rothi, 2008).

The spontaneous arousal power of cues is evidence that aphasia lies in lexical retrieval instead of being a loss of lexical storage (Howard, Patterson, Franklin, et al., 1985). Phonological cues are superior to semantic cues, possibly because the stimulus object already activates concepts in semantic memory. A person with aphasia, who knows what he or she wants to say, still needs help for accessing or retrieving the word (i.e., lexeme). One thought is that a stroke raises the thresholds for lexical activation and that form-related cues lower the threshold or raise the activation level.

With respect to the naming model (Figure 3.1), treatments have been designed variously for repairing the semantic system (Nickels & Best, 1996), the phonological output lexicon (Bastiaanse, Bosje, & Franssen, 1996; Miceli, Amitrano, Capasso, et al., 1996), or the route between semantic and lexical systems (Marshall, Pound, White-Thomson, et al., 1990). The therapies are classified as two general types: lexical treatment and semantic treatment. Both categories consist of a variety of tasks, and sometimes they are combined. Let us begin with the more deeply targeted semantic therapies.

Semantic Therapies

Semantic treatments are based on the assumption that concept activation precedes lexical access, and the therapy activates these concepts. Clients may not even be required to produce a word during the therapy, as if the semantic system is to be targeted by itself. One version, called **picture–word matching**, centers on word comprehension, sometimes supplemented with a semantic judgment task (e.g., Byng, et al., 1990). Progress in naming, especially regarding untreated items, has been mixed (Nickels & Best, 1996) if not disappointing (Pring, Hamilton, Harwood, et al., 1993). Studying a single case, Le Dorze and others (1994) alternated two versions of the therapy, one with production and the other without production. Naming improved for items drawn from the former procedure but not from the latter, indicating that including word production in a semantic task may be important.

In **semantic feature analysis** (SFA) a pictured object is placed in the center of a chart containing cues to various types of associations (e.g., *is used for ___, has ___, reminds me of ___*). After attempting to name the object, a client completes the phrases and perhaps writes answers in boxes surrounding the object. Then the client tries to name the object again. Clinicians believe that the procedure activates the semantic region around a word, making it easier to retrieve the word. Naming treated and untreated items improved in most cases, but spontaneous speech did not get better for those with Broca's aphasia (Boyle, 2004; Boyle & Coelho, 1995; Coelho, McHugh, & Boyle, 2000; Lowell, Beeson, & Holland, 1995).

More recently, SFA has been compared to or used with discourse-based therapy. The main goal was to improve discourse (see Chapter 10). At the University of Iowa, both therapies were effective for clients with agrammatism (Gordon, 2007). At New York University, Antonucci (2009) placed SFA in a group therapy that included storytelling activities. Beginning with an orienting SFA procedure, mildly fluent participants were prompted to provide features when experiencing word-finding difficulty in the discourse tasks. Word-finding and informativeness of discourse improved (see also Falconer & Antonucci, 2012). At Rush University Medical Center in Chicago, Peach and Reuter (2010) also integrated SFA into discourse and produced positive outcomes in more natural language production.

Lexical Therapies

Lexical therapies emphasize access and retrieval of *words per se*, either their phonologic or orthographic form (e.g., Carlomagno, Pandolfi, Labruna, et al., 2001). These therapies are commonly associated with conduction aphasia, in which impairment is located in phonology.

In an early **phonologic treatment** clients were given a package of word repetition and rhyme judgment cues for 4 days across 1 week or for 8 days across 2 weeks (Howard et al., 1985). Six weeks later, the superiority of treated items faded, raising a question of whether only a few sessions of lexical cueing is sufficient to restore the retrieval process for lasting use. Raymer and others (1993) administered a phonologic treatment for 15 to 20 sessions. As restimulation, the clinician tried a rhyming cue, then the initial phoneme, and then the word itself for repetition. Some clients improved in the naming of untreated items and in tasks not used in therapy (i.e., written naming).

Might a phonologic treatment be modeled after semantic feature analysis (SFA)? In Toronto, Leonard and others (2008) developed **phonologic components analysis** (PCA). Like SFA, a picture of an object is centered in a chart, and the object is surrounded by cues about sound features of the target word. From Table 8.6, we could guess what these features might be (e.g., first sound, rhymes, number of syllables, and so on). In the therapy, a client attempts to identify the phonologic components regardless of ability to name the object as if forcing a tip-of-the-tongue state. Most of the participants in Leonard's study maintained an increased ability to name objects four weeks after therapy was concluded.

Only a few clinical researchers have focused on orthographic cueing in which a clinician provides a printed or written cue to elicit a spoken word. In a study by Harris Wright and others (2008), written cueing was used as restimulation on failure to name a picture. The clients copied the word three times and again tried to produce the name orally. Both participants in the study improved in naming during the therapy. However, one client did not improve beyond the therapy. The other client generalized to untreated words and maintained naming with treated words 4 weeks after therapy.

Clinicians combined phonological and orthographic cues with some success when it was followed by a therapy using the same words in discourse (Greenwood, Grassly, Hickin, et al., 2010). Also, these therapies have been compared. Lorenz and Nickels (2007) found that first-sound and first-letter cueing were equally effective for one client. First-letter cues were superior for two others.

Phonologic treatments have been compared to semantic therapies. One comparison showed the two types of cueing to be equally effective for reacquisition of naming (Howard et al., 1985), and the two therapies were also equally effective with respect to a communication measure (de Jong-Hagelstein et al., 2010). There was a similar result for action naming therapy (Wambaugh, Cameron, Kalinyak-Fliszar, et al., 2004). These studies have not led us to prefer one type of cueing over the other. We are likely to try each, even in one session. Then we settle on what appears to be most productive for each client. Soon we shall consider combining lexical and semantic therapies.

Verb Retrieval

Noun and verb retrieval can be impaired differently, and verbs carry syntactic information for sentence structuring (Chapter 3). Like the variety of tasks used for nouns, a variety of tasks has been employed for verbs such as sentence completion and naming to definitions as well as action picture naming (Edwards & Tucker, 2006). Verb-oriented therapies have a long history mainly associated with agrammatism (Chapter 9). For now, let us stick with naming.

Whether eliciting verbs is more or less effective than eliciting nouns was examined by Conroy, Sage, and Lambon Ralph (2009b). Only the most severely impaired clients favored stimulation of nouns over verbs. These therapies did not lead to generalization for untreated verbs. In another study, these researchers compared word- and sentence-level cues in 10 sessions across 5 weeks. Word cues began with the spoken and written verb with a picture, then fading the word from its end to its beginning. Sentence cues were given for transitive and intransitive verbs, again fading the verb form (e.g., *He is ski-* for skipping). There were inconsistent differences between types of cues among clients (Conroy et al., 2009a).

Might we apply semantic feature analysis (SFA) to verb retrieval? In Australia, Miranda Rose directed a study of two individuals. In the main treatment, the clients practiced the production of features associated with a pictured action. The clients also practiced movements representing a pictured action (Rose, 2006). SFA was presented either alone or combined with the gesture practice. Clients improved their verb production in narratives and converstion with both approaches (Boo & Rose, 2011; see also Wambaugh & Ferguson, 2007). Gestures were also paired with verb retrieval by Rodriguez and others (2006), who found that a combined SFA and PCA treatment helped an individual with conduction aphasia to produce more verbs accurately.

Written Naming

Therapy to improve written naming often parallels therapy for spoken naming. However, writing poses its own challenges such as spelling and weakness of the usually preferred hand. At the University of Arizona, Pelagie Beeson has been studying orthographic therapy through the lens of CN models of word reading and writing. She has been particularly curious about severe expressive cases that may have more communicative capacity through writing than through speech (Beeson & Henry, 2008).

One procedure focuses on written word formation and is called **ACT** for Anagram and Copy Treatment. A clinician asks a client to write the word for a pictured object and presents scrambled letters for the word (e.g., *omnye*). The client puts the letters in order and then copies the word. The client may also be asked, "Make this spell *money*." Beeson supplements ACT with another therapy called **CART** for Copy and Recall Treatment. This therapy is conducted at home with pages of drawings accompanied by the associated printed word. The client practices copying the words and then recalling these words on pages of the pictures alone (Beeson, Hirsch, & Rewega, 2002).

Severely impaired clients improved with ACT and CART. One with Wernicke's aphasia failed to generalize to untreated words. Clients with global aphasia used some of the trained words for written communication. A moderately impaired client used trained words for e-mail. Similar outcomes were observed in a subsequent study in which clients could not generalize improved writing to speech (Ball, de Riesthal, Breeding, et al., 2011).

Other Naming Treatments

Because lexical and semantic therapies each have had mixed results, it has made sense to try a **combined lexical-semantic treatment**. Drew and Thompson (1999) were more impressed with the results of a combined phonologic and semantic treatment than with semantic treatment alone. Robson and others (2004) applied a mixed procedure to the treatment of proper nouns as well as common nouns. The treatment had a comprehension component and a lexically cued naming component. After five weekly sessions, 10 clients improved equally for naming both types of nouns, but they did not generalize to untreated items. Cameron and others (2006) found that four of five participants, who were trained in retrieving words from stories, exhibited "moderate" generalization to retelling these narratives.

In Philadelphia and Finland, Nadine Martin, Ruth Fink, and Mattie Laine introduced a slight variant of naming therapy called **contextual priming**. Object naming is preceded by having the client repeat the name. According to the theory of priming introduced in Chapter 3, this repetition is thought to activate the target in lexical memory prior to attempting retrieval. Of course, a client could be naming based on short-term memory. Nevertheless, the treatment occurs in the following sequence:

- Spoken word–picture matching
- Repetition of the name
- Independent naming ("delayed repetition")

Semantic context conditions focused on words from a category such as animals or professions, whereas phonological context conditions focused on a particular sound. In two studies, a few cases improved in naming during the therapy, but generalization to naming untreated items was inconsistent (Martin, Fink, Laine, & Ayala, 2004; Renvall, Laine, & Martin, 2007).

Hoping to obtain better generalization to untreated items, Kiran and Thompson turned task sequencing upside down. The approach has become widely known as the **Complexity Account of Treatment Efficacy** (CATE). This paradigm was originally developed for sentences and agrammatism (see Chapter 9). For now, let us consider how it works for naming.

We usually begin with familiar objects, assuming that they are the easiest to name. However, the investigators started therapy for a category (e.g., birds) with semantically more difficult or atypical items (e.g., *penguin*). For two clients with fluent aphasia, this more difficult treatment generalized to untreated typical items in the same semantic category (e.g., *robin*). Conversely, treatment with easy items failed to generalize to untreated difficult items in the same category (Kiran & Thompson, 2003b). This result was replicated elsewhere for one of two participants (Stanczak, Waters, & Caplan, 2006). It was thought that treatment with difficult items challenges word retrieval to a point that the process functions better when it comes time to try easy items that had not been practiced.

Later, Kiran and others (2009) applied CATE to the dimension of abstractness. Their therapy consisted of a variety of tasks that included category sorting, semantic feature analysis, and naming. In a category such as "hospital," concrete words were considered to be easy (e.g., *doctor*). Abstract words in the same category were considered to be difficult (e.g., *emergency*). Three of four participants were consistent with CATE. That is, improvement for trained abstract/difficult words generalized to untrained concrete/easy words. Conversely, the two individuals trained with concrete words did not generalize to untreated abstract words.

Summary and Conclusions: Word-Finding Treatments

One way to summarize the naming therapies, as if we were studying for an exam, is to consider them within the framework of the principles presented earlier. We would think of process-oriented goals, cognitive stimulation, and generalization. For stimulation, we may recall eliciting responses with an antecedent event and restimulating after errors.

Several clinical investigators identified the process as a two-stage semantic to lexical activation, and therapy packages were aimed at either stage. Semantic therapy contained comprehension tasks. Restimulation on error consisted of semantic or phonologic cues or both. Goal-related measures of generalization began with untreated words in the therapeutic naming task and stretched to untreated words produced in discourse activities not used in the therapy. It is essential to add, however, that **therapy for word-finding and retrieval goes well beyond naming things**. It includes divergent activities and attention to words when eliciting sentences and discourse and when maneuvering in conversation.

Those who have been studying theory-driven naming treatments have been well aware of their limitations. From her review of the literature, Hillis (2001) observed that diagnostics in case studies are time consuming and summarized the results as follows:

- Participants with the same diagnosis respond well to different treatments.
- Participants with different diagnoses respond well to the same treatment.
- Too often, the treatments fail to generalize to other items and other tasks.

Nickels (2002) was succinct: "We still cannot predict which therapy will work with which impairment" (p. 959). These conclusions continue to apply, especially regarding the frequent failure of naming therapies to produce generalization even a short distance to untreated words with the therapy task. There has been an indication that we should push for generalization by incorporating discourse-related tasks as part of the treatment (e.g., Antonucci, 2009; Cameron et al., 2006).

Computer-Assisted Treatment

Computers serve each of the main orientations to rehabilitation by delivering impairment-based practice and communication-based alternatives. Early programmed instruction was delivered in part by rudimentary "teaching machines" that provided automated stimulation and feedback (e.g., Holland, 1970; Sarno, Silverman, & Sands, 1970). The machines were reviled by Wepman (1968) as being a "devil's box" coming between a therapist and a client.

Richard Katz (2008) spent over two decades showing us how computers can supplement standard treatment of impairments. Computers become another stimulation delivery system. Companies such as Parrot Software and Bungalow Software have created programs for reading, typed naming, semantic categorization, visual attention, short-term memory, and reasoning. The software is capable of providing hints to improve response and data on performance over time. Computers provide auditory stimulation and spoken response playback.

For word-retrieval, a program called *MossTalk Words*® was developed in Philadelphia. It provides auditory and written cues for naming and can be clinician-assisted or self-guided (Fink, Brecher, Schwartz, et al., 2002). The software contains word–picture matching modules that allowed Raymer and her colleagues (2006) to study semantic naming therapy concentrating on comprehension. Participants acquired an improved naming ability during treatment phases, with treated words faring better than untreated words. Frequency of therapy sessions was a factor and will be discussed later in this chapter.

Computer-assisted stimulation becomes portable with **apps** for tablets and smartphones that deliver traditional clinical tasks (see Chapter 10 for communicative use). Up to the end of 2012, most were designed for young people. However, the "Language TherAppy" program by Tactus Therapy Solutions is friendly for all age groups (tactustherapy.com; see also constanttherapy.com).

One of the more recent innovations is the use of a **virtual therapist** created by Ron Cole of Boulder Language Technologies in Colorado. At the Rehabilitation Institute of Chicago, Leora Cherney inserted Cole's therapist into *Oral Reading for Language in Aphasia* (*ORLA™*). To the right of reading materials on the computer screen, culturally diverse avatars, "Pat" or "Anita," provide spoken cueing (Cherney, 2010). The virtual therapists are used for other interactive language programs (see Chapter 10).

It started as "remote therapy" over the telephone to accommodate a situation in which a clinician and a client must be in different locations. Now generally known as **telepractice**, we use the Internet to deliver services over a distance. It is either *asynchronous*, in which a clinician and client communicate at different times (e.g., e-mail), or *synchronous*, in which parties interact at the same time (e.g., live Internet). Mortley, Wade, and Enderby (2004) evaluated use of the Internet in which a client worked with software, and clinicians remotely updated the exercises. Clinicians have monitored and modified the aforementioned *ORLA* program in a similar fashion (i.e., Web-ORLA™). Now, Skype enables synchronous interaction for many types of therapy.

Efficacy of Impairment-Based Treatment

An SLP is minimally required to document a client's progress. In the few weeks or months poststroke, it can be difficult to detect whether language therapy boosts spontaneous recovery. Research replaces belief with fact regarding whether treatment matters.

The Meaning of Efficacy

Bloom and Fischer (1982) wrote of the "three *eff*'s" of accountability in clinical practice. *Effort* is documented as the number of client visits and the length of a visit. *Efficiency* is a measure of effort with respect to time (e.g., visits per day). However, working hard and efficiently does not guarantee *efficacy*, which is the effect of a treatment on recovery.

Some clinicians suggested that there is a difference between efficacy and *effectiveness*. However, this distinction is a bit tricky. Effectiveness may refer to whether treatment causes a change in functional abilities or in daily life, as opposed to a change in clinical measures (e.g., Brookshire, 1994). Yet Robey and Dalebout (1998) cut the distinction differently, with efficacy as the benefit of "treatment delivered under ideal conditions" and effectiveness as "treatment delivered under routine conditions" (p. 1227;

see also Wertz & Katz, 2004). What this tells us is that, in some circumstances, we should be clear on what we mean when making cause–effect claims. It would probably be good to distinguish between well-controlled conditions of an experiment and typical clinical conditions.

Measuring progress during a period of therapy does not, by itself, provide evidence for an effect of treatment. Any time postonset, other factors could account for this progress (e.g., neurological changes, medications, living environment, other stimulating activities). Demonstrating cause–effect requires control for other factors that could be present while treatment is being administered.

The efficacy research contributes to our ability to realize an **evidence-based practice** (EBP), a concept borrowed from evidence-based medicine (EBM). EBP ties diagnostic and therapeutic decision making to evidence. We would choose therapies for which *clinical trials* have been supportive, a clinical trial being any study of efficacy.

There are several systems for evaluating the **quality of evidence**, as well as for evaluating the quality of journal articles reporting this evidence (Agency for Healthcare Research and Quality, 2002). A common system of levels of evidence (strong to weak) is conveyed roughly in the following (see Murray & Clark, 2006, p. 248):

- **Level I**: at least one properly randomized controlled trial (e.g., large-group comparison)
- **Level II** (3 parts): for example, well-designed single-case experiments, preferably from more than one research group
- **Level III**: descriptive case studies, expert opinion or client testimonials

Among the variations of this rating system is the Oxford Centre for Evidence-Based Medicine Levels of Evidence. The strong and weak extremes are basically the same, but "most empirical evidence falls somewhere in-between, and the characteristics that distinguish among intermediate levels are not always transparent" (Dollaghan, 2007, p. 5). In 2009, the journal *Neurology* started requiring all therapeutic studies to include a level of evidence based on a similar scheme from Class I (strong) to Class IV (weak). A peer review determines the level for publication (Gross & Johnston, 2008). Now, the annual ASHA Convention has disclosure requirements for the presentations of therapeutic methods (e.g., any financial relationship to a clinical product).

Large-Group Comparisons

Chapter 1 introduced research as consisting of at least one comparison. We are probably familiar with the clinical trial in which a group receiving a treatment is compared to a similar group not receiving the treatment. Randomized placement maximizes comparability between groups (see medical treatments, Chapter 9). Also, a large size group improves the chance that results apply to anyone identified by that group (e.g., Morgan, Gliner, & Harmon, 2006). However, ethical concerns, such as randomly withholding therapy, have made it difficult to conduct such studies. Only a few have been done, and even fewer have appeared recently.

The largest study in terms of group sizes was carried out in Italy (Basso, Capitani, & Vignolo, 1979). Most of the participants had aphasia caused by stroke. The strength of this study would now be said to be below Level I because placement in the no-treatment group was not random; these participants "were prevented from attending therapy for extraneous factors, such as family or transportation problems" (p. 191). The study was still monumental, for it took 30 years to complete. The groups were similar in educational and socioeconomic levels and in distribution of types of aphasia, etiology, and gender.

Each of the treated and untreated groups were subdivided according to the time postonset that treatment was initiated. Some participants received treatment less than 2 months after onset. Others began treatment between 2 and 6 months postonset, and others did not start treatment until after 6 months (Table 8.7). At each period, the percentage of participants making substantial improvement was higher in the treated group. Therefore, people with aphasia that received treatment were more likely to improve than people with aphasia who did not receive treatment.

In Canada, Shewan and Kertesz (1984) compared three treated groups to an untreated group "who did not wish or who were unable to receive treatment" (p. 277). The group sizes ranged from 23 to 28 participants. The therapies consisted of an impairment-oriented treatment developed by Shewan and Bandur (1986), Schuellean stimulation-facilitation therapy, and an unstructured therapy provided mainly by nurses. The investigators reported few details about the procedures, and the first two were likely to have been similar. Treated participants received 3 hours of treatment per week for a year.

The investigators measured progress with standardized test batteries at intervals beginning within the first month and then at 3, 6, and 12 months postonset. Both treatments by SLPs had a better outcome than no-treatment, and there was no difference between the two language stimulation therapies. The unstructured group did not differ significantly from no-treatment. The treatment effect was most pronounced in

TABLE 8.7 Percentage of substantially improved patients in each of six groups (Basso et al., 1979). Groups were defined as treated or untreated and whether treatment was initiated within 2 months, 2–6 months, or after 6 months postonset.

	TIME POSTONSET		
	< 2 MONTHS	*2–6 MONTHS*	*> 6 MONTHS*
Auditory Comprehension			
Treated ($N = 107$)	88	65	50
Untreated ($N = 86$)	50	48	16
Oral Expression			
Treated ($N = 162$)	59	39	29
Untreated ($N = 119$)	33	9	4

the 6- to12-month period postonset. This study indicated that direct language stimulation may vary in style but not in effectiveness.

In Germany, Poeck, Huber, and Willmes (1989) followed the progress of 68 treated people with aphasia. The treated participants were compared to the spontaneous recovery of 92 individuals where aphasia treatment was not available. Treatment was reported to have been similar to Shewan's language therapy, but it was more intense. It was given in five 1-hour individual sessions and four 1-hour group sessions per week. Treatment periods lasted 6 to 8 weeks. The treated group was subdivided into an early group treated between 1 and 4 months postonset and a late group treated between 4 and 12 months postonset. A third group started therapy after 12 months.

Effects were determined by employing a statistical maneuver that accounted for spontaneous recovery. Significant treatment effects occurred for 78 percent of the early group and 46 percent of the late group, similar to the decline of proportional improvements in the Italian study. Poeck and his colleagues thought that their estimates were low because of the strictness of the statistical correction. No correction was made for the late-starting group, but 68 percent showed significant improvement.

These large clinical trials in Italy, Canada, and Germany indicated that a percentage of people with aphasia benefit from therapy beyond 6 or even 12 months, a result reinforced by Robey's analysis cited early in this chapter. In addition to Chapter 7's note of recovery beyond 12 months, this evidence should give hope to people with chronic aphasia who abhor the idea that they can look forward only to a "plateau" in their language abilities.

Treatment Comparisons

Comparing therapies is another approach to seeing if therapy has an effect. In the United States, a massive project was undertaken to compare individual treatment with a group treatment that consisted of informal discussion without direct language manipulation (Wertz et al., 1981). Several Veterans Administration Medical Centers participated in a fastidious effort to match treatment groups and assign participants randomly. For more than 3 years, over 1,000 patients were screened. Only 67 met the stringent criteria. Eight hours of treatment per week was started 1 month after onset. Each group received treatment until about 4 months postonset. Due to attrition, a total of 34 individuals were followed until about a year postonset.

Looking at the results, the only difference between treatments was that individual treatment had greater progress than group treatment. Otherwise, both methods were similar in being accompanied by significant progress. Treatment efficacy was implied by significant improvement after 6 months, the point at which spontaneous recovery is believed to have ceased.

The next Veterans Administration cooperative study addressed a comparison between two other categories of treatment (Wertz, Weiss, Aten, et al., 1986). One type was treatment in the clinic by an SLP. The other was a home-based treatment by a volunteer. The treatments began about 7 weeks after onset and lasted 12 weeks. A deferred-treatment group was added as a no-treatment control. This group had

12 weeks without treatment followed by 12 weeks of clinic treatment. The progress made by the clinic-treatment group was significantly greater than that made by the deferred-treatment group over the first 12-week period. The home-treatment group was between these groups, not differing significantly from either one. The three groups did not differ from each other at about 8 months postonset, indicating that delaying treatment for a while may not matter ultimately.

Intensity of Treatment

Intensity of treatment has received a lot of attention recently because of the rise of *constraint-induced language therapy* (CILT). More on this shortly. Two reviews of the literature preceded the arrival of CILT. Robey (1998) detected the strongest effects for moderate amounts (2–3 hours/week) in comparison to low (less than 1.5 hours/week) and high amounts (more than 5 hours/week). Basso (2005) factored in duration of therapy and examined the question of how intensive and prolonged treatment should be to produce the best results. Treatment was not effective when given 2 hours per week for an average of 23 weeks. Treatment was effective when provided about 9 hours per week for 11 weeks. Thus, more intensive treatment for a shorter duration had better outcomes.

Examination of therapy scheduling is occasionally incorporated into studies of treatment. One example is an aforementioned study of comprehension training to improve naming (Raymer et al., 2006). Each participant received one phase of therapy for one to two sessions per week and another phase for three to four sessions per week. The more intense phase was accompanied by more acquisition of naming ability during the treatment, but the more-intense phase did not differ from the less-intense phase when naming was assessed 1 month after treatment.

Constraint-induced language therapy (CILT) incorporates a very intensive schedule (see Chapter 10 for more about the interactive therapy). Most versions follow Pülvermuller's 3 hours per day for a few consecutive days (Pülvermuller, Neininger, Elbert, et al., 2001). Cherney and others (2008) analyzed a "paucity of studies" of intensity, including studies of CILT. They applied strict quality requirements to end up with 10 studies for review, including Raymer's study. Cherney found "modest evidence" favoring intense short-term scheduling over drawn-out scheduling for immediate gains (acquisition), depending on the outcome measure. Maintenance of effects for the long-term has hardly been studied at all.

Evaluation of the Efficacy Research

Only a couple of studies indicated that treatment has no effect. One targeted the most severe aphasias more than 2 years postonset (Sarno, Silverman, & Sands, 1970). The other study was poorly controlled, sparking some controversy (Lincoln et al., 1984; Wertz, Deal, Holland, et al., 1986).

A **meta-analysis** by Randall Robey (1998) at the University of Virginia is a specialized review that is "a mathematical means for synthesizing independent research findings scattered throughout a body of literature" (p. 173). In a tutorial, Robey and Dalebout (1998) suggested that "thoughtful reviews of salient literature" are insufficient. A meta-analysis determines the *weight of scientific evidence* bearing on a hypothesis. As noted early in this chapter, Robey (1998) concluded that recovery of treated patients is nearly twice the recovery of untreated patients when treatment is begun during the first 3 months. His analysis covered most of the large treatment studies that have been done to date.

Few studies have been replicated, and "as a result, many outcomes are singular observations and practically independent of all others" (Robey, 1998, p. 183). Group studies have particularly high hurdles to overcome. They are not like clinical drug trials in which people with the same disease are assigned randomly to two groups, one receiving the medication and the other receiving a placebo. In studies of aphasia therapies, the control group is likely to have differed from the treated group in ways other than just the absence of the treatment. Thus, the quality of evidence for aphasia treatment efficacy resides somewhere in Level II, not the best but not the worst either.

In addition, the treatments analyzed may not be typical of current clinical practice. Robey (1998) was concerned about the failure to report information. He noted that the most frequently reported type of therapy fit his category of "not specified." A present concern is *treatment fidelity* or the consistency of a therapy delivered by multiple research clinicians in a single study (Hinckley & Douglas, 2013).

Robey concluded that his meta-analysis of group studies substantiates the value of standard treatments and that the basic issue regarding efficacy has been settled. Yet a recent Cochrane review was only mildly impressed with the quality of treatment research (Brady, Kelly, Godwin, et al., 2012). Since 1998, small experiments have tackled more specific questions, such as the comparative efficacy of lexical and semantic treatments. A catalogue of efficacy research is maintained at PsycBITE™ (psycbite. com; McDonald, Tate, Togher, et al., 2006). In a search of the site for studies indexed for aphasia, 70 percent were single-case designs (Togher, Schultz, Tate, et al., 2009).

The Brain with Treatment

We pick up the story of the brain's adjustments to stroke with the question of whether therapy causes the brain to change. The story began in Chapter 2 and, later, we considered changes in the brain that may account for functional improvements without therapy (Chapter 7). The narrative wraps in the next chapter with medical treatments that may "re-wire" the brain more directly.

To determine the influence of our therapies, fMRIs are taken before and after a treatment while the participant is engaged in a generalization task. Such studies ideally would include two controls. A healthy group would help to identify stroke-related improvement. The other control is an untreated group with aphasia to determine if improvements are unique to receiving treatment. For a bilingual case in Italy, another control was to treat one language while withholding treatment from the other language (Abutalebi, Della Rosa, Tettamanti, et al., 2009).

Rochon and others (2010) used both healthy and brain-damaged controls. Brain activity for two people with aphasia was measured during phonologic and semantic tasks (without naming) before and after a phonologic treatment for naming. Two other people with aphasia and 10 healthy individuals received fMRIs under similar conditions but without treatment. The aphasias were at least 2 years postonset. One untreated patient showed no changes in brain activity. The other untreated control displayed an increase in right-hemisphere activity. The treated participants, along with improved naming during therapy, showed increased activity in the *left* hemisphere, differing from the untreated controls (see also Davis, Harrington, & Baynes, 2006).

Meinzer and Breitenstein (2008) reviewed the "first wave" of this research, most of which were case studies. The therapy was sometimes atypical, either very intense (Meinzer, Flaisch, Breitnestein, et al., 2008) or just 15 minutes per day (Raboyeau, De Boissezon, Marie, et al., 2008). It was often focused on naming. Some form of cerebral reorganization accompanied semantic therapy (Davis et al., 2006) and phonologic therapy (Abutalebi et al., 2009; Rochon et al., 2010). Changes, described as "perilesional," usually occurred in the damaged hemisphere (see also Kurland, Pulvermüller, Silva, et al., 2012).

At the University of South Carolina, Julius Fridriksson (2010) administered multiple fMRIs to a group of 26 people with varied aphasias. The participants received an intensive cueing therapy for naming, 3 hours per day for 2 weeks. For those who improved in naming, anterior and posterior ipsilateral regions increased in cerebral activation. The new wrinkle was finding that those who did not improve had damage in the posterior temporal region associated with word-retrieval. Therefore, positive outcomes occurred for those with other sites of infarction in the left hemisphere.

Health Care Topics

This section samples a few topics pertaining to the medical environment in which SLPs treat people with aphasia. It is not comprehensive, and further education on the issues comes with experience in these settings. The SLP in some way deals with Medicare, medical records, quality of care, and ethics.

The Third Party and Medicare

Chapter 1 introduced the general concept of payment for services that is mainly provided by a third party, public or private. In the United States before the age of 65, many of us rely on a **health maintenance organization** (HMO), which is a private insurance plan that contracts with a medical group or groups to provide a full range of health care. After 65, we rely on **Medicare**, a government-mandated insurance program. Congress approved this program in 1965 to be part of 1935's Social Security Act. At one rehabilitation program, reimbursement came from Medicare (58 percent), an HMO (23 percent), and Medicaid (4 percent), which is for certain groups with low incomes (Odell, Wollack, & Flynn, 2005).

Medicare consists of two main parts:

- **Part A** provides necessary inpatient medical and rehabilitation services within the first 90 days in a hospital and the first 100 days in a skilled nursing facility (SNF).
- **Part B** pays for subsequent physician-prescribed or "medically necessary" outpatient services in a hospital, clinic, or at home. A clinician submits a short *certification* form to the physician, noting planned visits per week and an anticipated maximum duration of treatment. Certification also requires a brief statement of *short-term goals* that are within a patient's immediate grasp and *long-term goals* for the duration requested.
- **Part C** is an optional *Medicare Advantage Plan* offered by Medicare-approved private companies such as an HMO. It covers Part A and B services and additional coverage for hearing and vision.

Most Medicare enrollees (75 percent) have the traditional Part A and Part B program, and 25 percent have a Medicare Advantage plan.

The Balanced Budget Act of 1997 changed Medicare reimbursement dramatically. For Part B, the significant change was the introduction of an annual cap on services per patient. One cap is shared by speech-language pathology and physical therapy, whereas occupational therapy has its own cap. It applies to inpatient rehabilitation, rehabilitation centers, and home health agencies. It does not apply to outpatient clinics in hospitals. The cap increases with inflation, and the figure in 2012 was $1,880.

In January 2006 Congress attached exceptions to the cap. Exceptions are automatic for certain conditions, including swallowing evaluations. Manual exceptions (not automatic) require a formal request supported by documentation. Staying abreast of legislation can be done by checking the Web site for the American Speech-Language-Hearing Association (asha.org). Local guidelines can be monitored by checking a Medicare contractor's Web site (Busch, 2007).

With managed care came a *prospective payment system* (PPS) in which payment is determined before provision of services. Emulating this concept, Medicare instituted the *Inpatient Rehabilitation Facility Prospective Payment System* (IRF PPS) (cms.gov/Medicare). Reimbursement rate changes and other pertinent information are announced regularly in *The ASHA Leader*. The IRF PPS utilizes information from a patient assessment instrument (IRF PAI), which relies mainly on the FIM (Chapter 6).

Medical Records

In 1996 the U.S. Congress enacted the Health Insurance Portability and Accountability Act, or **HIPAA** (pronounced "hippa") to standardize the exchange of all health care data. In April of 2003, the Secretary of Health and Human Services authorized "Privacy Rules" for safeguarding the confidentiality of a person's health information. These rules are intended to prevent someone from using or disclosing personally identifiable health information without the patient's consent. The rules also protect participants in research, and Horner and Wheeler (2005) published an article in *The ASHA Leader* explaining how the rules apply to our research practices.

We are familiar with the rows of color-coded paper records in doctors' offices, and these records are being transferred to less costly *electronic medical records* (EMR) stored in computers. Health care providers, including SLPs, have transitioned to software that addresses scheduling, documentation, and billing. ASHA developed documentation templates for volitional use in EMRs and encourages the use of the National Outcomes Measurement System (NOMS) in these templates (Chapter 6).

Quality of Care

As a member of a department in a hospital or rehabilitation center, an SLP participates in ongoing *quality improvement*. Quality is evaluated according to standards developed by each profession. One standard is the *care path* or critical pathway, which is a hierarchy of steps or protocols for rehabilitation of each disorder. For example, a hospital has a critical path for stroke with hemiplegia. Care paths guide decisions about diagnosis and treatment, and each decision is documented in a patient's records. Comparing the documentation to a care path is one basis on which a *utilization review* evaluates appropriateness of services at a health care facility (Table 8.8).

TABLE 8.8 Accreditation agencies.

LEVEL	AGENCY	MISSION	WEB SITE
Hospitals and other facilities	Joint Commission on Accreditation of Healthcare Organizations ("Jayco")	Improves safety and quality of health care through accreditation and related services; founded 1951	jcaho.org
Rehabilitation facility	Commission on Accreditation of Rehabilitation Facilities (CARF)	Provides accreditation for a variety of human services; founded 1966	carf.org
Speech-language pathology	American Speech-Language-Hearing Association (ASHA)	Quality indicators program (replaced Professional Services Board); since 1959	asha.org
Neurogenic disorders	Academy of Neurologic Communication Disorders & Sciences (ANCDS)	Promotes quality service by developing guidelines for training practitioners and standards for clinical practice; founded 1983	ancds.org

Ethical Practice

The Code of Ethics of the American Speech-Language-Hearing Association includes the following concerns (e.g., Bupp, 2012):

- Providing services with the appropriate clinical certifications
- Maintaining adequate records of professional services
- Engaging in any form of dishonest practice or misrepresentation of services or outcomes

Minimal documentation includes the basis for diagnosis and ongoing records of treatment objectives, procedures, and measures of progress. Possible misrepresentation includes diagnosis of a nonaphasic cognitive impairment as aphasia, prediction of recovery for a person with progressive disease, and documentation of progress when there has been no progress.

Beauchamp and Childress (1994) identified fundamental ethical issues, based on a construct developed in the 1970s by a national commission for the protection of human research participants (see also Strand, 1995). Conflicts can arise between three legitimate considerations identified in Table 8.9. Regarding patients' autonomy, patients have "a common law right to choose what care they will or will not accept" (Mariner, 1994, p. 43). A corollary to the clinician's beneficence or desire to "do good" is the need to prevent harm, called *nonmaleficence*. Third, there is society's need for justice or fairness in distribution of services given limited resources. Conflicts can be minimized by conducting a clinical practice with integrity and by following ASHA's code of ethics.

TABLE 8.9   **Food for thought: Framework for discussing ethical issues and conflicts.**

COMPONENT	DEFINITION	POTENTIAL CONFLICT
Client's autonomy	Or "respect for persons"; the right of an individual for self-determination	*Client vs. clinician*: A client does not want therapy that a clinician thinks is needed.
Professional's beneficence	The desire to contribute to another person's welfare and protect another from harm	*Clinician vs. client*: A clinician prescribes a communication board that a family member refuses to acknowledge
Social justice	Fairness in distribution of services given limited resources (third-party considerations)	*Clinician vs. third party*: An SLP prescribes care that a third party is unwilling to pay for *Third party vs. clinician*: A third party pays for services that are inappropriate or unnecessary

Summary and Conclusions

Deciding on appropriate treatment begins with an accurate diagnosis, in this case, of aphasia as a language disorder. This diagnosis includes recognition that it is a disorder acquired by a mature brain, affecting processing as opposed to erasing linguistic knowledge. In a doctor's office, a health magazine recommended that people with aphasia seek out smartphone apps that "display images of the mouth as it creates different letters and words" (Carr, 2011). This speech-oriented stimulation is unnecessary for the aphasia diagnosis (unless the person has Broca's apraxia of speech). The chapter cited a study showing that mouth shape cues improved naming significantly for only 3 of 16 participants, mostly with Broca's aphasia (Wunderlich & Ziegler, 2011).

Assessment should also produce a "problem list" of language difficulties, beginning with deficits in each modality. Each problem is translated into a goal. For example, when someone is impaired in reading words, a goal is to improve word reading. When someone is impaired in word-retrieval, a goal is to improve word-retrieval. At a patient's bedside, we may learn that naming can be stimulated with a phonologic or semantic cue. This is where treatment of word-finding might begin.

We choose tasks that stimulate the impaired process at a high level of accuracy. A different task may be used to measure whether a goal is being met. Our goals usually imply that we are looking for generalization, even a small "distance" away. For example, the therapy may be a cued naming task. The measurement is an unfettered naming task to see if the client is improving without therapeutic assistance.

In addition to the general principles of treatment and the examples in naming therapy, this chapter sampled other fundamental topics. Computers fulfill a wide variety of rehabilitative functions (Chapters 9, 10), but they started as simply another means of delivering cognitive stimulation. New imaging technology is blessing us with insights into whether our therapies really have an effect on the brain. Finally, all of our work is carried out in a health care system that influences some of what we do.

In the midst of these introductions, evidence was presented to show that treatment of language impairment makes a difference for people with aphasia. Moreover, treatment can help beyond 6 months postonset and even beyond the first year. Changes in the brain have been detected in association with therapy 2 years after a stroke. Our clients need not be fearful of a "plateau."

CHAPTER

9

Specialized Treatments for Impairments

The previous chapter introduced principles and methodologies for most people with aphasia. Clinicians extend menus of treatments by targeting a symptom or a hypothetical breakdown in cognitive processes of language use. Many of these therapies, the main topic of this chapter, are experimental in the sense that they are conducted in controlled conditions and are not yet widely deployed in clinics.

Clinical research is presented, as before. Depending on the demands of instructors, students are invited to think of the studies as not to be recalled for a test but rather as "pictures" that illustrate or explain a therapy that should be remembered. Procedural details are good therapy ideas. The studies also contribute to an evidence-based practice. About half of the literature and chapter addresses agrammatic aphasia (and, therefore, sentences). The chapter moves on to other symptoms and syndromes, including therapies for auditory comprehension, reading, spelling, and severe aphasia. The chapter concludes with medical treatments intended to change the brain.

Studying Individual Cases

Many studies of naming therapies and studies in this chapter were of individuals. Such studies, if they are to demonstrate cause–effect relationships, require special rules for the control of variables. These studies are commonly used to introduce experimental treatments and may often reach a Level II quality of evidence. A meta-analysis of single-case experiments indicated that treatment effects were large in the studies reviewed (Robey, Schultz, Crawford, et al., 1999). To understand further what goes into proving efficacy and to follow many conference presentations, it is useful to have a rudimentary understanding of single-case experiments.

Unlike group studies of efficacy, single-case or single-participant experimental designs enable a researcher to explore nuances of treatment procedures. Although clinicians have been encouraged to employ these designs while providing treatment, an adequate study usually requires external funding to pay for the time involved. Nevertheless, a general knowledge of these designs should help a speech-language pathologist (SLP) be an astute consumer of treatments that are purported to be evidence based.

A single-case experiment differs from a **case study**. The case study is meticulously, sometimes ponderously, descriptive of an individual's history, assessment, and treatment. It provides therapy-related test results from before and after the treatment, and it is at the lower end of evidence quality (Level III). A case study may inspire the planning of a single-participant experiment.

The hypothesis-guided experiment travels a sleek path. It controls variables of treatment on the way to providing a midrange quality of evidence (Level II). Like any experiment, a single-participant design contains the following components:

- Manipulation of an independent variable or treatment
- A measure of a dependent variable related to a goal of treatment

A participant is said to serve as his or her own control. That is, a comparison between the presence and absence of a treatment is performed with one individual, rather than one individual (or group) receiving treatment and another individual (or group) not receiving treatment.

The strategies of single-case experimentation have been summarized in research texts (Morgan, Gliner, & Harmon, 2006) and have been detailed in books for clinical and educational fields (Barlow, Nock, & Hersen, 2008; Franklin, Allison, & Gorman, 1996; Kazdin, 2010). Articles have explained their application for communication disorders (Kearns, 1986a; Willmes, 1995). The basic strategies are compressed in Table 9.1. Whereas group designs have tended to examine treatment within the first

TABLE 9.1   Summary of basic single-case experimental designs.

	DESIGN	NOTATION	DESCRIPTION
Single treatment effects	Pre-post treatment	ABA	Bordering a treatment (B) with extended baselines (A)
	Alternating phases	ABAB	Alternating periods of baseline (A) and a treatment (B)
	Multiple baseline	MB	A single treatment applied sequentially to different behaviors or settings; baselines for each are obtained throughout the study
Comparing treatments	Alternating treatments	ATD	Two treatments given within a single day; repeated in different orders for several days
	Crossover	BCBC	Alternating treatment periods (B & C phases); in different sequences for at least two participants (e.g., BCBC vs. CBCB)

year postonset, single-case designs have provided a look into treatment efficacy years following onset.

Let us start with the case study, which commonly includes measures before and after a treatment. Regardless of when they are obtained, these two data-points (or any two data-points) could be derived from random variation and, thus, are inconclusive as proof of how a client was doing through the period being measured. Uncovering real improvement involves collecting several probes across a period of time, rather than simply "bordering" a treatment phase. For future reference, these phases containing multiple probes are designated by a letter (e.g., **A** for baseline, **B** for treatment). The goal is to determine the *trend* across a phase. A trend could be flat, upward, downward, or random variation.

The minimal single-case design is an **ABA** in which baseline phases border a treatment phase. Let us assume that multiple measures (at least three) are taken during each phase, and we look for a flat baseline trend for the first **A**, an obviously upward trend for **B**, and at least maintenance of the improved performance in the second **A**. This design is often conducted beyond the reach of spontaneous recovery, making it tempting to attribute progress to the treatment. Indeed, the timing of the shifts may not be coincidental. However, other factors, such as new medication, may contribute to a change. A more complete ABAB design may be more convincing; however, because of the removal of therapy, this type of design may not be in the best interest of a client.

In clinical aphasiology, the more frequent strategy is a **multiple baseline**. A straightforward example is Thompson and Kearns' (1981) study of a cueing treatment for a naming deficit. The study was actually a series of ABA designs applied sequentially to four sets of words. A cueing treatment was applied to one list and then to a second, and so on in succession. During treatment of the first list (i.e., the first ABA), the initial baseline or A-phase for each succeeding list was extended until treatment began for the succeeding lists. Upward trends occurred only when treatment was instituted, indicating that the treatment had an effect. That is, there was only a small likelihood that the changes could have been caused by something else happening at those precise moments.

When comparing treatments given to a single client, one treatment must follow another. Two designs contain elements intended to control for sequence effects, namely the effect that one treatment might have on a subsequent treatment. The **alternating treatments design** (ATD) begins with a baseline of the dependent variable. Then, the treatments are administered on the same day (i.e., "simultaneous" treatments). Each day thereafter, the order of treatments is reversed, and the two daily sequences are randomly alternated across several days. Probes of the dependent variable are obtained for each treatment so that a graph of the treatment phase shows two sets of data (e.g., Avent, et al., 1995). **Crossover designs** are commonly used in Europe and require two participants (e.g., Springer, et al., 1991). For one participant, a treatment phase (B) precedes another treatment phase (C). The sequence is reversed with the other participant. A study may stop at this point or continue by alternating phases.

Sentence Production

Therapies for sentences are generally used to increase the verbal productivity of people with agrammatism. This section starts roughly with data-driven therapies derived mainly from observations of how people with aphasia respond to stimuli. Then we ponder more theoretically motivated treatments based on assumptions about the nature of sentence production. These treatments are mainly aimed at repairing an impaired process, and they offer clear examples of when the means differs from the ends in aphasia treatment.

Melodic Intonation Therapy (MIT)

Long ago clinicians made a startling observation that people with nonfluent aphasia, like people who stutter, sing better than they talk. Recently there has been a surge of publicity for a "music therapy" that was one of the aphasia treatments provided to Rep. Gabrielle Giffords by Nancy Helm-Estabrooks and others (Law, 2012a). The therapy was MIT, which has been the most studied and heralded form of music therapy for neurogenic language and speech disorders (Hurkmans, de Bruijn, Boonstra, et al., 2012). Although it does not target syntax per se, it is intended to help people produce sentences with less effort. Post hoc theorizing has suggested that the right hemisphere may be helping.

Robert Sparks crafted the program at the Boston Veterans Administration Medical Center in the 1970s. It was soon reported in explicit detail, making it easy for others to replicate (Helm-Estabrooks, Nicholas, & Morgan, 1989; Sparks, Helm, & Albert, 1974; Sparks & Holland, 1976). Candidates for MIT are clients with good auditory comprehension and minimal improvement in speech production by more standard clinical procedures. These clients are likely to have a severe Broca's aphasia.

The essence of MIT is to have an individual apply melody to an utterance. A client usually concentrates on the production of a few familiar phrases or sentences. Several steps lead into melodic production, and then additional steps involve fading the artificial melody from the production. Clients have proceeded through the program successfully, and performance by severely nonfluent clients can be spectacular (Albert, Sparks, & Helm, 1973). More recent results with the Persian language were encouraging (Bonakdarpour, Eftekharzadeh, & Ashayeri, 2003).

One case with Broca's aphasia 4 years postonset had received MIT previously with little success (Hough, 2010). One problem seemed to be a disruption of speech production by the rhythmic tapping component of the program, so tapping was omitted. The client was trained to produce lists of routine and personal phrases that had been used more spontaneously. Remarkable improvement was observed throughout the treatment program along with modest progress with untreated phrases. The investigator did not assess generalization to spontaneous production in natural contexts.

Reports have been elusive regarding generalization of these successes to communication outside the context of the program. In a review that did not include the more recent studies just cited, Hurkmans and others (2012) concluded that MIT and other music therapies should be considered cautiously. Using levels of evidence introduced in Chapter 8, they rated methodological quality of the studies as "low."

Sentence Production Program

The *Sentence Production Program for Aphasia* (SPPA; Helm-Estabrooks & Nicholas, 1999) started out as the *Helm Elicited Language Program for Syntax Stimulation* (HELPSS; Helm-Estabrooks, 1981). It is intended to increase the syntactic variety and complexity of utterances. For those familiar with HELPSS, the few changes were that the number of sentence types were reduced from 11 to 8, a male gender bias was removed, and *wh-* questions were added. The program is recommended for agrammatic clients with good comprehension and a minimum mean length of utterance of two to five words.

A clinician uses a short story completion to elicit sentences. Each story is accompanied by a picture. The program consists of two broad levels for training each type of sentence. In Level A, the target phrase is included in the story so a client can repeat it (e.g., *Whenever Shawna tries double jumps in ice skating, she falls. What happens when Shawna tries to do the double jumps?*). In Level B, the client is to complete the story with the target phrase (e.g., *When Shawna tries to do double jumps in ice skating, what happens?* seen in the picture). A response criterion of 90 percent accuracy determines movement up a sentence-type hierarchy within each level.

Most of the published studies so far have evaluated the original HELPSS. Helm-Estabrooks and Albert (2004) concluded that efficacy was demonstrated mainly in two pre-post studies showing progress in sentence production (Helm-Estabrooks, Fitzpatrick, & Barresi, 1981; Helm-Estabrooks & Ramsberger, 1986). In single-case experiments, HELPSS promoted some generalization to untreated items but little generalization to different conditions (Doyle & Goldstein, 1985; Salvatore, 1985). Later, a similar procedure was applied successively to several types of sentences. This multiple baseline study indicated that the procedure can influence production (Doyle, Goldstein, & Bourgeois, 1987).

A few years later, HELPSS was administered to four individuals with nonfluent aphasia in three sessions per week (Fink, Schwartz, Rochon, et al., 1995). The investigators observed generalization to stimuli designed to elicit specific types of sentences. Generalization did not occur in a storytelling task. More recently in Italy, improvements in sentence structure and informativeness of picture description followed a sequence of HELPSS and a functional therapy (Marini, Caltagirone, Pasqualetti, et al., 2007).

Response Elaboration Training

Clinical researchers tried behavioral training of a few specific forms, but it was not causing broad generalization (e.g., Kearns & Salmon, 1984; Thompson & McReynolds, 1986). So, the same researchers decided to modify the treatment. One change was called **loose training**, which introduced flexibility in stimuli and in the response to be reinforced (e.g., Thompson & Byrne, 1984).

One version of loose training is Kevin Kearns's *Response Elaboration Training* (RET). He suggested that "overly structured treatment programs may actually inhibit patients from using language creatively and flexibly by severely limiting their response options" (Kearns, 2005, p. 136). He wanted to expand a client's independence as a communicator by encouraging initiation of responses. In the procedure, "the clinician shapes and elaborates spontaneously produced client utterances rather than targeting preselected response" (Kearns, 1985, p. 196).

Kearns asked a client to describe a simple event (e.g., a man sweeping a floor) and then used modeling and shaping to encourage an expanded description. In an early step, let us say the initial description was "Man . . . sweeping," the SLP expands as restimulation ("Great. The man is sweeping"). In the next step, a question stimulates production of additional information ("Why is he sweeping?"). Then the SLP models a combination of the initial response and the response to the question. The client practices elaborated imitations ("The man sweeping. Wife mad"). The key is to avoid training a specific target response (Kearns & Scher, 1989; Kearns & Yedor, 1991).

RET was introduced with a client who had Broca's aphasia (Kearns, 1985, 1986b). Following a multiple baseline design, treatment was initiated for one set of 10 pictures and was delayed for another set. A treatment effect was observed in upward trends of performance beginning with each treatment. Some generalization occurred for a third set of pictures. Whereas the client's verbal score on the *PICA* had decreased over the 6 months prior to treatment, his score improved across this period of treatment.

Kearns and his colleagues concluded that RET promotes generalization and is also effective for conduction and anomic aphasia (Yedor, Conlon, & Kearns, 1993). Julie Wambaugh indicated that RET helps to increase amount and variety of content in utterances and discourse (Wambaugh, Martinez, & Alegre, 2001; Wambaugh, Nessler, & Wright, 2013).

Verb Production

Predicate-argument information is part of verb representation. It has been thought that if a person with agrammatism can retrieve verbs better, then more complete sentences should follow. After all, people with this symptom are already relatively good at retrieving nouns. Verb-retrieval treatment was introduced in Chapter 8, but now we should be thinking about the goal of expanding sentence production.

Perhaps, the first of the verb-oriented therapies was *cueing-verb treatment* or verbing strategy (Loverso, Prescott, & Selinger, 1988). It consisted of a hierarchy of tasks starting with producing an actor for a verb and culminating in producing a complete sentence when asked a question. Twenty years later, Edmonds, Nadeau, and Kiran (2009) experimented with a similar method that they called *Verb Network Strengthening Treatment* (VNeST). Moderately to mildly impaired clients were given a verb (e.g., *measure*) and, based on cue cards for various meanings (e.g., *chef/sugar, carpenter/lumber*), were asked to formulate different sentences around the verb.

Fink and others (1997) used a short story-completion task, much like Helm-Estabrooks's production stimuli. One example follows:

Clinician: Someone *carried* the sofa. It was the mover. Did I say the mover *dropped* the sofa?
Client: No, he *carried* the sofa.

Agrammatic individuals improved across six sessions in the use of trained verbs and verbs that were simply "exposed" during probing.

Other therapies emphasized verbs, and the goal of improving sentence production was reflected in the generalization probe. Clearly, the means (e.g., naming therapy) differed slightly from the ends (i.e., improving sentence production). Raymer and Ellsworth (2002) employed phonological and semantic therapies aimed at action-naming. Naming of trained verbs improved. Webster, Morris, and Franklin (2005) had a client associate nouns with verbs and retrieve nouns that serve thematic roles around a verb. In both studies, there was poor generalization to untreated verbs, but there was some improvement in sentence production.

At Northwestern University, Schneider and Thompson (2003) examined seven cases with agrammatism using a relatively complex combination of crossover and multiple baseline experimental designs. The crossover component accommodated a comparison between two treatments:

- *Semantic verb-retrieval treatment*, with extensive cueing of meaning for action naming
- *Verb-argument structure retrieval treatment*, with extensive cueing of thematic roles in pictures for action naming

Schneider and Thompson obtained a familiar result of improved verb-retrieval with both treatments, but little generalization to untrained verbs. Sentence production improved even though sentence production was not stimulated directly.

The laboratory in the Netherlands that has been studying verb impairments (Chapter 3) developed a therapy eventually called ACTION (Bastiaanse, Hurkmans, & Links, 2006). The method roughly consists of the following four steps with 30 transitive and 30 intransitive verbs:

- Lexical level: action naming
- Syntactic level: completing a sentence with a verb
- Morphosyntactic level: completing a sentence with an inflected verb
- Sentence level: describing an action with a sentence

The first step is omitted for agrammatic aphasia because the authors believe that training should be at the sentence level for these clients. In a more recent study, some untrained verb categories improved according to a multiple baseline design. Post-testing showed progress in spontaneous speech (Links, Hurkmans, & Bastiaanse, 2010).

Mapping Therapy for Production

Mapping therapy presumes a diagnosis of mapping disorder, which was originally posited as an explanation for asyntactic comprehension. For a theory of language production, some clinical researchers turn the comprehension process on its head. This is the idea that formulation begins with a meaning to convey and then proceeds to syntactic structure and then to insertions of lexicon into the sentence frame. The diagnosis for agrammatism was a faulty "mapping" in the early transition from semantics to syntax (Schwartz, Saffran, Fink, et al., 1994).

Candidates for mapping therapy usually fit the following profile:

- Agrammatic production (Broca's aphasia)
- "Good" grammaticality judgment ability
- "Poor" comprehension of reversible sentences

These criteria indicate that identification of asyntactic comprehension is crucial for diagnosing the impairment underlying expressive agrammatism.

Mapping therapy contributed an interesting twist to methodology that, later, was applied to semantic therapies for naming (Chapter 8). Let us consider the work of three research teams (Byng, et al., 1994; Marshall, Pring, & Chiat, 1993; Schwartz et al., 1994). Their slightly different techniques have certain common features that follow:

- The goal of improving sentence production
- **Therapy tasks that do not require production** (e.g., metalinguistic tasks)
- Thematic role cueing

Like the treatments of naming, mapping therapy is thought to stimulate a level of the sentence production process before production actually occurs. Again, the means differs from the ends. Producing utterances is not a key feature of mapping therapies. Versions of this method are summarized in Table 9.2.

Byng's group built a stage into their therapy intended to encourage generalization. This stage incorporated thematic cues to aid in the production of sentences during a structured conversation activity (for PACE, see Chapter 10). Other versions of mapping did not contain a generalization stage, indicating that clinicians hoped for a greater jump over the gap between the treatment and more functional sentence production.

The approach is similar to some verb-oriented treatments. Jane Marshall (1999a) presented the case EM for whom sentence and narrative production improved after a therapy that consisted of a variety of verb-related tasks not requiring sentence

TABLE 9.2 **Summary of mapping therapies for improving sentence production.**

INVESTIGATORS	LOCATION	TREATMENT STEPS	RESEARCH
Sally Byng Lyndsey Nickels Maria Black	Birkbeck College, London	Patient sorts color-coded phrases into sentence; patient describes same action (color cues); PACE therapy (color cues available)	Three cases improved in verb and sentence production
Jane Marshall Tim Pring	City Hospital, London	Present simple actions on video; ask questions about agent, recipient, and action	Spontaneous production did not improve in case studied
Myrna Schwartz Eleanor Saffran Ruth Fink	Moss Rehabilitation Hospital, Philadelphia	Present printed sentence; ask questions about agent, recipient, and action; patient underlines agent, recipient, and action (pens used as color cues)	Six subjects improved in comprehension and production

production. These tasks included analyzing the semantic properties of verbs and generating a verb when given a noun (see also Marshall, Pring, & Chiat, 1998). More recently, Harris, Olson, and Humphreys (2012) described their mapping therapy as one that employed thematic role queries around the verb. That is, after attempting to describe a simple action (e.g., *The boy follows the dog*), the client was asked to report the role of the boy, then the role of the dog.

Mapping therapy for sentence production takes different forms. It has emphasized metalinguistic tasks that do not elicit utterances. In this sense, this therapy has been thought to tap into a mental process leading to sentence production. Marshall and Cairns (2005) began talking about the mapping treatment as working on "thinking for speaking" or working at the level of the conceptualized event to be conveyed.

Treatment of Underlying Forms (TUF)

Since the early 1990s, Cynthia Thompson and Lewis Shapiro have been exploring a strategy called *treatment of underlying forms* (TUF; Thompson, 2008; Shapiro & Thompson, 2006; Thompson & Shapiro, 2005). The idea, like mapping therapy, is to stimulate knowledge of syntactic structure to facilitate sentence formulation. Both methods emphasize verbs. The story of TUF has three components, namely a method grounded in linguistic theory of movement, well-defined paths to generalization, and evolution of method utilizing efficient software and a virtual therapist named Sabrina.

The investigators were interested in the linguistic construct of *movement*, introduced in Chapter 3 in association with gap-filling (Thompson, Shapiro, Ballard, et al., 1997). For example, a *wh-* question is said to be generated from a kernel statement (e.g., *The woman followed the man*) by moving the slot for the direct object (e.g., *the man*) from its position after the verb to the front of the sentence (e.g., *Whom did the woman follow?*). In linguistic terms, a *trace* is left behind in the position vacated by the moved noun phrase (NP), enabling us to identify *Whom* as the direct object.

The short-term goal is to help individuals with agrammatism produce *wh-* questions (e.g., *What did the man send?*). Treatment contains steps that model movement. Using cue cards with the words of the sentence, clients start by repeating and reading a simple sentence such as *The man is sending flowers* (akin to deep structure). In early steps, the clinician provides additional cue cards containing *WHAT* and *WHO*. Subsequent steps include moving the correct *wh-* cue to the beginning of the sentence. All moves lead to a sequence of cues depicting the question (see Thompson, 2008).

Thompson and Shapiro were interested in whether linguistic theory predicts generalization of treatment effects across baselines defined according to type of *wh-* question. We might intuitively think that treatment of one type of *wh-* question should generalize to all other *wh-* questions. However, there are two types of movement with respect to *wh-* questions. One type underlies *who* and *what* questions, and another underlies questions beginning with *when* and *where*. After the treatment, progress in producing *who* questions generalized to *what* questions but not to the other type (Thompson, Shapiro, Tait, et al., 1996). In subsequent studies, generalization occurred within a type of movement but not across different types (Ballard & Thompson, 1999; Jacobs & Thompson, 2000; Thompson et al., 1997). Thus, types of movement seem to possess their own processing characteristics, and we cannot expect that treatment of one type of movement will generalize spontaneously to other types.

Later, Thompson and others (2003) applied their *complexity account of treatment efficacy* (CATE), introduced in Chapter 8, to the goal of improving sentence production. Multiple baselines followed production of complexity levels before and after TUF was instituted. Results for agrammatic participants showed that treating the complex structures first generalized to easier structures. However, for other participants, treating the easiest structures first did not generalize to the more difficult structures. Production of difficult structures began to improve only while being treated. Therefore, the combined results supported the complexity account (see also Stadie, Schröder, Postler, et al., 2008).

Regarding the study of brain changes across a period of therapy, Chapter 8 noted that most of the studies were of naming treatments. A study of syntactic treatment involved TUF and fMRI measures for a generalization task of sentence comprehension. In addition to indicating that cortical activation shifted posteriorly in the temporal lobe, the study provided more evidence of generalization to production of structures that were easier than those being treated (Thompson, den Ouden, Bonakdarpour, et al., 2010).

Are there characteristics of agrammatic clients that are predictive of efficacy and generalization outcomes with TUF? Dickey and Yoo (2010) inspected all the previous studies with respect to severity of aphasia, general auditory comprehension ability, and complex sentence comprehension. Acquisition was predicted by general comprehension ability. However, generalization seems more difficult to predict.

Thompson and her colleagues (2010) explained that TUF has not been widely used because "it requires considerable linguistic knowledge as well as a substantial amount of training" (p. 1244). Also, positive effects required up to 20 sessions per structure to achieve. To mitigate these circumstances, the investigators developed computer delivery software called **Sentactics**® (Thompson, Choy, Holland, et al., 2010). The software was created at the same center in Colorado where ORLA was produced. The client faces a computer screen containing a large workspace with Sabrina, the virtual therapist, to the right. The procedure had been studied earlier (Bastiaanse & Thompson, 2003). It differs from the stepwise movement programs.

The procedure, similar to a subtest in the *Northwestern Assessment of Verbs and Sentences* (Chapter 6), begins with a pair of drawings for a target sentence appearing in the workspace. The drawings are a slight variation of the same idea (e.g., *The mother is painting the girl, The girl is painting the mother*). Sabrina models a sentence for one drawing, and then that drawing disappears. This leaves the second drawing for the client to describe. Sabrina's utterance ("The mother is painting the girl") may serve as a syntactic prime for describing the remaining drawing ("The girl is painting the mother"). Printed word cues also appear at the bottom. Sentences of greater complexity are cued with additional word cards that can be moved about.

Thompson, Choy, and others (2010) conducted a study, first, to determine generalization effects of the treatment. Sentactics improved comprehension and production of trained and untrained sentences for six agrammatic participants in contrast to six control participants. Next, Thompson compared computer-delivered TUF to clinician-delivered TUF. Although both studies provided further support for the efficacy of TUF, the absence of differences between delivery mechanisms indicated that clinicians could consider adopting Sentactics for its logistic advantages.

SentenceShaper 2®

Some current methods flickered obscurely in the past. In the 1950s, Luria (1970) believed that agrammatic utterances result from a deficit in accessing structural representations or "schemas." His therapy, called *externalization of schemas*, was intended to raise structural representation to a conscious level of awareness. He presented visual cues to grammatical categories in syntactic order, such as stick figures of agent, action, recipient. While pointing to each cue, clients magically produced a complete utterance. This cueing of grammatical categories contributed to a system of color-coded lights (Davis, 1973) and was used in mapping therapy (Byng et al., 1994). Tapping movements were associated with colored squares on a table (Raymer, Rowland, Haley, et al., 2002).

Then, similar cueing was put on a computer screen. Marcia Linebarger, Myrna Schwartz, and colleagues in Philadelphia developed software called SentenceShaper®, which functions as a therapy tool and as a communication aid. The latter purpose is discussed in Chapter 10. The therapeutic component helps people with aphasia to create spoken sentences. A free trial version can be downloaded.

The main work screen for SentenceShaper can be inspected in publications and at the Web site (sentenceshaper.com). A person with aphasia says a word, which generates a unique shape (or cue) in a "sentence assembly area." The client can hear the recorded word by pressing the shape. Another part of a sentence is spoken, generating another shape, and so on. The user then moves the cues into an order that constitutes a sentence. Playback provides informative feedback. The client can drag unwanted items to a trash bin. A completed sentence can be labeled with a "bean," and the user can sequence beans above the assembly area to create a narrative.

Studies have shown that nonfluent clients, mostly with agrammatism, create sentences with SentenceShaper that are better than sentences attempted without the program (i.e., "aided effect"; Bartlett, Fink, Schwartz, et al., 2007; Fink, Bartlett, Lowery, et al., 2008). Also, some improve in spontaneous narration following a period of independent home practice with the program (i.e., "unaided speech"; Linebarger, McCall, Virata, et al., 2007). Luria would have been impressed.

Asyntactic Comprehension

For Broca's aphasia, treatment of language comprehension tends to start with sentences. General programming has consisted of manipulating length and structural characteristics of stimuli, without regard to internal process. Tasks, constructed to minimize linguistic demands in a response, have mimicked procedures used for assessment such as picture-choice and enactment with objects. Following principles of stimulation, we ask clients to respond to slightly challenging stimuli until these antecedent events become easy. Then the SLP increases the linguistic demands of the stimuli.

As with sentence production, Luria (1970) attempted to improve comprehension by heightening awareness of syntax. Clinicians paired diagrams that "differ little from those used in common grammar texts" with a spoken or printed sentence. The diagrams consisted of stick figures for actors, drawings of actions, and ideograms showing basic spatial relations. For example, *on* was represented as a ball on a plane, and *under* was represented as the ball beneath the plane. Phrases like *mother's daughter* were split into parts so a client could analyze structure. Two pictures represented the meaning of each word. A demonstrative was added for cueing the modifier (e.g., "*this* mother's daughter"). The purpose was "to externalize the meaningful relationships implied by the constructions and compensate for the inner schemata which the patient lacks" (p. 443).

For another explanation of asyntactic comprehension, Schwartz and others (1980) stipulated that the impairment exists *between* the syntactic parser and semantic interpretation, where a mapping operation superimposes "who is doing what to whom" on an accurate structure. This was called the *mapping hypothesis*. The robust ability to make grammaticality judgments suggested that the parser must be intact despite clinical evidence of difficulty with noncanonical sentences (Linebarger, 1990; Linebarger, Schwartz, & Saffran, 1983). This theory seems to have come about as a process of eliminating lexical and syntactic explanations (Chapter 3).

For instituting mapping therapy, Byng (1988) found two individuals who erred with reversible declarative (e.g., *The man kisses the woman*) and locative sentences (e.g., *The man is beside the woman*). She treated only locatives and measured comprehension of other types of sentences. In a therapy similar to externalization of schemas, comprehension was cued with a "meaning card" showing relations between noun phrases (NPs). Colors were also used to cue NP location in a sentence. One client's progress in understanding locatives spread to untreated reversible sentence types, which Byng interpreted as repair of a mapping mechanism that contributes to comprehending all sentences.

Wernicke's Aphasia

In addition to severe auditory comprehension deficit, Wernicke's aphasia presents some unique problems. The client may not have a clue that her discourse is a mystifying jargon. This leads to a poor "therapeutic set" (Sparks, 1978). The person with jargonaphasia lacks awareness of the reason for being in the clinic. The bimodal recovery discussed in Chapter 7 indicates that some clients with this aphasia recover a great deal of language ability, whereas others do not progress very much. Size of temporal lobe lesion may predict which is more likely. Early progress in treatment may also be an indication.

Auditory Comprehension

The first goal is to establish a therapeutic set or namely a responsiveness to stimulation. We begin simply by modeling the act of pointing to a picture. Numbers may be readily recognized with response cards showing simple quantities, and we start by using numerical sequence as a cue. When the client gets the idea of listening and pointing, we fade numerical sequencing and sneak in words as stimuli. We lean on familiarity with family names and photos. Following this path, we gradually work our way into a second goal of establishing reliable meaningful response to simple linguistic stimuli.

Treatment of comprehension is important with this type of aphasia for a couple of reasons. First, comprehension is a minimal requirement for communicative interaction. Second, stimulating auditory comprehension becomes a back door for production. Direct elicitation of production through modeling is often unsuccessful, because people with Wernicke's aphasia are terrible repeaters. Thus, comprehension training can be a means of setting up skills that can be used to gain control over expression.

The compulsion to speak or "press for speech" can interfere with auditory processing. We should direct attention to listening by inhibiting this tendency to talk. Whitney suggested a "stop strategy" in contrast to a "go strategy" for Broca's aphasia (cited in Holland, 1977). The idea is to keep the person with Wernicke's aphasia from talking during comprehension training. An alerting signal such as a raised hand may be invoked to remind the client to stop talking. As comprehension improves, we look for improved recognition of jargon and, thus, the initial sign that self-monitoring and control are possible.

We look out for the possibility that the client with Wernicke's aphasia has retained some ability to comprehend printed words. Some of these individuals possess an exceptional pattern of auditory comprehension depressed beneath a reading ability. Helm-Estabrooks and Albert (2004) considered word reading to be a starting point (see also Hough, 1993). Very quickly we begin to associate the printed word with the spoken word in a picture-choice task. Other tasks include printed word sorting and picking out the word that does not belong (Harding & Pound, 1999).

Mitchum and her colleagues (1995) provided mapping therapy for ML, a case who had moderate Wernicke's aphasia and who had been studied previously with other treatments. The SLP provided auditory stimulation through sentence–picture verification and picture-choice tasks. ML listened to versions of a message, and the clinician pointed out thematic components of a picture (i.e., agent and recipient). Progress generalized to auditory sentences with untreated verbs and to reading sentences. Progress did not generalize to understanding longer sentences or to sentence production.

Naming and Jargon

Therapy for auditory comprehension has a production objective in that, according to Schuell's guidance, auditory stimulation provides a gateway to other language processes. Self-monitoring may be important for getting control over unwieldy verbal expression but is not necessarily related to a client's comprehension.

Marshall and her colleagues (1998) studied four individuals whose comprehension ability had improved, but they could not recognize their own jargon. The participants did recognize neologisms when repeating words but not when naming. She tried a comprehension-oriented semantic therapy for object naming and supplemented pictured stimuli with printed words. The participants made no progress in naming. They improved in recognizing neologisms for treated items, though not for untreated items.

Wambaugh and Wright (2007) also looked at Wernicke's aphasia through a narrow window. They ignored spontaneous speech or jargon, concentrating solely on naming abilities. They presented semantic and phonologic cueing, supplemented with printed words, for action naming. In a multiple baseline design, each therapy was conducted three sessions per week for 5 weeks. Each treatment showed upward trends in naming the trained items at points when the treatments were instituted. However, similar to Marshall's results, there was no generalization to untrained verbs.

With the goal of improving naming, two single-case experiments bordered therapies with fMRIs to see if the brain changes. In Christine Davis and colleagues' (2006) study, with a participant 5 months postonset, the naming of treated and untreated items improved impressively along with some better word-retrieval in narration. Jacquie Kurland and colleagues (2010) studied an individual 3 years postonset. Treated naming improved, but untreated naming did not get much better. Both studies demonstrated increased left frontal lobe activation, and Davis also saw increased activation in the right hemisphere. Neither study addressed jargon explicitly.

Treatment of Wernicke's aphasia has been examined sparingly, mainly with a few case studies of naming therapies. Jargon appears to have been confronted by inhibiting speech during comprehension training. A direct assault on jargon may be discouraged by severe difficulty with repetition. For people with other syndromes, we use repetition to stimulate and control productions. For clients with Wernicke's aphasia, we watch for a spontaneous arrival of repetition during comprehension drills, and this may lead to intentional repetition. Exactly how this happens and how often it happens could be a fruitful area of clinical study in the future, when cases can be found in a timely manner.

Conduction Aphasia

Although it nails down the diagnosis of conduction aphasia, dissolution of repetition is the tip of the iceberg. For treating the definitive problems, investigators have focused on either short-term memory (i.e., repetition) or phonologic encoding (i.e., phonemic paraphasias). For the latter, it is useful to remember that this is not a motor speech disorder (Chapter 6). Because sentence comprehension problems were found to be similar to those in Broca's aphasia, making syntactic judgments and arranging words into sentences were embedded in a program designed mainly to treat phonemic paraphasias (Cubelli, Foresti, & Consolini, 1988). Kearns' RET program was also helpful (Yedor et al., 1993), and shortly, a reading therapy for this syndrome will be presented (Bowes & Martin, 2007).

The Buffer and Working Memory

In the 1980s, therapies consisted of repetition to improve repetition (e.g., Kohn, Smith, & Arsenault, 1990). Thinking of therapy for the underlying deficit, Peach (1987) treated memory span to improve sentence repetition. The client started by pointing to pictures in a sequence spoken by the clinician. Then, the client repeated words in order. Sentence repetition improved during the period of treatment. Later, sentence repetition as the therapy led to improved comprehension of simple sentences (Francis, Clark, & Humphreys, 2003).

Modern treatments are viewed in terms of working memory and phonologic representations in the short-term buffer. Methods are modeled after classic experiments in cognitive psychology. One is to present single words and place varying intervals (e.g., 5 seconds) between the stimulus and repetition. Nonwords are included for focusing on phonology rather than meaning (e.g., Majerus, Van der Kaa, Renard, et al., 2005). Progress was shown with a post-treatment battery of memory tasks (Kalinyak-Fliszar, Kohen, & Martin, 2011). A similar method consisted of sentences, and improvements were detected in memory span and sentence repetition (Koenig-Bruhin & Studer-Eichenberger, 2007). Yet some of these treatments were carried out for several weeks or months, and little attention was given to improvements in functional language abilities.

Phonological Production

Other clinicians focus on reducing phonemic paraphasias, often using lexical therapies (Chapter 8). Boyle (1989) instructed a client to look at a word, think about how it sounds, and then read the word aloud. In Italy, Cubelli and others (1988) had clients confront phonemic–graphemic structure with a few metalinguistic tasks. In one task, a client was shown a picture (e.g., table or *tavolo*) and cards containing each syllable of the word (e.g., *ta, vo, lo*). The client was asked to arrange the syllables in correct order and then read the word aloud. In another task, the clinician displayed a picture (e.g., table) and a letter (e.g., E). The client had to decide if the letter belonged to the word for the picture.

Later, Peach (1996) treated someone who had been diagnosed with Wernicke's aphasia and then took on some characteristics of conduction aphasia. The procedure was centered on an oral reading task. Restimulation included having the client write the word. If this did not improve the spoken response, a phonemic error was paired with the correct sound in the beginning of another word to read. In a multiple-baseline design, there was immediate generalization to an untreated baseline.

For a more recent attempt, Corsten and colleagues (2007) presented minimal phonemic contrast tasks. The drills were much like the assessments for speech perception noted early in Chapter 3. The client judged whether auditory word pairs were the same or different and identified a spoken word from printed choices. A third task consisted of word repetition. Significant improvement was observed within the confines of the treatment tasks, including improved naming.

A client diagnosed with reproduction conduction aphasia (severe deficit in non-word repetition) received a therapy for self-monitoring. The first phase consisted of phoneme-discrimination tasks, and the second phase contained three levels of monitoring. First, the client practiced recognizing a clinician's naming errors. Second, the client's naming responses were played back on a tape recorder, and she had to make the same kind of judgments. The third level involved building sentences. Self-monitoring did not get better, but the client improved in a variety of word-production tasks (Franklin, Buerk, & Howard, 2002). The method was followed with similar therapy for "phonological assembly difficulty," a fairly recent and unique diagnosis that appears to waver between phonemic paraphasia and apraxia of speech (Waldron, Whitworth, & Howard, 2011).

Anomic Aphasia

When thinking about impairment-based treatment for anomic aphasia, we should keep in mind that these individuals are good functional communicators. A few may not have the patience for naming drills and may want to proceed to group activities (Chapter 10). Still, the goal is to minimize word-finding frustrations in natural, conversational situations. Many believe that quiet concentration on word-retrieval activities is just what they need (Chapter 8). Only a few, explicitly described as having this type of aphasia, have found their way into the literature.

Early in the chapter, Thompson and Kearns's (1981) example of multiple baseline was a cueing treatment for a case of anomic aphasia. Linebaugh's (1983) Lexical Focus consisted of hierarchies of cueing for a convergent naming task and, for the mildest anomic aphasias, a divergent categorical word-fluency task. A hierarchy of difficulty was based on "width" of exemplars in a category. That is, an easy category was *sports*, and a more challenging, narrow category was *water sports*. At that time, we were accustomed to starting therapy with the easy and building to the more difficult. Now, we might consider Thompson's complexity or CATE principles by starting with the more difficult category.

In Finland, Renvall and Laine examined contextual priming for client PH, whose "spontaneous speech was fluent, well-articulated, and grammatically correct but lacked informational content and was frequently interrupted by word-finding difficulties" (Renvall, et al., 2007, p. 331). Introduced in Chapter 8, contextual priming consists of a repetition prior to presenting a picture to be named. For PH, progress in naming was modest and short-lived. The researchers were mainly interested in theoretical conundrums surrounding naming, so that any effect of such treatment on conversation in natural settings is left to our imagination. Compensatory strategies may be in order (Chapter 10).

Reading Impairments

Cognitive neuropsychology (CN) has dominated published treatments of reading. Therefore, much of the current literature addresses only the word level. Clinicians center therapies on diagnosis with respect to a word-reading model (review Chapter 6). Accordingly, clinicians suspect that therapy repairs an impaired component or compensates with an alternative route around the impairment. For functional reading, we are minimally interested in *comprehension* or namely activation of a concept on seeing a word (Beeson & Henry, 2008)

Phonological dyslexia has been diagnosed in a variety of aphasias. Key symptoms are a word superiority effect along with good word repetition. Consistent with the superiority of reading real words over nonwords, there is a particular problem with reading aloud unfamiliar letter strings. Because pronunciation of unfamiliar letter strings depends on grapheme–phoneme conversion rules (Figure 6.1), it is thought that a so-called orthographic–phonological conversion (OPC) mechanism is impaired.

Kendall, McNeil, and Small (1998) tried to repair the OPC for WT, a 42-year-old whose stroke occurred 17 years prior to the study. WT had a mild nonfluent aphasia with good reading comprehension. The treatment consisted of "systematic exposure" to two conversion rules over 6 weeks. The rules were as follows:

- *c-rule:* when *c* comes before *a, o,* or *u,* it is produced as /k/; otherwise, as /s/
- *g-rule:* when *g* comes at the end of words or just before *a, o,* or *u,* it is produced as /g/; otherwise, as /dz/

As with most stimulation therapies, the rules were not taught explicitly. WT practiced reading aloud words and nonwords embodying one of the rules (e.g., *cylecaber, girandole*). The clinician presented phonetic and morphological cues as restimulation. Progress in treatment generalized to pronunciation of words involving other conversion rules.

About 10 years later, Bowes and Martin (2007) reported a "bigraph-biphone sound-blending" approach to reading aloud for MQ, a 45-year-old female sportswriter diagnosed with a conduction aphasia that included phonological dyslexia. The study began nearly 3 years after her stroke while she was still employed at the newspaper with accommodations for her reading and writing. One stage of the treatment consisted of reading aloud syllables such as CA-ME-EL, then blending them to read CAMEL. The entire program took a couple of years. MQ progressed through levels of the therapy program to the point of being able to read and write phrase-length material.

A reading teacher with a similar diagnosis 8 years after a stroke had difficulty reading words when they were embedded in text. The treatment consisted of building a sentence context word-by-word as a cue or prime for reading particular words. She improved in reading untrained words and sentences (Lott, Sperling, Watson, et al., 2009).

Surface dyslexia has also been found in a variety of aphasias. Unlike phonological dyslexia, the OPC is intact, which is indicated by an ability to pronounce nonwords and function words. Irregular words are commonly mispronounced with a preference for regular pronunciation such as saying "sue" for *sew* (Table 6.1). The disorder is thought to occur primarily in the graphemic lexicon or in access to it.

Behrmann and Byng's (1992) aim was to repair the impaired component rather than compensate with the intact OPC route. One treatment consisted of reading aloud irregular words such as *bough* accompanied by a picture (e.g., a tree; see also Weekes & Coltheart, 1996).

Deep dyslexia has been diagnosed mostly in people with Broca's aphasia. They produce many semantic paralexias when reading aloud and have a strong word-superiority effect related to a seemingly agrammatic pattern of reading content words better than function words. The disorder has been identified either with OPC impairment (like phonological dyslexia) or with a lexical-semantic mapping problem.

de Partz (1986) studied a business executive who had progressed 3 months after an initial diagnosis of Wernicke's aphasia. de Partz wanted to repair the OPC process by using a spared lexicon as "a relay" between the written word and pronunciation. The treatment proceeded in three stages. First, the client worked on associating a letter with a word and reading aloud single syllables. Then, he associated letter combinations with words. Finally, he practiced word reading focused on certain conversion rules much like Kendall's procedure for phonological dyslexia. de Partz reported that one stage was laborious, and the whole program took several months (see also Davies, Cuetos, & Rodriguez-Ferreiro, 2010).

Treatment for **letter-by-letter reading** was studied with three clients who had chronic mild fluent aphasias and mild letter-reading deficits. These individuals had a bachelor's degree, a master's degree, and a law degree. Two phases of treatment were conducted. The first phase was a tactile letter-naming exercise consisting of tracing letters and copying them on the left palm. The second phase emphasized speed with rapid letter naming and then rapid word naming after naming each letter. Each participant improved in accuracy and speed of reading untrained words without the tactile cues, and two clients improved in reading aloud sentences (Lott, Carney, Glezer, et al., 2010).

Generally, the relationship between diagnosis and therapy has been less than straightforward. Similar to Hillis's critique of naming therapies (Chapter 8), reviewers noted that different approaches have been effective for one diagnosis, that a single approach has been effective for different diagnoses, and that a treatment may be successful for some clients but not others with the same diagnosis (e.g., Hillis & Heidler, 2005). Some of the therapies took months to reach a goal of reading words or phrases aloud, but many of the reported cases were highly educated and motivated. When we think of reading sentences and paragraphs, treatment follows traditional methods for listening (also see ORLA, Chapter 8; Lee & Sohlberg, 2013).

Spelling Impairments

For phonological-orthographic conversion (POC), let us think of a spelling bee. Think of words with the sound /f/. Spell "scarf." Spell "trough." Spell "phosphorus." Spelling is learned in school, and it is not easy. While riding an exercise bike in a gym with TVs overhead, the captions streaming beneath the news may show "pharmaceutical" spelled as "farm a sue tickle" or "Al Sharpton" translated into "a sharp ton." For a few people with aphasia, spelling is important. Direct treatment of POC consists of writing to dictation, often without regard for word meaning.

Homework practice of copying words, then writing with the model withdrawn, was reported in a study of a young man with agrammatic aphasia (Kumar & Humphreys, 2008). For minimal to moderate aphasia, Beeson and others (2008) targeted spelling more explicitly with an "interactive treatment." The report is unclear as to exactly what the clinician did in providing the stimulus. Nevertheless, clients first wrote phonologically plausible spellings (could be "sharp ton"), then made a decision regarding correctness, and finally attempted to correct errors. Spelling definitely improved.

A *graphemic buffer disorder* was detected in a 68-year-old British woman with a well-recovered stroke-related aphasia except for writing skills (Sage & Ellis, 2006). The graphemic buffer is a section of working memory that briefly holds graphemic representations while someone is writing. In the disorder, spelling errors increase with longer words. The client engaged in a 2-week program starting with word matching, then filling in missing letters, and finally finding a vertical, horizontal, or diagonal word embedded in a grid. Because the target word was always present, the therapy was considered to be an errorless learning paradigm. Results were mixed regarding improvement with untreated words.

Severe or Global Aphasia

Brookshire (2007) noted that "most globally aphasic patients are alert, task-oriented, and socially appropriate (which helps to differentiate the globally aphasic patient from the confused or demented patient)" (p. 303). However, "the presence of global aphasia in a neurologically recovered patient is an ominous prognostic sign for recovery of functional language" (p. 335). He suggested that having at least two of the following symptoms indicate that this person with aphasia may not have the capacity to become a functional verbal communicator:

- Stereotypic utterance along with severely impaired comprehension
- Inability to match objects
- Unreliable yes/no response to questions
- Jargon without awareness and self-correction

We should note that these projections pertain mostly to linguistic communicative capacity, not necessarily nonverbal communicative capacity (e.g., Edelman, 1987).

We have impairment-based and communication-based objectives for severe aphasia (Collins, 2005; Peach, 2008). Following principles of direct stimulation, we begin with the simplest levels of language using the simplest tasks. An example appeared briefly in Chapter 8 regarding ACT and CART for word writing (Beeson & Henry, 2008). A client in subacute rehabilitation is likely to improve some in auditory comprehension, but we should prepare for the likelihood that results for verbal expression will be discouraging. Even when improvement occurs across a period of treatment, it may take months or years to achieve (e.g., Samples & Lane, 1980). We establish or encourage any means of communication as soon as possible (Chapter 10).

Comprehension

Usually the least-impaired modality, auditory comprehension is stimulated by following the principles set forth in the previous chapter:

- Set a reasonable functional goal.
- Start with a task that has a high level of accuracy.
- Upon meeting a criterion of success, move to more demanding stimuli.
- Measure progress toward meeting the goal.

Methodology for comprehension can be similar to therapy for Wernicke's aphasia but without having to deal with press for speech.

Improved comprehension can have far-reaching consequences. A high level of accuracy in comprehending sentences is functional in the sense that comprehension can facilitate conversational interaction (e.g., answering another's questions). However, because treatment should begin at a level of high accuracy, it may have to

TABLE 9.3   A lesson plan for treating auditory comprehension for someone with global aphasia.

GOAL	TREATMENT	GENERALIZATION PROBE
Improve functional sentence comprehension from 10% to 70% accuracy	Point to pictures (2 choices) given common words and family names	10-item sentence comprehension test (e.g., yes/no biographical questions, functional commands)

begin with a task that is easier than the floor of initial assessment. For example, a word comprehension task may have two pictured choices instead of the six or eight in an aphasia test. To measure progress toward a goal of enhanced sentence comprehension, a brief test of sentence comprehension should be administered regularly. A lesson plan might include something like Table 9.3.

We should have the individual's attention for repetitive drills. In a hospital, a client may arrive at the clinic fatigued from physical therapy or in a state of depressed vigilance due to trauma. Alerting signals, such as the person's name or "Ready?" may be presented before each stimulus. Collins (1986) tried to heighten interest with playing cards in simple matching and sequencing tasks. Awareness may be heightened when content is individualized, as in pointing to pictures of family members.

For word comprehension, several variables can be manipulated to adjust difficulty. The stimulus may be repeated. Redundant verbal context may help in identifying an object. Pictures can differ markedly in semantic relatedness and can be labeled with printed words. However, despite the logical manipulations that could generate a brilliant stepwise program, a client should be progressing quickly to achieve functional comprehension. Stimulation should be awakening a process. If a client is not improving over a few sessions, then it is not likely that much repair of the language system is possible in an affordable amount of time. More data on this issue are needed.

At a slightly higher linguistic level, four people with severe aphasia were trained to follow simple verb–noun commands such as *take glove* and *cover fork* (Oleyar, Doyle, Keefe, et al., 1991). The clients had AQ scores from the *WAB* of 19.4 to 48.8. Treatment consisted of pairing a spoken command with a model of the action. The clinician also gradually increased the time between the command and the model. Two of the four participants responded favorably to the treatment by improving with trained commands without models and generalizing to untrained commands.

Language Formulation

Sarno and Levita (1979) noted that a few words could make a remarkable difference in the life of someone with severe aphasia. It may be valuable to begin with standard direct procedures free of anxiety and distraction. In principle, treatment begins with what the individual can do verbally. People with global aphasia easily produce verbal stereotypes with no relation to a situation. They can be prodded into counting to 10 or singing a song.

Clinicians have tried to harness whatever utterances are produced spontane-ously. If we can get these utterances under our control, then we may help someone to produce them more appropriately and in greater variety. Helm and Barresi (1980) for-malized this practice in a program called **Voluntary Control of Involuntary Utterances** (VCIU). It began with presenting the printed form of an utterance just heard. If the utterance was repeated as if read aloud, it was considered to be more volitional. If a different word was produced, the clinician went with the flow, and a stimulus card was written for that word. Treatment was not pursued further for any utterance that was difficult to elicit a second time. When reading or repeating elicited responses, an object picture was presented in a transition to naming tasks. Individuals improved in independent testing and used some of the words appropriately in conversational interactions.

Intensity of language treatment may make a difference. In one study, 17 par-ticipants received treatment of auditory comprehension along with some stimulation of multiple expressive modalities in conversation. Nine of the participants received 60 sessions over a 6-month period (2–3/week). The eight who received the more inten-sive treatment of 130 sessions over 6 months (5/week) made significant improvement (Denes, Perazzolo, Piani, et al., 1996).

We may think that the concentrated dose of therapy in constraint-induced treatments (Chapter 10) would be appropriate for severe aphasia. One of three cases studied by Kirmess and Maher (2010) was severely impaired across modalities and received 3 hours of treatment per day over 10 days, in the second month poststroke. The pre- post-test design did not control for spontaneous recovery (less likely in severe cases), but improvement in naming was substantial. Contrary to the other two less-impaired individuals, the one with severe impairment preferred more intensive treat-ment. Rewards of treatment intensity are showing up in other studies as well (e.g., Lee, Kaye, & Cherney, 2009).

Medical Treatments

Can something be done to change the brain directly? Family members inquire about drugs and unique procedures that they heard about from friends, television, or the Internet. Much of this section points to the future. We may be co-investigators in the research, or, along with physicians, we may be gatekeepers escorting clients through a garden of seductive offerings.

Pharmacotherapy

Similar to emergency administration of a clot-busting tPA within the first 6 hours after stroke (Chapter 2), a different thrombolytic treatment may be attempted in the first 24 hours or so. Informally called **induced reperfusion**, perfusion to regions surrounding the infarction is restored by an intravenous saline that increases blood pressure (Davis, Kleinman, Newhart, et al., 2008; Hillis, Ulatowska, Barker, et al., 2003). The increased blood flow was shown to improve comprehension and naming. Another study had a similar finding, but the patients had subcortical aphasias (Hillis et al., 2004).

For chronic aphasia, Steven Small (2002, 2004) of the University of Chicago has contributed to our understanding of medications and their impact on aphasia recovery. A group in France and Italy searched MEDLINE for reports on drug therapy for aphasia, which spanned 1970 to 2005 (de Boissezon et al., 2007). They evaluated results of a variety of chemical mechanisms with respect to the strength of experimental designs. We shall return to this review shortly.

Instead of exploring studies in too much detail, let us become familiar with the management of clinical drug trials so we can evaluate products and understand our clients' concerns as well as understand a fundamental approach to efficacy research. These trials are conducted in a series of phases, gradually building information that should advise and protect the public. In *Phase I*, researchers test a new drug in small groups for its safety (e.g., side effects). In *Phase II*, the drug is tested on a larger group mainly for its efficacy. *Phase III* continues to pursue previous concerns and adds comparison to other treatments in the determination of efficacy. After the drug has been marketed, *Phase IV* studies compare different populations and explore the safety of long-term use.

Efficacy is determined with at least one comparison involving the randomized placement of participants in one group receiving the drug and a control group receiving a sugar pill (i.e., placebo). To minimize bias, the strongest studies are *double-blind randomized placebo-controlled* trials (DRPo). In a double-blind study, neither the participant nor the doctor administering the drug knows who receives the drug or the placebo (e.g., Walker-Batson, Curtis, Natarajan, et al., 2001). A weaker study is an *open-label* trial in which both participant and experimenter know the drug and dosage (e.g., Berthier, Hinojosa, Martin Mdel, et al., 2003). Also, a drug may be compared to language therapy. It is feared that a desire for the drug to work can influence results in open-label studies and treatment comparisons.

Table 9.4 highlights analysis of 26 studies retrieved in the MEDLINE search. The investigators were not impressed with what they found. There were two types of drug-effects. One was an immediate improvement of language followed by return to baseline after drug withdrawal. The other was the possibility of an effect clouded by influences from language therapy and neuroplasticity. In conclusion, there were not enough definitive studies to be enthusiastic about pharmacotherapy at this time.

Following mixed results for widely studied *piracetam*, Güngör and others (2011) divided 30 people with stroke-induced severe aphasias randomly into one group receiving the drug and another group receiving a placebo for 6 months. Clinical assessments were repeated at the end of treatment, including the Gülhane Aphasia Test developed for Turkey by Oğuz Tanridağ (Mavis, Colay, Topbas, et al., 2007). Except for auditory comprehension, progress in varied language functions was the same for both groups, indicating that piracetam was largely not beneficial.

Neurorestorative drugs (or "regeneration therapies") present the possibility of inducing growth of new neurons in the brain (see Chapter 7). So far, research has been restricted to animals. Infusion of an "epidermal growth factor" into a rat model of

TABLE 9.4   Highlights mainly of a MEDLINE search for drug therapies for aphasia (de Boissezon, Peran, de Boysson, et al., 2007).

DRUG	CATEGORY	OUTCOME SUMMARY	SAMPLE STUDIES
piracetam	mixed	Mild positive effect or no effect for people with aphasia	Kessler et al. (2000) Güngör et al. (2011)
bromocriptine	dopaminergic	DRPo studies showed no effect for aphasia; earlier reports too anecdotal	Gupta, Mlcoch, et al., (1995) Sabe, Salvarezza, et al., (1995)
dexamphetam	amphetamine	Good subacute results; good when paired with therapy	Walker-Batson, Curtis, et al. (2001)
donepezil	cholinergic	Open-label effects need confirmation with a DRPo trial	Berthier et al. (2003)

stroke with motor impairment appeared to "mobilize endogenous adult neural stem cells to promote cortical tissue re-growth and functional recovery after stroke" (Kolb, Morshead, Gonzalez, et al., 2006, p. 1). Similar results for a rat model were discovered when using a different chemical system, reported with the ambiguous title "Long-lasting regeneration after ischemia in the cerebral cortex" (Leker, Soldner, Velasco, et al., 2007).

Let us consider what else a client might discover by searching the Internet for remedies. Moleac is a company in Singapore that produces a mixture of Chinese herbs called NeuroAiD™ (neuroaid.com). It is said that the herbs provide a "neurorestorative treatment" that enhances recovery from stroke in areas of walking, vision, and "speech." Evidence includes testimonials and placebo-controlled trials for safety and for effects on a scale for activities of daily living and a relatively unknown Diagnostic Therapeutic Effects of Apoplexy score. Other trials were conducted in Iran (e.g., Shahripour, Shamsaei, Pakdaman, et al., 2011). We would encourage our clients to search for independent confirmation about such products and to view evidence through the lens of the requirements for clinical trials.

In addition, Small and de Boissezon identified well-known medicines that have had deleterious effects for poststroke disorders. These include *diazepam*, which can cause anxiety, *haloperidol*, which can cause psychosis, and *phenobarbital*, which can cause seizures.

Brain Stimulation

Besides exploiting neurochemistry, investigators have recently explored methods for tampering with the electrical properties of brain activity. Electrical stimulation has a long history of application in psychiatry. Most of the techniques have been noninvasive with Phase I studies demonstrating that they are relatively harmless.

Repetitive transcranial magnetic stimulation (rTMS) began as a treatment for psychiatric problems. A handheld coil (or "wand") generates magnetic impulses, which modulate nerve cells in cortex. Two research groups, in different ways, have been exploring whether rTMS improves language functions for people with aphasia. Both target the right hemisphere and believe that the wand inhibits overactive perisylvian areas opposite the left-hemisphere language areas, possibly reorganizing bilateral language networks.

The first studies were reported by a team headed by Margaret Naeser and Paula Martin at the Harold Goodglass Aphasia Research Center in Boston. They were interested in immediate effects, much like a basic cueing study. After application of the wand to one area of the right hemisphere, eight cases of chronic nonfluent aphasia improved in naming accuracy and speed. Results were not as positive for another area, indicating that the target area is important (Naeser, Martin, Theoret, et al., 2011).

People with chronic nonfluent aphasia also participated in clinical trials in Australia. A team of Caroline Barwood, Bruce Murdoch, and Brooke-Mai Whelan distributed 12 participants randomly to an rTMS (i.e., active condition) and a blind *sham control* condition, which, like a placebo, makes it appear as if the participants received the experimental procedure. One article reported the immediate effect on naming. There was no difference between groups 1 week after stimulation. Naming was better in the active group after 2 months, indicating that it takes time for the brain to adjust (Barwood, Murdoch, Whelan, et al., 2011). Does the brain really change? Another article reported on an evoked-potential known for its relationship to lexical-semantic processing. Twelve months after the procedure, the EP response was better in the active group than the sham group (Barwood, Murdoch, Whelan, et al., 2012).

In another sham comparison for people with mild to moderate nonfluent aphasia, a research team in Philadelphia and Washington, D.C., measured effects of a 10 session/2 week rTMS treatment on Cookie Theft picture descriptions. Two months after the treatment, the active group had improved in number of words but not in sentence length, complexity, or grammaticality. The sham group did not progess in any of these measures (Medina, Norise, Faseyitan, et al., 2012).

Anodal transcranial direct current stimulation (A-tDCS, atDCS, or just tDCS) has also been used to treat depression. A weak electrical current applied to the scalp is thought to modulate cortical excitability and supplement the effects of behavioral therapies (Holland & Crinion, 2012; Schlaug, Renga, & Nair, 2008). Studies in South Carolina, using a sham control condition, indicated that A-tDCS may enhance effects of naming therapy by reducing naming time for participants with mild anomia (Fridriksson, Richardson, Baker, et al., 2011).

An invasive method, called **epidural cortical stimulation** (ECS), consists of an fMRI-guided implant of an electrode on the dura mater covering a targeted area of the brain. In a Phase I safety and feasibility study, two small groups with nonfluent aphasia received intensive behavioral therapy. One group received ECS activation above the ipsilesional premotor cortex during the therapy. Between-group differences in aphasia test change scores were not significant, but ECS seemed to augment improvements that accompanied aphasia therapy (Cherney, Erickson, & Small, 2010;

Cherney, Harvey, Babbitt, et al., 2012). Much more research needs to be done for a method that may be used, as with other surgeries, only when noninvasive interventions have failed (Meinzer et al., 2011).

Summary and Conclusions

Since Chapter 8's principles of cognitive stimulation, it has been noted repeatedly that a treatment is a means to an end. This underwhelming aphorism is a reminder that a therapy technique is likely to differ from a generalization probe used to see if a therapy accomplished what we wanted. There were several examples in this chapter:

- Melodic intonation (MIT) to get people to talk (Broca's aphasia)
- Response elaboration training (RET) to expand discourse (Broca's aphasia)
- Stimulating verbs to expand sentence production (Broca's aphasia)
- Metalinguistic tasks to promote sentence production (Broca's aphasia)
- Auditory comprehension training to spark some repetition (Wernicke's aphasia)
- Short-term memory training to improve comprehension (conduction aphasia)

For the reader, a good exercise might be to backtrack and look for more examples. Think of a goal. Jot down a relevant therapy procedure. Why this particular procedure and not some other procedure? Then, think of a generalization probe that reflects a functional goal (not the therapy). Debate the result.

The therapeutic techniques addressing specific symptoms and syndromes follow the fundamental principle of stimulating processes. In some instances, psycholinguistics and related cognitive sciences are being applied so that treatments may be focused on more clearly defined processes. Many procedures are experimental and hopefully encourage an appreciation for the effort to improve rehabilitation through an understanding of language functions and an application of rigorous experimental controls. Many of these procedures languish in their birthplaces. Their influence may be measured by the extent to which they are replicated and reported by others. This "fanning out" of new procedures takes time.

With theory-driven therapies, the relationship between the hypothetical impairment and the treatment may not be self-evident. That is, we are tempted to ask ourselves whether the treatment is a necessary result of the proposed impairment as opposed to being a treatment that would have been provided without having contemplated what lies beneath. Having an agrammatic client move an element from its trace position seems to be a logical treatment of a movement impairment. Establishing this kind of connection can be a challenge for theory-driven investigators.

The chapter ended with a few methods that seem out of the dark ages or science fiction. Current versions of elixirs, electrical stimulation, and brain implants offer hope for people who are discouraged by the burdens of aphasia and the work of rehabilitation. With human participants, investigators follow guidelines that have them begin by showing that the prospective methods are safe while producing effects that make prolonging exploration seem worthwhile.

10 Functional Rehabilitation and Participation

Repairing language addresses communication partially. We employ many strategies aimed at the consequences of aphasia. The strategies or approaches stem from the following goals:

- Maximize use of residual linguistic capacities
- Develop augmentative or alternative modes of communication
- Improve participation in communicative situations
- Improve the role of partners and settings in facilitating communication
- Maximize psychological and emotional adjustment to language impairment

These objectives, roughly in this order, comprise the main topics of this chapter. Late sections will be recognized as the "life participation approach." However, let us begin with modifications of impairment-based therapies.

The Clinical–Functional Gap

A neurologist wrote a letter to the former *Asha* magazine in which he referred to a contradiction between a speech-language pathologist's (SLP's) documentation of improvement in clinical tasks and an absence of progress when he conversed with a patient (Metter, 1985). The clinician saw acquisition, but the neurologist did not see generalization.

Researchers have, at the least, wanted to see acquisitions during a treatment generalize to content not used in the treatment. However, simple stimulus generalization has been limited with some of the treatments presented in Chapters 8 and 9. The study of naming therapy by Thompson and Kearns (1981) produced good news and bad news. The good news was that treatment had an effect on behavior. The bad news was that progress with a small list of words used in therapy was not transferring to very similar lists of words not being used in therapy. It seemed that the treatment would have to be applied to every word the client might use in daily life. This therapy was not improving the word-retrieval process, and such findings have persisted with modern naming therapies.

One reason for the absence of generalization may be some differences between the traditional treatment setting and real-life communicative situations. The clinic contains minimal distraction and supportive people who understand aphasia. Stimulation is designed to undercut deficits and ensure success. On the other hand, real life presents a rough road of communicative potholes. Distraction arises, and frustration is frequent. Partners had never heard of aphasia before. On the bright side, some partners are familiar with each other, and communicative content is often tied to the situation. The differences are indicative of a "clinical–functional gap."

Looking across the gap, Busch (1993) recommended three broad functional goals that would be acceptable to Medicare:

- The individual will communicate basic physical needs and emotional status.
- The individual will engage in social communicative interactions with others.
- The individual will carry out communicative interactions in the community.

These goals are suggestive of stimulus generalization. That is, we want to see someone with aphasia produce practiced behaviors in the presence of family. We want to see him or her produce trained key phrases whenever a need arises.

It has been said that we would "train and hope" (Thompson, 1989). That is, we would do our therapy and then hope that progress we observe transfers to a client's daily life. The assumption has been that impairment-based stimulation would improve mental processes that are useful anywhere. This sensible logic has been challenged by the aforementioned research, demonstrating a need to supplement hope with a bridge across the clinical–functional gap. Following behavioral principles, it has been argued that a footbridge can be built by programming for generalization (Stokes & Baer, 1977). However, Brookshire (2007) has suggested that "many do not pursue generalization in a systematic way" (p. 284).

We have bridged the gap with certain facilitators such as group therapies or activities related to daily life. Closing the gap systematically is accomplished by bringing attributes of natural situations into the clinic gradually. This careful approach has also been applied to rehabilitation for head injury: "For those who are making the transition to a home setting, guidelines establishing routines for spontaneous real-life situations should be developed and implemented prior to returning to independent living" (Starch & Falltrick, 1990, p. 28).

The gradual progression of programming for generalization has been fine in principle, but the time it consumes may be unrealistic. Its principles, as introduced in Chapter 8, direct our thinking as we begin treatment and look ahead. For example, we start with an individual who is maximally dependent on the clinician for improved language processing, and we move in the direction of increasing independence.

This chapter progresses along dimensions that might characterize a generalization program, first modifying impairment-based stimulation, then emphasizing activity limitation, and finally proceeding to participation limitation. There is a shift from dyadic clinical interactions to group activities. The setting progresses from the hospital to community centers and residential settings (Table 10.1). The pace and sequence

TABLE 10.1   Chapter topics for functional therapeutics organized according to the WHO levels used in this text. This sequence of topics proceeds from inpatient therapy to community-based group activity.

WHO CATEGORY	CHAPTER TOPIC
Impairment	Functional stimulation
Activity limitation (disability)	Adaptive language strategies Alternative & augmentative communication Interactive therapies
Participation limitation (handicap)	Situation-specific role-playing Group treatment Community reintegration Changing communities Creating communities

of this progression varies, depending on severity of aphasia for some clients and on a clinician's preferred approach for others.

For many clinicians, however, bridging the gap is a matter of jumping right in by providing authentic clinical interactions from the beginning. Kagan and Simmons-Mackie (2007) called it "beginning with the end . . . [with] 'real-life' outcome goals relevant to each individual's situation and related to life participation" (p. 309). Thinking of the aforementioned progression of rehabilitation as sequential, they offer a more simultaneous alternative by considering "relevant intervention in *all* areas at each stage of the healthcare pathway" (p. 310). These areas include impairment-based therapies. Their framework for establishing "personally relevant end goals" is A-FROM (*Aphasia: Framework for Outcome Measurement*), which was briefly introduced at the end of Chapter 6.

Functional Stimulation

People with aphasia want to work on language, and impairment-based exercises can be more functional than they appeared in the previous chapters. If stimulation is to provide "functional repair," progress should extend beyond the therapeutic situation. Brookshire's principle of aiming treatment at a process rather than a specific word or sentence is an essential strategy for creating conditions that can achieve some degree of generalization. If word-finding is genuinely improved, then it should be better with a wide variety of words in a number of circumstances. After reviewing impairment-based therapies, Carragher and others (2012) found that naming therapies per se can lead to improvements in conversation.

Functional repair begins with maximizing the likelihood of generalization beyond the therapy when employing traditionally targeted stimulation tasks. Reviewing generalization research, Thompson (1989) concluded that a few features of treatment should maximize the possibility of transfer, including the following:

- A sufficient number of training responses
- A sufficient number of training conditions
- Activities that incorporate aspects of the natural environment

In the single-subject experiments that did not show much generalization, treatment tended to consist of drilling a small sample of language with one task.

Brookshire (2007) expanded Thompson's suggestions, relying on behavioral programming and generalization principles set forth by Stokes and Baer (1977). The idea of "training sufficient exemplars" fits well with the goal of stimulating a process. Instead of naming 5 foods repeatedly, a client practices naming 20 or 30 foods. Brookshire recommended training in a variety of stimulus conditions, including changing participants and settings. Flexibility in response expectations corresponds with the strategy of "loose training" (see RET in Chapter 9). Another principle is to train behaviors that elicit favorable consequences in a client's daily life (e.g., greetings). Finally, Brookshire recommended that we use a more realistic intermittent or delayed reinforcement.

Once we loosen stimulation activities, we enhance functionality further by molding semantic content according to a client's world and interests. On the one hand, standard or commercial materials are constructed to be universally familiar. Their functionality stems from being objects and events that are common in daily living. On the other hand, content may also be unique to an individual, demanding that we investigate each client's individuality. We can conduct **contextual inventories** (Simmons-Mackie & Damico, 1996) or *Thematic Language Stimulation* (Morganstein & Certner-Smith, 2008). The client names photos of family members and objects in the home. We enlist preferred activities, television programs, movies, and so on.

Personally relevant content is often chosen the first day of treatment. Wallace and Canter (1985) compared self-oriented and nonpersonal content for people with severe aphasia. Tasks included auditory comprehension (e.g., *Is your birthday in December?* vs. *Is Christmas in December?*) and naming object drawings (e.g., *television vs. chicken*). Personal material was better understood than nonpersonal content. Freed, Celery, and Marshall (2004) asked clients to come up with their own semantic cues to be used in naming therapy. They asked someone where he listens to the radio, and then the location became a cue. Later, with this treatment, two clients showed generalization of trained words to natural settings but no generalization to untrained words (Olsen, Freed, & Marshall, 2012). Goral and Kempler (2009) injected content related to a client's work in construction and handiwork at home. An example of when content may not be personally relevant was when Congresswoman Gabrielle Giffords was asked to name celebrities and comment on their clothing (Giffords & Kelly, 2011).

We may also do a **functional analysis** of targeted situations (e.g., restaurant, airport, bridge club, sporting events). What are the language functions and levels used in these situations? A situation may require some reading, some talking, or some writing.

What are elements of reading the phone book (e.g., searching, scanning)? Driving a car involves reading simple signs quickly. Panton and Marshall (2008) described a spelling therapy that concentrated on note-taking needed in a client's work as a counselor. Job-related vocabulary was chosen, and tasks included recording phone messages and writing to dictation. In the case study, writing strategies and accuracy generalized to an independent task of note-taking.

Morris and colleagues (2011) described a progression of dependence to independence for a person with mild aphasia who wanted to return to a complex job at a large insurance company. Tasks were constructed around auditory processing (e.g., listening with background noise) and reading and writing (e.g., working with e-mails). The SLP fostered confidence-building. Moreover, during therapy, the client appeared at the workplace, which increased the comfort level for colleagues. The client returned to work in a modified role for about 19 months. Afterward, he volunteered at an aphasia group.

Adaptive Language Strategies

With compensatory behaviors we embark on a journey through the domain of communication-based rehabilitation. Like using a wheelchair for mobility deficits, compensatory communication implies a realistic acceptance of chronic impairment and a search for other means of conveying messages. An individual with aphasia possesses residual resources identified previously (Chapters 4 and 6). These include some language abilities.

There is more than one way to convey a meaning or message linguistically. In principle, when someone with aphasia has difficulty constructing one linguistic form to convey an idea, another linguistic form might be attempted to convey the same general idea. So-called positive symptoms are indicative of spared language skills that can serve as adaptive mechanisms. Holland (1978) argued that it is okay for a client to be "in the ball park, rather than pitching a verbal no-hitter." With a familiar situation and partner, an approximation of an intended verbalization, including a semantic error, can get an idea across.

Residual language capacities are most evident in anomic and Broca's aphasias. People with either type of aphasia tend to make adjustments on their own. Someone with anomic aphasia uses sentence fluency to produce circumlocutions around words that cannot be found at the moment. The very nature of circumlocution points to the intended meaning (and word). People with agrammatic aphasia access semantic and lexical stores to produce structurally simplified versions of an idea. Thus, saying "girl tall and boy short" is pretty close to saying that the girl is taller than the boy.

Focusing on agrammatism, Kolk and Heeschen (1990) mused that morphosyntactic omissions are adaptive (e.g., a telegraphic strategy). **Telegraphic adaptation** may be preventive (before formulation is started) or corrective (after mistakes are made). A client's ellipsis (e.g., "more milk," "too late") appears to be intended to avoid a computational overload that would occur when trying to formulate a complete sentence (Kolk & Heeschen, 1992; Sahraoui & Nespoulous, 2012).

Kolk and his colleagues believed that some people with agrammatism learn preventive adaptation on their own. For those who do not adopt this strategy, Springer and colleagues developed *Reduced Syntax Therapy* (REST), which trains the use of reduced utterances or ellipses (Springer, Huber, Schlenck, et al., 2000). Their research unearthed a tendency for previously nonpreventive adapters to use trained ellipsis more than those who were already using reduced utterances on their own. So, REST encourages simplified structures with grammatical morphemes omitted such as "yesterday granny station" and "wash car" (see also Beeke, et al., 2007).

Shifting to word-finding, Tompkins and others (2006) wondered if spontaneously **self-generated cues** during failed attempts might themselves be communicative. If someone with aphasia can be in a tip-of-the-tongue (TOT) state, then some resources are available, let us say, to produce the first sound of the intended word. If the self-cue were effective, the client could be more independent of the clinician. It was a good idea first suggested long ago by Berman and Peelle (1967). Marshall has asked clients to recall predetermined personally relevant cues in a naming activity. When an individual could not produce the cue, the clinician would provide it (e.g., Olsen et al., 2012).

Bruce and Howard (1988) studied possibilities with 20 persons who had Broca's aphasia, only half having been helped by clinician-generated phonemic cues. Only six clients could point to first letters when failing to name objects. None retrieved words when identifying the first letter. Only two sounded out letters, and none displayed all three abilities. Attempts to train "sounding out" were laborious.

Other clinical researchers in England speculated that circumlocution might lead to improved word-finding in addition to serving as a communicative substitute (Francis, Clark, & Humphreys, 2002). In a naming task, they asked a client with anomic aphasia to "talk around" the word until the name came to her. Improvement generalized to untrained words, and errors nudged closer semantically to the target. By the way, semantic information generated during semantic feature analysis therapy (Chapter 8) is considered to be a form of self-cueing (Tompkins et al., 2006).

Unassisted self-correction, like self-repairs (Chapter 4), occurs in conversation when the person with aphasia "unprompted by the clinician, illustrates that he is unable to retrieve a word and initiates some effort to do so without assistance" (Marshall, 1976, p. 445). As examples, we look out for related paraphasias, circumlocution, indefinites (e.g., *that one, stuff*), and, most frequently, taking or requesting more time. Self-correction consisted of cued corrections (i.e., a related response prior to the target), effortful corrections (i.e., partial responses leading to the target), and immediate corrections. Low-verbal clients engaged in as much self-correction as high-verbal clients but were less successful (Marshall & Tompkins, 1982).

A listener might discourage some of these behaviors as undesirable symptoms and insist on the intended or correct word. This may lead someone with aphasia to shut down functional subsystems of language production. Our job is to encourage and reinforce communicative cues, circumlocution, and sentence simplification for conversation and, also, to educate others regarding their value. Recognizing the positive is a hallmark of Holland's (2007) approach to counseling people with aphasia, discussed later in this chapter. This counseling includes modifying the behavior of significant listeners.

AAC: Alternative and Augmentative Communication

Alternative communication *substitutes* for dysfunctional verbalization, and augmentative communication *supplements* effortful verbalization. AAC consists of low-tech and high-tech options (Beukelman, Yorkston, & Garrett, 2007; Hux, Weissling, & Wallace, 2008). Low-tech options include drawing, pointing to pictures, and other body movements. High-tech options generally rely on computers with digitized speech output. For many clients, the recovery process entails learning something new in addition to stimulating something already there.

A review of all options revealed disappointments in the ability of people with aphasia to carry acquired communicative modes over to functional situations. Purdy and Koch (2006) thought that this limited generalization has something to do with cognitive flexibility. There was a correlation between a common measure of cognitive flexibility and strategy usage in a functional communication task. Therefore, cognitive flexibility is considered to be a criterion for predicting functional AAC use.

Joanne Lasker at Florida State University and Kathryn Garrett at Duquesne University felt that it is important to distinguish those who can employ AAC strategies independently from those who depend on partners to limit the response set and provide cues and instruction. They developed a screening for the ability to identify symbols. Those with the least accuracy and requiring the most cueing were partner-dependent communicators. Those needing the least cueing were the most independent (Lasker & Garrett, 2006; Lasker, Garrett, & Fox, 2007).

Low-Tech AAC

Communication boards may be introduced early for severe motor speech disorders. Soon after a stroke, the boards provide a means of communicating until speech or writing become functional. With minimal language impairment, printed words and phrases can be used freely without pictures or symbols. Pointing to letters provides flexibility for forming any word or phrase, but it is much slower.

Bellaire and others (1991) studied acquisition and generalization of communication board use for two people with Broca's aphasia. The boards contained 15 line drawings of items for a coffee hour to be used for social greetings, requesting food, and providing personal information. Treatment started with a client responding to requests from a clinician. Generalization training consisted of role-playing coffee hour situations in individual sessions, and in the next phase, the clinician accompanied the client to a social hour. The participants acquired requests and personal information responses but did not readily generalize use of the boards to the social setting. Instead, they relied on vocalization or head nods that had been used before training.

The investigators suggested that communication boards may be more useful for individualized content that cannot be readily expressed through natural gesturing.

The communicativeness of gestures depends on their intelligibility and a client's willingness to use them. Those with Broca's aphasia may spontaneously use more left-handed gestures than usual. Those with Wernicke's aphasia gesture the way they talk and may require some training if they are to clarify some of their spontaneous gestures (Le May, David, & Thomas, 1988).

People with severe aphasia may rely on pointing or natural gesturing to convey basic needs. Severely nonfluent individuals have enough comprehension for pointing to words without much training. Those with more severe comprehension deficits require some training to use simple printed material. In the Netherlands, Visch-Brink and others (1993) trained clients to use a "Language Pocket Book," which consisted of word lists and pictures organized by category or situation. Part of the training included conceptualization such as sorting words into functional categories. Any individual, along with frequent communication partners, may need some practice in the functional use of boards or notebooks.

Pointing behavior is a valuable communicative tool, and some real-life settings may be more communicatively accessible than others. Menus are communication boards. For ordering in a restaurant, one need only read and point to an item. Some menus have mouth-watering pictures of the food. At home, a client can tear out catalog pages as a shopping list and use them for asking about the location of a product. Bus stations and travel agencies have brochures. Functional analysis of a situation includes identifying compensatory materials and strategies that are accessible in the situation.

Training has been designed for pantomime, defined in Chapter 4. **Visual Action Therapy** (VAT) takes an individual through steps of object manipulation to train the use of pantomimic gestures (Helm-Estabrooks, Fitzpatrick, & Barresi, 1982). The program begins with matching tasks for perception and recognition of objects and proceeds to gesturing of function with the object in hand and then without the object.

If a pantomime is to replace speech as a communicative mode, it should be intelligible to most people without having to educate them. Flowers and Wyse (1985) examined intelligibility of pantomimes produced by normal adults mimicking paralysis by using only their nonpreferred hand. A receiver, familiar to the sender, wrote the name of an object that was demonstrated. Participants' gesturing was highly variable, with a 46 to 91 percent level of intelligibility. In data available for the Duffys' referential abilities test (Chapter 6), four normal participants were 97 percent accurate (Duffy et al., 1984).

At one time, American Indian sign language (Amer-Ind) was enticing because it is descriptive of referents and can be used with one hand (Skelly, 1979). Amer-Ind proved to be much more transparent than American Sign Language (Daniloff, Lloyd, & Fristoe, 1983). From reports on training of Amer-Ind, Skelly (1979) decided that "there was almost universal dissatisfaction expressed concerning transfer from the cued retrieval/replicative stage to self-initiated use" (p. 40). Following a couple of attempts at training in Amer-Ind, Coelho (1990) concluded that "the production of sign combinations from previously acquired single signs does not occur spontaneously—that is, without training—and that even with training, at least within the context of the present experiment, the maintenance effect is weak" (p. 399).

Looking at combining low-tech techniques, Purdy, Duffy, and Coelho (1994) trained use of gestural symbols and a communication board. They found that participants did not use as many gestures in a structured conversation task as they used in direct training, and participants continued to prefer verbal over nonverbal response. Would a client spontaneously switch to one modality when an attempt with another modality failed? The participants switched modalities only 39 percent of the time, but they were successful in conveying messages 73 percent of the time when they did switch. Despite effectiveness, use of gestures is a matter of choice.

Some believe that gesture inhibits speaking, but gesturing may draw out verbalization when stimulation fails. Rosenbek and his colleagues (1989) argued that "verbal expression can be improved by the appropriate pairing of performances or with the systematic use of unique sensory inputs" (p. 218). Naming was better when paired with gesture for nonfluent clients (Hanlon, Brown, & Gerstman, 1990; see also Rodriguez, et al., 2006). In Rosenbek's method, the first step is to teach gesture recognition. The next step involves modeling a gesture and a word for imitation. If a client should spontaneously start talking while gesturing, it is likely that he or she can benefit from other treatments for language production. The challenge is to maintain the verbal response after the gesture is faded.

Drawing may be attempted after traditional language treatments prove to be unsuccessful (Hunt, 1999; Lyon, 1995; Rao, 1995). Morgan and Helm-Estabrooks (1987) instituted "Back to the Drawing Board" with two cases of nonfluent aphasia. Lyon and Sims (1989) provided "expressively restricted" individuals with a cued training program for three months. Then, transfer to communicative use was encouraged with an interactive procedure. The clients improved as a group. Holland (1995) tried to teach drawing for a variety of aphasias. She encouraged self-motivated use of natural drawing abilities; but blaming her own poor drawing skills, she concluded that her attempts were "notably unsuccessful." Drawing may stimulate spoken word finding (Farias, Davis, & Harrington, 2006).

High-Tech AAC

The high-tech option actually began when chimpanzees were trained to use cutout paper symbols for communicating with humans (Glass, Gazzaniga, & Premack, 1973). People with aphasia were trained to comprehend statements, questions, and commands constructed out of such symbols arranged in syntactic order. This gave Gardner and others (1976) the idea to create a similar system for people with aphasia called VIC, which stood for Visual Communication.

For over a decade, a team of researchers led by Michael Weinrich at the University of Maryland fashioned Computerized Visual Communication, shortened to C-VIC. At first, people with global aphasia displayed knowledge of syntactic relations through this system (Shelton, Weinrich, McCall, et al., 1996). C-VIC had limitations as a communicative device, partly because learning the system took up to

2 years. Two people with severe Broca's aphasia were trained to create basic sentences with varied tense marking on the computer. Their spoken sentence production was improved after the training (Weinrich, Shelton, Cox, et al., 1997).

Lingraphica®, developed by Richard Steele, took C-VIC a lot further (aphasia .com). Its program contains a hierarchically organized picture vocabulary of over 6,000 words, each represented by icons. Verbs are animated to smooth comprehension. The software has an extensive store of prebuilt sentences, or a client can arrange nouns around verbs without regard to syntax. A sentence looks like a row of picture cards. The clinician makes a statement on one row, and the client responds on a second row. Selected icons can be turned into spoken words or sentences. Speech-generating devices include *AllTalk*™ as a laptop and *TouchTalk*™, a tablet.

Another program for severe verbal impairment is *C-Speak Aphasia*, which is also based on C-VIC, available from Mayer-Johnson. Pictures appear on-screen and can be combined to create novel messages conveyed by computer-generated speech. Nicholas and others (2005) reported on at least 6 months of training five people with severe nonfluent aphasia. Three of them became better at conveying information with the computer than without it. However, some clients were unable to use the system for communicating, and the investigators attributed this difficulty to a deficiency in problem solving.

Portable devices have been produced for communicative disorders. One is *MessageMate*™ with prefabricated words and phrases that can be spoken with the press of an icon (words-plus.com). A person with severe nonfluent aphasia completed a 3-month training program with *Dialect* (now *Dialect 3*; zygo-usa.com), a touch-screen device with speech output (Hough & Johnson, 2009).

To help someone with conduction aphasia to have writing available, Estes and Bloom (2011) tried out dictation software (voice recognition), called *Dragon NaturallySpeaking*©. Ten sessions of instruction led to improved basic computer skills as well as better functional writing that depended on speaking skills. Handwritten picture descriptions also improved slightly.

Cost has limited the wide scale use of high-tech AAC. Beukelman and others (2007) noted that funding has improved but also that, in the United States, it is not always easy to obtain, varies from state to state, changes regularly, and may be beneath the radar of medical service providers. Nevertheless, they cited three sources: Medicare Part B for those older than 65 years with disabilities of more than 2 years, Medicaid for those who meet financial limitation guidelines, and vocational rehabilitation for those who can return to work. The Lingraphica Web site, for example, has a section explaining insurance and other funding. To keep up with policy, we can check the Web site for the Rehabilitation Engineering and Research Center in Communication Enhancement (AAC-RERC).

Apps

Most everyone knows that "app" refers to applications or software available for hand-held computers and smart phones. A few apps are aphasia-dedicated, and many others can be adapted for a multitude of purposes such as stimulation, communication, and memory. Lingraphica has *SmallTalk*™ for Apple's mobile devices with a selection of phrases and videos for use in everyday situations. With earphones, people with aphasia can cue themselves for key phrases.

TouchSpeak™, differing slightly from C-VIC, was designed for people with aphasia. It is based on a vocabulary and ready-made messages related to everyday scenarios such as shopping and answering the phone. After training, some individuals used a handheld device creatively in everyday situations, and others did not use it. Two factors predicted positive functional outcome. Younger individuals were more proficient, and so were those with intact semantic processing (van de Sandt-Koenderman, Wiegers, Weilaert, et al., 2007).

Gus Communications makes *TalkTablet* for the iPad (gusinc.com). A client can use a touch screen of symbols to produce speech. Another product from Gus, *EZ Speech* for Apple mobile devices, requires some reading skill and is advertised for motor speech disorders. *EZ SpeechPro* is also text based and can be used with Android devices.

Although not an app per se, *SentenceShaper 2*® runs on a desktop or laptop computer and helps people with aphasia to create spoken sentences (Chapter 9). It was evaluated as an augmentative option for someone with nonfluent aphasia and achieved limited use for e-mail (Albright & Purves, 2008). *SentenceShaper To Go*, on the other hand, is a version of the original software that allows someone with aphasia to download spoken messages, created in SentenceShaper, to a handheld device (True, Bartlett, Fink, et al., 2010).

Let us keep thinking about e-mail. The story of *Tapgram* illustrates how useful apps are likely to be developed in the future. Chad Ruble's mother had suffered a stroke and was severely nonverbal. Chad also had some knowledge of software. He created an app so that she could tap simple e-mails to family and friends. Now, he is making the app available to others (tapgram.com).

Interactive Therapies

We can transform the traditionally didactic clinical interaction so that it has some of the unique components of conversation, helping to bridge the clinical-functional gap. We do not have to teach conversational structure for people with aphasia (Chapter 4). Instead, a more conversational interaction is an opportunity to apply strategies that were practiced in impairment-based training. In doing so, people with aphasia may become emboldened with confidence in their communicative abilities, a goal of the life participation approach (Babbitt, Heinemann, Semik, et al., 2011). Because conversation is a collaboration between partners, someone with aphasia may come to realize that he or she does not have the sole responsibility for the success of communication. This section covers a range of topics beginning with the structured interaction of PACE therapy and then proceeding to the training of language in conversation, and finally conversational partner training.

PACE Therapy

The basic naming task can be transformed to incorporate features of face-to-face conversation. One strategy for doing this is called **Promoting Aphasics' Communicative Effectiveness (PACE;** Davis, 2005; Davis & Wilcox, 1985). It was developed in a unique graduate student training program at the University of Memphis, supported by the Veterans Administration. The procedure follows four principles and is described in Table 10.2 (read first). Any one principle suggests a change from traditional tasks, but the four together approach conversation as intended by the authors. The principles are elastic and are used to shape group therapies (Beeson & Holland, 2007).

Having read the basic procedure in Table 10.2, let us consider a few tips. For example, with the new information condition, a message sender need only convey what is necessary to get an idea across. Message stimuli can be pictures of objects or events or anything else a client or clinician wants to explore. Turn-taking should discourage us from being directive by placing us on equal footing with the client. Our turns as sender are opportunities for modeling communicative behaviors that a client is capable of using but may not be choosing. Direct instruction is different activity in the session. In PACE, we provide an atmosphere in which an adult can decide on the use of modalities. The clinician's modeling shows that gesture or drawing is a

TABLE 10.2 The four principles and essential procedures of *Promoting Aphasics' Communicative Effectiveness* (PACE; Davis & Wilcox, 1985).

PRINCIPLE	DETAILS
1. The clinician and client exchange new information	Instead of having a picture of an object or event (called the message) in simultaneous view of the clinician and client, a stack of *message stimulus* cards is placed facedown to keep the messages from view of a receiver. A client selects a card and, hiding its content, attempts to convey the message. A "Brussels modification" is to place a screen between participants, and the message receiver chooses the message from options (Clérébaut, Coyette, Feyereisen, & Seron, 1984).
2. The clinician and client participate equally as senders and receivers of messages	This principle inserts *turn-taking* into the interaction. The clinician and client simply alternate in drawing a card and sending messages.
3. The client has a free choice as to the communicative modes used to convey a message.	Contrary to training one modality such as gesture, the client is left to choose the mode that is used for any message. We do not tell a client to perform in a particular way.
4. The clinician's feedback as a receiver is based on the client's success in conveying the message.	The new information condition should make this inevitable for both participants. Our feedback should let the client know if he or she got the idea across. If we already know the message, we should respond as if we did not know.

respectable option for getting the idea across. We can measure a client's communicative success according to a listener's receipt of the message.

The client can also practice a few skills that are unique to conversation. One is responsiveness to a listener's attempts to interpret what the client is trying to convey. Another skill is responsiveness to one's own communicative failure, provoking the use of repair or revision to get a message across.

Investigators have compared progress in different functions and have compared PACE with other procedures. After PACE therapy, communicative abilities improved but not language skills (Carlomagno, Losanno, Emanuelli, et al., 1991). For someone with conduction aphasia, PACE was compared with traditional stimulation for improving naming, and more progress in naming was shown during the PACE phases of treatment (Li, Kitselman, Dusatko, et al., 1988). Some investigators have distorted the procedure, calling it PACE-like, usually by turning it into a nonverbal therapy (e.g., Avent, et al., 1995).

Other studies focused on responsiveness to a clinician's modeling. Glindemann and others (1991) examined the influence of modeling names or descriptions. Participants with mild aphasia were more likely than others to switch between names and descriptions as a function of what the clinician does as sender. Greitemann and Wolf (1991) found that modeling has an influence across modalities and that the use of speech does not necessarily disappear as gesture increases. Glindemann and Springer (1995) were unimpressed with the modeling function for severe aphasia. They recommended direct training for compensatory behavior. However, modeling might have been misunderstood. It was intended to help a client become comfortable with modalities trained in other activities.

More recently, PACE has been employed for different purposes. It has been a component of evaluating candidacy for AAC by exploring "the natural tendencies of the person with aphasia to use alternative modalities or the person's stimulability for learning to use them" (Lasker et al., 2007, p. 174). In efficacy research, it has been a component of communication-based therapies that have been compared to impairment-based therapies (de Jong-Hagelstein et al., 2010). It was used as a functional comparison to syntax stimulation (Marini, et al., 2007) and to constraint-induced treatment. In the latter case study, both an intensive speech-focused treatment and an intensive phase of PACE were accompanied by improvement in language production (Kurland, et al., 2010, 2012).

In Milan, Italy, Anna Basso (2003) critiqued PACE in the context of a more general critique of pragmatic therapies. She noted that the procedure is not as authentic as conversation because a client is merely describing things. Certainly the claim of artificiality is true, but PACE was never claimed to be authentic conversation. It is simply one of a long menu of procedures, including natural conversation as employed by Basso (2010). The structure of PACE makes it easier to analyze elements of the interaction.

Another concern was that the new information feature is diluted when a clinician selects the cards and, therefore, anticipates what a client is likely to be conveying.

This, too, has been acknowledged, and the problem can be minimized when the clinician, being aware of the problem, pretends not to know what is on a stimulus card or has someone else, including the client, provide a stack of cards (see Davis, 2005).

Constraint-Induced Therapy

Some may be surprised that this well-known approach is presented in a section on interactive therapies. However, this placement should become clear. It is known as constraint-induced aphasia therapy (CIAT) in Germany (Barthel, Meinzer, Djundja, et al., 2008) or constraint-induced language therapy (CILT) in the United States (Kirmess & Maher, 2010). Regardless of label, there are two salient components. Mostly in a communicative and interactional activity, an unimpaired function is constrained so that a client must attend to the impaired function. The other component is the intensity of treatment, involving the number of hours in a day and the number of days that it is administered (Chapter 8; Cherney et al., 2008).

We may understand the constraint component by contrasting it with approaches, such as PACE, that encourage compensatory response to impairment. The contrast is clear with respect to the origin of CIAT in the physical therapy of Edward Taub at the University of Alabama, where patients were observed to become discouraged in trying to use an impaired extremity. This discouragement evolved to **learned non-use** (Taub, Crago, Burgio, et al., 1994). For upper limb hemiparesis, for example, an individual works on using the affected side of the body while the unaffected side is put in a sling or glove (i.e., constrained). Physical therapy is straightforward, but without a distinct left and right, constraints in language therapy can be less clear. In general, constraint is applied to easy communicative modalities, whereas treatment is applied to an impaired modality.

The first application of CI therapy to aphasia was reported by Friedemann Pulvermüller and his colleagues in Germany (Pulvermüller, Neininger, Elbert, et al., 2001). The therapy was interactive, and his constraints consisted of adjustments in a card game that focused a client on making requests across a barrier, creating a new information condition similar to PACE. Unlike PACE, a client communicated without gestures, drawing, or writing. The idea of "constraint" has been viewed broadly as anything that narrows context and restricts communicative behavior (Pulvermüller & Berthier, 2008), and the method has been detailed more recently as "intensive language-action therapy" (Difrancesco, Pulvermüller, & Mohr, 2012).

Also in Germany, Gabriela Barthel and Marcus Meinzer tried to separate type of therapy from intensity by comparing CIAT to traditional treatments with the same schedule of 3 hours per day for 10 consecutive days (Barthel et al., 2008). CIAT consisted of card games restricted to speech. Maintenance of improvements six months later were more varied with the traditional treatment than with CIAT.

Pulvermüller's barrier game was extended in the United States. Faroqi-Shah and Virion (2009) constrained behavior to the speech modality for people with agrammatic aphasia. There was little improvement for these individuals. Goral and Kempler (2009) directed participants to aim for verb production in sentences, a kind of linguistic constraint. Intensity of treatment was less than the schedule employed in Germany. Twenty hours of therapy were provided within 4 weeks. Goral and Kempler discovered generalization of increased verb production to narratives.

A few years earlier in Houston, Lynn Maher had started a research program comparing CILT to PACE. The main difference between the therapies was that PACE encouraged communication with multiple modalities, whereas the CILT interaction allowed only spoken expression. Both therapies were associated with improvements, but CILT appeared to produce more progress with speech. In some incarnations, CILT has the appearance of PACE without the multimodality principle (Maher, Kendall, Swearingin, et al., 2006; see also Rose, 2013).

Maher contributed to Melanie Kirmess's studies of a few individuals in Norway. Kirmess strove to provide the original 10-day/3 hours per day regimen, but stamina and other therapies forced reductions so that treatment ranged from 20 to 30 hours total. The therapy maintained the interactive quality of Pulvermüller's card game, and we can only assume, based on reviewed literature, that the interaction was confined to spoken production (Kirmess & Lind, 2011; Kirmess & Maher, 2010). Pre-post testing was suggestive of some improvements in verbal expression.

Conversational Coaching

Conversational coaching was developed by Audrey Holland (1991), who provides a client with a short script. The client should be able to read aloud simple sentences, but a script may consist of few words and some pictures. The script also incorporates communicative strategies that were previously trained or suggested more directly. Strategies include "conversational management," such as asking a listener to slow down. We may recall the clinical–functional gap introducing this chapter as Holland noted that the approach is another "bridging framework to initiate transfer of strategy use to patient-generated conversation" (p. 204).

Clients choose the topics for their scripts. In a study of 33 people with aphasia, Holland, Halper, and Cherney (2010) found that by far the most frequent choice for monologues was personal stories. Dialogues were more varied with conversation with family comprising 21 percent, followed by seeking or providing information (18 percent) and discussion of outside interests (14 percent).

The first step procedurally is that the client and clinician practice following the script. The client reads the script one sentence at a time. The clinician's job is to evaluate communicative effectiveness and suggest ways of conveying the information differently. The client then may practice with another listener, often a family member. The clinician reminds the client of strategies and sometimes coaches the listener (e.g., "If you don't understand, it's probably better to ask him to say it another way"). This activity is videotaped, and the participants get together to view and discuss it. The entire procedure may be repeated with a stranger as the listener (Hopper, Holland, & Rewega, 2002). Two individuals with nonfluent aphasia learned to produce the scripts naturally, and this ability generalized to some extent to novel conversation partners (Youmans, Holland, Muñoz, et al., 2005).

A client may learn to utilize strategies for managing a conversation. For example, someone with mild aphasia may not be able to process conversation at its normal rate. The individual starts to get lost and is too embarrassed to say so. However, instead of allowing others to restrict his or her ability to comprehend and respond, the person with aphasia can ask people to reduce their rate of speech or repeat every now and then. Holland (1991) called these "comprehension strategies," and they included asking others to simplify or elaborate their messages.

More recently, conversational coaching was reborn as **AphasiaScripts**™, a program developed at the Rehabilitation Institute of Chicago with the help of Leora Cherney (see Web site for Boulder Language Technologies). The software is also known as *Computerized Conversational Script Training for Aphasia* (C-CoSTA). An individualized script appears to the left, and one of two culturally diverse virtual therapists appears to the right (i.e., Pat or Anita). The client listens to the script, then practices each sentence of his or her turn, and then finally practices the conversation taking turns with the virtual therapist. Segments of script may be highlighted as they are spoken by Anita or Pat, and the cues are gradually removed. Investigation of progress occurring across a 9-week period of treatment showed that amount of treatment per week was related to progress (Cherney, Halper, Holland, et al., 2008; Lee, Kaye, & Cherney, 2009; Mannheim, Halper, & Cherney, 2009).

In Germany, Bilda (2011) developed a "video-based script training programme" modeled after AphasiaScripts. The difference was that people with aphasia viewed video scenes of amateur actors engaged in simple conversations filmed in real-life locations, considered an alternative to actually going to a setting. Bilda was interested in the massed drilling feature of the training for five individuals more than 6 months poststroke. Each participant practiced five levels of response to the dialogues, concluding with saying his or her part of the full conversation. Improvements were noted in a loosely constructed pre- and post-test experimental design.

Conversation as Therapy

Simmons-Mackie (2008) encouraged the incorporation of natural conversation to enhance the authenticity of treatment. Her method, however, is not just "having a conversation." It is "goal directed and individualized" (see also Basso, 2010; Fox, Armstrong, & Boles, 2009). The SLP sets out to help someone transfer compensatory strategies, such as drawing or gesture, to an interaction. The client uses residual strategies that might have been practiced in PACE or conversational coaching.

Simmons-Mackie also advocated the use of *scaffolded conversations*, in which the clinician provides cues or facilitators within the flow of an interaction. We may quickly write a word that a participant was gesturing. Cues may be aimed at initiation of a conversational turn or conveying a message (e.g., Garrett, Staltari, & Moir, 2007). Another activity, known as supported conversation, is provided at the Aphasia Institute in Toronto, featured later in the chapter.

Holland (1998) was concerned that some clinicians may be uncomfortable conversing with people who have aphasia, and she detected a bias against conversation as a therapeutic medium. She asked "what relegates conversation to some sort of sleazy, shady, unreimbursable Neverland that must . . . follow the real goods—the therapy?" (p. 845). Chapter 4 indicated that conversation is often studied with interviews. Thus, clinicians who think they are engaged in conversation are really engaged in something that is more like traditional therapy. Holland (1998) stated that "interview models" emphasize a receiver function over a participant function, and she provided examples of the difference from a chat about "my most embarrassing moment" (p. 846):

- *Interview model:* "Today we are going to talk about the most embarrassing thing that ever happened to us. Why not begin, Joe?"
- *Conversation:* "You're not gonna believe what happened to me yesterday . . . Can you top this?"

Conversational Partners

People with aphasia comprehend better when their spouses make adjustments in their utterances (Linebaugh, Margulies, & Mackisack-Morin, 1984). A spouse may increase pauses and redundancy, give a person more time to talk, and minimize "speaking for" behaviors (Chapter 4). Training spouses to modify their behavior may lead to a reduction of interruptions of their partners with aphasia (Simmons, Kearns, & Potechin, 1987). Training programs appeared that helped caregivers or friends improve communication with their partners (Cunningham & Ward, 2003; Purdy & Hindenlang, 2005). Turner and Whitworth (2006) evaluated studies available at the time and found methodological weaknesses that are characteristic of the initial stage of a line of research.

Wilkinson and others (2010) reported a case study regarding the conversation training of married retired teachers, one with Broca's aphasia. Clinicians used the qualitative data of conversation analysis (CA) for therapy planning and evaluation. Therapy for the spouse without aphasia aimed at reducing restrictive initiations (e.g., yes–no questions) and increasing the use of encouraging paraphrases. Postintervention observations showed that the spouse with aphasia changed little in formal aphasia testing but produced conversational turns containing more sentences. The investigators produced materials called *Supporting Partners of People with Aphasia in Relationships and Conversation* (SPPARC). It provides the clinician with "the necessary tools to run support and conversation training programmes" (Lock, Wilkinson, & Bryan, 2001).

Efficacy of Communicative Treatment

Although communicative therapies usually supplement impairment-based therapies, clinical researchers in the Netherlands pitted the two strategies against each other in a comparison of their effectiveness (de Jong-Hagelstein et al., 2011). Their impairment-based therapy was called *cognitive-linguistic treatment* (CLT), consisting of the semantic and phonologic therapies described in Chapter 8 (38 participants). *Communicative treatment* encouraged compensatory strategies practiced in PACE therapy, role-playing, and conversational coaching (42 participants). These treatments were compared mainly for their effect on a functional communication test, namely the *ANELT* (see Chapter 6). Semantic and phonologic lexical tasks were also administered.

Therapy for each group began within 3 weeks poststroke and continued for at least 2 hours per week for 6 months. This intensity was less than the large studies reported in Chapter 8. There was no difference in *ANELT*-measured progress for the two treatment packages. With the semantic and phonologic measures, significant improvement favoring CLT occurred only with the fluency tasks. The conclusion was that there is little reason to favor one treatment over the other in the first 6 months after stroke. Because there was not a no-treatment control, especially during spontaneous recovery, efficacy of the treatments was undetermined. It would also be interesting to do a comparison that includes a group receiving the two treatments at the same time.

Life Participation

Some graduate students may be taken aback by the specter of tampering with someone's quality of life. *Doesn't the social worker do that?* Of course, the stroke and aphasia have already intruded, and an SLP sees that communication is important for daily living. SLPs with this vision have created some life-affirming programs that seem to reinforce and extend gains in communication-oriented therapies.

The social or life participation approach has been finding its way for a couple of decades. Some offered it as a "client-centered" alternative to a "medical model" that emphasizes impairments (e.g., Davidson & Worrall, 2013; Hilari & Cruice, 2013; Simmons-Mackie, 2008). Generally, however, social concerns are reasons to do impairment-based treatment (Kagan & Simmons-Mackie, 2007). Work explicitly on improving quality of life may occur in stages, beginning with preparations in the rehabilitation setting and then targeting a person's individual circumstances.

The principal architects of life participation approaches have been eloquent about the difficulties faced by people with aphasia and their families (Lyon, 2001) and have articulated most of the strategies introduced here (Elman, 2005; Kagan & Simmons-Mackie, 2007). Interviews with clients revealed that living successfully with aphasia involves four core themes, namely doing "as much as you can," having meaningful relationships, being positive, and talking better (Brown, Worrall, Davidson, et al., 2010). To illustrate this consequence-based approach, this section features some of the group programs and community centers that have inspired or been inspired by the life participation concept. Continuing our stroll across the bridge over the clinical–functional gap, let us begin with preparatory activities that can be carried out in a hospital or clinic.

Situation-Specific Role-Playing

Real-life situations and activities can be models for clinical activities. This differs from the earlier mentioned functional analysis of situations, leading to more traditionally structured treatments of functions and processes. Now, we consider constructing the situations themselves.

Role-playing induces varied speech acts such as advising, warning, and arguing. We create a situation in which conflict is likely. The clinician and client may disagree over what to have for dinner or how much to spend for a vacation. The clinician plays other partners, such as a helper at a market. Like people, settings influence language behavior to the extent that they are familiar and demanding of the language processor. A client could pretend to take care of business after standing in line at a bank.

To give us an idea of how we can vary simulated life situations, Schlanger and Schlanger (1970) divided them into nonstress situations such as planning a picnic and stressful situations such as going out to dinner. We would begin with nonstress situations. Then, stressful situations could be pleasant (e.g., going out to dinner) or unpleasant (e.g., dealing with an emergency). For various situations, the clinician and client anticipate communicative problems and work together, like conversational coaching, to figure out how a functional goal could be achieved with retained communicative resources.

One characteristic of other persons in a communicative situation (e.g., a cab driver, a telephone operator, the minister), is the lack of knowledge of aphasia. By pretending to be ignorant of aphasia, the clinician exposes communicative frustrations that a client is likely to face. Then, strategies for dealing with these frustrations can be developed.

Let us suppose a mildly impaired client is going through a divorce and must deal with a future ex-spouse and a lawyer over the phone. In the clinic, we play the roles of these persons so the client can become comfortable with instituting some control such as asking the spouse or the lawyer to explain slowly, repeat, or be available if a question should come up later. If the spouse and lawyer cannot agree to these conditions, then the conversation should be at another time. This dress rehearsal may strengthen confidence and the likelihood of using these strategies outside the clinic.

In training two nonfluent individuals to use symbolic gestures, Coelho (1991) first provided direct treatment in producing a gesture to a picture of a food item and then had the client practice in a contrived restaurant. The clinician played the role of waiter, asking questions such as, "What kind of sandwich would you like?" Generalization probes included waitresses asking similar questions in a restaurant. One client transferred gestures to a natural setting, but a more severely impaired client did not.

Hopper and Holland (1998) contrasted such situation-specific training with approaches, such as PACE, which are applicable to any situation. Managed care has moved treatment toward activities that establish functional independence in real-life tasks. The investigators reported training two individuals with Broca's aphasia to report emergencies over the phone. Treatment consisted of three steps:

- Describe a pictured emergency situation.
- If the description was incorrect, answer *wh-* questions about components of the situation.
- With the picture present, role-play the scenario with the clinician asking, "What is your emergency?"

Six pictured emergencies were trained, and four other pictures were used for a generalization probe. The participants improved over 10 sessions in responding to treated and untreated scenarios.

Jacqueline Hinckley, at the University of South Florida, has referred to situation-specific role-playing as a context-based approach (Hinckley & Carr, 2005). Ordering from a catalog over the telephone is one example. A few years ago, she compared this approach to impairment-based treatment with two groups of people with nonfluent aphasia. The two approaches appeared to lead to mixed effects not strongly related to either treatment. That is, context-based treatment was associated with improved naming but no change in scores with a functional battery. Nevertheless, the authors felt that they found improvements that were related to the treatments (Hinckley, Patterson, & Carr, 2001). Now, some clients are working on ordering on-line rather than over the phone.

Group Treatment

To maximize efficiency, a great deal of treatment during and after World War II was conducted in groups (Huber, 1946; Sheehan, 1946; Wepman, 1951). Then, group treatment came to be viewed as a valuable supplement to one-on-one therapy. Most clinicians recognize that groups possess dynamics that are absent in individual treatment (Elman, 2007; Kearns & Elman, 2008; Simmons-Mackie, Elman, Holland, et al., 2007), and there is evidence that group treatment is efficacious (Elman & Bernstein-Ellis, 1999; Wertz, et al., 1981).

When someone reports only that group therapy was conducted, we can assume only that it consisted of two or more clients. For people with aphasia, groups usually fit in the following categories:

- *Treatment* of cognitive and psycholinguistic impairments
- *Maintenance* of communicative gains achieved in prior treatment programs
- *Transition* from a treatment program to real life
- *Support* for clients and/or families

Group therapy for aphasia has evolved from mainly providing impairment-based stimulation sequentially around a table to providing creative interactive and communicative problem-solving opportunities.

Groups provide experiences for graduate students in university clinics. Garrett, Staltari, and Moir (2007) employ the aforementioned scaffolded discourse at Duquesne University. At the University of Arizona, Beeson and Holland (2007) emphasize conversation through application of PACE therapy and role-played simulations. The groups have discussions of current events, card and board games, and a book club. Students do not start off running groups alone but participate as assistants for several weeks. Later in a term, students assume a larger role in managing a group.

In a study of group therapy, Simmons-Mackie, Elman, and others (2007) observed sessions that satisfied their vision of conversational groups. First, communicative opportunities were distributed equally among participants. Second, interactions consisted mainly of peer exchanges rather than clinician-directed therapeutic tasks. Third, multimodal communication was encouraged. Fourth, clinicians functioned as "translators" between participants with aphasia. Fifth, as in the stimulation therapy of Chapter 8, errors were rarely corrected explicitly. Finally, clinicians promoted participation by soliciting contributions, using gaze to signal a speaking turn and minimizing the length of their own contributions.

Cynthia Busch (2007) has advised SLPs regarding Medicare and other third-party payers: "Group treatment services must fulfill the basic Medicare requirements for coverage of any SLP services" (p. 64). The service must be reasonable, necessary, specific, effective, and skilled. It must be appropriate for the diagnosis and be related to treatment goals. Part B service guidelines include group size of four or fewer members and a proportion of no more than 25 percent of total therapy. Justification should be explicit. Busch also advised that "the inherent functional aspect of group treatment should be explained in the supporting documentation" (p. 65).

After Medicare, whether group members pay for services can be related to the philosophy of the group. One support group in Arkansas, sponsored by the American Stroke Association, does not charge a fee. Any suggestion of payment is avoided "because that would define the group as treatment and underscore the medical model of care, rather than a social model . . ." (Shadden, 2007, p. 124). Clinicians at the University of Arizona have a different interpretation of out-of-pocket consequences. Beeson and Holland (2007) reported that "our group members hold the view that long-term rehabilitation is a service worth paying for" (p. 154). Group treatment could be considered to be comparable to other expenditures on quality of life such as fitness center memberships or continuing education classes.

Community Reintegration

Before going to a nearby restaurant with a group, a woman with severe Broca's aphasia practiced pointing to items on a menu in a role-playing activity. She pretended to order while a clinician gave her feedback. Then, seated at the restaurant, the client was stymied because the waitress was at the other end of the table out of view for practiced pointing. Although role-playing might have anticipated the need to motion for the waitress to come over, there is no guarantee that role-playing and other clinical activities will anticipate everything that happens during the real thing.

After training gestures for food items, Coelho (1991) concluded that there are aspects of real-world settings that cannot be simulated, such as conversations stopping, persons staring, waitresses' embarrassment, all as the person with aphasia struggles to communicate. "These need to be overcome by the aphasic patient for true generalization to occur" (p. 217).

How might resumption of activities be facilitated, especially when clinicians do not have time to accompany clients outside a rehabilitation center? Jon Lyon's (1992) **Communication Partners** is one program in which an adult volunteer from a client's community "serves as the vehicle with which activities of the patient's choice are introduced, either at home or in the community where they naturally occur" (Lyon, Cariski, Keisler, et al., 1997, p. 694).

The program has two phases. The first occurs in the clinic for 6 weeks. Supervised by an SLP, the volunteer and client become comfortable with each other in plausible situations. The volunteer practices several communicative strategies such as the following:

- Listen for a general theme rather than specific words.
- If a spoken message is not clear, encourage use of gestures.
- Draw your best guess as to what the client is trying to say.
- Verify what you think you know every 1 or 2 minutes.

The 14-week second phase of Communication Partners consists of outside activities. In the first of two weekly sessions, an SLP assists in reviewing the previous week's activity and planning the next activity to be carried out as the week's second session. In the second session, the person with aphasia and the volunteer engage in activities in the home or at a community site. Activities include a favorite from the past (e.g., gardening, card playing, grocery shopping), an activity considered but never tried before (e.g., learning computer skills), and volunteering in the community (e.g., visiting a day-care center).

Losing the ability to drive can be more distressing than losing the ability to speak. It creates an overwhelming sense of dependence. In the United Kingdom, Mackenzie and Paton (2003) interviewed people with aphasia and rehabilitation professionals regarding a return to driving after stroke. Those with aphasia showed some reduction in the recognition of road signs. They reported driving less, more carefully, and for shorter distances. Mackenzie and Paton indicated that training in road sign recognition has definite implications for reentering the community.

Changing Communities

In addition to adjusting to a community as it is, we consider modifying a living environment with respect to its **communicative accessibility**. It was already noted that a person with aphasia is not solely responsible for communication. Chapter 4 presented research that revealed barriers in three categories, namely other people, the physical environment, and society (Howe, et al., 2008). Others have pursued strategies for organizations to become more communicatively accessible for people with aphasia (Pound, Duchan, Penman, et al., 2007; Simmons-Mackie, Kagan, O'Neill Christie, et al., 2007). Three areas are presented here: emergency responders, physical environment, and reading materials.

Emergency responders (or "first responders) are a readily targeted group. The National Aphasia Association sponsors a training program for police, firefighters, and medical technicians (aphasia.org). In addition to reducing mistaken "diagnosis," the training modules increase sensitivity to comprehension difficulties and the need for time to speak. Elsewhere, a training program for medical students improved their interviews of patients with aphasia (Legg, Young, & Bryer, 2003), and another program for nursing staff of a large hospital improved their knowledge of aphasia and awareness of their interactions with patients (Sorin-Peters, McGilton, & Rochon, 2010).

Barriers in the physical environment have been addressed by Lubinski (2008) with her long advocated *environmental language intervention*. A "communicatively impaired environment" has the following characteristics, especially considering residential institutions for the elderly:

- Rules restricting communication
- Few places for a private conversation
- A staff that devalues communication involving residents
- Many residents with multiple problems, including dementias
- Poor physical conditions for communication, such as linear or distant seating and poor lighting and acoustics

Diplomatic and persuasive skills may effect modifications of these conditions. New and remodeled nursing homes include spaces for private meetings with family and friends, attractive areas for social gatherings, and circular seating in the dining room that facilitates face-to-face interaction.

Environmental intervention contributes to making an **aphasia-friendly** environment (Howe, Worrall, & Hickson, 2004). The first step is to identify both barriers to communication and the characteristics that are facilitative. For people with aphasia who are commuters, a public transportation system in Australia was examined by Worrall's group (Ashton, Aziz, Barwood, et al., 2008). Barriers included unsupportive interpersonal transactions and complexity of printed material. Turning these around became goals such as educating transportation personnel, improving printed materials, and encouraging the person with aphasia to travel with a caregiver and to carry routing cues and other aids.

A movement gaining traction is to help businesses become aphasia-friendly. One program is being conducted by the Snyder Center for Aphasia Life Enhancement (SCALE) in Baltimore, Maryland. Like other centers to be introduced shortly, SCALE is a support community for people with aphasia and their families. One of their projects is to create tools (e.g., picture boards of product options) to make it easier for people with aphasia to navigate restaurants, pharmacies, and shoe stores (Polovoy, 2012).

Changing communities also entails improving access to information. Linda Worrall and her colleagues in Australia have advocated successfully for the use of aphasia-friendly printed material in health education literature and beyond, including Web sites (see also Kerr, Hilari, & Litosseliti, 2010). Accessible language and formatting includes simplified text, familiar words, large font, lots of white space, and helpful illustrations (Aleligay, Worrall, & Rose, 2008; Brennan, Worrall, & McKenna, 2005; Worrall, Rose, Howe, et al., 2005). It does not matter if illustrations are line drawings or photographs (Rose, Worrall, Hickson, et al., 2011).

Creating Communities

When formal treatment has concluded, people with aphasia may become socially isolated. One remedy has been weekly aphasia groups, many of which are provided at university clinics. Vickers (2010) compared 28 people with aphasia who attended a weekly aphasia group to 12 people with aphasia who did not attend a group. She used a social network analysis to compare networking status before and after a stroke. For those attending aphasia groups, there was an increase in social participation and feelings of connectedness. For those not attending groups, there was a reduction of networking and an increased sense of isolation.

Another remedy for isolation is community centers staffed primarily by volunteers. There has been a stream of inspiration for development of these centers, beginning with Aura Kagan in Canada. Her colleagues say that she inspired the social and life participation movement in the United States (e.g., Elman, 2007). Web sites for community centers often refer to the social and life participation concepts as guiding their efforts. Many people with aphasia and their families now have a new life inspired by their participation in these centers. The centers are listed at the Web site for the National Aphasia Association. The story begins in Toronto.

In 1979, Pat Arato recognized a need for a program for her husband and others after discharge from therapy. She founded an aphasia center that was eventually named for her and became part of the Aphasia Institute in Toronto. Aura Kagan became the center's director (Kagan, Black, Duchan, et al., 2001; Kagan, Cohen-Schneider, Sherman, et al., 2007). It has been recognized for its orientation to group activities and has been a model for the activities provided in other centers.

An atmosphere of normality is fostered at the Aphasia Institute by referring to participants as "members" instead of patients or clients. The program has two phases. A 12-week introductory program is for educating members and their families, improving communication, and providing psychological support. Then a 16-week program offers conversation groups, music therapy, art classes, caregiver groups, and other options. Volunteers, such as graduate students, serve as conversation partners.

The communication intervention at the Institute is called *supported conversation for adults with aphasia* (SCA), with a focus on severe language impairment (Kagan, 1998). SCA is based on the premise that working on the skills necessary for conversation, such as a PACE activity, is not the same as actually having an adult conversation. There are a couple other key assumptions:

- Access to conversation is denied people with aphasia because of a perceived lack of competence.
- Competence is achieved with a "communication ramp" (i.e., skilled partner) to conversation opportunities.

Volunteers are trained in a workshop that includes an instructional video, role-playing, work with a group of members with severe aphasia, and an apprenticeship with experienced volunteers.

Kagan (1998) claimed that emphasis on "natural-sounding conversation . . . differentiates the SCA approach from other similar-sounding approaches" (p. 820). Members with aphasia still practice communicating by any means. Particular attention is given to an extensive manual of pictographs used to identify conversational topics and support getting a message across. Later, Kagan developed rating scales of partner participation (Kagan, Winckel, Black, et al., 2004; see also Correll, van Steenbrugge, & Scholten, 2010). Others in the United Kingdom developed a similar volunteer training program that increased the confidence of people with aphasia while extending long-term communicative rehabilitation (McVicker, Parr, Pound, et al., 2009).

Roberta Elman visited Kagan's center in 1989 and decided to open the *Aphasia Center of California* in 1996. It was the first independent nonprofit organization in the United States that provides direct services to people with aphasia (Bernstein-Ellis & Elman, 2007). It is housed in a senior center and offers conversation groups, a group for caregivers, reading and writing groups, and an art class.

Near New York City in New Jersey, Mike and Elaine Adler created the Adler Aphasia Center in 2003. Mike Adler had been the CEO of a global mail order company with 1,000 employees. In 1993 he suffered a stroke and aphasia. He was depressed and was not comfortable with speaking. His wife Elaine felt frustrated and helpless. They sought support from people who had a similar experience but found that professionals in their region could not direct them to a program. Wanting to help others, they investigated model support programs at aphasia centers in the United States, Canada, and England.

Like the Aphasia Institute in Toronto, the Adler Aphasia Center depends on volunteers to be communication partners, computer partners, and creativity partners for art, music, and cooking. One activity is Adler's Court, in which members take on all the key roles for trying a case that may have recently been in the news. SLPs spend a great deal of time preparing cue pages for the judge, attorneys, and witnesses. The center has a store, "Something Special," that sells jewelry crafted by members whose biographies are included in the packaging. Also, members perform a popular Broadway musical every August, spending the summer rehearsing and designing the set. On a single day, graduate students from nearby universities may observe 50 to 60 people with aphasia and related disorders engaged in a variety of activities. The Adlers' goal is to help people with aphasia and their loved ones live a fuller life (adleraphasiacenter.org).

A small "community" within a community can be created by pairing two people with language impairments in communicative interactions. Initiated by the Medstar National Rehabilitation Network in Washington, D.C., a confidence-building mentoring program pairs one person who has lived with aphasia for a few years with another person who is beginning to adjust. They get together for an hour one day per week. They talk on the phone, meet in person, or engage with each other over Skype (Law, 2012b).

In the United Kingdom, Connect is a Web-guided "charity for people living with aphasia" (ukconnect.org). It sponsors "Access to Life" services, including peer volunteer-led conversation groups and training for health care workers. Another service is "befriending," in which volunteers with aphasia offer support for others with aphasia in the hospital or home. Volunteers without aphasia also provide Toronto-inspired supported conversation for relatively isolated people in the home (Pound et al., 2007; McVicker et al., 2009).

For something unique, there is Théâtre Aphasique in Montreal (theatre-aphasique.org). After taking theater workshops, people with aphasia perform comedic productions with aphasia-related themes for service-providers and conferences. One theme tackles isolation. Another story is about a postman who suffers a stroke and, with the help of others, takes on a new life.

Psychosocial Adjustment

Meeting the goals of rehabilitation depends on the well-being of the person with aphasia and family members. Reciprocally, psychological adjustments depend on the success of communicative rehabilitation. Audrey Holland (2007) articulated a "wellness perspective" or *life coaching* approach to helping families with aphasia cope with significant change (see also Lyon, 1998; Worrall, et al., 2010). Holland exhorts SLPs to embrace communication counseling fearlessly to provide a positive atmosphere for rehabilitation.

Clinician Characteristics

It has long been realized in our profession that the relationship between a clinician and a client can invigorate rehabilitation. Rapport and trust are two bonding elements. Cyr-Stafford (1993) suggested that "the serene attitude of the knowledgeable professional who is familiar with these situations is reassuring to the person with aphasia" (p. 108). Our technical skills are not enough for a therapeutic relationship to flourish. Our "people skills" are just as vital. If a person with aphasia is uncomfortable with a clinician, that person quits.

Wulf (1979) commented on the first contact with her therapist: "And this was the first miracle speech therapy wrought for me. No word was needed—it was the magic of a look—an instantaneous rapport partly because my innermost messenger had told me that it would be that way" (p. 50). Ackerman (2011) observed "irresistible" Kelly enter her husband's hospital room "upbeat and hopeful, her smile always appeared genuine" (p. 91). **Unconditional positive regard** creates a positive climate for therapeutic change. The influential clinical psychologist Carl Rogers (1951) defined it as "an outgoing positive feeling without reservations, without evaluations" (p. 62). Depression, frustration, and anger are allowed in the clinical setting without reservation or evaluation by the clinician.

Yet studies have shown that clients and their families are likely to express more optimism than SLPs (e.g., Herrmann & Wallesch, 1989). The person with aphasia detects body language and prosody conveying negative attitudes. Sacks (1985) stated that "one cannot lie to an aphasic person." In a survey by Skelly (1975), people with aphasia "cited numerous subtle signs of impatience from those around them which were deeply discouraging—audible sighs, tightening of the mouth muscles, shoulder and eye movements, and drumming fingers" (p. 1141). A few SLPs may confuse professionalism with aloofness and exude a coolness that intimidates family members.

Wulf (1979) also wrote that an SLP's rare talent is "being able to hop on anybody's wavelength and stay there until the aphasic has learned how to climb the unending tortuous crag facing him" (p. 50). In a survey of clients who evaluated attributes of a good clinician, "empathetic-genuineness" ranked second to technical skill (Haynes & Oratio, 1978). **Empathy** is a capacity to sense the feelings and personal meanings that another person is experiencing at each moment. We cannot walk in a client's shoes, but we can convey that we understand the problems created by brain damage.

An example of empathy is the soothing of frustration that comes with statements like "I know—you know what you want to say but just can't think of the words to say it." An SLP may be the first person to convey this understanding. A patient discovers someone who knows that he or she is not stupid and believes there is someone in the hospital who can help with the exasperation of trying to talk. A client is inclined to accept the rigors of clinical advice when he or she knows that the helper understands the problem.

Rogers (1951) advised that "it is the counselor's function to assume, in so far as he is able, the internal frame of reference of the client . . . to lay aside all perceptions from the external frame of reference while doing so, and to communicate something of this empathic understanding to the client" (p. 29). An external frame of reference includes stereotypic conceptions according to gender, age, race, or religion. Ageism, for example, may entail a fear of the elderly that interferes with addressing a client as an individual (Davis & Holland, 1981). Prospective clinical aphasiologists should evaluate any inkling of stereotypic attitudes so they can keep them out of clinical interactions and can attain unconditional positive regard and empathy for their clients.

A third clinician characteristic is **patience**. A family member, who is accustomed to a certain pace of conversation or who feels compelled to help a loved one, may jump in quickly when the person with aphasia is slow to respond. An experienced clinician, on the other hand, knows that the goal is to increase the client's independence and allows some time for generating a response. Family members, who are used to speedy cures for diseases, may become distressed over the relatively slow rate of progress that is common with stroke-related dysfunction. An experienced clinician knows that progress moves in small steps and takes some time, and educates family members accordingly.

Finally, **openness** contributes to responsiveness to the client. Writing about her husband's recovery, Ackerman (2011) reported on difficulties that some SLPs had in relating to her husband Paul's career as an author and his extensive vocabulary. One therapist was showing him postcards, one being a famous painting of two baby angels. "Chair-oo-beem," he responded. "No," the therapist replied, "these are angels,

AINGELS" (p. 191). There is not much this therapist, by herself, could have done; but, if the spouse were in the room, we may want to check first to see if the effort is a real word.

Holland (2007) posed several questions for SLPs to ask themselves. Here are some of them:

- Are you a good communicator?
- Can you listen comfortably to people who have trouble talking?
- Can you listen to ideas that conflict with your values?
- Are you sensitive to cultural differences?
- Do you have a good sense of humor?
- Are you flexible?

Let us pause for a moment to consider flexibility. Plasticity of feedback was introduced earlier in the chapter with respect to accepting the use of any linguistic form that conveys an idea. This sensitivity to the essence of communication might have modified the response to "cherubim."

The Person with Aphasia

Adjusting to stroke and aphasia is more often than not a grueling process (e.g., Ackerman, 2011; Hale, 2003). Counseling-oriented SLPs have relied on the grief response as a model for stages of psychological adjustment to sudden "loss" of natural language abilities. Tanner and Gerstenberger's (1988) four stages were denial, frustration, depression, and acceptance. Whether people with aphasia actually go through this sequence has not been clearly established (Lyon, 1998).

Denial of impairment can be a psychological defense mechanism in contrast to the absence of awareness to be introduced in Chapter 11 on right hemisphere dysfunction. Not all individuals deny their aphasia, but for some, it may be a premorbid coping style, and it "allows patients to borrow time while they come to terms with reality" (Sarno, 1993, p. 325). After patience grants this time for just a few days, the SLP helps the person with aphasia and family members accept the relevance of rehabilitation.

Depression, or discouragement, is common after a stroke. Depression is more common with good comprehension and nonfluent aphasia than with other types of aphasia (Starkstein & Robinson, 1988). Physicians have advised that depression may not be just a stage of coping that a person passes through. Herrmann, Johannsen-Horbach, and Wallesch (1993) suggested that it is likely to be an unavoidable neurochemical consequence of stroke. The spectrum of poststroke depression includes *emotional lability*, which is sudden laughter or crying for no apparent reason. Treatment of severe depression or pathological crying has included antidepressant medication (Andersen, 1997).

Someone with aphasia thinks, "I want to be me again." Brumfitt (1993) noted that motor and communicative disabilities batter someone's **sense of self**. Holland and Beeson (1993) added that "as clinicians, we will be involved with individuals and family members as they mourn the insult to the pre-stroke identity, and as they make adjustments to the sense of self" (p. 581). Fundamental to identity is a client's adulthood. Caring family may start to treat the member with aphasia like a child or a "patient," especially with respect to communicative style (Le Dorze & Brassard, 1995). Everyone, including the clinician, can shift to the adult mode by involving the client in establishing goals and evaluating outcome (Kagan & Simmons-Mackie, 2007). Mainly the person with aphasia wants to be treated like an adult.

A person with aphasia may quickly exhibit **unproductive coping mechanisms** as a shield (Eisenson, 1984). Parr (1994) found that people with aphasia deal with disabilities differently. One person was resigned to his impairments but pursued an active life. His relationship with his wife improved. Yet another individual responded to his condition with "angry fatalism." He was unwilling to discuss many things about his condition, including possibilities for functional progress through rehabilitation. People with aphasia below age 65 were more likely than older individuals to take control in their situation.

Holland (2007) had some suggestions for how to be a counselor. She recommended acting as a guide, advocate, and interpreter. We should help an individual feel like a "person," instead of a "patient." She noted that a client's needs and the counseling role changes somewhat through the phases of recovery: the acute phase (e.g., provide information, encouragement), the subacute or rehabilitation phase (e.g., explain the rehabilitation process, expectations), and the chronic or living-with-aphasia phase (e.g., point out resources). An important component of any phase is to include the family.

Family Adjustment

A spouse may say, "I want someone to help me." Porter and Dabul (1977) applied transactional analysis to help us and spouses understand the situation. A spouse responds to shifts in Adult, Parent, and Child ego states by the client. "He acts like a child." In the person with aphasia, the Adult state is often weakened and turned into the dependent state of the Child. "He just sits around all day and watches TV." The childlike ego is impulsive and turned to "me, me, me." The Parent state diminishes. Other people with aphasia expand the Parent by becoming overly protective of the spouse, constantly monitoring his or her activities. A spouse, in turn, can become overly protective of a client. Examples of these shifting roles can be found in stories told by spouses of people with aphasia (e.g., Ackerman, 2011; Giffords & Kelly, 2011; Hale, 2003).

Holland (2007) discussed the importance of providing family members with information, in particular, keeping them posted on progress in therapy. She discussed leading a counseling group of people with aphasia and family members. She asks members to share stories, especially stories that would be meaningful to others in the group. As new members join the group, the more experienced ones share stories of conquering difficulties. Each member discovers that he or she is not alone. Finding support is facilitated by organizations such as those in Table 10.3.

TABLE 10.3   A sample of organizations providing information for persons with aphasia, their families, and professionals.

ORGANIZATION	UNIQUE FEATURES	WEB SITE
National Aphasia Association	Founded by Martha Taylor Sarno in New York City. Promotes universal awareness of aphasia and encourages creation of support groups for people with aphasia and their families; sponsors conferences and theatrical productions.	aphasia.org
Aphasia Hope Foundation	Founded in 1997. Provides a forum where anyone can have questions answered by professionals; lobbies Congress for research funding.	aphasiahope.org
AphasiaHelp	A charity in the United Kingdom; people can write to each other as "penpals."	aphasiahelp.org

Summary and Conclusions

Communicative rehabilitation is aimed at helping an individual with aphasia maximize retained capacities to comprehend and convey messages through any means. The internal and external contexts of Chapter 4 suggest a menu of variables that we consider in providing a functional or pragmatic treatment program. The goals of functional rehabilitation have expanded to embrace social or life participation by a person with aphasia. Community centers now offer both impairment-based and communication-based activities, called "intensive comprehensive aphasia programs" (ICAPs).

A great deal of functional or pragmatic treatment does not repair damaged language processes or teach something new. It reduces fear of communicative situations and increases confidence in the use of retained capacities or processes partially repaired by cognitive stimulation. We walk clients to the end of the diving board and ask them to look down. With confidence comes participation.

CHAPTER
11 Right-Hemisphere Disorders

In 1974, Associate Supreme Court Justice William O. Douglas suffered a stroke. Because he could talk and write, he appeared to recover rapidly. He checked himself out of rehabilitation and was anxious to resume work, claiming his weakened left arm was injured in a fall. Returning to the Court, he insisted he was the Chief Justice. In court "he dozed, asked irrelevant questions, and sometimes rambled on." After being asked to resign, "he came back to his office, buzzed for his clerks . . . asked to participate in, draft, and even publish his own opinions separately; and he requested that a tenth seat be placed at the Justices' bench" (Gardner, 1982, p. 310).

For a long time, people with right-hemisphere strokes were not referred to speech-language clinics, because their preserved verbal abilities make them appear to be functionally intact, and they are disinterested in sticking around for rehabilitation. Now, they may be referred for the following reasons:

- The patient has a swallowing problem or motor speech deficit.
- Someone with an old right-hemisphere infarct has recently suffered a left-hemisphere stroke.
- The patient may have communicative difficulties.

Justice Douglas's rambling talk and failure to appreciate situations might have put him in the third category.

Two speech-language pathologists (SLPs) have been prominent in the study of *right-hemisphere dysfunction* (RHD). Penelope Myers-Duffy of the Mayo Clinic and Connie Tompkins of the University of Pittsburgh have studied the pertinent cognitive and communicative problems extensively (Myers, 1999; Tompkins, 1995). One of Tompkins's students, Margaret Lehman Blake, has followed at the University of Houston (Lehman Blake, 2007; Myers & Lehman Blake, 2008). Together they reviewed medical charts of 123 individuals with RHD. Only 45 percent had been evaluated by an SLP (Lehman Blake, Duffy, Tompkins, & Myers, 2003). This situation is similar in other countries (e.g., Brady, Armstrong, & Mackenzie, 2005).

This chapter begins with an introduction to clinical neuropsychology and general assessment. Then, the cognitive impairments of RHD are reviewed followed by secondary implications for linguistic and communicative functions. This reentry into the SLP's scope of practice proceeds with the pragmatic language difficulties of RHD and the possibilities for rehabilitation.

Clinical Neuropsychology

The wider cognitive territory of these final three chapters corresponds to the domain of clinical neuropsychology. In many settings, an SLP collaborates with a clinical neuropsychologist and may skirt the borders of this domain. *Clinical* neuropsychology is a specialization in clinical psychology and, thus, is different from *cognitive* neuropsychology. Initially as clinical psychologists found themselves working increasingly with brain injury, they applied available tools, such as tests of intelligence, to the assessment of neurologically impaired populations. Currently clinical neuropsychologists supplement their assessments with cognitive-behavioral and psychotherapeutic interventions.

The most widely applied comprehensive battery is the **Wechsler Adult Intelligence Scale** (WAIS) now in its fourth edition (Wechsler, 2008). Starting in the 1950s, the WAIS has been used to measure general intelligence, called *g*, represented by the Full Scale IQ (FSIQ). The FSIQ has been interpreted with respect to the famous mean of 100 and the surrounding bell curve. The test continues to be divided into verbal and performance scales, which conveniently, but not ideally, correspond to LH and RH functions.

Beginning with the WAIS-III in the 1990s and a desire to consider contemporary constructs of working memory and processing speed, developers added and modified subtests as summarized in Figure 11.1. Modifications were intended to reduce test time, clarify presentation, and minimize cultural biases. The WAIS-IV is now divided into four scales fitting into the traditional dichotomy. General intelligence is still represented by the FSIQ based on 10 core tests (i.e., buttons in Figure 11.1). A General Ability Index (GAI) is comprised of the six subtests of Verbal Comprehension and Perceptual Reasoning.

The difference between the traditional VIQ and PIQ, called the *discrepancy score*, is of interest when there is unilateral brain damage. A person with left-hemisphere damage was likely to have a lowered VIQ relative to the PIQ, and someone with RHD was likely to present the reverse (Hom & Reitan, 1990). The discrepancy has occurred more for men than women, who tend to have little difference between the VIQ and PIQ no matter which side of the brain is damaged (e.g., Sundet, 1986).

One performance subtest, called **Matrix Reasoning**, was new for WAIS-III. Its origins are in Raven's (1938/1965) *Progressive Matrices*, which are familiar to SLPs as a predictor of intelligence. One segment of Raven's test, called the **Coloured Progressive Matrices** (CPM), consists of figuring out geometric patterns to identify a missing piece. People with moderate-to-mild aphasia were comparable to those with RHD. People with severe aphasia were substantially deficient (Kertesz & McCabe, 1975). In WAIS-IV, the new test **Visual Puzzles** requires similar spatial reasoning skills in which a person must find three of six parts that combine to make a whole.

FIGURE 11.1   Evolution of the Wechsler Adult Intelligence Scale. Core subtests are designated with dots. Supplemental tests are in italics. New subtests are in boldface.

WAIS-R (1981)			
Full Scale IQ (FSIQ)			
Verbal IQ (VIQ)		Performance IQ (PIQ)	
WAIS-III (1997)			
Verbal Comprehension Index (VCI)	Working Memory Index (VMI)	Perceptual Organization Index (POI)	Processing Speed Index (PSI)
WAIS-IV (2008)			
Verbal Comprehension Index (VCI)	Working Memory Index (VMI)	Perceptual Reasoning Index (PRI)	Processing Speed Index (PSI)
• Similarities • Vocabulary • Information *Comprehension*	• Digit Span • Arithmetic *Letter-Number Sequencing*	• Block Design • Matrix Reasoning • **Visual Puzzles** *Picture Completion* **Figure Weights**	• Symbol Search • Coding *Cancellation*

The Processing Speed Index (PSI) is of interest with respect to visual attention and concentration. Each test is "timed," namely for the time it takes to complete the task. This area used to be assessed with the classic digit-symbol test in which a person matches a long series of digits and symbols. For WAIS-IV, a similar test is renamed as **Coding**. For **Symbol Search**, the task is to find a target symbol among a row of symbols. In the new and supplemental **Cancellation** task, the examiner records the time it takes to mark a recurring colored shape in a page of colored shapes.

A clinical neuropsychologist can choose from several other tests that are for specific cognitive functions. The array of assessment options can be appreciated by inspecting a handbook covering the landscape (e.g., Lezak, Howieson, Bigler, et al., 2012; Snyder, Nussbaum, & Robins, 2006).

In their review of records for patients with RHD, Lehman Blake and others (2002) found that deficits of attention, perception, memory, and reasoning were reported most frequently. These diagnoses tended to be made by clinical neuropsychologists and others. SLPs were the professionals who would identify deficits of communication, which were noted in fewer than 20 percent of the charts (Lehman Blake et al., 2003). The investigators concluded that the same deficit may be viewed differently by different professionals and that other professionals do not tend to recognize communication deficits in patients with RH stroke. Some in-service training may be in order.

Primary Cognitive Impairments

The primary cognitive impairments of RHD are manifestations of functions that are largely unique to the right hemisphere. They may be classified as "nonlinguistic deficits" (Myers & Lehman Blake, 2008). Technically they lie outside the scope of practice in speech-language pathology. Yet as will be shown later, these impairments spill over into communicative skills such as conversing and reading, and they interfere with rehabilitation. Occasionally an SLP will do an informal assessment.

Anosognosia for Deficits

Justice Douglas's insistence on returning to the Supreme Court was indicative of **anosognosia**, which is a lack of awareness or recognition of disease or disability (McGlynn & Schacter, 1989). It is associated with brain damage. Clinicians use other terms such as *lack of insight* or *imperception of disease*. Anosognosia is often distinguished from **denial** of impairment, which is a psychological defense mechanism. Denial is a conscious strategy for avoiding problems and is unrelated to brain damage.

Unawareness of disease is usually observed as anosognosia for hemiplegia (AHP; Kortte & Hillis, 2009; Orfei, Robinson, Prigatano, et al., 2007; Vocat, Staub, Stoppini, & Vuilleumier, 2010). We may see someone with left hemiplegia who makes plans to play golf (Tompkins, 1995). Another person may not recognize his paralyzed limbs as his own. Unawareness of right hemiplegia by people with aphasia is rare (Cutting, 1978).

Myers and Lehman Blake (2008) suggested that AHP may be part of hemi-inattention or left neglect (see also Bisiach, Vallar, Perani, et al., 1986). They also described an individual who will "deny a need for rehabilitative services, refusing to take his physical limitations seriously. . . . He may talk about returning to work next week, yet be unable to transfer himself from bed to wheelchair" (p. 963). The belief that nothing is wrong is dangerous, and the person's safety is a major issue for discharge planning.

Impaired Way-Finding

Some patients are likely to get lost in the unfamiliar maze of hospital corridors on their way to the speech-language clinic. SLPs either do their assessment in the person's ward or room, or a transportation service brings the individual to the clinic. Persons with RHD, in particular, suddenly cannot find their way around. Informally this is known as a way-finding problem, and formally it is called **topographical disorientation** (Aguirre & D'Esposito, 1999).

With topographical disorientation, an individual fails to orient to the immediate environment. The person has difficulty reading maps, remembering familiar routes, and learning new ones. The deficit may be attributed to an inability to recognize landmarks, but it also occurs when object recognition is preserved (Ellis & Young, 1988).

This type of disorientation differs from *geographic disorientation*, in which an individual relates to immediate surroundings but fails to conceptualize general locale (e.g., *What state do you live in?*). Lehman Blake and others (2003) found orientation problems in 43 percent of their reviewed records.

Left Neglect

We may see a patient in the hospital who is "only half made-up, the left side of her face absurdly void of lipstick and rouge" (Sacks, 1985, p. 74). Neglect of one-half of space is caused by damage in the parietotemporal region. It is more frequent and/or obvious with RHD, so that left neglect is more common than right neglect. People with posterior RHD bump into things on their left, leave food on the left side of the plate, and dress only the right side. Left neglect was noted in 63 percent of the cases reviewed by Lehman Blake and others (2003) and, similarly, in 58 percent of cases reviewed in South Korea (Lee, Suh, Kim, et al., 2009).

Clinical neuropsychologists use functionally nonspecific paper-and-pencil tests to identify hemispatial neglect. One is a **crossing out test** of marking lines through circles scattered about a page. Similarly, a **line cancellation test** has lines scattered about a page. A person with left neglect crosses out circles or lines on the right, ignoring the items on the left. Severity of neglect is measured by the number of omissions. In a **line bisection test**, a person is asked to mark the center of a horizontal line. Ignoring the left end of the line, someone with left neglect marks to the right of midline. Computerized assessment of neglect reduces some of the bias of the traditional tests (Erez, Katz, Ring, et al., 2009).

Myers (1999) used a test of scene copying to measure left neglect. The scene consists of a simple house, a fence, and trees to the left and the right. She provided a *copy-scene scoring system*, whereby a client gets a point for each detail of the drawing.

Neglect is thought to be a disorder of selective or focused attention and may be called *hemi-inattention*. Posner discovered that *covert attention*, or a "cognitive spotlight," is impaired, rather than overt shifts of eye movement (Posner, Walker, Friedrich, et al., 1987). A sense for the internal spotlight was provided by Bisiach and others (1981) in Milan, Italy. In the clinic they asked people with RHD to imagine the Piazza del Duomo, a large square commanded at one end by a spectacular cathedral. Pretending to look out from the front of the cathedral and asked to report buildings on each side, participants could report buildings on the right but not on the left. However, intact memory for the neglected buildings was exhibited when the participants imagined the piazza facing the opposite direction. Now, the previously neglected buildings were reported from the right side, whereas the previously reported buildings (now on the left) were ignored.

Might the neglected space still be processed at an automatic level? In a priming task, the prime was a pictured object (e.g., a bat) presented 400 milliseconds before a semantically related target (e.g., *ball*; McGlinchey-Berroth, Milberg, Verfaellie, Alexander, & Kilduff, 1993). A twist was that the prime was shown in either the left or right visual field. To avoid attentional adjustments, a nonsense drawing was always presented in the other field. Four participants with left neglect displayed normal semantic priming from either visual field. Thus, the picture to the left was processed apparently at a subconscious level, leading to the conclusion that neglect is a disruption of controlled or intentional processing.

In a study of functional implications, RHDs either with or without neglect drove through an obstacle course of folding chairs in a rehabilitation center. Both groups sideswiped more chairs on the left than the right, and participants with obvious neglect made more direct hits than those without obvious neglect. Some RHDs were taught to scan the course before starting and while driving. The training reduced their direct hits but not their sideswipes (Webster, Cottam, Gouvier, et al., 1988; see also Punt, Kitadono, Hulleman, et al., 2008; Turton, Dewar, Lievesley, et al., 2009).

An SLP should watch for the influence of neglect when dealing with language test materials. Neglect can affect any test requiring the scanning of a visual array from left to right. Word comprehension errors disappeared for many RHDs when clinicians controlled for neglect of the left side of picture displays (Gainotti, Caltagirone, & Miceli, 1983). The clinician can arrange pictures vertically to the right side or can verbally cue a client to shift gaze leftward.

Both left hemianopia (see Chapter 2) and left neglect interfere with processing stimuli in the left hemispace. The former is a sensory impairment affecting the ability to see left of center. Individuals are aware of the problem and try to compensate with eye movement on their own. Left neglect, on the other hand, is an attentional impairment. "Patients fail to report stimuli in the neglected area, not because they cannot see them, but because they do not *notice* them" (Myers, 1999, p. 30). These individuals are often unaware of the problem and have to be prompted to compensate.

Constructional Apraxia

Impairments of visuospatial motor functions, such as drawing or building something, are called *constructional apraxia*. In general terms, it is an impairment of building a whole from its parts, usually caused by damage to the right parietal lobe. The most convenient clinical test is a drawing task. Copying is preferred over drawing on command because the former is less culturally biased. A person may be asked to draw a house, flower, or clock, the latter being central to Cahalan's (2012) mysterious tale of *Brain on Fire*. Clinical neuropsychologists sometimes present a Picasso-like abstraction called the Rey-Osterrieth figure to be copied. The **Block Design** subtest of the WAIS, in which blocks are arranged to match a design, is also used as a test of constructional skill.

Might motor impairments interfere with constructional abilities? Anteriorly damaged RHDs are likely to have left hemiparesis, but the unimpaired right side is usually preferred for writing and drawing. Also, limb apraxia is rare with RHD. Estimates vary from no patients with this disorder to 27 percent, whereas 68 percent of LHDs may be impaired (DeRenzi, Faglioni, & Scotti, 1969; Duffy & Duffy, 1989). In general, RHDs are less likely than LHDs to have praxic interference with visuospatial skills.

In early comparisons of RHDs and LHDs, there was a higher prevalence of constructional apraxia in RHDs than LHDs (e.g., Arrigoni & DeRenzi, 1964; Grossman, 1988). In other studies, the two groups turned out to be similar with a 30 to 40 percent prevalence of drawing deficiency in each group (e.g., Carlesimo, Fadda, & Caltagirone, 1993). Despite similar test scores, there are qualitative differences. For example, RHDs neglect the left side and are more likely to have poor spatial relationships among parts. LHDs are more deliberate, simplify, and preserve spatial relationships among parts (Gainotti & Tiacci, 1970). Gardner (1982) described RHDs' artistry as "fragmented and disconnected drawing, whose parts, while often recognizable, do not flow or fit together into an organized whole" (pp. 322–323). In general, parietal RHDs draw details incoherently, whereas parietal LHDs omit details in a coherent structure.

Problems with Sound

People with RHD generally recognize common sounds like a hissing teapot or flushing toilet (Faglioni, Spinnler, & Vignolo, 1969). Like visual object agnosia, it usually takes bilateral brain damage to cause agnosia for environmental sounds (Bauer & Rubens, 1985). It is music that makes us think of the right hemisphere. Impairment in the recognition, production, and reproduction of melodies is called **amusia**. It may also be called *music agnosia* (Peretz, 2001).

The right temporal lobe seems to be responsible for storing and activating familiar melodies. When neurosurgeons used tiny electrodes to stimulate this region before surgery, the patients reported hearing an orchestra or a choir (Penfield & Perot, 1963). Sacks (1985) described an elderly woman with a right temporal infarction. In the early months after her stroke, she woke up to hearing familiar songs even though she was nearly deaf and no radio was on. She would ask, "Is the radio in my head?" Sacks called it a "musical epilepsy."

We should differentiate *melody* and *lyrics*. RHDs can be impaired in pitch pattern perception but not speech perception, whereas people with aphasia have difficulty with speech but not tones (Sidtis & Volpe, 1988). In one study, LH damage caused more problems than RH damage in recognizing music with familiar lyrics. However, RHDs did worse than LHDs in recognizing music without familiar lyrics such as "Hail to the Chief" (Gardner & Denes, 1973). This study indicated that familiar lyrics are encoded when listening to melodies, a mental skill that helps RHDs but hinders LHDs (Winner & von Karolyi, 1998). With RHD, deficit is purely with melody.

People with RHD and LHD also differ with respect to *pitch* and *rhythm*. Early research indicated that pitch processing is more susceptible to RH damage and, to a lesser degree, rhythm processing is more susceptible to LH damage (Shapiro, Grossman, & Gardner, 1981). Years later, Alcock and her colleagues (2000) found that pitch and rhythm differentiated RHD and LHD more clearly with production than with perception. RHDs were impaired in producing pitch and melody, whereas LHDs were impaired in producing rhythmic sequences (see also Prior, Kinsella, & Giese, 1990).

A well-known test of musical skills is the **Seashore Rhythm Test** (*SRT*). It requires clients to discriminate between pairs of musical beats. In clinical circles, it was believed that this test is sensitive to unilateral RH damage, but two studies demonstrated that LH- and RH-damaged groups do not differ with the SRT (Karzmark, Heaton, Lehman, & Crouch, 1985; Sherer, Parsons, Nixon, & Adams, 1991). RHDs do appear to have more difficulty than LHDs when asked to discriminate between longer pairs of three- to five-note melodies.

A more recent assessment is the **Montréal Battery of Evaluation of Amusia** (*MBEA*), developed by Isabelle Peretz, a psychologist specializing in the cognition of music at the University of Montréal (Peretz, Champod, & Hyde, 2003). The MBEA contains six subtests. The first four subtests require discrimination of two short melodies. In the fifth subtest, clients classify melodies as a waltz or a march. Recognition memory for previously presented melodies is the final subtest. The MBEA may be critiqued for not separating pitch and rhythm (e.g., adding a monotonic rhythm test such as tapping).

The French composer Maurice Ravel illustrates a double dissociation in musical skills. He was stricken by a left-hemisphere stroke that caused Wernicke's aphasia. Despite language comprehension deficit, he continued to recognize melodies. Yet Ravel was no longer able to compose because he could not read notes or perform from a score (Gardner, 1982). Although individuals with aphasia can have a music-processing impairment, generally people with aphasia retain purely musical competencies; whereas RH damage causes problems with melodies while retaining the ability to deal with symbolic codes (Botez, Botez, & Aube, 1980).

Another type of sound has implications for communicative interaction. A person's voice helps us recognize who we are talking to, especially over the phone. Two tasks were used to study *speaker recognition* by brain-damaged people. In one test participants were asked to tell if two voices were the same or different. The other task involved recognition of famous voices (Van Lancker, Kreiman, & Cummings, 1989). Temporal damage in either hemisphere caused voice discrimination deficit. Impaired recognition of famous voices was linked to right parietal lobe damage. Even people with global aphasia were able to recognize the voices of Johnny Carson or John F. Kennedy.

Emotion

The neurology of emotion is complex. It is a feeling in the gut of limbic and autonomic nervous systems and is a message recognized in cognitive cortex. Both hemispheres have been shown to contribute to emotional qualities of behavior, but the RH is dominant (Silberman & Weingartner, 1986). Persons with RHD may display a flat affect or indifference that often accompanies left neglect (Gainotti, 1972). Based on physiological measures, RHDs have demonstrated **hypoarousal** to tactile stimulation (Heilman, Schwartz, & Watson, 1978) and emotional pictures (Morrow, Vrtunski, Kim, et al., 1981). In their chart review, Lehman Blake and others (2003) found a diagnosis of "hyporesponsive" in about 40 percent of the cases.

RHD and LHD transform mood differently with respect to positive or negative valence. RHDs tend to joke and laugh excessively, a change in a "positive" direction. LHDs with aphasia can be depressive and may cry excessively (Gainotti, 1972). In one study, depression was greatest with anterior LHD. Some RHDs react to cartoons with excessive hilarity, and others are unresponsive (Gardner, Ling, Flamm, et al., 1975). Posterior RHDs may be more depressed than anterior RHDs, who can be "unduly cheerful" and apathetic about their disorders (Robinson, Kubos, Starr, Rao, et al., 1984). Cheerfulness may go along with unawareness of impairment.

Recognition and expression of emotion are important ingredients of communicative exchanges. We convey feelings through facial expression, speech intonation, or the semantic content behind words. As we look for common threads through different tasks (Chapter 5), a deficit in all of these modes would be evidence for a central impairment of emotion.

At the cognitive level, clients are usually examined for recognition of happiness, sadness, and anger in faces. RHDs have difficulty recognizing facial expressions and the emotional significance of pictured situations, and this deficit is not necessarily related to hypoarousal (Dekosky, Heilman, Bowers, et al., 1980; Zoccolotti, Scabini, & Violani, 1982).

RHDs had more pronounced difficulty than LHDs for identifying emotional language (Borod, Andelman, Obler, et al., 1992). In another study, RHDs and LHDs participated in three recognition tasks. Emotive sentences conveyed sadness (e.g., *I'm going to miss you when you leave*), happiness (e.g., *I can hardly believe I passed the test*), and anger (e.g., *I want you to stop harassing me*). The same emotions were presented also in facial expressions and with prosody. Response consisted of pointing to words for the emotions. Participants with only cortical lesions performed these tasks without difficulty. Those with additional subcortical lesions had deficits, but only the RHD subcortical group was impaired in recognizing emotion of facial expressions (Karow, Marquardt, & Marshall, 2001).

With RHD, expression of emotions is unrelated to recognition of emotion (Borod, Koff, Perlman-Lorch, & Nicholas, 1986). In formal testing, facial reactions were inaccurate to pictures of familiar people and to pleasant and unpleasant scenes (Buck & Duffy, 1980). RHDs demonstrated less facial expressivity than LHDs in interviews (Blonder, Burns, Bowers, et al., 1993). Sherratt (2007) asked participants to produce positive and negative personal narratives (i.e., tell a funny or frightening experience). RHDs were similar to a control group when telling the funny experience. However, in the negative narratives, the RHDs tended to be evaluative without expressing feelings.

Tests of facial affect recognition have arisen out of concern for brain trauma as well as RHD. The **Florida Affect Battery** (FAB) assesses discrimination, matching, and naming the emotion in faces or utterances. The manual contains results from the research, such as RHDs performing worse than LHDs on most of the tasks, including naming the emotion in a semantically neutral utterance (Bowers, Blonder, & Heilman, 1999; Blonder, Bowers, & Heilman, 1991). Subtests in the **Diagnostic Assessment of Nonverbal Affect-2** (DANVA-2) rely on photographs and voices (Nowicki & Carton, 1993).

Secondary Impairments

As we think about an individual's anosognosia and flat affect, we may begin to anticipate unusual behavior in communicative situations. Left neglect, constructional
apraxia, and hypoarousal appear to affect language modalities. This section deals with
the simple proposition that primary disorders affect specific skills that are within the
scope of practice in speech-language pathology.

Neglect Dyslexia

"A *rose* is a *rose* or a *nose*" (Patterson & Wilson, 1990). Some people with RHD misread the beginning of words (Riddoch, Humphreys, Cleton, et al., 1990). Others
misread words on the left side of a page. Some have both types of problems (Ellis,
Flude, & Young, 1987; Young, Newcombe, & Ellis, 1991). Misreading the left side of
words or the left side of a page are symptoms of *neglect dyslexia*, also classified as a
peripheral dyslexia (Chapter 6). Neglect dyslexia was found in only 38 percent of the
neglect cases reviewed in South Korea (Lee et al., 2009). Therefore, we cannot say
that hemispatial neglect necessarily "causes" neglect dyslexia. Also, rare cases of right
neglect dyslexia with LHD have been reported (e.g., Warrington, 1991).

   One test is to present words that can still be words when the first letter is omitted
or substituted (e.g, *blight*). Case VB understood these words according to the errors
(e.g., *blight* as "light"), indicating that the impairment was in an early point in the process, such as perception or recognition. Of the errors, 66 percent were clear left-side
errors, usually substitutions of the first one or two letters irrespective of word length
(e.g., "slain" for *train*, "pillow" for *yellow*; Arguin & Bub, 1997). There are very subtle
variations of neglect dyslexia (Hillis, Newhart, Heidler, et al., 2005).

Aprosodia

Along with facial expression, we express emotions through voice. The present discussion is oriented to the effect of primary RH impairments on prosody, introduced in
Chapter 4. Does recognition impairment occur with auditory input as well as the look
on faces? Is hypoarousal revealed in speech? There is another possibility, however.
Might the primary disorder of amusia seep into the melodic qualities of talking?

   At the University of Texas and then at the University of Oklahoma, Elliott Ross
(1981) proposed receptive and expressive forms of *aprosodia*, modeled after posterior
and anterior aphasias. It is unclear whether this dichotomy is common with RHD.
Some RHDs speak with a flat contour or monotone (Ross & Mesulam, 1979). Some
are deficient in identifying emotional tone in mundane sentences, detected in tasks
requiring pointing to a happy, sad, or angry face (Heilman, Bowers, Speedie, et al.,
1984; Schlanger, Schlanger, & Gerstman, 1976). More recently, Ross and Monnot
(2008) marshaled evidence for the conclusion that affective prosody is a specialized
function of the right hemisphere.

Along the way, Ross developed a brief **Aprosodia Battery** (Ross, Thompson, & Yenkosky, 1997). For comprehension, clients indicate if a pair of intoned stimuli are the same or different, and they identify emotional intonation by pointing to a vertical array of faces. For production, clients repeat six emotions, and utterances are analyzed acoustically (see also Ross & Monnot, 2011).

Other research has been centered at Marc Pell's Neuropragmatics and Emotion Lab at McGill University in Montréal. He compared RHDs and LHDs with three emotion-recognition tasks. Both had deficits but for different reasons. LHDs had difficulty recognizing emotion in linguistic meanings, whereas RHDs had a more pervasive deficit for recognizing emotional prosody (Pell, 2006). RHDs also had diminished ability to recognize speaker attitudes of confidence and politeness, providing hints at how someone with this stroke location might participate inappropriately in conversation (Pell, 2007).

Returning to a question for aphasia, we may ask again whether affective and linguistic prosody can be dissociated by brain damage. It has been expected that RH stroke would spare linguistic function. Indeed, in two studies, RHDs interpreted lexical stress normally (e.g., *blackboard, black board*), and most had no problem producing lexical stress (Behrens, 1988; Emmorey, 1987). Yet in another study, RHDs were impaired in comprehending and producing lexical stress (e.g., *con*vict, con*vict*) and in discriminating and recognizing sentence contours (Bryan, 1989). Compound words may be easier. The Geigenberger and Ziegler (2001) study mentioned in Chapter 4 indicates that processing linguistic prosody depends on how it is tested. In general, RHDs have had more difficulty comprehending emotional and pragmatic prosody than sentence-level linguistic prosody.

Studies emphasizing production had mixed results. Some RHDs were successful, and others were impaired in reading sentences aloud with declarative, interrogative, and imperative contours (Behrens, 1989; Cooper, Soares, Nicol, et al., 1984; Shapiro & Danly, 1985). Inconclusive research reduces our expectations and reminds us to evaluate each client objectively, being on the lookout for problems with linguistic prosody that could be distracting in communicative situations.

Returning to the questions opening this section, it should be noted that nearly all the secondary deficits cited here pertained to emotion in prosody. The present author observed monotonic speech in a client who had severe amusia and no difficulty recognizing emotions, but investigators have not been very curious about a link between amusia and aprosodia.

American Sign Language (ASL)

A fair question would be whether visuospatial or constructional impairments affect the use of ASL, especially the spatially configured syntactic component. In one study, three RH-damaged signers were impaired in recognition of syntax but not other components of the language (e.g., "lexical"). However, they were "flawless" in production of syntactic and other features of ASL (Poizner, Klima, &

Bellugi, 1987). Like hearing individuals, RHD spares many aspects of the use of a language.

One person with RHD "correctly uses the left side of signing space to represent syntactic relations, despite her neglect of left hemispace in non-language tasks" (Klima, Bellugi, & Poizner, 1988, p. 323). What is the effect of left neglect on "reading" American Sign Language? JH was working for an aircraft manufacturer when he suffered a stroke in his right hemisphere. Corina, Kritchevsky, and Bellugi (1996) compared his lateralized sign identification with object recognition. His recognition of objects was strongly affected by neglect, but recognition of signs was not affected. The intact left hemisphere's linguistic system appears to have overridden the visual attention deficit.

Cognitive Pragmatics of RHD

Conversation is an exchange of *speaker meanings* (Chapter 4). Figuring out a speaker's message or intent involves relating an utterance to an external or internal context. Disciplined explanations of any linguistic communication begin with theories of language processing. We use the same cognitive system when talking to each other in an everyday setting. Pragmatically speaking, a cognitive system operates in context, and *inference* is the mechanism that utilizes context to extract conveyed meaning from an utterance.

Nonliteral Interpretation

Researchers study speaker meaning in contexts where it is likely to differ from literal meaning. Chapter 4 introduced metaphor as a means of studying differences between literal and conveyed meaning. Contrary to people with aphasia, people with RHD preferred literal meanings over nonliteral meanings (Winner & Gardner, 1977). People with RHD had more difficulty understanding idioms (Van Lancker & Kempler, 1987). Many people with RHD take on a trait of "extreme literalness" in their reactions to others. Looking at automatic processing, Tompkins (1990) found that people with RHD are able to make metaphoric interpretations of individual words (e.g., associating *sharp* with *smart*). Thus, automatic activation appears to be intact, and difficulty shows up in slower strategic tasks.

Hiram Brownell, a psychologist at Boston College, added **indirect requests** and **sarcasm** to the study of metaphor. Using off-line methods, his research team presented situations called "vignettes," and participants made judgments about concluding statements. In one study, vignettes ended with an indirect request (e.g., "Can you . . . ?"). RHDs made a few mistakes but still used context to comprehend an indirect message (Weylman, Brownell, Roman, & Gardner, 1989). In another study, vignettes ended with a comment that, depending on the context, could be interpreted literally or sarcastically (e.g., *You sure are a good golfer*). RHDs had difficulty detecting sarcasm and thought, literally, that a sarcastic positive statement makes a person feel better (Kaplan, Brownell, Jacobs, et al., 1990). Later in this chapter, we shall return to this insensitivity to the beliefs and desires of others, restated as impaired "theory of mind."

Tompkins and others (1994) saw the sporting acceptance of sarcasm as requiring revision of an initial interpretation, and they wondered if this heightened demand on processing is related to working memory capacity. To understand this notion of **inference revision**, introduced for aphasia in Chapter 4, let us examine two versions of a short story presented to participants:

> (1a) Nan invited her new neighbor, Mark, to a party.
>   He told hilarious stories, and everyone enjoyed listening.
>   Nan's husband said to her, "Good decision. He's really fun to have around."
> (1b) Nan invited her new neighbor, Mark, to a party.
>   He told boring stories, and no one enjoyed listening.
>   Nan's husband said to her, "Good decision. He's really fun to have around."

Story *1a* is congruent in that the second and third sentences convey a positive mood, whereas *1b* was incongruent in that the second and third sentences are inconsistent with respect to mood. Yet *1b* is coherent when the husband's comment is interpreted as sarcasm (thus, requiring revision of an initial interpretation).

Tompkins tested comprehension with yes/no questions after each story, and she also measured working memory capacity. Results showed that incongruent sarcasm (*1b*) was more difficult to comprehend than the other stories for all groups. For RHDs, working memory had its highest correlation with the incongruent condition. It appeared that inference revision is strenuous for people with RHD.

Some people with RHD also have difficulty inferring the implications of situations. This deficit was suggested by a content analysis of descriptions of the Cookie Theft picture. Myers (1979) looked for literal content (e.g., a woman) and interpretive concepts (e.g., "She is the mother"). RHDs produced fewer interpretive concepts than normal. In another study, RHDs omitted inferences that fill in transitions between frames of cartoon stories (Joanette, Goulet, Ska, & Nespoulous, 1986). However, Tompkins (1995) warned about going overboard in expecting that all people with RHD will be insensitive to situations (e.g., Stemmer, Giroux, & Joanette, 1994).

How RHDs deal with pictured situations may be indicators of how they would handle natural communicative situations. What if we could present videos of professional actors in conversation? This is the stimuli contained in ***The Awareness of Social Inference Test–Revised*** (*TASIT-R*) developed by McDonald, Flanagan, and Rollins (2011) in Australia. Part 1 involves interpreting emotional displays. Parts 2 and 3 are for social inference by distinguishing literal and nonliteral intentions. First, there are questions about sincere and sarcastic enchanges. Then other vignettes assess the utilization of situational cues to discern true intentions. Psychometric properties of validity and reliability were reported for the first version of the test (McDonald, Bornhofen, Shum, et al., 2006).

Bridging Inference

Two investigations focused on inferring relations between propositions. McDonald and Wales (1986) presented sentence-triplets. Upon hearing *The bird is in the cage* and then *The cage is under the table*, would people think they also heard an inferred *The bird is under the table*? RHDs recognized true inferences as often as true facts. However, another presentation of triplets exposed a deficit. Participants first heard *Barbara became too bored to finish the history book* and then *She had already spent five years writing it*. Would the third sentence be considered to be true (i.e., *Barbara became bored writing a history book*)? RHDs made more errors with inferences than with factual statements (Brownell, Potter, Bihrle, et al., 1986). Such inferences became known as a *bridging inference*, involving recognition of a meaningful connection between sentences.

Using a cross-modal priming task to explore automaticity of inferencing, Beeman (1993) concluded that RHDs are slow or fail to activate concepts necessary to build the bridge, which became known as *activation theory*. Tompkins and her team followed with a strictly auditory priming task in which the target word was presented after a short story. Example *2* shows the last two sentences of a story about Roger going to a lake for a swim:

> (2) Roger did not know that there was a lot of glass there.
>   The lifeguard came running when Roger called for help.

One target pertained to the bridging inference that Roger stepped on the glass (e.g., *cut*). Another target was semantically related only to the second sentence (e.g., *drown*). RHDs were primed by the presumed activation of bridging inferences, leading to rejection of Beeman's theory of failed activation. Yet the semantically related targets were not primed, indicating a preference for the bridging inference. Bridging inference dominated interpretation of the final sentence, and alternative meanings were suppressed (Tompkins, Fassbinder, Lehman Blake, et al., 2004).

Discourse

Although there was a hint of linguistic context in discussing cognitive pragmatics, the emphasis was on the mechanism of inference. This section takes broader aim at strings of sentences. With their clinical test of discourse comprehension (see Chapter 6), Nicholas and Brookshire (1995a) found that RHDs recalled explicit information better than implied information. However, people with aphasia and neurologically intact controls had the same pattern, indicating that this strategy of assessment may not detect differences between brain-damaged groups.

Thinking of the level of discourse, Brownell (1988) contrasted RHDs with LHDs according to a simple but powerful framework. He suggested that "aphasic patients often appear to understand more of a conversation or story than one would expect given their impairments with words and sentences, and RHD patients appear to understand less than one would expect given their intact linguistic skills" (p. 249). Once clinicians and researchers started paying attention to people with RHD, it was noticed that they "miss the point" of proverbs and narratives and tend to "wander from the point" when telling a story.

Comprehension

We usually depend on cohesion and coherence for following discourse. Bridging inference is a top-down mechanism for detecting cohesion. Assessment, however, is usually limited to reading paragraphs and asking questions about what someone can remember. Conclusions are limited to diagnosing areas of difficulty. The study of RHD in this regard is not highly developed, and we must be satisfied for now with a few courageous but disjointed attempts.

Jokes were an early device used to study detection of general coherence in stories. A conclusion becomes a punch line because of surprise relative to expectations in the body of a joke and coherence relative to a theme. In their first study, Brownell and others (1983) tried to separate surprise from coherence. After hearing the body of a joke, participants selected a conclusion from choices containing a punch line, a surprising nonsequitur, and two coherent conclusions (e.g., *3*). When RHDs fail to choose the correct punch lines, do they err in favor of surprise or coherence?

> (3) BODY: The neighborhood borrower approached Mr. Smith on Sunday afternoon and asked if Mr. Smith would be using his lawnmower. "Yes, I am," Smith answered warily. The neighborhood borrower then replied:
> CORRECT: "Fine, then you won't be needing your golf clubs. I'll just borrow them."
> SURPRISE: "You know, the grass is greener on the other side."
> NEUTRAL COHERENCE: "Do you think I could use it when you're done?"
> SAD COHERENCE: "Gee, if I only had enough money I could buy my own."

Asked to pick the funny conclusion, RHDs chose the punch line 60 percent of the time. Neurologically intact controls got the joke 81 percent of the time. Therefore, RHDs were deficient but not devoid of a sense of humor. In their errors, they chose surprise over coherence, indicating that RHDs may have a problem with the coherence feature of a narrative (see also Bihrle, Brownell, Powelson, & Gardner, 1986).

A few studies addressed sensitivity to overall macrostructure of a discourse. RHDs had difficulty arranging sentences into a story (Delis, Wapner, Gardner, et al., 1983) and sequencing frames of cartoons (Huber & Gleber, 1982). In one study, the crucial thematic statement for a story was put at its usual position at the beginning or at an unusual position at the end. Participants were tested for recalling main ideas (Hough, 1990). For normal controls, there was no effect of delaying the theme. However, RHDs scored much better when the theme was early than when the theme was delayed. Hough decided that the RHDs were "unable to utilize the macrostructure as an organizer in apprehending the paragraph" (p. 271). Another possibility is that RHDs recognize familiar story structure, and exceptions create hardships for top-down application of common macrostructure.

Discourse Production

The earliest descriptions of discourse production after RH stroke were swift and general. Eisenson (1962) characterized it as "empty." Picture descriptions and narratives were not as informative as we would expect normally (Joanette et al., 1986). Some individuals were verbose, whereas others exhibited a paucity of utterance. Some were extremely literal and focused on detail (Trupe & Hillis, 1985). The following example starts a lengthy description of the Boston Exam's Cookie Theft picture:

> Well, it's on $8\frac{1}{2} \times 11$ inch paper overall covered by plastic. Looks like it may have been done with drawing pens and India ink on white paper. It's less than 20 pound paper. Else you wouldn't have used black to keep it from shining through . . . (p. 94)

Soon investigators wanted to be more specific than noting that discourse is verbose, literal, and empty.

The evaluation of discourse production has two key elements, namely the method of eliciting a sample and the method of analysis (Chapter 4). We can elicit a type of discourse without analyzing the features that make it coherent. The study of RHD has been quite varied. For a while, picture elicitation was used more often than spontaneous conditions. Narrative was the most frequently studied type of discourse, and content analysis was used more than cohesion or macrostructural analyses (Davis, O'Neil-Pirozzi, & Coon, 1997).

RHDs have been said to wander from the point or theme when telling stories. In several studies, autobiographical stories and story retelling included what researchers classified as event-sequence errors, confabulations, digressions, and embellishments (Gardner, Brownell, Wapner, et al., 1983; Rivers & Love, 1980). In script production, some were tangential, and others terminated too soon (Roman, Brownell, Potter, et al., 1987). RHDs were deficient in cohesion and number of episodes (Uryase, Duffy, & Liles, 1991). On the other hand, Bloom and others (1995) found that RHDs were not deficient in telling stories with respect to completeness, logic, and having a beginning, middle, and end. Perhaps, different definitions of discourse characteristics took investigators down roads to different conclusions.

Some difficulties were exposed when telling a story from cartoons. One cartoon, the "Flower Pot Story," shows a man walking his dog when a falling flower pot hits him on the head. He gets angry and storms into the building where the pot came from. After rapping on a door, a female culprit appears. She is nice to his dog, and he tips his cap gentlemanly without mentioning the bump on his head (from Huber & Gleber, 1982; see also Snow, Douglas, & Ponsford, 1995). Here are two versions from individuals with RHD (Davis et al., 1997):

> It looks like the man is out walking his pet dog, and it looks kinda like he's lost, and he's looking for help. So he goes banging on one of the doors, and a lady opens her door, and out runs her pet. Looks like he's asking her for directions, and she gives 'em to him (pp. 202–203).

> The first one it looks like he's returning home with a stray dog. He takes him in. The third one. Fourth one, he's banging on the door. Fifth one, he's giving the dog a bone. Sixth one, he seem to be pleased with him. And the dog is taking off with his bone (p. 204).

The first one is a good story with a theme, characters, and related resolution. Yet it is the wrong story with an incorrect detail about the pet. The second version is also the wrong story and has inaccurate details and missteps with pronouns. The pictures are treated as independent entities leading to less logical coherence than the first story.

Davis was concerned that the participants with RHD had problems with visual stimuli. These individuals were more accurate when retelling a story than when narrating from cartoons (see also Marini, Carlomagno, Caltagirone, et al., 2005). Our picture of discourse with RHD may depend on our choice of methods for elicitation as well as on our level of analysis. Like assessment of naming objects or any other linguistic skill, we are cautious about diagnosing based on one story or one type of task.

Conversation

A few impairments discussed so far anticipate problems in conversation, such as recognizing the emotions of others and failure to infer meanings and intentions. RHDs even had difficulty deciding whether a speaker should refer to someone formally (e.g., *Mr. Smith*) or informally (e.g., *Bob*; Brownell, Pincus, Blum, et al., 1997). Do people with RHD wander from the point in conversation? Brady and her colleagues (2003, 2005) examined interviews in addition to other discourse production. There were no consistent or widespread differences between RHDs and control participants in topic coherence or management. There was minimal tangential utterance. Although an interview is more structured than other types of conversation, Brady considered the findings to be a striking contrast to the prevailing impression that veering off topic is common in those with RHD.

Kennedy (2000) wondered if irrelevant information or tangential utterances would occur in a more natural type of interaction. RHDs engaged in a *first-encounter conversation* with a stranger. Because conversation frequently becomes an interview in the clinic, Kennedy's instructions are of interest:

- *For the RHD participants:* "I would like you to meet someone that you have not met before . . . This is not an interview, so she doesn't have a list of questions to ask you . . ."
- *For the SLP partner:* "This is not an interview. Converse as you would with anyone you have met for the first time. Allow the participant to initiate topics . . . Do not take notes . . ." (p. 76)

Analysis divided conversation into three phases, namely initiation, maintenance, and termination.

Some RHDs could not be distinguished from controls. Only two of eight RHDs' topics could be coded as off-list or misplaced. Four of the RHDs produced more off-list and misplaced topics in the termination of conversation. These four had difficulty terminating the interaction, especially after their partners attempted termination.

Humor energizes social interaction. Heath and Blonder (2005) wondered if the laboratory findings of Brownell and others might be observed in natural settings. The researchers compared people with RHD and LHD in semistructured interviews, and then independent raters coded humor events. The raters did not come up with a problem in the participants with RHD, but spouses rated them as being different in the telling of funny stories following their strokes. Heath and Blonder interpreted these mixed results as pointing to limitations of their interview rating methodology, rather than a lack of evidence for humor reduction in RHDs' interactions at home.

Taking the point-of-view of others is essential for effective communication. It helps a speaker to encode new information relative to old or known information. It helps a listener decode a speaker's intent. This well-known ability has been labeled as **theory of mind** (ToM). Initially conceived as a construct for understanding autism, ToM is defined as the ability to infer another person's mental states (Tompkins, Scharp, Fassbinder, et al., 2008; Weed, McGregor, Nielsen, et al., 2010). Because facial expression and prosody are cues to a person's mental state, it has been predicted that RHD should include a weakened ToM (e.g., Brownell, Griffin, Winner, et al., 2000; Martin & McDonald, 2003). *The Awareness of Social Inference Test* (*TACIT*) contains tests of ToM (McDonald et al., 2011).

A failure to take the point-of-view of another was demonstrated when RHDs had difficulty with recognizing the beliefs of one character about another when telling lies or ironic jokes (Winner, Brownell, Happé, et al., 1998). A well-known test is the Sally-Ann marble-in-basket scenario in which children are asked where Sally will look for a marble that had been moved by Ann. The answer could be from Sally's or Ann's perspective. In Italy, RHDs and LHDs were given a "Smarties test." The participant was shown a Smarties candy box filled with pencils and then was asked what a third person entering the room would say is in the box. From the (egocentric) viewpoint of the participant, it would be pencils. Recognizing the viewpoint of the third person, the correct answer is candy. LHDs were nearly normal in recognizing the other viewpoint. RHDs were worse than the other groups. RHDs were tagged as having a theory of mind deficit (Cutica, Bucciarelli, & Bara, 2006).

Clinical Assessment

Once someone with RH stroke agrees to be evaluated, the first stop is likely to be clinical neuropsychology and maybe the WAIS-IV. Hopefully, the clinical neuropsychologist and SLP have agreed on the importance of looking for communicative difficulties, and the client is referred to speech-language services. An SLP is likely to begin with familiar tests of language ability that were designed for assessing aphasia. Having read this chapter, clinicians would spend some time with discourse-level subtests and would take notes on how the client interacts in conversation and in testing.

Traditional Language Assessments

Standardization samples for some aphasia batteries included people with RHD. The *Western Aphasia Battery* (*WAB*) was given to 53 of these individuals (Kertesz, 1979). This group had an average Aphasia Quotient (AQ) of 92.9, which is slightly beneath the cutoff score of 93.8 for impairment and well above the 53.5 average for stroke-related aphasia. Many were normal, but others were somewhat below the cutoff. On the *Porch Index of Communicative Ability* (*PICA*), RHDs had an average overall score of 13.03 compared to 11.12 for people with aphasia (Wertz & Dronkers, 1994).

For those who enjoy the *PICA*'s numbers, Porch and Palmer (1986) produced percentile conversion tables based on 94 RHDs (see also Davis, 2007a). Some differential diagnostic impressions can be drawn from comparing the RHDs to LHDs. First, as severity of deficit increases, the difference between aphasia and RHD becomes more pronounced, at least, quantitatively. Above the 60th percentile, RHDs' spoken language falls into the normal range of 13.48 to 15.03, whereas LHDs are impaired (i.e., 12.30). The gap is a bit wider at the 25th percentile (RHD 12.56, LHD 6.04), showing that severe RHD maintains substantial language production ability.

Second, relative to aphasia, comparative deficit is reversed for the test of copying shapes in which RHDs have scores lower than writing. RHDs' drawing difficulty is especially striking, considering that these individuals are not likely to have paralysis of their preferred (right) hand, whereas many people with aphasia attempt to draw with their weakened right hand.

Long ago, research gave us an idea of how people with RHD would do on an aphasia test. Starting with comprehension, people with RHD understand words but with a hint of semantic difficulty (Coughlan & Warrington, 1978; Hagoort, Brown, & Swaab, 1995). We need not expect people with RHD to be limited in short-term memory (Tanridag, Kirshner, & Casey, 1987) nor in taking the Token Test (Hartje, Kerschensteiner, Poeck, et al., 1973). Judgment tasks indicated that grammatical knowledge is intact (Grossman & Haberman, 1982; Schwartz, Linebarger, Saffran, et al., 1987). Off-line sentence comprehension difficulty may appear when we test RHDs for thematic roles in passive sentences (Heeschen, 1980).

For language production, we should find that naming common objects is within or close to the normal range (e.g., Germani & Pierce, 1995). Word-finding aberrations appear with divergent word fluency tests (e.g., Wertz, Dronkers, & Shubitowski, 1986).

Difficulty with word-stream generation across clinical populations led to the inclusion of this task in the cognition pretest of the *Comprehensive Aphasia Test* (Chapter 5).

A close look at word fluency deficits with RHD showed that reduction of productivity occurs after the first 30 seconds, when a person becomes more strategic or contemplative (Joanette, Goulet, & Le Dorze, 1988). Compared to people with aphasia, RHDs generated more clusters of related items, but many items were more peripheral to a category. For example, SPORTS elicited "waterskiing, sailing, swimming," instead of *baseball* or *football* (Grossman, 1981). For word production, people with RHD appear to live on the edge of semantic fields.

RHD does not allow people to escape difficulty with some language-related activities, especially when overall dysfunction is severe. However, we realize that a low score on an aphasia-dedicated test does not necessarily mean that the person has aphasia. This chapter has indicated how someone with RHD can make mistakes on language tasks for reasons other than having a language disorder or aphasia (e.g., neglect dyslexia).

RHD-Dedicated Assessment

A few SLPs hurried to provide us with assessments for RHD during the nascent stage of the experimental study of this population. First published in 1985, the ***Rehabilitation Institute of Chicago Evaluation of Communication Problems in Right Hemisphere Dysfunction*** (*RICE*) was modified for a second edition (Halper, Cherney, & Burns, 1996). Its Pragmatic Communication Skills Rating Scale consists of 10 four-point ratings for nonverbal and verbal communication (e.g., facial expression, turn taking, topic maintenance). Another scale addresses awareness of illness, attention, orientation, and recent memory.

Soon after in 1988, the ***Right Hemisphere Language Battery*** (*RHLB*) was published, also later in a second edition (Bryan, 1995). The test assesses lexical-semantic comprehension, inference generation, and comprehension of metaphor and humor. Other components are for production of emphatic stress and conversational discourse. Independent researchers used the test to study people with RH tumors. An absence of differences pre- and postoperatively led the investigators to decide that they could not recommend this battery for diagnosis or measuring recovery (Thomson, Taylor, Fraser, et al., 1997b).

The ***Mini Inventory of Right Brain Injury*** (*MIRBI-2*) first appeared in 1989 (Pimental & Knight, 2000). It is a brief screening for primary cognitive impairments and pragmatic abilities with affective language, humor, and metaphor.

Two psychologists developed the ***Right Hemisphere Communication Battery*** (*RHCB*; Gardner & Brownell, 1986). Its subtests are distributed within four parts: Humor (Pictorial Humor, Verbal Humor, Humor Production), Emotion (Prosody), Nonliteral Language (Indirect Requests, Pictorial Metaphors, Verbal Metaphors, Inferences), and Integrative Processes (Sarcasm, Alternative Word Meanings, Narrative Comprehension). A Hebrew adaptation was given to RHDs, LHDs, and healthy controls. Only two subtests distinguished clinical groups, and it was the LHDs who did worse. Scores correlated better with the *WAB*'s Cortical Quotient (CQ) than the Aphasia Quotient (AQ; Zaidel, Kasher, Soroker, et al., 2002).

Zaidel's results pose some problems for the RHCB and, perhaps, other batteries for the RHD population. Although the research forming the basis for the RHCB had shown deficits for RHDs, the test may not tap into problems unique to RHD. The test may more likely be a measure of general cognitive functions performed by the LH as well as the RH. The study of this elusive population, some of whom do not believe they have problems, is still fresh and scattered. Test developers may have, idiomatically speaking, jumped the gun a little bit.

Supplemental Assessments

Given that many people with RHD have pragmatic impairments, we can marshal the pragmatic supplements of Chapter 6 and draw from the research presented throughout this chapter. The latter is the source of content for the RHD-dedicated batteries. Reviewing the previous sections, we find assessment strategies for visuospatial neglect, constructional apraxia, amusia, neglect dyslexia, aprosodia, and situational inferencing.

With respect to supplemental tests in Chapter 6, we would be most interested in those oriented to the communicative difficulties in RHD. The *Discourse Comprehension Test* (*DCT*) has been used for this population, but its validity as a measure of inferencing has been challenged (Tompkins, Meigh, Gibbs Scott, et al., 2009). Tompkins and others (2012) have used story retelling subtests of the *Arizona Battery for Communication Disorders in Dementia* (see Chapter 13). *Communication Abilities of Daily Living* (*CADL-2*) contains components relevant for RHD such as contextual communication and brief tests of metaphor and humor. The *Communicative Effectiveness Index* (*CETI*) and the *Amsterdam-Nijmegen Everyday Language Test* (*ANELT*) may supplement McDonald's *TASIT-R* in assessing situation-related communication.

Myers (1999) was particularly concerned about measuring severity and recovery, exemplified by her scene coding for left neglect. She also applied a narrative analysis to descriptions of the Cookie Theft picture that comes with the Boston Exam. We can identify the client who produces literal concepts to the exclusion of interpretive concepts, and then we can count interpretive concepts for documenting recovery.

Treatment

Treatment for RHD is an underdeveloped territory (Lehman Blake, 2005, 2007). Authors suggest that research paradigms *may* become therapies. As Tompkins and others (2012) put it, "the RHD treatment literature contains a gaping hole where an evidence base should be" (p. 703). Lehman Blake (2007) suggested that "in the absence of evidence for treatments designed for communication deficits associated with RHD, treatments may be derived from hypotheses or theories of right hemisphere processes"

(p. 333). Recommendations usually follow the logic of aphasia rehabilitation so that each problem area of RHD would be treated in two ways:

- Stimulation/facilitation of an impaired process
- Teaching compensatory strategies to bypass an impairment

Consistent with our traditional scope of practice, stimulation might focus on metaphor and discourse level functions. Compensatory strategies capitalize on the language abilities of the undamaged hemisphere.

Like therapy for aphasia, SLPs emphasize improvement in communication and strive to select activities that are important in an individual's daily life (i.e., client-centered approach). Anita Halper, Leora Cherney, and Martha Burns have been particularly active in the Chicago area in developing treatments for RHD (Halper et al., 1996; Cherney & Halper, 2007). Rehabilitation begins with having an awareness of difficulty.

Awareness and Orientation

We tend to provide language treatment only for those who want it. A patient should be aware of a communication problem to make sense of a referral to an SLP. A number of people with RH stroke are aware of their difficulties. Mildly impaired individuals become aware of a problem, such as mechanical prosody, once it is defined for them (Myers, 1999).

Our first thought might be to consider self-monitoring tasks that we try with Wernicke's aphasia and lack of awareness of jargon. Kortte and Hillis (2009) cited a similar approach for anosognosia for hemiplegia. A therapist provided video feedback of a motor assessment for an individual with AHP persisting 3 weeks poststroke (Fotopoulou, Rudd, Holmes, et al., 2009). Spontaneous recovery of awareness was noted, but Kortte and Hillis recommended further research.

Regarding disorientation, an SLP may assist rehabilitation staff in providing language-oriented compensatory aids (see also Chapters 12 and 13). Improving orientation is important for a person's **safety**. Clocks, calendars, and schedules are prominent in rehabilitation facilities. Hospital staff is trained to remind patients of the date and time. Cherney and Halper (2007) wrote about orientation groups for patients with RHD during acute and subacute rehabilitation.

Spatial Attention and Reading

Let us start with the stimulation treatments and then consider the compensatory strategies. Stimulation for neglect dyslexia is likely to begin by addressing left neglect in general. Application of assessment tasks includes some practice with crossing out items in an array. *Leftward search-and-find activities* are designed to encourage subconscious perception of left space. We ask a client to locate certain colored cubes in a small array. The idea is to set up a simple condition for volitional attention without external cueing, which Myers (1999) believed increases the likelihood of generalization.

Another suggestion is the use of *contiguous stimuli* for picture description or "search and find." These stimuli are coherent only with both sides across the midline (e.g., a couple holding hands). A client is likely to realize that recognition requires shifting attention leftward. For reading, we should remember that the hunt for linguistic meaning is not impaired. Clients read aloud words (e.g., *school*) and sentences (e.g., *Our hats were off to them*) that make sense only with leftward attention.

Compensatory cues encourage leftward scanning, although Myers and Lehman Blake (2008) were not enthusiastic about this strategy for restoring attention. They noted that "verbally cuing the patient to look to the left, highlighting stimuli on the left . . . are rarely effective because while they may improve performance in therapy, they rarely translate into internal self-cues or generalize to more functional tasks" (p. 966). Yet if attention improves slowly, compensatory cues may be helpful. For reading, **anchors** such as colored lines or arrows may be placed on the left side of a page. Letters or numbers may be printed to the right and left of text, and the client is occasionally told to read the letter or number. Some clients may resort to tricks, such as "imagine a little green man on my shoulder, tapping me to remind me" (Andrewes, 2001).

In a *cued line-bisection test*, some lines have letters at the right end, others have letters at the left end, and other lines have these anchors at both ends (Harvey, Milner, & Roberts, 1995). Clients are instructed to name the letters and then bisect the line as accurately as possible. There is a bias toward the cued end, even for people without neglect. Harvey was interested in the effect of these cues for those who already have a tendency to bisect to the right. Unilateral left cues decreased the extent of rightward error as if "dragging" attention leftward. Unilateral right cues did not increase the rightward error.

Prosody

A mildly impaired individual may have a vague sense that he or she does not sound like him- or herself (Myers, 1999). As with most research, most of rehabilitation assumes that aprosodia is linked to emotion. We educate and counsel the client and family regarding the role of prosody in communication and the fact that the flat tone and affect are due to the stroke rather than indifference. A heightened awareness can lead to compensatory strategies by family members who begin to encourage the production of linguistic cues to feelings and meaning.

Comprehension deficits can also be dealt with by linguistic compensatory strategies. We advise families to identify their own moods and emotions verbally and, perhaps, use more words with emotional meaning (e.g., saying "I am happy" in addition to sounding and looking happy). Stimulation drills might begin with a pitch discrimination task, then moving on to identifying melodies and listening to sentences for meaningful pitch variation (e.g., questions versus statements).

Regarding production, restorative practice may begin with imitation of emotionally expressed, semantically neutral sentences. In another task, sentences may represent an emotion in wording, and a client must express the emotion with prosody. A higher-level activity consists of reading a story in which the client identifies and conveys the moods and emotions of the characters. This activity is likely to overlap with working on inference and narrative coherence. A client could follow a script for a play. Acting the parts is analogous to role-playing situations in which certain emotions are common. Also, clients are encouraged to follow the advice given to families with respect to verbal identification of feelings, perhaps, with some role-play in the clinic with the therapist.

Rosenbek and several colleagues (2006) compared two stimulation treatments classified as imitative and cognitive-linguistic for 14 participants mostly with RH stroke. Both therapies targeted prosody for *happy, sad,* and *angry,* and they contained six steps of cueing that were faded from maximal to minimal stimulation. The imitative therapy started with repeating a clinician's model and ended with independent production. In the cognitive-linguistic therapy, participants produced intonation based on the emotion's name, a description of the tone, and a picture of the facial expression. The therapist gradually removed the cards, asking for the same productions. *Fear* was an emotion that was not treated but was measured for generalization.

Because there have been so few studies of communicative therapy for RHD, let us consider some more of the details. The researchers used an ABAC single-case design to determine whether the therapies had any effect on prosody (B = one treatment, C = the other treatment). Each treatment phase was 1 month of 20 sessions, and the second baseline (A) separated the treatments by 1 month. Order of the therapies was balanced across participants. The investigators were also interested in maintenance of effects 1 and 3 months after the therapy.

Twelve of the 14 participants had significant response to at least one of the therapies, and the treatments did not differ in effectiveness. Only four participants were available for follow-up, and each had maintained gains after 1 and 3 months. Unfortunately the effects did not generalize to the untreated emotion. The investigators concluded that the treatments are promising but looked forward to improved experimental designs with multiple baselines or randomized group comparisons. Also, in the future, Chapter 10's principles for maximizing generalization may be applied to the therapies.

Inference and Discourse

Contextual Constraint Treatment consists of two procedures originating in experiments suggestive of two processing impairments that may be related to inferencing and discourse comprehension (Scharp & Tompkins, 2013; Tompkins, Blake, Wambaugh, et al., 2011). To appreciate these procedures, let us backtrack for a while to the experiments that exposed the impairments being addressed. To understand the experiments, we must return to the semantic priming paradigm of Chapter 3.

Tompkins, Fassbinder, and others (2008) indicated that RHDs have difficulty activating the edges of a word's meaning. With a short prime-target interval permitting only automatic processing, primes such as *potatoes* facilitated response to both the closely related target *skin* and to the distant *fluffy*. However, RHDs departed from controls by making more errors for the distant targets. Tompkins began referring to this subtle weakness as a **coarse coding deficit** (Tompkins, Sharp, Meigh, et al., 2008).

Thinking about the pragmatic implications of lexical-semantic deficits, Tompkins compared coarse coding in semantic priming to two assessments of discourse comprehension. The coarse coding task did not correlate with the two discourse tasks. However, a subgroup that was poor at sustaining activation of distant meanings was also poor at comprehending implied information in narratives. So, in some cases, lexical-semantic deficit may be related to inferencing difficulty (Tompkins, Scharp, Meigh, et al., 2008).

The other process is the context-driven selection of an appropriate meaning, which Tompkins calls suppression (of the inappropriate meanings). Immediately on contact with an ambiguous word, people automatically activate multiple meanings. In her lab at McGill University, Baum inserted short intervals between ambiguous primes (remember *fan*?) and multiple targets (e.g., *breeze, sport*), and RHDs activated multiple meanings automatically (Klepousniotou & Baum, 2005). Another study considered that a biased context normally leads to inhibiting inappropriate meanings. Contrary to LHDs, who activated both meanings immediately regardless of context, RHDs activated only the most frequent meaning immediately regardless of context, and given more time, only the most frequent meanings remained active (Grindrod, 2012; Grindrod & Baum, 2003). The investigators concluded that RHDs can be impervious to context and rely on lexical familiarity to activate meanings selectively.

Tompkins and her colleagues (2000; Fassbinder & Tompkins, 2001) studied the inhibition of meanings activated by ambiguities like *spade* (e.g., playing cards, garden tools). The task was different, not the familiar lexical decision. RHDs made judgments as to whether a target (e.g., CARDS) was related to the meaning of the preceding sentence:

(4a) He dug with a *spade*. CARDS
(4b) He dug with a *shovel*. CARDS

The correct judgment was *no* for both conditions. With a short interval, the *no* should take longer with *4a* than with *4b* because an ambiguous word like *spade* activates its multiple meanings automatically. These meanings should delay the judgment. Suppression of inappropriate meanings requires more time and, therefore, should show up with a longer interval through equal response times between conditions.

So, how did the RHDs do? They activated meanings automatically, as in one of Baum's studies. Yet contrary to healthy controls, RHDs also had a longer response with ambiguous primes at the longer interval. Thus, multiple meanings continued to be active, indicating that many of the RHDs failed to suppress alternate meanings when given time to do so. A second deficit became known as faulty suppression of inappropriate meanings or, simply, **suppression deficit**. Kennedy (2000) entertained the possibility that suppression deficit may cause tangential or off-topic utterance. Faulty suppression is somewhat inconsistent with Baum's other finding of frequency-based selectivie activation and with the previously mentioned study of bridging inference in which alternative meanings were suppressed (Tompkins et al., 2004).

Based on the priming experiments, Tompkins concluded that, depending on site of lesion, RHDs can have either a coarse coding disorder (parietal lesion) or a suppression disorder (frontal lesion). The procedure for coarse coding deficit consisted of computer controlled *priming* of semantically related targets for lexical decision. The procedure for stimulating suppression, like the experiment, consisted of making a quick *relatedness judgment* about a target and a prime. Strength of contextual bias was manipulated. Participants improved on the treatment tasks, but only one was evaluated for generalization. That individual improved in narrative comprehension but not in metaphor interpretation (Tompkins et al., 2011, 2012).

"There is no test yet for use in clinical practice to distinguish a coarse coding deficit from a deficit in . . . suppression" (Tompkins et al., 2012, p. 690). Probably before we worry about this, the inconsistencies between priming and inference should be resolved, and the deficits need to be validated by investigators in other laboratories. Yet Tompkins and her colleagues have provided an intriguing look into the application of contemporary psycholinguistic science. The treatments require software that is not beyond modern clinical practice.

Assuming that activation of multiple meanings and inhibition of inappropriate meanings are processes that contribute to inference, Myers (1999) had some suggestions that are more strategically explicit than Tompkins's implicit tasks. So-called activation tasks are intended to stimulate the generation of alternate meanings. One example is to have a client provide two meanings for semantically ambiguous words such as *bank*. Investigators were particularly worried about the ability to revise an initial interpretation that turns out to be inappropriate for the context. So-called suppression tasks are intended to stimulate inhibition. We instruct a client to produce one meaning for an ambiguous word as quickly as possible, particularly words for which two meanings are equally common.

Metaphor helps us get a handle on inference for comprehending nonliteral expression in general. Brownell's research group in Boston tackled therapy with five RHDs. The goal was to comprehend novel metaphors such as *The project is a monster*, and *A family is a cradle*. These metaphors are deconstructed so that that the subject noun (e.g., *family*) is a topic and the predicate (e.g., *cradle*) is a vehicle for the metaphor. Understanding comes from linking shared characteristics such as [*comforting*]. This common analysis of novel metaphors provided the basis for a "structured semantic training."

The training was a series of tasks for constructing nonliteral interpretations. Stimuli were shown in a diagram containing a central bubble linked to surrounding satellite bubbles. The first task oriented a client by showing a word like *father* in a solitary central bubble, then asking the client if other words might be related in any way (e.g., *strong*). In the third activity, like Myers's activation task, clients generated associate words to put in the satellite bubbles. The fourth task added a second central bubble that contained a vehicle following the first bubble's topic. The client would generate more associations. This set up the final task in which possible shared features of the topic and vehicle were shown, and the client picked the best one. All clients improved in novel metaphor comprehension (Lundgren, Brownell, Cayer-Meade, et al., 2011). Simplified, we can take advantage of retained language skills with a **let's**

TABLE 11.1   **Examples of inference and discourse tasks (Myers, 1999).**

SKILL	TASKS
Inference generation	Create titles for pictures or stories Provide the ending to a story Tell what a cartoon is about Discuss the meaning of a painting
Integration/organization	Identify fragmented objects Puzzles Arrange pictures or sentences into a story

discuss activity. What could "this project" (or any topic) and "monster" (or any vehicle) have in common?

With other manifestations of inferencing, a client can contemplate the implicit meaning of a Rockwell drawing. The client can work on recognizing and explaining what is funny about a cartoon or written joke. Then we can shift to narrative, which has an apparent macrostructure that is often implicit and, thus, has to be inferred. A client can figure out the global theme of a news story in an attempt to think of a headline, or the client can generate a news story when given a headline. A few suggestions are listed in Table 11.1.

Some therapy consists of conversation. In aphasia treatment, conversation is an authentic context in which to build confidence in improving language processes or adaptive strategies. For RHDs, the same principle holds for generalization of task-related improvements of prosody. On the other hand, elements of conversation, such as turn-taking or staying on topic, also become targets of treatment. Cherney and Halper (2007) reported on how this is done in various groups (i.e., high-level cognitive group, life skills group, and pragmatics group). The pragmatics group, for example, begins with identifying turns and topics in videotaped conversations. The life skills group takes on problem solving and self-monitoring in everyday situations.

Recovery and Outcomes

General characteristics of recovery with RHD follow the path that is typical for stroke, namely a period of spontaneous recovery for a few weeks or months followed by a slowing of the rate of progress. However, we do not have a picture of changes in key communicative functions with RHD. Some of the tests for communication deficits in RHD may not be built for measuring recovery in the way that the *PICA* and *WAB* were constructed for aphasia (Thomson et al., 1997b).

Although little outcome research has been reported for RHD, experienced clinicians tend to recommend using currently available tests and scales for documenting general functional status and quality of life. SLPs specializing in the right hemisphere also borrow from the cognitive rehabilitation of traumatic brain injury, partly because areas of deficit are similar. Is the person functioning independently at home? Has the individual returned to work and maintained employment?

Odell and others (2005) noted that studies of RHD focus on the relationship between left neglect (or hemi-inattention) and outcome. People with left neglect have had lower outcomes than those without neglect (e.g., Cherney, Halper, Kwasnica, et al., 2001). Odell studied Functional Independence Measures (FIMs) administered at the discharge of 101 persons with RHD. The RHDs had received treatment in a rehabilitation unit of a hospital. Neglect was not a significant predictor of outcome. The best predictors were initial severity and age. Motor items showed more recovery than cognitive items but were also more severely impaired.

Summary and Conclusions

Right-hemisphere dysfunction (RHD) is an umbrella term for numerous cognitive impairments that do not necessarily occur with each other. This chapter provided brief encounters with deficits of self-awareness, visuospatial attention, orientation to surroundings, constructional skills, melody processing, and emotion processing. Some language behaviors, such as aprosodias, are a result of these disorders. Difficulties in activation of alternative meanings and in taking the perspective of others may be the basis for pragmatic deficits in inferencing (getting the point) and managing conversation (staying on point). Supporting information is found elsewhere. It begins with cognitive pragmatics in Chapter 4, includes functional assessments of Chapter 6 as well as principles of treatment beginning in Chapter 8.

The recognition of communication disorders with RHD may create an expectation that these individuals would be referred to SLPs more often than they are. Hospitals may refer all stroke cases to the SLP for swallowing evaluation and to ensure personal safety before discharge. An individual's nonchalance may make us reluctant to check for communication problems.

This nonchalance may also be making treatment research for RHD hard to find. Tompkins and Rosenbek referred to their experiments as Phase I (or Level 1) studies. Regarding their own therapies, "clearly, systematic replication and group studies with random assignment are necessary before confident treatment recommendations can be made" (Rosenbek et al., 2006, p. 386). Most of the suggestions for RHD treatment in this chapter, although they make sense according to traditional therapeutic logic, have not even reached Phase I scrutiny. There is lots of research to be done in this area.

The lack of real rehabilitation stories is more troubling. We might be more confident if we could fall back on a substantial body of case studies illustrating exactly how it went with clients. What convinced an individual to participate in treatment? How was awareness dealt with? What were the goals? What were the pitfalls? What was the outcome?

CHAPTER 12

Traumatic Brain Injury

It was kind of a freak accident. I was on a motorcycle and I didn't have my helmet buckled. I just put it on, you know, and didn't buckle it. I was comin' down the road, and there's like an island in the road, you know, there was an island with two telephone poles in the middle, and I bounced off both those poles. Bounced off and flew forty feet through the air and lost my helmet in the meantime. And my brains were leaking out on the ground, and then I got to the hospital, and I was in a coma for four months. I was supposed to croak but I didn't. I fooled them all.

Traumatic brain injury (TBI) impairs cognitive functions that have a broad reach. These general cognitive systems include attention, memory, and a resource management capacity called the executive system. After 18 years of examining 2,500 head-injured cases, Hagen (1981) sorted them into three general diagnostic categories:

- Residual cognitive impairment without language dysfunction
- Disorganized language secondary to cognitive impairments
- Predominant language-specific disorder, or aphasia

These possibilities indicate TBI can cause aphasia or, like right-hemisphere stroke, can result in language difficulties that are expressions of other cognitive impairments, or an individual can possess an unruly mix of both. The clinician's job is to figure out which is which. One clue is the nature of the trauma.

Head Trauma

TBI is brain damage that is caused by external forces (Ylvisaker, Szekeres, & Feeney, 2008). Another label is acquired brain injury (ABI). Let us stick with "TBI," the most common cause of death for those under age 40 in the United States. The evening news reverberates with stories of trauma from politicians' gunshot wounds to athletes' concussions. Using real cases of TBI, public service announcements warn of the dangers of texting while driving (see Recinto, 2012).

Around 1.4 million TBIs of all kinds occur in the United States annually, leaving over five million living with related disability (Corrigan, Selassie, & Orman, 2010; Langlois, Rutland-Brown, & Wald, 2006). The most typical head-injured person is male, single, with a high school education or less, and between the ages of 15 and 19 years. More than half of the injuries are caused by motor vehicle accidents ("MVA" in the medical report). Falls are the next major cause. The most common contributing factor is alcohol use, and most injuries occur in summer or fall. In one study, 12 percent of head injuries were precipitated by interpersonal violence, most of which were self-inflicted or stemmed from domestic problems (Rimel & Jane, 1983).

If the human skull is placed on the ground and weight is slowly piled on, it can support three tons (Rolak, 1993). It takes violent forces to damage the skull, and the brain can be damaged without harm to the skull. These head injuries have been broadly classified according to whether the skull is displaced, meninges are torn, or cortex is violated. A traditional approach is to distinguish **open** (i.e., penetrating) from **closed** (i.e., nonpenetrating) head injuries. Mechanisms of injury are quite variable (Table 12.1).

Large samples of war-related open head injuries revealed a great deal about cerebral dysfunction. Studies followed World War I (Goldstein, 1942), World War II (Luria, 1966; Newcombe, 1969; Russell & Espir, 1961), and Vietnam (Mohr, Weiss, Caveness, et al., 1980). Small-caliber weapons provided Luria (1970) with "cleanly punched out" lesions to study. High-velocity injuries from modern weapons can be quite devastating, causing extensive *laceration* (i.e., tearing) of brain tissue. Low-velocity traumas are like closed head injuries, except for the laceration of brain tissue when skull fracture is severe. Well-known examples of open head trauma were from bullets that befell Ronald Reagan's press secretary James Brady in 1981 (right-hemisphere dysfunction

TABLE 12.1   A classification of head traumas.

TYPE	DEFINITION	SUBTYPE	DESCRIPTION	CAUSES
Open	Skull fragments penetrate brain tissue	High velocity	Projectiles perforate or pierce the skull, bringing hair and skin with them	Gunshots Explosions
		Low velocity	Concentrated blunt trauma causing skull fracture rather than perforation	Blows to head MVAs
Closed	Foreign substances do not penetrate brain tissue	Acceleration	Unrestrained head struck by moving object or moving head strikes stationary object	Blows to head Falls MVAs
		Nonacceleration	Fixed head struck by moving object	Blows to head

[RHD]) and Arizona congresswoman Gabrielle Giffords in 2011 (left-hemisphere dysfunction [LHD] and aphasia).

Most of this chapter is devoted to **closed head injury** (CHI), including many studies identifying probable closed injuries as "TBI." The damage tends to be **bilateral** and the consequences are unique, contrasting with disorders in previous chapters. Table 12.1 distinguishes acceleration and nonacceleration injuries. The latter are usually less severe than acceleration traumas. Nonacceleration causes *contusion* (i.e., bruising) of the brain's surface at the point of impact, called impression trauma.

The **primary effects** of acceleration traumas occur at the moment of impact. Linear acceleration causes contusion of the cortex both at the point of impact (i.e., *coup* injury) and opposite the point of impact (i.e., *contrecoup* injury). Angular acceleration, however, creates twisting forces and produces more severe injuries. These violent movements damage certain regions consistently. These regions are the **prefrontal area** ("orbital" area behind the forehead) and the anterior and inferior **temporal lobes** (above the sharp bony floor of the skull). Because the lateral walls and roof of the skull are smooth, laceration is uncommon in the superior frontal lobes and the parietal and occipital lobes.

In addition, twisting or stretching forces cause **diffuse axonal injury** (DAI). This stretching (or "shearing") of white fiber tracts within the cerebrum and brain stem occurs more with high-speed traffic accidents than with blows or falls.

The brain's responses to primary trauma are called **secondary effects**. Accumulation of fluid (i.e., edema) over the first few hours causes swelling and pressure. Laceration of blood vessels causes hemorrhages. Pulmonary weakness can reduce blood flow to the brain, causing ischemic damage. A person may be conscious for a while before lapsing into a coma, signifying severe secondary trauma. At a hockey game in Columbus, Ohio, in 2002, a 13-year-old spectator was struck in the forehead by a puck. She was alert when entering the hospital but died 2 days later (SI.com, 2002).

Now, we know what a hospital's trauma unit faces. When a hospital is notified that a trauma patient is on the way, the beepers of the Trauma Team activate simultaneously with a trauma code. All members not occupied with patients proceed immediately to the booth in the emergency room for trauma victims. The trauma surgery attending physician is the team leader. The team includes a senior trauma surgery resident, resuscitator, airway manager, primary nurse, nurse assistant, and X-ray technician.

On the resuscitator's count of three, the team and paramedics transfer the patient from a transport litter to a gurney. The nurse assistant removes clothing and obtains vital signs. The resuscitator directs the team to establish an airway and access to intravenous fluids. The oropharynx and nasopharynx are suctioned for blood, secretions, and foreign matter. When the patient is stabilized, the senior resident develops an evaluation plan. An unstabilized patient is taken immediately to an operating room. Depending on the nature of trauma, the surgeon evacuates subdural hematomas and/or repairs the skull and removes foreign matter. Now, we know what a patient goes through.

The chain of services is similar to treatment for stroke (Ylvisaker et al., 2008). Following stabilization in the emergency room, patients are transferred to intensive care for a short time. Then, they may move to a neurological care ward where they receive early rehabilitation, or depending on the size of the hospital, they may proceed to the hospital's rehabilitation facility for more intensive therapies. Following in-patient rehabilitation, the individual may be discharged to home and may continue treatment as an outpatient or may participate in a community support group.

Mild traumatic brain injury (MTBI or mTBI) is signified by alteration or loss of consciousness for less than 20 minutes. It is a closed head injury and is synonymous with **concussion**. Often there are no findings with neuroimaging. Hospital stay is likely to be no more than 48 hours. MTBI is a hazard in many sports. Subtle cognitive deficits resulting from MTBI are known as *postconcussion syndrome* (PCS) (Barth, Broshek, & Freeman, 2006; Salvatore & Sirmon Fjordbak, 2011).

MTBI has also been a "signature wound" in the wars in the Middle East. It was not until 2011 that the U.S. Purple Heart could be awarded for concussion. Early in 2012, the U.S. Army and the National Football League (NFL) teamed up to promote awareness of this type of injury (Vergun, 2012). MTBI can occur with **blast-related trauma** (or simply "blast injury") caused by improvised explosive devices (IEDs) and other explosives. *Primary blast injuries* are caused by pressure waves in the atmosphere. Fragmentation and other objects in motion cause *secondary blast injuries*, and being hurled against solid objects results in *tertiary blast injuries* (Taber, Warden, & Hurley, 2006; Warden, 2006). These injuries are not well understood, partly because soldiers give the appearance of a quick recovery.

Neuropsychological Assessment

An army of neuropsychological assessments can be brought to bear on the consequences of TBI, including tests mentioned in the previous chapter. Only a small number are likely to be used by a speech-language pathologist (SLP), but it is useful to know something about them in staff meetings and in reports. Also, the tests give us an idea of what clinical professionals believe the mental processes to be. Let us begin with broad assessment of cognition, with more specific tests to follow in sections on attention, memory, and other functions.

Richardson (2000) reviewed several studies of the *Wechsler Adult Intelligence Scale* (*WAIS*) given to people with CHI and found variation in Full Scale IQs among the groups, from 76.3 in one study to 98.0 in another. In the middle, a sample of 263 cases had a mean Full Scale IQ of 83.0, with a Verbal IQ of 85.8, and a Performance IQ of 81.3 (Cullum & Bilger, 1986), which is indicative of a general finding that the performance section is more deficient than the verbal section (Crawford, et al., 1997). With the recovery that is common with CHI, individuals often approach normal or average IQ within 2 years (Table 12.2).

For a quick test of cognition, the *Neurobehavioral Cognitive Status Examination* (*NCSE*) or **Cognistat** assesses intellectual functioning in language, construction, memory, calculation, and reasoning/judgment. It takes 20 to 30 minutes to administer to cognitively impaired patients (Kiernan, Mueller, Langston, et al., 1987). Although

TABLE 12.2   Comparison of 20 persons with closed head injuries (CHI) and 20 matched controls on selected subtests of the WAIS-R. The CHIs had incurred severe injuries at least 18 months prior to testing (Schmitter-Edgecombe, Marks, Fahy, et al., 1992).

		CHI	CONTROLS
Full Scale IQ		95.60	102.80
Verbal IQ	Arithmetic	9.10	9.90
	Similarities	9.35	10.30
	Digit span	9.40	11.35
	Vocabulary	8.40	10.25
Performance IQ	Digit symbol	7.80	12.05
	Block design	10.20	11.40

recommended for the elderly, it may be better suited for younger adults because of its difficulty relative to other screening tests mentioned in the next chapter (Nabors, Millis, & Rosenthal, 1997).

SLPs developed two tests for head injury. One is the **Scales of Cognitive Ability for Traumatic Brain Injury** (*SCATBI*), which contains 41 subtests for perception, orientation, organization, recall, and reasoning. Administration can take 10 to 45 minutes, depending on which tests are given (Adamovich & Henderson, 1992). The other is the **Brief Test of Head Injury** (*BTHI*), which is a screening test that, like Cognistat, can be administered at bedside in 20 to 30 minutes. It contains more subtests for language, such as reading comprehension and naming (Helm-Estabrooks & Hotz, 1990).

For overall functional measurement, the FIM or FIM + FAM are commonly used in rehabilitation settings at admission and discharge in the manner described in Chapter 6. In a study of 965 patients with CHI, seen in several rehabilitation settings, the physical and cognitive sections were found to be reliable (Hawley, Taylor, Hellawell, et al., 1999).

The **Rancho Los Amigos Scale** (*RLA*) has been a popular rating of cognition and behavior (Hagen, 1981). Researchers in speech-language pathology often use the *RLA* to identify the severity of deficit in experimental participants. The scale points range from Level I (unresponsive to all stimuli) to Level VIII (capable of new learning; good remote and recent memory; supervision not needed). In between, for example, Level IV is labeled with the fairly severe portrait of *Confused-agitated* (bizarre behavior, incoherent utterance, short attention span, uncooperative). The scale is sometimes a frame of reference for characterizing phases of recovery. It is accessible with an Internet search and is available as an app for Android (Sutton, 2012).

Sports neuropsychologists developed a cognitive screening approach for MTBI known generally as *computerized response time-based assessment*. At the University of Virginia in the 1980s, researchers started with the "Sports as a Laboratory Assessment Model" (SLAM). In 1993, the Pittsburgh Steelers instituted a similar program

(Lovell, 2006). The goal was to develop a protocol for quickly identifying postconcussion syndrome and determining whether a player should return to a contest (i.e., return-to-play; also return-to-classroom). Premature return to play can result in a serious outcome known as *second impact syndrome* (SIS). Policies regarding concussion management were instituted in 2007 for Major League Baseball and the National Football League. Other professional leagues have policies as well.

Computerized testing, like the widely used **ImPACT** (impacttesting.com), allows large numbers of athletes to be examined at one time. ImPACT, standing for "Immediate Post-Concussion Assessment and Cognitive Testing," was developed in the early 1990s. It takes about 20 minutes and has six subtests ("modules") addressing memory, attention, problem solving, and response time (Iverson, Lovell, & Collins, 2003). Another protocol is **CogSport**. It consists of five tasks covering the same areas but delivered on the computer screen with familiar playing cards (Collie, Maruff, Darby, et al., 2006).

The ***Sport Concussion Assessment Tool*** (*SCAT2*) was developed as a collaborative effort after a conference in Prague in 2004. In addition to guidelines for return-to-play, it contains guidelines for removing an athlete from play. *SCAT2*, available as an app for iPhone and iPad, consists of various techniques such as an athlete interview, Glasgow Coma Scale (introduced shortly), and cognitive tasks for orientation, short-term memory, and delayed memory. Normative data for high school athletes in Seattle, Washington, have been reported for *SCAT2* (Jinguji, Bompadre, Harmon, et al., 2012; for SLP's role, see Salvatore & Sirmon Fjordbak, 2011).

Primary Cognitive Impairments

Specific neuropsychological tests will be introduced in the following presentation of classical cognitive impairments in the areas of attention, memory, and executive function. In relating general dysfunctions to sites of damage with CHI, we can attribute disorders of attention and executive functions to the frontal lobes, and memory problems stem from temporal lobe damage.

Attention

Impaired attention/concentration is the factor found to be most responsible for difficulties with the *WAIS* (e.g., Crawford, et al., 1989). Attention is multifaceted, overlapping with working memory and necessary for resource allocation (Carr & Hinckley, 2012). Attention is a very gross level of awareness, as well as a strategic spotlight (Table 12.3). Some assessments are said to emphasize only one aspect of attention, but it is difficult to test one component without others being involved.

The base level of attention coincides with a physician's first concern, as an emergency patient may be classified quickly as a "talker" or "nontalker." The physician prefers to hear a victim screaming when entering a hospital, but around 25 percent of head-injured people are nontalkers at admission (Rimel & Jane, 1983). These

TABLE 12.3   **Levels and types of attention, applicable to any discussion of this function throughout this text.**

LEVELS AND TYPES	FUNCTION	ASSESSMENT
Arousal	State of consciousness; primitive wakefulness	Gross motor response to sensory stimulation
Awareness	Assumes arousal; from stupor to clear perception of surroundings	Answer questions
Selective attention	Focus; resistance to distraction; managing limited resources by selection	Two stimuli or tasks; response to one (e.g., dichotic listening)
Sustained attention	Vigilance or concentration; maintaining focus on one stimulus for a period of time	A series of stimuli; response to each or a target
Divided attention	Allocating limited resources to multiple processes or tasks	Two stimuli or tasks; response to both (dual-task paradigms)

conditions are initial rough indicators of a person's state of consciousness. Any reduction of consciousness is called a *coma*.

Acute care decisions are based partly on depth of coma, which is commonly assessed with the **Glasgow Coma Scale** (GCS; Jennett & Teasdale, 1981). For a non-talker, pupils are checked for size and reaction to light. A thumb pressed next to an eyebrow might elicit a motor response. Does eye gaze respond to commands? Is respiration abnormal? The talking patient is questioned for awareness of surroundings. Ratings are obtained for eye opening, motor response, and verbal behavior. The maximum "coma score" is 15 (Table 12.4). Depth and duration of coma are rough estimators of severity of injury. Mild traumatic brain injury (MTBI) would produce a GCS rating of 13 to 15. A hospital's protocol may specify that a medically stable patient with a GCS less than 12 should get a CT scan before surgery.

Cortical arousal to any environmental stimulus depends on the reticular activating system (RAS). Axons of the RAS course through the brain stem and then spread evenly to all areas of the cortex. Loss of consciousness is usually attributed to diffuse axonal injury. Once a patient is aroused or conscious, levels of awareness vary from

TABLE 12.4   **Bases for estimating severity of traumatic brain injury (Hannay & Levin, 1989; Jennett &Teasdale, 1981).**

	GCS SCORE	DURATION OF COMA
Mild	13–15	Less than 20 minutes
Moderate	9–12	
Severe	8 or less	More than 24 hours

stupor (or "obtundation") to alertness. An alert patient can still be distractible or can have difficulty focusing attention.

Selective or focused attention may be studied with a **Stroop interference task** in which someone is presumed to suppress a distraction. In color-naming tasks, printed color names are shown in different colors, so that the word *red* might be printed in the colors red or blue. When a participant names an incongruent color (i.e., *blue*), response time can be slowed or misnaming can occur because the person was distracted by the conflicting word. A group with severe CHI 1 to 3 months postinjury was as accurate as controls, indicating that focused attention was intact (Ponsford & Kinsella, 1992).

For assessing focused attention, clinical neuropsychologists may use the Symbol Search subtest in the *WAIS* (Chapter 11) or the ***Trail Making Test*** (*TMT*; Reitan & Wolfson, 1995). In the *TMT*, the simpler Part A consists of randomly displayed, circled numbers that must be connected in sequence. Part B looks like Part A, but a client alternates between circled numbers and letters.

For assessment emphasizing sustained attention, a client may be asked to concentrate on a boring task for 20 or more minutes. In Ponsford and Kinsella's (1992) study, participants watched lights go on and off and pressed a button whenever a target light appeared. The CHI group was again slower but not less accurate than controls, and performance did not deteriorate over duration of the task. The Digit Symbol subtest of the *WAIS* has been used as a measure of concentration, and it produced the largest deficit in Table 12.2.

Divided attention is thought to be evaluated with Letter–Number Sequencing in the *WAIS*, which entails alternating focus. The ***Brief Test of Attention*** (*BTA*) presents lists of alternating letters and numbers, increasing in length from 4 to 18 units, via audiocassette. Form N for numbers asks clients to ignore the letters and count the numbers. Form L poses the reverse problem for letters. The challenge is to ignore certain units while counting the others (Schretlin, Bobholz, & Brandt, 1996).

The ***Test of Everyday Attention*** (*TEA*) contains tasks for assessing varied aspects of attention (Robertson, Ward, Ridgeway, et al., 1996). Its simulations include finding symbols on a map and tracking stimuli associated with an elevator. Also, Sohlberg and Mateer (2001) use an *Attention Questionnaire* that asks clients to rate the frequency of general problems in everyday life, such as "my mind keeps wandering" or "difficult to pay attention to more than one thing at a time" (p. 155).

Memory Systems: Storage and Process

Before memory is broken down into its major components, let us consider what may be the best known neuropsychological measure, namely the ***Wechsler Memory Scale-Fourth Edition*** (*WMS-IV*; Wechsler, 2009). The current *WMS*, influenced by contemporary theory of memory systems, contains several modifications of earlier versions. It retains the Logical Memory subtest, which we would call "short story recall," but it no longer includes the classic digit span test of immediate memory. It makes use of eight core subtests, some having both immediate and delayed recall versions. Like the *WAIS*, the *WMS* was rebuilt to be more user-friendly.

The subtests can be configured into various batteries such as a Standard Battery of six of the subtests and an Older Adult/Abbreviated Battery of four subtests. The subtests are also grouped according to four main functional indexes, yielding index scores (e.g., immediate memory, delayed memory, auditory memory, visual memory). Two subtests are thought to measure visually oriented working memory. Performance on the *WMS* is not necessarily related to overall intelligence. A case whose frontal lobe was penetrated by a billiard cue was impaired on an earlier version of the *WMS* but had a Full Scale IQ of 123 (Kapur, 1994). In addition, formal tests may not be predictive of CHIs' everyday memory (e.g., where they put something, names of familiar people, what was just said; Sunderland, Harris, & Baddeley, 1983).

The ***Rivermead Behavioural Memory Test*** (*RBMT*), which can be given by "qualified speech therapists," is used to predict the status of everyday memory (Wilson, Cockburn, & Baddeley, 1985). Subtests entail learning someone's name, finding an object that has been hidden from view, recalling a route, and recalling a sequence of actions. It evaluates *prospective memory*, in which a client is asked to remember to do something at a prearranged time or signal (i.e., "remember to remember"). Research indicated that the RBMT is predictive of functional independence in the community (Wilson, Baddeley, Cockburn, et al., 1989).

Now, let us consider the main components of the memory system. The Digit Span subtest of the *WAIS* has exposed a deficiency of **short-term buffer capacity** in people with CHI (see Table 12.2). An individual can be left with only an STM deficit 6 months after injury (Van der Linden, Coyette, & Seron, 1992). In a study of adolescents with CHI, Hannay and Levin (1989) found that short-term recognition memory varied as a function of severity of injury. Those with mild head injuries were like normal controls, whereas moderately and severely injured participants were impaired.

Sternberg's (1975) classic **short-term memory scanning** procedure provides a precise picture of processing speed and style. The Symbol Search subtest in the *WAIS* appears to have been modeled after this procedure. The Sternberg task is a subspan recognition test in which response time is measured. A short series of digits is presented, followed immediately by a test digit. A person indicates whether the test digit was in the preceding list. Length of the digit series is varied to determine scanning speed and type of search (i.e., terminating at recognition or exhaustive no matter when the match is found). Severe CHIs were slower than controls, but they scanned exhaustively like the controls (Schmitter-Edgecombe, Marks, Fahy, et al., 1992). Considering the timed Digit Symbol test from the *WAIS* (Table 12.2), slow information processing can be said to be a general consequence of head injury.

People with CHI have trouble remembering the past or **long-term memory** (LTM). There are two types of difficulty:

- **Retrograde amnesia** involves forgetting memories acquired *before* injury (e.g., "remote memory")
- **Anterograde amnesia** involves forgetting experiences occurring *after* injury (e.g., "recent memory")

FIGURE 12.1   Time periods of forgotten information relative to the moment of injury.

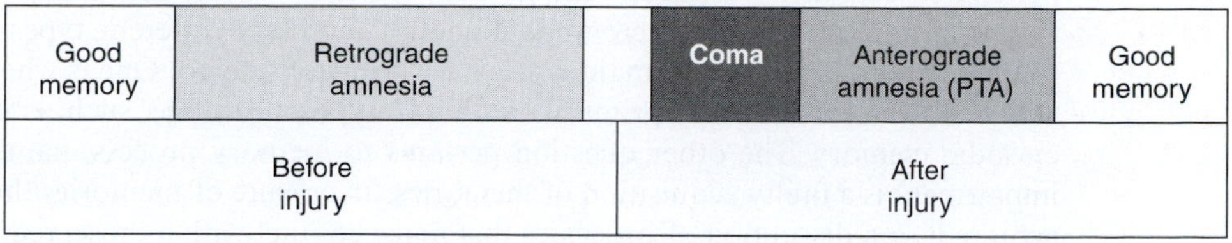

Good memory	Retrograde amnesia		Coma	Anterograde amnesia (PTA)	Good memory
	Before injury			After injury	

The time periods of the original memory formation are illustrated in Figure 12.1. Because remembering depends on storage and related processes, we would be astute in suspecting that these amnesias are different types of disruption of the memory system.

Severity of retrograde amnesia increases as the memory gap extends further into the past, going backward from the time of injury. An interview may explore recollections from contemporary life to childhood (e.g., Van der Linden, Brédart, Depoorter, & Coyette, 1996). Memory of impersonal world events might be quizzed with questions organized according to periods of time (e.g., Beatty, Salmon, Bernstein, et al., 1987). During recovery, the amnesic gap shrinks toward the time of injury. A mild gap comprises 30 minutes prior to injury but is usually long lasting.

One assessment for retrograde amnesia is the ***Autobiographical Memory Interview*** (*AMI*), a test of "personal remote memory" (Kopelman, Wilson, & Baddeley, 1989). An interview focuses on three time periods of a patient's life. Each recollection is scored for amount of information and vividness. In general, anyone's memory of the distant past is spotty, so an evaluator should check with a family member or friend for confirmation.

Anterograde amnesia, along with disorientation, is a significant component of what is widely known as **posttraumatic amnesia** (PTA). With anterograde amnesia, the client does not remember events that occurred after awaking from coma, such as meeting hospital staff or what was for breakfast earlier that day. The client also experiences retrograde amnesia, but day-to-day recording of postinjury events is more prominent and problematic. PTA usually lasts much longer than the duration of coma. It is said to end when a patient "remembers today what happened yesterday and does not begin each day with a blank mind" (Jennett & Teasdale, 1981, p. 89).

A brief assessment of PTA is the ***Galveston Orientation and Amnesia Test*** (*GOAT*; Levin, O'Donnell, & Grossman, 1979). Eight of its 10 questions assess orientation to person, place, and time. The other two questions ask a patient to recall the first memory after the injury and the last memory before the injury.

Claudia Osborn (1998), a physician at New York University, was riding a bicycle when she was struck by a car and sent flying into the air. She was diagnosed as having postconcussion syndrome (i.e., MTBI). Yet she insisted on returning to work, where other doctors had to keep reminding her of things such as a patient she had seen earlier in the day. She forgot appointments. Visiting one patient, she asked, "Where's her chart?" Her intern replied, "You have the chart in your hand" (p. 37).

Do retrograde and anterograde amnesias represent different types of damage to the memory system? Two main issues have been considered. One is whether people with CHI have a difficulty primarily with one type of storage, such as semantic or episodic memory. The other question pertains to memory process, namely whether impairment is a faulty acquisition of memories, an erasure of memories that had been acquired, or a disruption of processes that make contact with a preserved LTM.

Several case studies have addressed the question of whether memory deficit is specific to one type of information. Gene, who suffered a severe head injury in a motorcycle accident, could not recall day-to-day events and could not remember specific events from any period in his life (Schacter, 1996). The deficit was with episodic memory, not semantic memory. He could not recall motorcycle trips with his friends or a train derailment near his home. Yet he could remember facts such as the floor plan of his childhood home and names of friends and schools. He could discuss the nature of his work prior to injury but could not recall events that had occurred while on the job.

Assuming pretraumatic memories were acquired normally, then retrograde amnesia can be either a destruction of stored memories or a retrieval problem. The spontaneous return of remote memories is indicative of preserved storage, leaving a damaged retrieval mechanism as the explanation.

Because anterograde amnesia involves memories that should have been acquired after the injury, research has focused on new learning. One example is a paired-associate learning task, similar to one *WMS* subtest (Schacter & Graf, 1986). A list of word-pairs is presented for study (e.g., *window-reason*). Then, recall is tested two ways. An **explicit test** consists of presenting the first word to see if the paired word is remembered. A participant is aware that memory is being tested. Prior to the explicit test, the participant is also given a word-stem completion task (e.g., *rea____*). **Implicit learning** is detected if stems from the list are completed more accurately or faster than stems not in the list.

Schacter and Graf found impairment with explicit testing but not with implicit testing. Implicit recall indicates that new information can be acquired and retained for a while. Thus, impairment lies in explicit or effortful retrieval processes. Distractibility and a stimulus encoding problem in the first year after injury can also make it difficult to acquire new information, thus, making anterograde amnesia appear falsely to be a loss of memories (Freedman & Cermak, 1986).

A severe retrograde amnesia can be devastating for a person's **sense of self**. Schacter (1996) commented on the aftermath of Gene's motorcycle accident: "A life without any episodic memory is psychologically barren . . . Nothing much happens in Gene's mind or in his life. He has few friends and lives quietly at home with his parents . . . he thinks little about the future. It does not occur to him to make plans . . ." (pp. 149–150). Another amnesic individual could not remember most of what happened in his life prior to a bilateral stroke, but he could remember details about his service in the navy during World War II nearly 50 years before. His identity became so attached to that period that he believed he was still in active service and would have to return to his ship soon (Hodges & McCarthy, 1993).

Executive Functions

In 1848, an iron rod was blasted into the frontal lobes of Phineas Gage, who wandered America fitfully for the rest of his life (Damasio, Grabowski, Frank, et al., 1994). His central executive, now impaired, was supposed to manage his cognitive resources to keep him on track (Baddeley, 1986). The executive is like "a little person in the head to direct behavior" (Andrewes, 2001, p. 135); and like a good business executive, it performs no specific function, yet makes sure things get done. Baddeley (1996) worried that his initial definition was "so vague as to serve as little more than a ragbag into which could be stuffed all the complex strategy selection, planning, and retrieval checking that clearly goes on . . ." (p. 6). This ragbag is filled by additional or overlapping notions of shifting sets, cognitive flexibility, problem solving, inhibition, and self-regulation.

The general assumptions begin with the idea that routine or skilled actions are carried out quickly and efficiently in the automatic processing mode. A person invokes the executive system intentionally for novel or difficult actions or when errors occur. It regulates resources to reach a goal. One goal may be getting to work. According to Duncan (1986), executive function starts with *goal lists* such as taking a shower, getting dressed, and eating breakfast. An *action list* is the mental operations and overt actions engaged in meeting these goals. *Self-monitoring* compares current states and goal states, ensuring that goals are being met (see Table 12.5).

Impaired executive control produces what is known as **dysexecutive syndrome**. Because executive control applies to any information-processing domain, the syndrome should be manifested in a wide variety of tasks. The **Wisconsin Card Sorting Test** (*WCST*; Grant & Berg, 1948) is often used to test executive function. It is said to test abilities to identify abstract categories and shift cognitive set. In one study,

TABLE 12.5   **Components of the executive system and impairments pertaining to grocery shopping.**

NORMAN AND SHALLICE (1986)	SOHLBERG AND MATEER (2001)
Initiation and drive	Does not go to the grocery when the refrigerator is empty
Inhibition	Shops impulsively
Task persistence	Does not get all items on a shopping list
Organization	Does not use aisle headings
Generative thinking	Does not think of a substitute for an unavailable item
Awareness	Is not concerned about a need for groceries

CHIs exhibited fewer card sorts and more perseverative errors than normal controls (Gansler, Covall, McGrath, et al., 1996). In general, clients have difficulty shifting response sets and evaluating their own performance.

A few batteries give us an idea of what neuropsychologists think the executive system is. The **Delis-Kaplan Executive Function System** (*D-KEFS*) examines integrity of the frontal lobes (Delis, Kaplan, & Kramer, 2001). Its nine tests include trail making, verbal fluency, and proverb interpretation. A sorting test (like the *WCST*) and a tower test were used in a study of CHI (Mozeiko, Lê, Coelho, et al., 2011). Tower tests (e.g., Tower of Hanoi, Tower of London) entail moving rings strategically across three pegs according to rules to end up with a particular configuration. The **Behavioral Assessment of the Dysexecutive Syndrome** (*BADS*) tests planning and problem solving (Wilson, Alderman, Burgess, et al., 1996). Also look into **Functional Assessment of Verbal Reasoning and Executive Strategies** (FAVRES; MacDonald, 1998).

Personality and Behavior

After a boat accident on a family vacation, Alan Forman went through "an extreme disinhibited phase" (Crimmins, 2000). He threw things and called the nurses "bitches" and "assholes." Professionals refer to this as a social skills deficit.

A person with CHI appears to have taken on a different personality. There is an absence of self-regulation. The individual becomes easily agitated and embarrassingly impulsive. These **challenging behaviors**, according to Sohlberg and Mateer (2001), may be reactive factors associated with feelings of loss and frustration. A person "acts in ways that appear selfish, rude, or otherwise unmindful of others" (p. 338). These behaviors may be piled on to the natural distress of sudden disability and are disruptive of attempts at rehabilitation. Stambrook and others (1991) found that severely impaired CHIs were more bewildered, depressed, and hostile than moderately impaired CHIs and a group with spinal cord injuries. Wives rated the severe CHIs as being more belligerent, helpless, and withdrawn than the others.

Denise was 42 years old when her truck was broadsided by a bigger truck. When she arrived at rehabilitation, she had no energy for therapy. She was bored and surly, and she preferred to stay in bed. She was impatient. "Why are you asking all these questions? I'm 24." She screamed for no apparent reason. After four items of the SLP's testing, she shouted "I'm overloaded right now!" With the SLP's easy and steady tone, Denise calmed down but could not continue with the assessment. The goals for the first week of her rehabilitation were to tolerate the presence of her therapist and to interact for 20 minutes without agitation.

Two weeks later, Denise was in physical therapy joking around with the therapists and her husband, who was on his cell phone telling his friends how well she was doing. "We take so much for granted," he was saying. She stood three times for 3 minutes each and then got dizzy. With support, she walked 5 feet. Denise turned, smiled, and declared, "OK. The bitch is back." Therapists are patient and wait until early agitation disappears.

Insight

People with CHI are often unaware of their behavior or personality changes, an anosognosia that is linked to frontal lobe damage (McGlynn & Schacter, 1989). Family members become stressed by the individual's anxiety and bad temper, but the person with CHI denies such disturbances. Persons with CHI also may not complain of physical disabilities. Neuropsychologists say that people with CHI have a **posttraumatic insight disorder** that is observed as an underreporting of the severity of impairments (also, referred to as "unawareness").

Dr. Osborn's friend Marcia knew that Claudia was different, but Claudia insisted on returning to work soon after the accident. At work, she had trouble following conversations. She recognized that a particular conversation was difficult, but she did not recognize that this was a general problem. "My family perceived my problems more clearly than I did" (Osborn, 1998, p. 32). Another doctor told her that she had a head injury and insisted she have therapy before returning to work, but she replied, "I still know medicine . . . It's only the little pieces causing trouble." When asked what she meant by "the little pieces," Claudia replied, "Memory problems, according to them" (p. 40).

Several studies show that people with head trauma, like Claudia, often underestimate memory impairments (McGlynn & Schacter, 1989). They realize their memory is worse but are not aware of the severity of deficit. Family members feel that the memory impairment is more serious than the person with CHI does (e.g., Van der Linden, et al., 1996). An individual might admit to a slight memory problem when questioned. Training of compensatory strategies may be accompanied by an increase of self-awareness during training, but this insight sometimes does not carry over to the work setting.

Insight improves over time. At 1 to 3 years postinjury, people with CHI demonstrated greater insight than those at 6 months postinjury (Godfrey, Partridge, Knight, et al., 1993). However, this progress was accompanied by increased emotional dysfunction. Depression and anxiety were found to be less in the first 6 months than later, and these problems peak between 7 and 12 months after injury (Lezak & O'Brien, 1988). The delayed onset of depression may be the result of a gradually increasing awareness. In general, clients may be difficult to engage in rehabilitation during the first year because of unrealistic treatment goals, whereas a later challenge is the negative reaction to an emerging understanding of impairment (Prigatano & Klonoff, 1998).

Language

At the beginning of this chapter, Hagen (1981) was cited for suggesting that CHI in some cases causes cognitive disorders without language problems and in other cases causes language problems that are secondary to cognitive disorders. Wertz (1985) referred to the secondary deficits as "language of confusion" (e.g., McDonald, 1993).

Some people with CHI have a clear-cut aphasia. Before considering broader cognitive-communicative deficits, let us focus on the most familiar territory for SLPs, namely the areas of language that are implicated in aphasia.

Clinical Tests and Diagnosis

What proportion of CHIs have a clear-cut aphasia? Heilman, Safran, and Geschwind (1971) administered an unspecified aphasia examination to 750 patients with CHI and concluded that only 2 percent had aphasia (see also Schwartz-Cowley & Stepanik, 1989). In another study, 50 participants had minimal deficits on language tests except for 40 percent who had naming difficulties (Levin, Grossman, & Kelly, 1976). Among Heilman's 13 diagnosed with aphasia, 9 had anomic aphasia, and 4 had Wernicke's aphasia. Hartley and Levin (1990) said that acute CHIs can display language behavior similar to Wernicke's aphasia, which evolves to anomic-like aphasia as orientation improves.

Sarno, Buonaguro, and Levita (1987) examined 25 CHIs nearly 4 months after injury with tests of naming, sentence repetition, word fluency, and the Token Test of sentence comprehension. The participants were impaired in all tasks to levels found in stroke-related aphasia. Sarno decided that they had found "parallel aphasias which characterized both CHI and CVA aphasic patients" (p. 336). Earlier, Sarno (1980) had concluded that 32 percent of a head-injured group had aphasia, whereas others had a "subclinical aphasia" with no apparent deficit in conversation but still an impairment in word fluency.

Thirty Italian severe CHIs received a test for aphasia plus more naming tasks and tests of other cognitive functions (Luzzatti, et al., 1989). Sixteen participants had unilateral lesions according to CT scans. On the aphasia test, CHIs scored in the range for mild language deficit. Of 18 diagnosed with aphasia, 11 had Broca's aphasia according to test criteria. However, the presence of dysarthria influenced classification of six of these nonfluent cases.

These studies indicate that some people with CHI exhibit deficits on language tests. The studies also leave an impression that clinical investigators differ with respect to diagnosing these deficits as aphasia. However, even if everyone agrees on what aphasia is, findings are going to differ when one sample size is 750 and another is 25. Yet there is an impression that "language of confusion" has been diagnosed as aphasia or, at least, as "subclinical" aphasia. Holland (1982) did not mince words: "If the language problems seen in closed head injured patients don't look like aphasia, sound like aphasia, act like aphasia, feel, smell or taste like aphasia, then they aren't aphasia" (p. 345).

The debate has implications for treatment. Sarno and others (1987) concluded that "the traditional language rehabilitation approaches implemented with CVA aphasic patients are appropriate for the management of aphasia in CHI patients as well" (p. 336). On the other hand, Holland (1982) stated that CHI patients "will not be terribly responsive to the traditional methods by which we have come to treat aphasia" (p. 345). This apparent disagreement dissolves if we agree that CHI is not a homogeneous condition and is similarly diverse in its consequences, as Hagen suggested. It is possible that CHI clients with secondary language deficits may not be responsive to traditional aphasia methods, whereas CHI clients with aphasias caused by more focal insults may be responsive to these methods.

What are the effects of MTBI (i.e., concussion)? In Australia, a battery of tests was given to four people who had suffered mild traumas from an assault, a fall, and bicycle and motor vehicle accidents. The tests were in the categories of general language (i.e., aphasia battery, Boston Naming Test), high-level language (e.g., inferences), and cognition (e.g., *SCATBI*). A case with a longer loss of consciousness than the others had naming and word-fluency deficits and several cognitive deficits. Deficits in the other cases were hard to find, but high-level language, such as inferencing, was suspect. The investigators concluded that more sensitive detectors are needed (Wong, Murdoch, & Whelan, 2010).

Language Comprehension

The experimental study of language comprehension with CHI is a barren landscape compared to the study of aphasia caused by stroke. To examine lexical contact with semantic memory, Haut and others (1991) presented a unique priming task in which participants made rapid judgments about whether a second word is a member of the semantic category of the first word. The CHIs were primed, indicating that semantic organization was preserved. However, they were also slow. This result is consistent with preservation of semantic memory (while access to episodic memory is impaired) and is consistent with the robust finding that CHI reduces the speed of information processing.

People with CHI were compared to people with stroke-related aphasia on Caplan's *Thematic Role Battery*. The battery tests "final interpretation" of canonical and noncanonical sentence structures and employs the enactment strategy of manipulating toy animals. Pattern of difficulty among sentence types was similar between groups, leading to the conclusion that LH stroke and CHI cause qualitatively similar sentence comprehension impairments (Butler-Hinz, Caplan, & Waters, 1990).

Language Production

Anomia is "the primary linguistic deficit" with CHI (Hartley & Levin, 1990). As with RHD, deficit is most frequently evident in word-fluency tasks. Several investigators studied CHI with a letter-fluency task (e.g., Crowe, 1992; Gruen, Frankle, & Schwartz, 1990; Wertz, et al., 1986). Lohman and others (1989) found that the number of words per letter increased as Rancho Los Amigos (RLA) cognitive level increased from V to VII. There were also reductions in words produced for nine categories such as clothes, furniture, and birds. Typicality of words was unusual for only two categories, which is again consistent with the retention of fairly good semantic organization.

King, Hough, and others (2006) compared object and action naming (nouns vs. verbs) with 10 people who had MTBI. These cases fit the usual criteria including a negative CT scan, GCS of 13–15, and loss of consciousness under 30 minutes or

PTA under 24 hours (Table 12.4). The researchers found that response time was more indicative of deficit than accuracy. For the MTBIs, there was no effect of word category. Hough (2008) continued this research with an expanded group of TBI caused by motor vehicle accidents. She considered most naming errors to be "fleeting" or isolated occurrences, as opposed to clustered or extended errors.

In discussing misnaming, Holland (1982) argued that impaired language behavior need not be indicative of aphasia. Errors with CHI may be perceptually based or confabulatory. Boles (1997) found that people with TBI and Alzheimer's disease make more visual misperception errors than people with stroke-related aphasia (e.g., "can" for *drum*).

We may analyze words and sentences in discourse. Severe CHIs at various times postonset were deficient in content units per minute when describing a picture (Ehrlich, 1988). In interviews, nine CHIs at RLA Levels V to VII produced paraphasias but did not produce more indefinite or generic words than normal controls. They made some syntactic errors but spoke at a normal level of syntactic complexity (Glosser & Deser, 1991). In all, word-finding appears to be a function of severity of injury, and initial testing should guide an SLP as to whether improving this function is going to be a goal of rehabilitation.

Discourse

Audrey Holland's (1982) educated hunch was that "it is in the area of language pragmatics that aphasia and head injured language most vividly contrast" (p. 347). Communicative difficulties are likely to be secondary consequences of cognitive impairments, and pragmatics has consisted of mainly the study of discourse. We may suspect that retrograde amnesia and dysexecutive syndrome influence storytelling. Anterograde amnesia and apathy are likely to affect interpersonal interactions. Skye McDonald of Sydney, Australia, and Carl Coelho of the University of Connecticut have been gathering data regarding Holland's hunch and some of the cognitive explanations.

Discourse Comprehension

McDonald has examined the pragmatic use of language with TBI extensively. Like the study of RHD, the comprehension of sarcasm seemed to be a good vehicle for studying inferencing and theory of mind (ToM) in persons with CHI. The frequently injured frontal lobes may be important for representing the intentions or beliefs of others (e.g., Gallagher & Frith, 2003).

McDonald and Pearce (1996) studied a group of 10 with varied TBIs, each having frontal lobe damage. Participants read snippets of a conversation between Mark and Wayne and then answered questions about what they meant:

(1a) Mark: *What a great football game.*
(1b) Wayne: *Sorry I made you come.*

Mark must have thought it was a lousy football game. The head-injured group comprehended literal meaning (i.e., When Wayne said *You are glad I asked you to come*) but had difficulty with sarcastic intent (i.e., *1a*). The same results were found when speakers provided sarcastic prosody. In the same report, five of seven TBIs had difficulty interpreting the emotion conveyed with semantically neutral utterances. Together, the experiments indicated that some individuals with frontal lobe damage have a problem with nonliteral interpretation.

Channon and others (2005) decided to try a slightly different approach that entailed making a distinction between direct and indirect sarcasm. One story had Alex burning toast and then asking Mary, "Am I a good cook?" With direct sarcasm, she replied, "The best cook in the world." With indirect or more subtle sarcasm, she replied: "I'll hire you in my restaurant." Direct sarcasm requires a simple inference of opposite meaning, whereas indirect sarcasm requires a longer inferential chain. A group of 19 with CHI was deficient in comprehending both types of sarcasm relative to sincere literal remarks. The type of error was detected in these studies by asking participants to explain the meaning of target statements. In Channon's study, errors were mostly a variety of incorrect nonliteral interpretations. This showed that the CHIs had some appreciation for nonliteralness but had difficulty with getting the correct inference. Also, a difficulty across multiple tasks was evidence for a general deficit in theory of mind.

Martin and McDonald (2005) compared two explanations of comprehension impairment in a study involving ironic jokes. One was ToM deficit. The other was executive dysfunction. The particular executive function in this case was thought to be a cognitive flexibility in adjusting interpretations according to context. The theories were evaluated with ToM tasks and tests of executive functioning, and the investigators looked for links between these tests and irony comprehension. There was no correlation between ToM tasks and joke comprehension, nor between executive tasks and joke comprehension. Tests of inferential reasoning were correlated with each other, however, which is an indication that inferencing is likely to be a unique function, apart from ToM and the executive.

Clinical examination of discourse comprehension has been different. Nicholas and Brookshire (1995a) gave their *Discourse Comprehension Test* to a group with TBI, who performed like RHDs and people with aphasia. If there is a special influence of attention deficit or other primary impairments on this level of language comprehension, asking about main ideas and details in stories does not seem to tap into it (Kennedy & Nawrocki, 2003).

Discourse Production

Compared to RHD, research with CHI has had a different style with regard to elicitation methods and types of analysis. For a while, at least, study of CHI relied less on pictures to elicit discourse, and it relied more on cohesion analysis and less on information analysis (Davis, et al., 1997).

The Coelho group, focusing on CHI, began their research program with four participants telling stories from a filmstrip (Liles, Coelho, Duffy, et al., 1989). The CHIs tended to use fewer cohesive ties than normal controls. On the other hand, Glosser and Deser (1991) found nine mid-level CHIs to be unimpaired in referential cohesion in interviews. These early results varied as a function of severity of injury and elicitation methods.

Early studies of macrostructure also consisted of few participants and focused on storytelling (Coelho, Liles, & Duffy, 1991; Glosser & Deser, 1991; Hough & Barrow, 2003; Liles et al., 1989). One analysis emphasized completeness with respect to the presence of an initiating event, actions, and a consequence. Another analysis targeted thematic coherence by judging topic maintenance through an entire discourse. CHIs were impaired, contrary to good cohesion and sentence form. Thus, deficit was greater for "global" or macrostructural coherence than for "local" or microstructural cohesion. Yet the opposite was found for one participant who had poor cohesion but good story structure.

Coelho (2002) continued to accumulate narrative transcripts. His work began to stand out for the size of his groups from rehabilitation hospitals in New England and the coverage of multiple levels in analysis. He elicited stories in two conditions, namely retelling a story from a filmstrip and generating a story from a Norman Rockwell painting (*The Runaway*). Analysis addressed cohesion (i.e., number of complete cohesive ties) and content (i.e., number of episodes, T-units within an episode). Fifty-five CHIs differed from controls in all measures. Cohesion and story content were better for retelling than for generation, indicating that story generation is more likely to expose difficulties.

The research team in Connecticut added 15 minutes of conversation for comparing CHIs and non-brain-injured adults. Conversation required a different analysis that tracked speaker-initiations, speaker-responses, and topic initiations. The goal was to determine whether discourse can be diagnostic. A statistical analysis identified CHI 70 percent of the time for narratives and 77 percent of the time for conversation. The misdiagnosed CHIs and controls overlapped considerably. The researchers concluded that the use of discourse for diagnosis is risky, mainly because of variability in storytelling among people without brain injury (Coelho, Youse, Lê, et al., 2003; Youse, Coelho, Mozeiko, & Feinn, 2005).

Later, Coelho employed his *goodness of narratives* measure (Chapter 4) to study 171 Vietnam War veterans. These participants, 50 to 70 years of age, had suffered a variety of open or penetrating head injuries. They were asked to retell a story seen on a filmstrip. "Goodness" addressed completeness relative to components of story grammar as well as the aforementioned story content. The statistical analysis was fancy (e.g., multivariate analysis of variance), but the simple conclusion was that the goodness analysis detected deficits, even 30 years after an injury (Lê, Coelho, Mozeiko, et al., 2011; Grafman, 2011; Coelho, Lê, Mozeiko, et al., 2013).

It is logical to think that executive dysfunction (e.g., disorganization) interferes with storytelling. Conversely, some problems with storytelling have been used to diagnose executive dysfunction. To see if there is a relationship, Coelho's team returned to the Vietnam veterans and administered the sorting and tower tests from the *D-KEFS* battery introduced earlier. The group with TBI did not differ from a control group in executive abilities despite the finding that the sorting task was correlated with the TBIs' impaired narratives. What do sorting and storytelling have in common? The researchers suggested it might be goal-setting, having a plan, and self-evaluation. What do we make of the absence of executive impairment? Instead of explaining, the authors pointed to a need for assessing story grammar (Mozeiko et al., 2011).

Let us finish storytelling with some examples. Davis's study of narrative with RHDs was also conducted with a small group of people with CHI (Davis & Coelho, 2004). It was a rare comparison of the populations with the same procedures. Two mildly impaired participants told the Flower Pot story (Chapter 11) differently. One gave the following fairly accurate version:

> Looks like the guy got hit on the head with a flower pot, and he's probably swearing or something. He's gonna go up and paste the guy one. He's banging on the door, and the woman goes up, "Oh, nice doggie." And he's all sucked in. And he's showin' her the bump on his head. She gave the dog a bone.

Technically, *the woman* has no antecedent in the narration as an instance of signaling lexical co-reference. Also, there are no inferences connecting the events, and the order of the last two events is reversed. However, it is more accurate and detailed than another version produced by an individual with the same overall rating of cognitive impairment:

> The apartment of the Mrs. Jones or Mr. Jones each waving his cane up her, cause he was watering the plants and fell out the window.

Conversation

Conversation has been investigated more frequently with CHIs than RHDs. Some of these interactions are bolstered by a series of questions called "semi-structured conversation" (Snow, Douglas, & Ponsford, 1995). The *La Trobe Communication Questionnaire (LCQ)*, developed in Australia for adolescents with TBI, consists of 30 items exploring the client's and "close-other's" perspectives on current communicative abilities (Douglas, et al., 2000; Douglas, Bracy, & Snow, 2007).

Dr. Osborn's experience illustrates the influence of attention impairment and lack of insight on discourse comprehension and conversation. When she returned to work unaware of her impairments, she could not stay focused on the presentations by residents. "I lost track of the conversation . . . I faked understanding because I couldn't believe I didn't understand" (Osborn, 1998, p. 32). We ask people with CHI if they forget things they were just told or forget what they had just said.

Coelho and his colleagues (1993) compared five people with mild aphasia to five mild CHIs in conversations. Both clinical groups had difficulties initiating and sustaining conversation, and it was difficult to discern differences between them. Partners had to assume more communicative burden than in interactions with intact partners (e.g., topic and turn initiation). The CHIs were described as especially subdued or requiring prompting to talk. Like efforts to apply Conversation Analysis to aphasia (Chapter 4), subsequent research has been devoted to developing ways of measuring conversational behavior that is particularly characteristic of CHI.

With an expanded sample of 32 CHIs engaged in 15-minute conversations, Coelho created an "Appropriateness" system for classifying pertinent behaviors. Relative to controls, the clinical group took less responsibility for initiating topics. Also, this group produced information that did not contribute to the flow of conversation. One individual embarked on tangents as if a topic made him think of something about himself (Coelho, Youse, & Lê, 2002). Later, Youse and her colleagues (2011) decided that the appropriateness method was insensitive to subtle difficulties. With one participant, she indicated that a more detailed modification uncovered more deficiencies in facilitating conversation.

McDonald was interested in the influence of disinhibition on conversation. In one study, she had two people with CHI explain how to play a game to a blindfolded listener. Both CHIs were disorganized and ineffective. One was repetitive, and the other had too little detail. Statements were irrelevant or badly sequenced, making instructions very confusing (McDonald, 1993).

A study of politeness was more to the point. McDonald and van Sommers (1993) asked the two people with CHI how they would respond in situations like asking to borrow a car and hinting that you want to leave a dinner party. The participants had difficulty formulating requests indirectly (i.e., politely). They ended up being impulsively direct. The investigators concluded that "impaired problem-solving ability and poor behavioural control also disrupt normal social communication skills" (p. 313). Later, they had similar findings with a group of 15 mostly with CHI (McDonald & Pearce, 1998).

Also in Australia, researchers studied *service encounters* in which information, goods, or services are exchanged in face-to-face interaction or over the telephone. One encounter was to call a bus service for information that would be helpful for organizing a group outing. Another was to call the police to find out how a brain-injured person gets a driver's license reinstated. Transcripts were assessed with a Generic Structure Potential (GSP) analysis, which began with dividing the conversations into speaking turns. The turns were classified as to the presence of obligatory elements, such as a greeting, service request, service enquiry, closing, and goodbye. The investigators also looked for incomplete, unrelated, or inappropriate responses, and they found that people with TBI differed from controls engaged in the same encounters (Togher, Hand, & Code, 1997).

A research team in Illinois and Iowa used a barrier task to examine referential communication by people with amnesia, some with CHI. The job of a person with amnesia was to instruct the partner across the barrier in arranging 12 abstract figures. The descriptive study was intended to see how the CHIs would do across attempts, and they displayed a normal rate of increased referential efficiency but some lack of creativity in their expressions (Duff, Hengst, Tranel, et al., 2008, 2009).

One area of concern, as it was with RHD, is the ability to infer the mental state of another (i.e., ToM). TASIT, the test of social inference introduced in Chapter 11, was given to head-injured people and familiar partners. The participants with TBI had difficulty interpreting facial expressions in the TASIT and, thus, were anticipated to have misunderstandings in social encounters (Watts & Douglas, 2006).

Cognitive Rehabilitation

Speech-language pathologists have built on the pioneering work of Yehuda Ben-Yishay (1980), George Prigatano (1999), Barbara Wilson (1987), and certainly others, in part, by integrating principles of clinical aphasiology with cognitive rehabilitation (e.g., Cappa, Benke, Clarke, et al., 2011; Johnstone & Stonnington, 2001; Ponsford, Sloan, & Snow, 1995; Sohlberg, Turkstra, & Wilson, 2011; Wilson, Herbert, & Shiel, 2007; Ylvisaker et al., 2008). Rehabilitation in the United States has been supported on a large scale by the National Institute on Disability and Rehabilitation Research (NIDRR) with a data-collection program called the Traumatic Brain Injury Model System (TBIMS). An additional boost was provided by passage of the federal Traumatic Brain Injury Act of 1996.

These days we find few clinicians focusing only on direct treatment of impairments, and most employ strategies that combine the targeting of impairment and the training of compensatory strategies, all with functional activities and within a realistic milieu (e.g., Hartley, 1995).

Ylvisaker and others (2008) mapped out a *context-sensitive, everyday, routine-based approach* (Table 12.6). Like Kagan and Simmons-Mackie's (2007) "beginning

TABLE 12.6   Stages of cognitive rehabilitation, drawn loosely from Table 33-9 in Ylvisaker, Szekeres, and Feeney (2008).

STAGES	THERAPEUTIC SUPPORT	SAMPLE GOALS
Early	Maximum	■ Increase alertness ■ Improve focus ■ Increase recognition of people and objects ■ Improve basic communication
Middle	Moderate	■ Increase duration of attention ■ Improve recent memory (with prosthetics) ■ Improve organization of functional tasks and discourse ■ Improve awareness of deficits
Late	Minimum	■ Increase independent use of compensatory strategies ■ Decrease reliance on cues for organization ■ Improve language functions related to vocational and avocational goals

with the end," Ylvisaker preferred functionality and authenticity as soon as possible. Their emphasis on *routine* "suggests normal activities of life, motivating clinicians to move beyond commercial therapeutic materials, generic therapeutic activities, and exclusively clinical intervention settings . . ." (p. 896). The approach is compatible with Sohlberg and Mateer (2001), who recommended that SLPs should "actively facilitate generalization from the start of treatment" (p. 137).

Coma Management

A few specialists acknowledge a controversial treatment generally known as *coma stimulation therapy* (or coma arousal therapy), which need not be conducted by an SLP. The purpose is to improve responsiveness to environmental events (e.g., Chamberlain, et al., 1995; Gillis, 1996). There are multiple approaches (e.g., multisensory, familiar routines, and structured stimulation). They are supported with complex neurological rationales and animal studies, but evidence of efficacy for humans is hard to find.

The general procedure, similar to the Glasgow Coma Scale, consists of brief stimulation and passive motion exercise to prevent muscle atrophy. Senses are stimulated with smells, tastes, and touch. The sensations may be related to daily activities such as drinking coffee or brushing teeth. There may be a progression from unisensory to multisensory stimulation. Eager to do whatever they can, family members or caregivers may learn to perform these simple tasks.

Challenging Behaviors and Fatigue

Rehabilitation cannot proceed on all cylinders until (a) posttraumatic amnesia (PTA) has passed and the client recognizes the therapist and can remember goals and strategies, and (b) acute agitation subsides, as illustrated by the case of Denise earlier in this chapter. How do we deal with acute agitation? We wait patiently until it subsides. Alan Forman's story is instructive. "Nurse Megan . . . doesn't cringe when he yells obscenities at her or throws food" (Crimmins, 2000, p. 87). It was also helpful for Alan and his wife to realize that this rudeness was the result of brain injury and was certainly not Alan's natural personality.

Intervention may be necessary when the challenging behaviors persist and time for rehabilitation is running out. Strategies include altering the environment to minimize irritants, counseling caregivers, and providing behavioral treatments that reinforce good behavior and discourage bad behavior. However, "the ultimate goal . . . is internalized self-regulation of behavior" (Sohlberg & Mateer, 2001, p. 360). This begins by training individuals to become more aware, leading to monitoring and evaluating their own behavior.

Instituting therapeutic measures may also be stalled by a patient's fatigue in combination with the lack of initiation associated with executive dysfunction as well as some depression. A general lack of energy or extreme lethargy is a common consequence of brain damage, particularly traumatic injury (Stoler & Hill, 1998). Fatigue may be dealt with through medication, dietary modifications, and a midday nap. Compensatory strategies also include rationing time for strenuous activities and reducing distracting stimulation. Feelings of strength and cognitive energy should return with encouragement and patience from caregivers, as well as successes in treatment.

Insight (Awareness)

Do we remember Dr. Osborn's return to work too soon? A client's cognitive rehabilitation can proceed smoothly with a heightened awareness of the impairments caused by the head injury. Sohlberg and Mateer (2001) advised that an *awareness-enhancing program* is likely to benefit clients who have a little recognition that some abilities have changed and who have sufficient cognitive resources to integrate information. It is not likely to benefit clients who have an intense global unawareness and weak cognitive resources.

An awareness-enhancing program begins by providing information about the nature of deficits. Structured exercises, such as situational role-playing, allow the individual to experience difficulties that may await when leaving the hospital. Eventually, the client should be asked to predict performance on a particular task and then compare actual performance with the prediction.

Orientation and Attention

Management for low-level attention (e.g., arousal, alertness) is usually instituted *after* a patient comes out of a coma and while the patient is experiencing problems with orientation and attention during PTA. Goals of increasing alertness or arousal are important in the early stage of rehabilitation, and procedures should emphasize stimulation and managing the environment as opposed to anything that requires new learning or puts demands on memory.

Although there is some spontaneous diminishing of PTA, clinicians should still help patients orient to personal identity, time, and place. Orientation programs are similar to those that might be instituted for RHD or dementias. Training begins immediately postcoma with *passive drills* consisting of repeating orienting information and pointing out cues that are posted on the bulletin board and walls of a patient's room. Large clocks and calendars, names of hospital staff, and other reminders are part of a rehabilitation center's décor. *Active orientation training* consists of activities aimed at recognition of people, place, and time.

Various approaches to treating attention are organized around the types of attention. Perhaps the most well-known system is **Attention Process Training** (APT) by Sohlberg and Mateer (1987), which is now available on computer software as its third edition (APT-3; Sohlberg & Mateer, 2011). The kit includes flash drives containing exercises for clients to use at home. A skeleton view is provided in Table 12.7. General tasks are modeled after basic assessment procedures and are aimed at a process stripped of functional identity. In principle, they exercise a cognitive process that would be used in any real-life activity.

TABLE 12.7   Treatment of attention in language- and communication-related activities, mainly following Sohlberg and Mateer's (2001) *Attention Process Training* (*ATP*).

GOALS		PROCEDURES	
		General	*Functional*
Focused	Decrease response to distraction	Crossing-out task with distracting designs	Conversation in a busy physical therapy gym
Sustained	Increase duration of concentration on a simple task	Raise hand whenever a digit is heard in a list	Read newspaper for increasing lengths of time
Alternating	Improve allocation of attention to multiple stimuli	Crossing-out task with letters, then numbers	Conversation about news simultaneously on TV
Divided	Improve ability to perform two tasks at once	Sustained-attention activity along with a simple computer task	Read a newspaper while listening to music; later asked about each

A client should identify meaningful problems: "I cannot concentrate when preparing dinner because of the noise of the children playing. I forget ingredients or parts of the meal. I get frustrated and blow up at the children" (Sohlberg & Mateer, 2001, p. 156). The approach includes (1) practicing elements of a task (e.g., recall recipes, prepare meals in quiet, gradually increase artificial distractions); (2) anticipating and discussing difficulties; (3) when at home, managing the environment by having children play somewhere else while dinner is being prepared. Sohlberg and her colleagues (2000) felt that the effectiveness of APT was demonstrated in structured interviews where clients reported changes in specific real-life situations (e.g., "I can drive and listen to music"). For a review of evidence for attention training efficacy, see Sohlberg, Avery, Kennedy, and others (2003).

We used to search for computer software with games that force focus, require concentration, and divide attention. Expectations of technology are high, and there are apps for smartphones and tablets that are compatible with any objective for cognitive training or "brain fitness." The *Attention Training Game* (Mindware Consulting, Inc.), an app for Android, is based on a classic experimental method in cognitive psychology called the Eriksen *flanker task* (Eriksen & Eriksen, 1974; Schmidt & Dark, 1998). In the task or game, a central arrow is flanked by distractors that are other arrows pointing in the same or different directions, and a person responds to the direction of the central arrow. The idea is to ignore the other arrows.

Memory

Let us consider basic memory rehabilitation, which comes up again in dealing with language and communication. Two general approaches parallel work with other disorders, including aphasia. That is, treatment is oriented to restoration of memory and compensation for memory deficit (Wilson, 2009). We consider retrograde and antero-grade amnesias. Relatively less emphasis is placed on improving remote episodic memory, but we keep track of its progress. More emphasis is placed on anterograde amnesia as it contributes to the client's functioning in the here and now. Although the conditions for rehabilitation are more favorable when PTA appears to be over, certain compensatory strategies are instituted early.

A logical restorative tactic is to use *memory drills* or the repetitive practice of remembering lists and other things, suggesting that, according to Sohlberg and Mateer (2001), "memory can be strengthened as if it were a mental muscle" (p. 177). Although Sohlberg and Mateer found no empirical support for memory drills, they also found numerous computer programs and workbooks devoted to them. Another possibility is commonly taught to neurologically intact people who want to improve their memory. A *mnemonic strategy* is an internal self-cueing technique that entails associating important information with a visual image or some other link, but there is little indication that using mnemonics in the clinic generalizes to real life for head-injured individuals.

Clinicians have had some success with training prospective memory, which is remembering to do something in the future, such as taking medication or shaving. Prospective memory has practical implications, and a Prospective Memory Process Training (PROMPT) appears to generalize across contexts and tasks (Raskin & Sohlberg, 1996; Sohlberg, White, Evans, et al., 1992). The basic task is to carry out a target activity in a specified number of minutes (e.g., in 5 minutes, go open the door), and the training proceeds as follows:

- Gradually increase the interval between request and execution
- Start with a simple one-step task, then make the task more complex
- Introduce self-cues such as an alarm
- Introduce a distracting task during the time interval

The prospective memory task should also model real-life target tasks such as return-ing a phone call, shutting off an appliance, or paying the bills.

Rehabilitation specialists have become interested in a couple of learning techniques:

- **Spaced practice**, which entails gradually increasing the interval between tasks or trials (also referred to as spaced rehearsal or spaced retrieval)
- **Errorless learning**, or using tasks and cues so that the client makes no mistakes

Errorless learning (Baddeley, 1992) is similar to the success principle in aphasia rehabilitation. We shall return to these concepts in the management of dementias (Chapter 13).

Compensatory strategies tend to be preferred and are incorporated into osten-sibly restorative tasks, such as prospective memory activities. These strategies consist of the use of **external memory aids** because the individual with CHI cannot rely on his or her memory alone. All of us use memory aids such as calendars and lists, both with smartphone apps. We just do not need them for remembering to shower or turn off the stove. Examples for clients include notebooks, environmental props, alarms, and paging systems in computers (Hersh & Treadgold, 1994; Sohlberg & Mateer, 1989). Some time is spent in the clinic for training to remember to use the memory aids, and caregivers are alerted that the individual should be using them. Establishing awareness of memory difficulty is important because the individual must recognize a problem when it occurs or, even better, anticipate a problem before it occurs.

Remote memories (i.e., retrograde amnesia) may be targeted incidentally in topics for group therapies that form the core of communication or community-based rehabilitation programs. Retrograde amnesia may involve episodic and semantic memory to some degree. Conceptual knowledge becomes a component of domain-specific training, when we are working within an avocation or a vocational problem. Perhaps the most common activity is the creation of an *autobiography*, which may consist of a scrapbook, written memoir, résumé, or pages in a memory book.

Executive Function

Rehabilitation of the executive system addresses initiating, planning, organizing, and executing. Like the general tasks for treatment of attention, some precedents have consisted of neutral assessment tasks, such as the Tower of London puzzle of transferring rings across pegs (Cicerone & Giacino, 1992). More functional activities include tasks of daily living (e.g., doing laundry, paying bills, making a reservation, going somewhere) or work activities (e.g., using a computer, ordering supplies). Treatment emphasizes the use of organizing aids as well as environmental structuring and supports (e.g., Kennedy, Coelho, Ylvisaker, et al., 2008; Togher, 2012). One such aid is *SymTrend*, a "portable guidance system" for smartphones (symtrend.com). For more, go to the application of this function to storytelling a bit later in the chapter (see Table 12.8).

Group Therapies

Gillis (2007b) noted that group therapy is widely employed for cognitive rehabilitation and, in many facilities, may be the only form of treatment. Criteria for selecting members include (a) choosing those with a deficit shared by all and (b) limiting numbers so enough professional staff are available in case a member becomes verbally or physically unruly. There are two types of groups. For economic reasons, *therapy in a group* consists of a cognitive therapy administered to several people at one time. It is as if we are providing individual therapies in sequence or simultaneously. In *group therapy*, on the other hand, interactions are a means to achieve communicative and social goals that only a group can provide. There are certain familiar recommendations, such as encouraging group members to establish their own goals and plan their own programs. Both types of groups are common for CHI.

Groups oriented around particular cognitive functions are conducted in different stages of recovery and tend to have a "therapy in a group" structure. Gillis (2007b) described an *orientation group* that is helpful in addressing and monitoring the early

PTA phase. Another early intervention theme is *attention.* One category of activities is to present lists or lots of information and have members listen for a target item. This may produce some motivating friendly competition. *Memory and organization groups* tend to be offered in later recovery and/or for higher-level clients.

Communication: Discourse and Conversation

Here is where the SLP's role is most dominant. As with RHD, pragmatic theory and pragmatic assessments certainly give us some direction for coverage. Yet one reason for doing research is to see if people with CHI have particular pragmatic difficulties that may help us narrow our focus for assessment as well as treatment. Three general targets stand out:

- Theory of mind or the ability to take the perspective of another for making inferences
- Global or thematic coherence of discourse-level formulation
- Conversational management and social skills

Regarding perspective taking, the clinician may borrow situations from the research on sarcasm and irony and then discuss them with the client. For each of these areas, we consider restorative and compensatory strategies, often operating in tandem. Also, certain components of functional communicative treatment for aphasia and RHD are applicable, such as conversation therapies and situation-specific role-playing.

Telling a story might not be considered to be the most useful activity per se, although it may be important in some families. Conversation is often about the story told in a movie. Storytelling can also be a means by which the SLP contributes to team rehabilitation of attention and executive disorders. This task requires sustained attention. It has a familiar structure, and Table 12.8 is suggestive of a relationship to the

TABLE 12.8 Elements of an activity for executive functions, including elements of storytelling. May also be useful for RHD.

	GENERAL THERAPEUTICS	STORYTELLING
Initiating	▪ Treatment of fatigue ▪ Set up reminders	Initiating event (What gets the story started?)
Planning	▪ Articulate the goal ▪ Anticipate subgoals and steps ▪ Use calendars and notes ▪ Get help from caregivers	Goal is to tell a story (What is the story about?)
Organizing	▪ Sequence the steps (organizational aids) ▪ Simplify the task ▪ Organize the environment for a task ▪ Self-monitoring (look for and correct mistakes)	Setting first (Who? Where? When?) Episode sequence (What happens? In what order?) Conclusion (Happy ending?)

executive function. It contains question cues for helping someone tell stories that are initially in view (e.g., cartoon sequences), then in a recall activity of retelling a story, and finally in telling a favorite story from recent memory (the day before) or long-term memory (childhood).

Although conversation and role-playing have a general similarity to aphasia treatment, the problems and objectives are different. Some of the cognitive difficulties that have been found to interfere with conversational interaction are noted in Table 12.9. Consistent with the logic of a primary disorder (e.g., inattention) infiltrating a communicative function (e.g., conversation), Youse and Coelho (2009) attempted a treatment of attention that had weak effects on conversation. This try with just two individuals should not discourage more attempts. Meanwhile, a session may be designed to focus on one or two of the problems in Table 12.9. An overarching objective is to increase self-awareness. Awareness activities include viewing oneself on videotape, looking for what is good as well as for what might interfere with the smooth exchange of information.

The clinician and client should agree on specific objectives, such as improving concentration on a topic or reducing the number of interruptions. Some treatment may consist of instruction and discussion concerning the components of a conversation, which should heighten awareness of aspects of everyday interaction that had previously been taken for granted. Then, we want to see if this work generalizes to real-life situations by role-playing phone skills, a job interview, or conflict resolution with a family member or fellow employee. Favorite real-life group activities can be anticipated with a game of poker or a simulated group tour of an art gallery.

In a study of a problem-solving interaction, people with severe TBI performed so well that the task appeared to be a therapeutic opportunity. The task was an interaction between a person with TBI and a friend in which they were to figure out a name and function of an unfamiliar object (e.g., a tap turner, an assistive device for water faucets and door knobs). There was no significant difference between the participants with and without TBI in the quality of their discourse (Kilov, Togher, & Grant, 2009).

TABLE 12.9   Target problem areas, finding areas of primary disorder in conversation. May also be useful for RHD.

Controlling emotions	Disruptive turn Interruptions
Focusing attention	Not listening to conversational partner
Sustaining attention	Unexpected topic shifts
Recent memory	Forgetting topic-related experiences
Executive initiation	Not starting a conversation Not raising a new topic Not taking a turn
Thematic coherence	Off-topic, tangential talk
Theory of mind	Missing the point of others

Genuine group therapy is devoted to communicative and social skills. Adamovich (2005) recommended several types of groups that may be incorporated into a single, ongoing communication group. Her groups were for interpersonal interaction, social skills, empathic abilities, personal and social adjustment, and life skills. Peers in a group may encourage initiation of speaking turns. Groups are a good place to work on reducing the impulsivity of talking out of turn.

Community Reintegration/Reentry

Community reentry programs provide the boost for achieving **long-term goals** of cognitive rehabilitation. They are often conducted in groups and by rehabilitation teams, and Gillis (2007a) provided guidelines for conducting and evaluating reentry groups. Much of the work is conducted in the community and has some similarities to Jon Lyon's Communication Partners program for aphasia (Chapter 10).

The demographics of people with TBI dictate that **return to work** is a frequent individual goal and an indicator of successful rehabilitation outcome (Penn & Jones, 2000), and a little work on politeness may help with the job interview (McDonald and Pearce, 1998). At the Office of Vocational Rehabilitation (OVR) in Pennsylvania, Alan Forman was advised that the goal of community reentry is not necessarily to return to one's old job but rather to find a way to contribute to society (Crimmins, 2000). However, Alan wanted to return to his job at a bank.

Vocational rehabilitation offers **supported employment** in which a rehabilitation counselor, or *job coach*, works with the individual and employer (Wehman, Bricout, & Targett, 1999). OVR partially funded Alan's counseling through a community training program. Bill Gardner, a graduate student in neuropsychology, was Alan's job coach. The bank agreed to allow Alan to work part-time. Bill came to Alan's house 3 days a week, 4 hours each day. In the beginning, Alan had to work on selecting, initiating, and completing work-related tasks. Bill also had to help Alan with strategies for managing irritability and impulse control, which, among other things, drained Alan's energy.

A job coach, like Bill Gardner, negotiates with employers to make accommodations. Thus, like one strategy for aphasia, we try to change communities. In Australia, SLPs evaluated a program for improving police recruits' telephone inquiries from people with TBI before and after a 6-week training program. Training for the recruits included instruction about TBI and role-playing. The prospective police officers improved in establishing the nature of the inquiry and providing information. Moreover, the callers with TBI improved in staying on topic (Togher, McDonald, Code, et al., 2004). In South Africa, similar training for sales assistants proved to be successful (Goldblum & Alant, 2009).

Several organizations provide support for clients and education for employers and service providers (Table 12.10). The Brain Injury Association of America (BIAA) successfully advocated for reauthorization in 2000 of the Traumatic Brain Injury Act of 1996. The original legislation provided for state-based grant programs to improve the care of persons with TBI. In addition, the Traumatic Brain Injury Model System (TBIMS) coordinates innovative research at 17 sites on all aspects of

TABLE 12.10   Organizations providing support for research and people with TBI.

ORGANIZATION	DESCRIPTION	WEB SITE
Brain Injury Association of America (BIAA)	Advocacy and support for brain-injured people and their families (chartered affiliates in states)	biausa.org
Traumatic Brain Injury Model System (TBIMS)	National data-gathering center, supporting a variety of programs at 17 rehabilitation centers in the United States (many are university affiliated)	tbindc.org
Center for Outcome Measurement in Brain Injury (COMBI)	Resource for information on measures; includes details about outcome scales	tbims.org
National Resource Center for Traumatic Brain Injury (NRC for TBI)	Provides information for professionals, brain-injured people, and family members	neuro.pmr.vcu.edu

care and contributes results to the TBI National Data Center at the Kessler Medical Rehabilitation Research and Education Center (e.g., Seel, Kreutzer, Rosenthal, et al., 2003; Sherer, Sander, Nick, et al., 2002).

Recovery and Outcomes

This final section examines cognitive recovery, functional outcome, prognosis, and the influence of rehabilitation. For characterizing functional outcomes, researchers and clinicians rely on general scales, judgments of psychological status, or whether the individual has returned to school or work.

Phases of recovery are summarized in Table 12.11 and parallel the rehab stages of Table 12.6. Posttraumatic amnesia (PTA) concludes when a patient begins to remember day-to-day events and conversations from a few hours earlier. In more than 90 percent of cases, this phase lasts more than a week and more than 4 weeks in 60 percent (Jennett & Teasdale, 1981). The longer PTA lasts, the more difficult it is to recognize when it ends. Identification of the end of PTA can be 1 or 2 weeks off.

The *WAIS* has been used to measure cognitive recovery beyond PTA. Becker (1975) tested 10 head-injured individuals 2 weeks after their accident and then 10 to 11 weeks later. The head-injured participants improved significantly, but so did the IQ-matched controls, indicating that test-related improvement can be attributed to practice or experience with the test. Stretching assessment to 2 years after injury, Bond and Brooks (1976) found that most recovery occurs in the first 6 months. Verbal IQ returns to normal levels before Performance IQ, consistent with the greater severity of deficit with Performance IQ (e.g., Mandelberg & Brooks, 1975). Basic language

TABLE 12.11   Phases in recovery from closed head injury (CHI; Cripe, 1987).

PHASE	DESCRIPTION	TREATMENT ORIENTATION
Coma	Loss of consciousness lasting hours to months	
Posttraumatic amnesia (PTA)	Beginning when consciousness is regained and ending when a patient can remember day-to-day events	Assistance with attention and orientation; complex cognition is avoided
Rapid recovery	Significant progress over 3 to 6 months depending on severity	Focus on basic skills; minimize unrealistic expectations
Long-term plateau	Persisting residual deficits; progress is painstakingly slow	Emphasis on adjusting to disabilities

functions progress impressively within the first 6 months (e.g., Levin, Grossman, Sarwar, et al., 1981; Luzzatti et al., 1989). Also, the recovery of linguistic and cognitive functions is correlated during this period (Vukovic, et al., 2008).

Two general scales have been used to characterize outcome. The **Glasgow Outcome Scale** (GOS) offers general levels defined by severity of disablement and amount of social support required (Jennett & Bond, 1975; Wilson, Pettigrew, & Teasdale, 1998). A sketch of the five-point scale follows:

- *Death*
- *Persistent vegetative state:* unresponsive
- *Severe disability* (conscious but disabled): dependent for daily support
- *Moderate disability* (disabled but independent): can work in a sheltered environment
- *Good recovery:* resumption of normal life despite mild deficits

The other general indicator is the **Disability Rating Scale** (DRS; Fryer & Haffey, 1987; Rappaport et al., 1982). The DRS consists of eight general ratings for eye opening, communication, motor response, feeding, toileting, grooming, level of functioning, and employability. It was determined to be more sensitive to recovery than the GOS (see also Hall, Cope, & Rappaport, 1985).

Clinicians may turn to proxy reports of outcomes, which usually consist of family members' perceptions of how a head-injured individual is doing (Brooks, Campsie, Symington, et al., 1986; Brooks, McKinlay, Symington, et al., 1987). Dawson and Chipman (1995) conducted a survey of 454 persons with TBI 13 years after injury. Most still needed help for daily living activities and were unemployed. Ninety percent were unhappy with social integration. Ponsford and others (1999) studied outcomes of over 1,200 people between 2 and 10 years after injury. One-third still needed help for shopping, finances, and home maintenance, but over 90 percent had attained independence performing more basic activities of daily living. Around 50 percent were working by 2 years postinjury, but many did not sustain their employment. More than half were depressed and anxious, and many of these were socially isolated (also, Johnson, 1998).

Can these outcomes be predicted? Duration of PTA has been used for prognosis. There is some evidence that recovery to normal levels of cognitive function within 6 months to a year is predicted by PTA of under 6 weeks. If PTA lasts longer than 3 months, outlook is not promising. A Glasgow Outcome Scale obtained at 3 months may predict a GOS measure of function at 1 year postinjury (King, Carlier, & Marion, 2005). Investigators have tended to be more interested in predicting return to work than a level of cognitive function (e.g., Prigatano, 1999).

In a follow-up study of severe head injury based on proxy reports, Brooks and others (1987) found that communication deficits were significant predictors of failure to return to work. The following highlights other predictors of a return to school or work (Boake, Millis, High, et al., 2001; Crepeau & Scherzer, 1993; Ip, Dornan, & Schentag, 1995; Ruff, Marshall, Crouch, et al., 1993; Sherer, Sander, Nick, et al., 2002):

- Preinjury substance abuse history
- Information processing speed
- Executive function ability
- Early neuropsychological test performance

Technically sufficient **efficacy** data is rare (Jordan, 2000). Support for rehabilitation consists mainly of follow-up outcomes for large rehabilitation programs or pre-post assessments of specific treatment procedures for individuals, with some small-group studies in between. The state of the science was demonstrated by Carney, Chestnut, and others (1999) in a review process that started with over 3,000 articles that might have something to say about cognitive rehabilitation. Eventually, 600 addressed the key question of whether cognitive rehabilitation affects outcomes. Only 32 of these satisfied criteria for an adequate study. Only 15 included a control group. Only six measured real-life outcomes.

Hall and Cope (1995) found general support for cognitive rehabilitation. They reviewed 28 studies published between 1984 and 1994. Acute rehabilitation reduced postacute rehabilitation by two-thirds. Postacute rehabilitation (e.g., outpatient programs) was beneficial for functional outcomes even after a reasonable period for spontaneous recovery. There is some evidence that early intervention is more effective than later intervention (e.g., Rappaport, Herrero-Backe, Rappaport, et al., 1989).

Coelho, DeRuyter, and Stein (1996) sampled studies of rehabilitation programs and training for specific cognitive functions. These studies provided documentation of improvements. The investigators also gathered their own retrospective outcome data from five inpatient rehabilitation programs across the United States. The average length of stay was 46.3 days, ranging from 32.5 to 58.4 days (or about 2 months). Most clients demonstrated improvement with functional status measures. An average of 84 percent were discharged to home, and 11 percent were discharged to long-term care facilities.

Another literature search was conducted for articles published between 1998 and 2002. The team of investigators' broad sweep of "cognitive rehabilitation" included stroke as well as TBI and concentrated on seven areas including language and communication. Conclusions were similar to Robey's in Chapter 8. There is satisfying evidence to support cognitive rehabilitation of attention, memory, and executive function. "Future research should move beyond the simple question of whether cognitive rehabilitation is effective" (Cicerone, Dahlberg, Malec, et al., 2005, p. 1681). The results were supported later by another meta-analysis (Rohling, Faust, Beverly, et al., 2009).

Summary and Conclusions

This chapter covered the range of topics that were included for aphasia in the previous 10 chapters, namely impairments, assessment, rehabilitation, and recovery. This chapter may have seemed refreshingly light on technical research, especially for language, mainly because this research is rare. Cases with closed head injury (CHI) can be quite different from cases with stroke. The condition of the brain is quite different. Cognitive impairments can also be quite different. Furthermore, the needs of a younger population differ from an older population with stroke. Parents are more likely to be involved, and clients are more likely to have concerns about returning to school, work, and parenting.

People with CHI have deficits of attention, episodic memory, learning new information, and behavioral organization. Sometimes their personalities seem to change as they become irritable or impulsive. Some seem to be unconcerned or unmotivated. On the other hand, older adults with stroke can concentrate for long periods, remember their past, absorb new information, and structure their daily routines. They tend to maintain their prestroke personalities and have normal reactions to sudden disability. Many are highly motivated to improve their language abilities. Thus, CHI presents a special challenge for rehabilitative teamwork among neuropsychologists, psychologists, and speech-language pathologists.

Except for the cases in which a focal trauma causes a nearly classic aphasia, a striking difference between the effects of stroke and CHI is the level of residual or chronic language ability. People with CHI are likely to be able to retrieve words and formulate fluent sentences. Many have such mild and subtle impairments that they seem ready to return to school or work. Upon returning, some succeed but many fail because of demands that exceed their concentration or patience. Communicative difficulties appear in the organization of discourse and in pragmatic aspects of conversation.

An SLP's contribution to rehabilitation consists of assessing and treating the communicative consequences of cognitive impairments. We take into consideration the impact of communication and participation limitations on a young adult's educational and vocational objectives. Again, treatment is consistent with the two fundamental approaches to aphasia and RHD, namely some stimulation activities for impairments and extensive training of compensatory strategies to bypass chronic impairments.

Dementias and Progressive Aphasias

Thomas DeBaggio, a journalist and coauthor of books about growing herbs, wrote, "I am alone and I can hear water running somewhere in the house. I don't remember going to the bathroom. Who else turned on the water?" (2002, p. 5). A few months after his 57th birthday, he was diagnosed as having Alzheimer's disease.

In the past, dementia was thought to sweep across the entire domain of cognition. Dementias, however, are varied and are considered to be a group of disorders with multiple cognitive deficits (American Psychiatric Association, 2013). This chapter introduces a few causes, but, for the sake of efficiency, it focuses on the most well-known cause, namely Alzheimer's disease. Finally, the chapter takes us back to Chapter 2's introduction to *primary progressive aphasia* (PPA).

Diagnosis and Assessment of Dementia

In 1992, the Agency for Health Care Policy and Research, part of the U.S. Public Health Service, sponsored a panel of experts to develop a clinical practice guideline on screening for Alzheimer's and other dementias. Regardless of the neuropathology or cause, diagnosis of dementia is based on a medical history, a physical examination, informant reports, and a mental status evaluation. The general criteria for diagnosis of dementia are as follows (Ballard, 2000; Fields, 1998; see also *DSM-5*, American Psychiatric Association, 2013):

- A change from a previous level of cognitive function
- No disruption of consciousness
- A disruption of daily functioning
- Cannot be explained by situational stress

Doctors have begun to screen their elderly patients for cognitive impairment or dementia (Dash & Villemarette-Pittman, 2005).

A clinical neuropsychologist may administer a comprehensive evaluation. DeBaggio (2002) was given the National Adult Reading Test (NART), the *WAIS-R* (Chapter 11), and the *WMS-R* (Chapter 12). "It was numbing and took about six hours" (p. 15). The NART consists of 50 irregular words to pronounce (Nelson & O'Connell, 1978; see also Grober & Sliwinski, 1991) and has been used to estimate intelligence either premorbidly or without having to give an entire *WAIS* (e.g., Crawford, Parker, Stewart, Beeson, & DeLacey, 1989). DeBaggio's estimated premorbid IQ was 124. The results of his assessment showed that his postonset IQ was 91, and his memory test scores indicated severe impairment.

The most widely employed screening test for cognitive deterioration is the ***Mini-Mental State Examination*** (*MMSE*; Folstein, Folstein, & McHugh, 1975). As will be seen several times in this chapter, it is commonly used to identify participants in research. The *MMSE* is a 10-minute bedside assessment of six areas, namely orientation for date and location, "registration" (repeating three words), concentration (counting backward by sevens), short-term or recent memory (repeating the previous three words), language (naming, following instruction), and visuospatial (copying shapes). The best score is 30. The *MMSE* has been criticized for being sparse, and extended versions were created in which each of the six areas was expanded (Ashford, Kumar, Barringer, et al., 1992), and in a version called the *3MS*, the range of scores was stretched to 100 (Teng & Chui, 1987).

The ***Global Deterioration Scale*** (*GDS*) consists of seven levels, with Level 1 representing no cognitive decline and Level 7, very severe cognitive decline (Reisberg, Ferris, de Leon, et al., 1982). Levels 2 and 3 are identified with mild cognitive decline. Diagnosis of dementia begins with Level 4 (Table 13.1). The *GDS* is supported by two other scales, namely the *Brief Cognitive Rating Scale* (*BCRS*) and the *Functional Assessment Staging Test* (*FAST*), which focuses on the last area of the *BCRS* (Reisberg, Ferris, & Franssen, 1985).

At the University of Cambridge in the United Kingdom, physicians and psychologists developed ***Addenbrooke's Cognitive Examination*** (*ACE*; Dudas, Berrios, & Hodges, 2005). The ACE is used east of the Atlantic for identifying participants in studies. The test takes about 30 minutes to evaluate a variety of cognitive and linguistic functions. In one study, it was more sensitive than the *MMSE* in detecting dementia (Mathuranath, Nestor, Berrios, et al., 2000).

The ***Mini-Cog Rapid Assessment Battery*** (*MRAB*), not to be confused with *Cognistat* or *CogSport* in Chapter 12, is a self-assessment that can be used anywhere (Shephard & Kosslyn, 2005). It was originally designed for astronauts and mountain

TABLE 13.1   *MMSE* and GDS scale definitions of severity levels ("stages").
MMSE scores are commonly used to identify the stage or stages of dementias being studied.

STAGE	*MMSE* SCORE	GDS LEVEL
Mild	20–26	4
Moderate	10–19	5
Severe	<10	7

climbers to wear on their wrists (i.e., "a blood pressure cuff for the mind"). More generally, the *MiniCog* can be administered with a handheld or desktop computer. It is intended to provide an "early warning" for someone who is suffering from stress-related deficits that may affect performance. The *Mini-Cog* proved to be as effective as the longer *MMSE* in detecting dementia (Borson, Scanlan, Chen, et al., 2003).

Other brief tests and rating scales were created partly for drug research, and most can be found on the Internet (e.g., Blessed, Tomlinson, & Roth, 1968; Mattis, 1988; Rosen, Mohs, & Davis, 1984). Mental status tests are not by themselves diagnostic. Certain "biomarkers," to be discussed later, now supplement cognitive tests.

Alzheimer's Disease

Let us switch from diagnosis of dysfunction to the most recognized cause. In Frankfurt, Germany, in 1906, Alois Alzheimer wondered about the progressively deteriorating memory of a 52-year-old patient known as Frau Auguste D. Following her death, the young physician performed an autopsy and discovered some unusual tangles and a "peculiar substance" spread over the entire cortex that others later said was neuritic plaques (Shenk, 2002).

Until the 1950s, Alzheimer's disease (AD) was thought to be a rare affliction of middle age, whereas "senile dementia" was thought to be simply a severe form of aging. Then Neumann and Cohn (1953) found plaques and tangles in the brains of elderly individuals. They established that Alzheimer's disease causes dementia at any age and, therefore, that dementia in old age can often be the result of a disease rather than a manifestation of aging.

Neuropathology is observed at two levels. At the macroscopic level, a physician can see the atrophy of certain areas of the brain indicative of the death of brain cells (or neuron loss). Sulci appear wider as convolutions become smaller. Atrophy is attributed to what can be seen microscopically with nerve cell stains. A Congo red stain exposes **neurofibrillary tangles**, which are triangular and looped fibers located *within* nerve cell bodies. These tangles, containing a protein called *tau*, appear early in the disease. A silver stain detects granular deposits and remains of degenerated nerve fibers called **neuritic plaques** located *outside* neurons. The plaques contain a *beta-amyloid* protein (i.e., "amyloid plaques").

The disease spreads. It begins with tangles in the *hippocampus*, a structure within the temporal lobe that is important for memory. It then infiltrates frontal, parietal, and temporal lobes (Petersen, 2002). Tangles are pronounced in the *inferior temporal lobe* and accumulate in the *parieto-temporal juncture*. Studies of cerebral blood flow and metabolism reveal bilateral reduction in parietal and posterior temporal lobes. There can be more hypoperfusion in one hemisphere than in the other in early stages. Locations of pathology result in fairly specific impairments, especially of memory and language in the early stage.

Because there is no definitive diagnostic criterion for AD short of autopsy, diagnosis is usually a careful process of elimination of other possible causes. In the logic of elimination, AD is likely in the absence of depression, multiple infarcts, excessive medication, alcoholism, and malnutrition.

Three **biomarkers**, related to the aforementioned plaques and tangles, are now available to improve earlier diagnosis of Alzheimer's disease. This trio, found in cerebro-spinal fluid, is technically known as (1) low levels of beta-amyloid protein, (2) high levels of total tau protein, and (2) elevated phosphorelated tau. Markers can be found with structural MRI and molecular PET neuroimaging (Dubois, Feldman, Jacova, et al., 2007; Sohrabi, Weinborn, Badcock, et al., 2011). Some markers may also be detected in biopsy-derived tissue and in blood samples (Hye, Lynham, Thambisetty, et al., 2006).

Once thought to be rare, Alzheimer's disease is now recognized as the most frequent cause of dementia in adulthood, responsible for over 50 percent of cases. A history of AD is summarized in Table 13.2. The long period of archaic terminology, such as *presenile dementia* and *senile dementia*, coincides with the time in which cognitive problems after age 60 were considered to be simply old age. Use of the term *senile* and its variants has been dwindling rapidly but has still lingered. Labels for specific versions of Alzheimer's disease are becoming common:

- *Early-onset Alzheimer's disease*, before age 65, like basketball coach Pat Summitt
- *Late-onset Alzheimer's disease*, after age 65, like former President Ronald Reagan
- *Familial Alzheimer's*, multiple members of the same family
- *Sporadic Alzheimer's*, only one member of a family

TABLE 13.2 Historical sketch of Alzheimer's disease and dementia. Some events are discussed later.

YEAR	EVENT
1906	Alois Alzheimer finds plaques and tangles in a patient's brain
1910	Alzheimer's mentor Emil Kraepelin mentions "Alzheimer's disease" in his *Handbook of Psychiatry*
1953	Neumann and Cohn recognize Alzheimer's disease as a pathology that can occur in middle and late adulthood
1975	*Mini Mental State Examination* (*MMSE*) introduced
1984	Diagnostic criteria for probable Alzheimer's dementia established by NIH-NINCDS
1996	FDA approval of Aricept®
2001	Medicare funding for AD rehabilitation authorized
2007	Dubois and others' suggested revision of NINCDS criteria, to include biomarkers
2012	Medicare revises criteria for rehabilitation reimbursement; improvement not required

An extended family of 5,000 people in Medellín, Colombia, is the world's largest example of familial Alzheimer's. It is participating in a prevention study (Lasprilla, Iglesias, & Lopera, 2003).

Other Causes of Dementia

The pattern of an individual's dementia depends on etiology. Pathologies may be classified as progressive or nonprogressive, or as nonreversible or reversible (Table 13.3). Alzheimer's disease is one of several progressive and nonreversible pathologies with a gradual onset and relentless deterioration. Regarding the other pathologies, this section briefly cites some characteristic dysfunctions, leaving details of dementia to be represented later by Alzheimer's.

Primary location of pathology is another basis of classification (e.g., cortical or subcortical). For example, AD is concentrated in the cerebral cortex, whereas

TABLE 13.3   Neuropathologies that cause dementias.

	DIAGNOSIS	SITE OF DAMAGE	DISEASE PROCESS
Progressive	Alzheimer's disease	Bilateral parietal and temporal lobes (including hippocampus)	Accumulation of neuritic plaques and neurofibrillary tangles
	Pick's disease	Frontal lobe degeneration and more temporal lobe atrophy than in Alzheimer's disease	Absence of plaques; presence of tau protein ("Pick's bodies")
	Lewy Body disease	Frontal and temporal lobes; basal ganglia	Protein deposits (i.e., Lewy bodies) in neuronal cells
	Chronic traumatic encephalopathy (CTE)	Bilateral cortical and/or subcortical atrophy	Repeated blows to head; Neurofibrillary tangles and other microscopic material
	Parkinson's disease	Subcortical dementia; caudate nucleus of the basal ganglia	Cell loss reducing production of the neurotransmitter dopamine
	Huntington's disease	Subcortical dementia; caudate nucleus of the basal ganglia	Inherited atrophy of the caudate
Nonprogressive	Vascular dementia (e.g., multiple infarcts)	Any location	Arteriosclerotic reductions of blood supply
	Herpes simplex viral encephalitis (HSVE)	Medial temporal areas extending into orbitofrontal regions; usually bilateral	Infection causing acute necrosis, edema, and hemorrhage

pathology in Parkinson's disease is beneath the cortex. We may hedge with phrases like "primarily located" because white matter pathology has been found with AD, and frontal lobe hypometabolism has been detected in some subcortical pathologies.

What if it's not Alzheimer's? asked Lisa and Gary Radin (2003) with regard to *frontotemporal dementia* (FTD). The pathology is usually **Pick's disease**, consisting of tangles that differ from those in Alzheimer's disease. Pick's disease does not include the amyloid plaques of AD. Personality change is an early sign, such as inappropriate disruptive behavior prompting psychiatric evaluation (Cycyk & Harris Wright, 2008; Davis, Price, Moore, et al., 2001).

Lewy body disease occurs alone, or it can occur with around 20 percent of cases with AD. Lewy bodies are abnormal protein deposits that progressively destroy brain cells. They are widespread throughout the cerebral cortex and hippocampus, but they are also found in the brain stem. As a result, a person with Lewy body disease can have a symptom complex that appears to be a combination of Alzheimer's and Parkinson's diseases. Problems with focusing attention and memory usually appear before the rigidity and tremors of motor dysfunction (e.g., McKeith, Fairbarn, Perry, & Thompson, 1994).

The story of the mild sports concussions or MTBIs of Chapter 12 can be much worse. A newly discovered and highly publicized degenerative disease, **chronic traumatic encephalopathy** (CTE), can be caused by repeated blows to the head, mainly in football and boxing, but also from blast injuries. Atrophy of both hemispheres, including the medial temporal lobe, has been seen with macrostructural imaging. Microstructural laboratory analysis has exposed a variety of tau-related tangles and other trespassing structures (e.g., McKee, Cantu, Nowinski, et al., 2009).

With **reversible dementias**, causes can be treated to restore normal or nearly normal cognitive function. This treatability is why early diagnosis of dementia is so important. The most frequent causes are depression, alcohol abuse, and drug toxicity. In particular, *polypharmacy*, or the simultaneous use of multiple medications, can promote declining intellectual function. Medications with cognitive side effects include anticholinergics such as Elavil and Benadryl, narcotics such as Vicodin and Percocet, and sedatives such as Xanax and Valium.

Depression is common in the elderly, is often ignored (i.e., "underdiagnosed"), and may even be mistaken for Alzheimer's disease. People who appear to have Alzheimer's dementia but really have only depression are said to have *depressive pseudodementia*. In fact, people with depressive pseudodementia are considered to be different from those who are simply depressed because the former have problems that show up in cognitive testing. Physicians recommend that older adults with depression be evaluated regularly for cognitive decline and that people with AD be evaluated regularly for depression (Dash & Villemarette-Pittman, 2005).

Dementia of Alzheimer's Type (DAT)

Having considered neuropathology of the disease, let us turn to its consequences for cognition. A variety of cognitive functions have been studied. After a general discussion of diagnosis and progression, this section concentrates on memory. Other aspects of cognition will be touched on in later discussions of language, communication, and rehabilitation.

Criteria for Diagnosis

What if the dementia is Alzheimer's? **NINCDS-ADRDA criteria** for diagnosis of *probable dementia of Alzheimer's type* (pDAT) were drafted in the early 1980s at the National Institute of Neurological and Communicative Diseases and Stroke–Alzheimer's Disease and Related Disorders Association (McKhann, Drachman, Folstein, et al., 1984; see also Blacker, Albert, Bassett, et al., 1994). Accordingly, pDAT is diagnosed when, along with medical history, there are two or more declining functions from the following areas (or memory impairment and one other area):

- Language (e.g., misnaming)
- Memory (e.g., forgetting appointments)
- Orientation (e.g., getting lost in familiar settings)
- Judgment (e.g., not wearing a coat in freezing weather)

Dubois and others (2007) recommended revision of NINCDS-ADRDA criteria to take into account early signs of memory difficulty and biomarkers of the disease.

In the study of cognition and language with dementias, experimental participants have usually been identified according to both the NIH criteria and *MMSE* scores. Also, participants are beginning to be identified according to the Dubois revision (e.g., Sajjadi, Patterson, Tomek, et al., 2012). Healthy control participants are matched according to age and education. Because more women than men have AD (women live longer), most participant groups have more women. The following discussion of DAT starts with its progression in stages and then focuses on memory.

Stages

The onset of Alzheimer's dementia is invariably identified with the date of *diagnosis* because the beginning of the subterranean disease cannot be determined. ". . . [I]t is not uncommon for a person to have already been in the early phase of AD by the time a family member first feels memory lapses are an actual problem" (Dash & Villemarette-Pittman, 2005, p. 20). For Burton Wheeler's (2001) wife, "there was no evident trigger, no first domino" (p. 3). Early warnings include a noticeable increase of forgetting, disorientation, erratic changes in mood and personality, and difficulty finding words. "Researchers are attempting to clarify the boundaries between what we consider the effects of normal aging and the onset of Alzheimer's disease" (Petersen, 2002, p. 31).

A transitional area between normal aging and DAT is **mild cognitive impairment** (MCI) and is assigned the Level 3 in Reisberg's GDS scale. It falls short of NIH criteria for DAT and is characterized by recent memory impairment greater than what one would expect for the person's age. Other cognitive skills decline at a faster rate than for people without MCI but at a slower rate than those with DAT. In fact, people who had been diagnosed with MCI did not decline in discourse production 6 months later (Fleming & Harris, 2009). People with MCI may never progress to Alzheimer's disease but do have an increased risk for it (Peterson, Smith, Tangalos, et al., 1993).

With the goal of detecting trouble as soon as possible, the **Montréal Cognitive Assessment** (*MoCA*) is a 10-minute screening for mild cognitive deficit and is accessible at its Web site (mocatest.org). Like the *MMSE*, best score is 30 derived from several quick tests of attention, constructional skills, memory, orientation, and language production (Nasreddine, Phillips, Bedirian, et al., 2005). The *MoCA* can detect dementia in individuals scoring above 25 on the *MMSE* (Smith, Gildeh, & Holmes, 2007).

Even before MCI, there is an acknowledgement of a "preclinical" phase by the National Institute on Aging (nia.nih.gov) and the Alzheimer's Association (alz.org). For research purposes, this phase consists of the initial "subterranean" formation of Alzheimer's tangles and plaques but without overt symptoms.

The course of Alzheimer's disease is a continuum of changes often parsed into stages. When discussing someone with DAT, clinicians often identify if they are referring to an "early stage" or "late stage" condition. There are different depictions of the progression, but three stages are summarized here to get the idea across (Table 13.4; also Table 13.1). Following MCI, the person in *Stage I* (*MMSE* 20–26) of diagnosed DAT conducts household chores carelessly but can follow routines. Apathy, not forgetfulness,

TABLE 13.4   **Stages in the progression of dementia of Alzheimer's type (DAT).**

	OTHER TERMS	SYMPTOMS	LANGUAGE
Predementia	Mild cognitive impairment (MCI)	Forgetful	
Stage I	Early Mild	Forgetful Disoriented Careless Apathetic Irritable	Usually comprehends Word-finding difficulty in conversation Word fluency impaired Good repetition
Stage II	Middle Moderate	Recent events forgotten Math skills reduced Unprovoked agressiveness	Comprehension reduced Paraphasias, jargon Irrelevant talk Naming becomes wordy Poor self-monitoring
Stage III	Late Severe	Recent events fade fast Remote memory impaired Family not recognized Incontinence	Becomes unresponsive Becomes mute

was the first sign of trouble for Burton Wheeler's (2001) wife. He wrote, "She became listless; the brightness of her eyes dimmed. She lost interest in going to concerts, plays, and movies. Her enthusiasm for travel vanished" (p. 3).

Stage II (*MMSE* 10–19) is characterized by an increasing burden on family members. The spouse is becoming a parenting caregiver. Memory deficits are more obvious and disruptive. Shoes are put on before socks. There is frequent pacing and staring into space. Irritability changes to outbursts of aggression. Sensory and motor deficits appear. Motor disability arises in *Stage III* (*MMSE* <10). The individual sits motionless in a corner and becomes totally dependent on others for tasks of daily living.

Episodic Memory

Daniel Schacter (1996), who has written a great deal about memory impairments, played two rounds of golf with Frederick, who was in the early stage of Alzheimer's dementia. It was a test. One round was on a familiar course, and the other on an unfamiliar course. Retaining procedural memory, Frederick could still play. He also retained perfect use of golf strategy and terminology, indicative of intact semantic and lexical stores. He chose the right club, knew who should putt first, and evaluated slopes on the green before putting. However, he forgot the shots he had just hit. He could not remember where his ball went after being the first to tee off, probably because of a delay between hitting and walking to the ball. Unlike most golfers in the clubhouse, he could not recall a single shot from the round. Frederick had a problem with personally experienced events or episodic memory.

Although episodic memory is easily identified with autobiographical memory (Chapter 12), the study of episodic memory in ageing and progressive dementias has frequently relied on naming. The research emphasizes the object to be named, with naming being an indication of memory for the object. As a result, there is an acknowledged intersection between episodic and semantic memory. In particular, an influence of episodic memory on semantic memory is suspected with respect to a person's experience with an object to be named.

The success of recall follows a **temporal gradient** observed as remote memories (e.g., objects from the distant past) being remembered better than recent memories (e.g., contemporary objects). This gradient is common in healthy elderly people who have an uncanny recollection of distant events (Sagar, Sullivan, & Corkin, 1991; Westmacott, Freedman, Black, et al., 2004).

In one study, participants in an *MMSE* range of 10 to 27 named objects that were used uniquely early in their lives (i.e., dated), such as a *washboard* and *milk can*, and objects uniquely in use after the 1970s (i.e., contemporary), such as a *computer* and *microwave*. In addition, objects like a *camera* were compared in their dated and contemporary forms. Giving the objects a period identity was considered to imbue concepts with an episodic quality. Whereas younger adults had no difference in naming dated and contemporary objects, both healthy older adults and those with DAT favored the dated objects. The best naming for the two older groups occurred with common dated objects (e.g., *stove*) (Small & Sandhu, 2008).

We began to learn about the neurological basis of episodic memory from HM, who underwent a bilateral medial temporal lobectomy in 1953 at the age of 27 to relieve intractable epilepsy (Scoville & Milner, 1957). HM's memory and language have been thoroughly investigated (e.g., Milner, Corkin, & Teuber, 1968; Skotko, Andrews, & Einstein, 2005). Two years after the surgery, HM had an IQ of 112 but did not recognize hospital staff and forgot when he had eaten a recent meal. Besides his anterograde amnesia, he also had retrograde amnesia for events years prior to his operation. Now we know his name. Henry Gustav Molaison passed away in 2008.

Like the association of Broca's area and speech nearly a century before, it is thought that HM provided the first direct evidence that the medial temporal lobe, the *hippocampus* in particular, plays an important role in memory. Noted earlier in the chapter, Alzheimer's disease usually begins in the hippocampus. This structure appears to be responsible for sorting the parts of new or recent memories and then reassembling them for recall. MRI studies have shown substantial neuron loss or atrophy in the hippocampus. Later we shall consider a related deficiency in the production of acetylcholine (ACh), a neurotransmitter in the region of the hippocampus that is important for memory.

Semantic Memory

Semantic memory is the long-term storage of general conceptual knowledge and is presumed to contain the meanings of words. When there is a deficient semantic memory, more specific issues arise pertaining to whether there is a problem with storage (i.e., degraded conceptual representations) or with the processes of activation or access. Also, there is the question of whether word-finding difficulty is related to deficiencies of semantic memory. For some investigators, unsuspecting of what aphasia tells us about a distinct lexical memory, words are part of semantic memory.

Clinical researchers have assessed semantic memory with effortful tasks, such as meaningful and meaningless phrase repetition (Bayles, Tomoeda, & Rein, 1996) and production of definitions (Harley, Jessiman, MacAndrew, et al., 2008). Cognitive psychologists have also used a variety of effortful tasks to see if deficits are category-specific (e.g., object similarity judgment, object classification). There has been a frequent finding of more difficulty with living things such as animals than nonliving things such as tools (e.g., Daum, Riesch, Sartori, et al., 1996; Chan, Salmon, & De La Pena, 2001), but people with DAT have also displayed the opposite pattern (Montanes, Goldblum, & Boller, 1996).

Some cognitive psychologists have preferred implicit methods such as semantic priming (Chapter 3) in which semantic memory is accessed more purely, with minimal conscious manipulation. Initial results in several studies were mixed, partly due to differences of procedure, but semantic priming with short stimulus onset asynchronies (SOAs) detected some preservation of semantic memory (Giffard, Desgranges, & Eustache, 2005).

One phenomenon unique to some people with DAT is **hyperpriming**, when the robust effect of semantic relatedness is larger relative to healthy controls (i.e., response to related targets is much faster than to unrelated targets). Sometimes hyperpriming occurs when conditions promote strategic processing (Bell, Chenery, & Ingram, 2001). Researchers have been deconstructing this phenomenon, digging into the mind of someone with Alzheimer's dementia. Explanations include cognitive slowing and a degrading of storage.

How might the general slowing of cognitive processing lead to hyperpriming? General slowing is seen in the fact that all response times by people with DAT are longer than those by control groups. In particular, "baseline" responses are much slower (e.g., unrelated prime-target conditions), which ends up exaggerating the advantage of related prime-target conditions (Chertkow, Bub, & Seidenberg, 1989; Nebes, Brady, & Huff, 1989).

The evidence for degradation of storage is varied and extends the cognitive slowing explanation. In one study, people with a mild clinical semantic impairment exhibited priming for both animate (i.e., animals) and inanimate (i.e., artifacts) categories. Those with the more severe moderate deficits exhibited a selective absence of priming for inanimate concepts, indicating that a category-specific deficit becomes part of the decline in semantic memory (Hernández, Costa, Juncadella, et al., 2008). This pattern diverges from living and nonliving comparisons with explicit or strategic tasks, underscoring the need to study both automatic and strategic levels of processing.

Findings may depend on the type of relationship between the prime and target. For example, an associative relationship (e.g., *cottage-cheese*) is based on common experience, whereas categorical associates (e.g., *peach-plum*) are related purely to the conceptual structure presumed to characterize semantic networks. One study found that participants with DAT were primed for associates but not for categorical relationships, suggestive of a degraded semantic network (Glosser, Friedman, Grugan, et al., 1998; see also Perri, Zannino, Caltagirone, et al., 2011).

Another relatedness manipulation compares categorical relationships (e.g., tiger-lion) to attribute relationships (e.g., tiger-stripes) with the assumption that category coordinates and attributes reflect different levels of conceptual structure. Coordinates are *between* concepts (i.e., two animals), and attributes are *within* concepts (i.e., of one animal). In a priming task with a short, 250 millisecond SOA, people with DAT exhibited hyperpriming, due to cognitive slowing, for coordinates but not for attributes. A general conclusion was that a partial loss of semantic information accompanies the cognitive slowing of dementia (Giffard, Desgranges, Nore-Mary, et al., 2001).

Language with DAT

As speech-language pathologists (SLPs), we are especially concerned with language in Alzheimer's dementia. Some people with DAT appear to have aphasia, usually mixed with other cognitive deficits. Most studies have been done with mild-to-moderate dementia. People with mild dementia correspond to early-stage DAT, and those with moderate dementia correspond to those with midstage DAT. People with early-stage dementia are able to participate in some of the sophisticated experiments.

Clinical language assessment was carried out with the *Western Aphasia Battery* (*WAB*). In one study, all 25 participants with DAT were below the AQ's 93.8 cutoff for aphasia or language disorder (Appell, Kertesz, & Fisman, 1982). Later, a discriminant analysis showed that the *WAB* had difficulty distinguishing DAT from stroke-related aphasia (Horner, Dawson, Heyman, et al., 1992). Thus, people with DAT have clinical language deficiencies.

Comprehension

Clinical tasks, such as sentence–picture matching, have revealed a slight decline of sentence comprehension in the early stage (e.g., Bickel, Pantel, Eysenbach, et al., 2000; Rochon, Waters, & Caplan, 1994). MacDonald and her colleagues (2001) studied 11 persons with mild-to-moderate DAT (*MMSE* 16–24). The group had a deficit in making explicit grammaticality judgments. Yet when the investigators measured time to read aloud a word that either appropriately or inappropriately completed a spoken sentence, the group with DAT was just as quick as matched controls. The implicit task indicated that individuals with DAT understand sentences.

Murray Grossman, at the University of Pennsylvania, directed a series of studies of language comprehension with dementia (Lee, Grossman, Morris, et al., 2003). Price and Grossman (2005) had 15 individuals with mild-to-moderate DAT (ave *MMSE* 21.7) engage in an on-line word-monitoring task. Semantic and syntactic aspects of verbs were examined, namely semantically oriented information about actions and their agents and syntactically oriented information about whether a verb can take a recipient (i.e., transivity). Like healthy matched controls, the group with DAT was sensitive to transivity. Unlike matched controls, however, the group with DAT was insensitive to thematic appropriateness. This result reinforced a view that people with early DAT are more impaired for semantics than for syntax.

Does **working memory** influence comprehension with DAT? First, let us consider whether there is a decline of working memory per se. In a *digit-ordering* task, participants repeated randomly presented digits (e.g., 7–2–4–9–1) in ascending numerical order (e.g., 1–2–4–7–9), requiring a mental conversion in addition to simple retention. Those with "questionable dementia" were similar to controls, but those with mild or moderate DAT were impaired (MacDonald et al., 2001).

Waters, Caplan, and Rochon (1995) followed their comprehension study with one in which people with mild or moderate DAT remembered digits presented while doing a sentence-picture matching task. These participants were more affected than matched controls by the digit load, leading the researchers to conclude that people with DAT have a reduced working memory capacity for language processing. Later, employing a variety of picture-matching formats, Waters and her colleagues (1998) found no evidence of a syntactic deficit. Difficulty arose with heightened processing demands of the task.

The pragmatics of comprehension with DAT was introduced with an investigation of metaphor. The metaphors were idiomatic (conventional), depending less on context, and novel (nonconventional), depending more on context (Chapter 4). The items were uniquely Italian, but translated, novel metaphors included *Investors are squirrels gathering nuts* and *Shoppers at sales are ants at a picnic*. Participants with mild-to-moderate DAT understood conventional metaphor normally but were deficient with novel metaphor. With some additional testing, including Theory of Mind tasks, difficulty with novel metaphor was traced to deficits of reasoning and executive function (Amanzio, Geminiani, Leotta, et al., 2008). If we try to be creative in conversation, people with DAT may not get it.

For discourse comprehension, let us first consider the ability to connect pronouns to antecedents across sentences. MacDonald and her colleagues (2001) used a cross-modal word-naming procedure to find that people with DAT are sensitive to pronoun appropriateness. However, these participants did not have as strong an effect as controls, indicating that people with DAT process pronouns less effectively.

Welland, Lubinski, and Higginbotham (2002) administered Brookshire and Nicholas's *Discourse Comprehension Test* to persons with mild or moderate DAT. Both groups scored significantly worse than matched controls. People with DAT had the same pattern of performance as the controls, namely better scores for recalling main ideas than details and better scores for recalling explicit content than implicit content. This comprehension test has a strong episodic memory component, as it entails answering questions about a story just heard, so it was not surprising that comprehension was correlated with a measure of episodic memory.

Word-Finding and Retrieval

We have already dealt with word-finding for the study of episodic and semantic memory. For standardized clinical assessment, we should recall that the best score on the *Boston Naming Test* is 60. Persons with mild DAT are only somewhat different from age- and education-matched controls (e.g., 45.7 vs. 51.5), but deficit is pronounced with moderate DAT (e.g., 26.5; Nicholas, Obler, Au, et al., 1996; see also Williams, Mack, & Henderson, 1989). Another naming test showed a considerable reduction in naming accuracy over a 2-year period. Type of error changed from semantic errors to "I don't know" responses, a common observation in naming studies (Cuetos, Gonzalez-Nosti, & Martinez, 2005).

As indicated in Chapter 3, a category-specific difficulty points to degraded semantic memory as the culprit. Naming studies have consistently pointed to category-specific deficits, but like the semantic memory studies earlier, they have been exasperatingly inconsistent on whether the deficit is with living things (e.g., Montanes et al., 1996) or nonliving things (e.g., Whatmough, Chertkow, Murtha, et al., 2003). Sometimes there is no difference (Moreno-Martinez & Montoro, 2010). Other methodologies indicated that the naming deficit is more a problem of lexical retrieval than a degrading of semantic memory (Astell & Harley, 1998; Moreaud, David, Charnallet, et al., 2001; Nicholas et al., 1996).

The study of categories was expanded to actions or "verb naming," and people with mild-to-moderate DAT were found to have more difficulty naming actions than objects (Druks, Masterson, Kopelman, et al., 2006). However, it was merely an exaggeration of a pattern exhibited by matched controls. The difference between nouns and verbs was unimpressive in a subsequent study, which tested a variety of semantic categories of nouns and verbs. In types of errors, the investigators found evidence of a gradual loss of semantic features underlying declining word retrieval, which they called a *graceful degradation* for nouns and verbs (Almor, Aronoff, MacDonald, et al., 2009).

Word fluency is likely to be reduced, as it is with other types of brain damage. In a semantic task even in mild DAT, participants with moderate dementia were less accurate and produced more atypical exemplars than those with mild dementia. Use of production strategies such as clustering was also weakened, even in mild DAT (Hough & Givens, 2004). In other studies, deficits were more severe for semantic categories than letters (e.g., Barr & Brandt, 1996; Crossley, D'Arcy, & Rawson, 1997). The greater problem with semantic categories and the nature of responses are consistent with a hypothesis that degraded semantic memory influences word fluency in DAT.

When tip-of-the-tongue (TOT) states were induced, individuals with a wide range of dementia (*MMSE* 8–22) were unable to produce information about the word. This was indicative of a serious deficit in accessing the lexicon. The people with DAT produced semantically related errors, indicating access to the appropriate region of semantic memory. The investigators speculated that the impairment is a *weakening of connections* between semantic and lexical stores (Astell & Harley, 1996).

Sentence and Discourse Production

Research over the years has led to the broad characterization of language production with mild-to-moderate DAT as declining mainly in the area of lexical-semantics, whereas phonology, morphology, and syntax remain well preserved (e.g., Appell et al., 1982; Kempler, Curtiss, & Jackson, 1987). These individuals tend to hold on to a fluent conversational ability long after the initial diagnosis. Lexical retrieval begins to decline early, whereas syntactic features of utterances become problematic at later stages (Bates, Harris, Marchman, et al., 1999).

The role of the verb has been of great interest in clinical sentence production research. Kim and Thompson (2004) compared a group with moderate-to-very-mild DAT to a group with agrammatic aphasia on action naming, sentence completion, and narrative production. The syntactic complexity of verb argument structure influenced those with aphasia but not those with DAT. On the other hand, semantic complexity affected the DAT group but not the group with aphasia. The authors considered that these results add to the support for a deficit in semantic representations.

A few studies of discourse production have relied on information analysis, such as counting small information units (e.g., Arkin & Mahendra, 2001). In hunting for a trigger of incipient dementia, Giles, Patterson, and Hodges (1996) elicited spoken descriptions of the Cookie Theft. A deficit of information units and syllables distinguished early or minimal dementia (*MMSE* 24–29) from healthy adults.

Researchers began to find trouble with syntax in discourse. Bates and others (1995) found simplification of structure and reliance on certain common forms in action descriptions by people with mild-to-moderate DAT. Oral and written descriptions of the Cookie Theft were elicited in a study of 22 persons with mild-to-moderate DAT (Croisile, Ska, Brabant, et al., 1996). In general, these individuals produced fewer words than healthy controls, and syntax was simplified. Picture description may be more sensitive to lexical-semantic deficits than an interview, which seems to be sensitive to morphological and syntactic deficits. There may be more difficulty with syntax than had been suspected in the past (Sajjadi et al., 2012).

Inappropriate intrusions and reduction of subordinate clauses made writing seem to be more sensitive to the presence of dementia than oral descriptions (Croisile, et al., 1996). Even so, DeBaggio's (2002) testimonial provides another perspective: "Some days it seems I live in two worlds . . . gasping as words slip through my lips with effort and imprecision. . . . In the other, slower world where I write on paper or directly on the computer, vocabulary is more fluid and I often surprise myself . . ." (p. 180).

Conversation

Watson and others (1999) employed conversation analysis (CA) to describe 10 conversations between persons with DAT and strangers. The experimental participants had a fairly wide range of dementia, including some with moderate-to-severe impairment. CA targeted trouble indicators, repair trajectories, repair types, and success of repairs. Unimpaired partners shouldered much of the burden of indicating trouble and initiating repairs. Some inappropriate repair behavior by those with DAT, such as veering off topic, was accepted by partners, apparently to preserve the self-esteem of the experimental participants (see also Guendouzi & Müller, 2006).

Elsewhere, researchers studied use of self-monitoring tags (e.g., . . . *didn't I?*) during interviews occurring over 12 months of a drug study. Those who continued to use these tags showed better cognitive test scores than those who did not, suggesting that attention to self-references may be a useful way of evaluating responsiveness to treatment (Asp, Song, & Rockwood, 2006).

As discussed in previous chapters, conversational interaction thrives when a participant considers the point-of-view of the communicative partner. Also called theory of mind (Chapter 11), ToM has been tested artificially in adults by presenting a story of two individuals and then asking questions about what one of the individuals may or may not know about the other (e.g., Gregory, Lough, Stone, et al., 2002). In a *first-order false belief test*, Person A (P-A) places an object in a location observed by Person B (P-B). Then P-A leaves the room, and P-B moves the object. P-A returns to the room. An individual with DAT is asked questions about the story, one of which is about where P-A thinks the object is. A *second-order false belief task* is more complicated. After leaving the room, P-A peeks to see where P-B places the object. Someone with DAT is now asked where P-B thinks P-A thinks the object is. Whew!

In one study, people with DAT had difficulty, not surprisingly, only with the second-order test. They also did well with a *faux pas test* in which they were asked if anyone in a short story said something they should not have said (Gregory et al., 2002). In another study, people with mild-to-moderate DAT were like controls when memory support (i.e., printed story in view) was withdrawn during questioning. Deficit for both orders of false belief arose when the printed story remained in view, interpreted as a mild reduction of ToM possibly due to the distraction of reading (Youmans & Bourgeois, 2010).

Communicative and Cognitive Interventions

Teaching compensatory strategies and improving quality of life comprise the main orientations to cognitive intervention (Bourgeois & Hickey, 2009). People with DAT may receive clinical assistance in a variety of settings (Table 13.5). Some large facilities combine all the components of independent retirement living, assisted living, and nursing home care. "The most appropriate facility for someone with advanced and terminal stages of the disease would be a nursing home with a dedicated Alzheimer's care program" (Dean, 2004, p. 246).

The first or "archetypal" approach was Reality Orientation, which is thought to have begun in U.S. Veterans Administration Hospitals in the 1960s. Reality Orientation was the repetitive presentation of date, time, and place, which were posted in residents' rooms, rehearsed with staff, and rehearsed again in group meetings. Its notoriously rigid and occasionally harsh implementation led to a reduction of popularity in the 1980s, but kinder renditions of the program continue in rehabilitation and residential settings as components of cognitive stimulation and other approaches (Spector, Orrell, Davies, et al., 2001). Now, testimonial-supported brain- or mind-exercise

TABLE 13.5   Settings of Alzheimer's care programs.

Retirement homes with assisted-living programs	Has licensed personal care programs along with independent living; often for couples when one has early stage or mild AD
Assisted-living facilities (ALFs)	Usually smaller than retirement homes; provide health care for those who need assistance in daily living; includes community living spaces
Licensed residential-care home	A home setting for a maximum of six residents with moderate to severe AD; provides basic care but not skilled nursing
Alzheimer's dedicated-care facility	Currently rare, larger residential-care facility for severe-stage AD
Nursing homes	Provides skilled medical care for those in a wheelchair or those who are bedridden; often the "final stop" for someone in advanced or terminal stage

regimens are freely available on the Internet, such as "The Serper Method" and its *Brain Storming* (serpermethod.com).

Communication Assessments

As with other disorders, intervention begins with identifying weaknesses that suggest goals and strengths that comprise compensatory adjustments. In addition to the general tests and scales reviewed earlier, dementia-oriented tests and scales for language and communication have been developed by SLPs. Any evaluation begins with a check of hearing and vision and of hearing aids and glasses.

At the University of Arizona, Kathryn Bayles and Cheryl Tomoeda (1993) developed probably the best-known assessment of mild-to-moderate deficit, namely the ***Arizona Battery for Communication Disorders of Dementia*** (*ABCD*). The battery consists of 14 subtests addressing the following five areas of cognition:

- Linguistic expression
- Linguistic comprehension
- Verbal episodic memory
- Mental status
- Visuospatial construction

An SLP can compute summary scores, which are converted for determining the status of the five cognitive areas. Hopper and Bayles (2008) suggested that the Story Retelling subtest is an effective screening tool.

A second battery was developed for middle- and late-stage DAT. The ***Functional Linguistic Communication Inventory*** (*FLCI*) consists of 10 components covering everyday language and communicative behaviors and takes less than 30 minutes to administer. Tasks include greeting, naming, comprehending signs, and reminiscing (Bayles & Tomoeda, 1994).

Scales for communicative abilities have also appeared. Caregiver and self-assessments are employed for *Communication Adequacy in Daily Situations* (*CADS*; Clark & Witte, 1995). It relies on five-point frequency scales for 26 items of functional communication. For moderate-to-severe dementia, the *Pragmatic Assessment of Communication-Dementia* (*PAC-D*) allows SLPs to rate the adequacy of communicative behaviors with 10 common objects (England, O'Neill, & Simpson, 1996).

Assessments expand to the activities of daily living (ADLs) introduced briefly near the end of Chapter 6. Coverage also includes instrumental activities (IADLs) such as using the telephone, preparing food, housekeeping, shopping, and managing money and medications (Lawton & Brody, 1969). The **Texas Functional Living Scale** (TFLS) was developed recently for people with Alzheimer's disease and later was found to be useful for people with TBI and intellectual disabilities (Cullum, Weiner, & Saine, 2009). The TFLS contains 24 items with questions to answer and activities to demonstrate (e.g., making a peanut butter and jelly sandwich). Its subscales deal with time, communication (i.e., functional reading and writing), and memory for previous activities. Average administration time is under 15 minutes.

Efficacy of Intervention

Before getting into treatments, let us first consider whether cognitive and communicative treatments are helpful. Moore and others (2001) demonstrated that a memory training program improved recognition and recall. Another program, called procedural memory stimulation, trained 13 activities of daily living (e.g., personal hygiene, telephone, dressing) for 1 hour per day, 5 days per week, for 3 weeks. A group with an average *MMSE* of 20 showed significant improvement over an untrained control group in the time it took to complete the activities (Zanetti, Zanieri, Di Giovanni, et al., 2001).

Arkin (2001) studied student-administered training in a community program. She compared two groups with an *MMSE* range of 15 to 29. Both groups received physical fitness and volunteer work sessions, but one group received additional memory and language exercises for two semesters (28 weeks). The cognitive training group improved in a few of the cognitive measures, whereas the other group did not improve in any of the measures. Discourse was reexamined, and there was no difference between the groups. The fitness program with some conversation was enough for maintenance of discourse abilities (Arkin & Mahendra, 2001).

Chapman and her colleagues (2004) evaluated a 2-month cognitive stimulation program for 54 people with DAT (*MMSE* 12–28) who were receiving the drug donepezil (Aricept). Roughly half received the stimulation along with Aricept, and the other half received Aricept alone. The stimulation consisted of discussions and some homework. After 12 months, the stimulation-Aricept group was performing better on discourse and quality of life measures. The authors concluded that "this study adds to growing evidence that active cognitive stimulation may slow the rate of verbal and functional decline and decrease negative emotional symptoms" when combined with medication (p. 1149).

Many studies have indicated that rehabilitation services can be helpful, especially for mild-to-moderate DAT (Grandmaison & Simard, 2003; Lawton & Rubinstein, 2000). Also, earlier diagnosis means that more people have an opportunity to benefit from the treatments that are effective during the early stage. Treatments do not restore functions, but they do stave off progression temporarily or slow it down. Because of advances, the Bush administration authorized Medicare coverage for the treatment of DAT in 2001, including speech-language therapies.

In the fall of 2012, the Alzheimer's Association announced a change in Medicare policy from its "Improvement Standard" for supporting rehabilitative services including speech and language therapy. Instead of having to demonstrate improvement to receive benefits, a person with progressive dementia may now receive benefits if the SLP can show a client is maintaining a current level of performance or is reducing the rate of decline.

Language and Communicative Therapies

Impairment-based therapies for language begin with word-finding. Ousset and others (2002) provided a "Lexical Therapy" for a group with mild DAT. The therapy consisted of naming from definitions and reading narratives. Half of the definitions were from the narrative and half were not. The therapy was assessed with a pre-post naming test with some of the items from the narratives, others from the nonnarrative definitions, and others that were not part of the treatment. The group improved only for the treated items.

For discovering a treatment that considers degraded semantic memory, the trail begins with semantic memory research and then passes through naming studies. Based on a debatable assumption that people with DAT have a category-specific deficit with living things, Mahendra, Arkin, and Kim (2007) structured a study to examine generalization of therapeutic gains from a naming task and a question-answering task, both dealing with animal names. Although short-term progress occurred with the trained category, longer-term gains were better for the nonliving category of things people wear. The implications were not clear, and future research will try to sort out the various factors.

One common objective of lexically oriented treatment is to improve people recognition and naming through the practice of face–name associations. **Errorless learning** has been applied to such tasks (e.g., Clare, Wilson, Carter, et al., 2001). In Chapter 12, it was suggested that minimizing mistakes is essentially the same idea as the principle of success that is so essential to stimulation treatment for aphasia. Accuracy is maximized by using the most familiar materials, providing plenty of cues, and repeating the successes.

The Breakfast Club was a conversational group for nursing home residents. It centered around planning, preparing, and eating breakfast. The SLP used a 10-step program for facilitating interpersonal interaction with visual cues, conceptual associations, and questions with two-choice answers. Santo Pietro and Boczko (1998) compared this group with a pared-down discussion group in which the clinician provided a topic and questions were open ended. The Breakfast Club displayed many more improvements in language and functional independence than the other conversational group, indicating that the type of conversation group can make a difference (see also Hopper, 2007).

One strength of memory can be a source of content for conversation. The temporal gradient of episodic memory is a theoretical foundation for **reminiscence therapy** (RT) consisting of discussion of activities and experiences that occurred in the distant past. An SLP, as group leader, may include prompts such as photographs and music (Harris, 1997; Woods, Spector, Jones, et al., 2005).

Hopper and Bayles (2008) explained Medicare reimbursement for speech-language therapy provided to people in skilled nursing facilities. The main approach is **functional maintenance therapy** (FMT) based on a functional maintenance plan (FMP). The FMP consists of evaluation and a short-term diagnostic treatment program for people who demonstrate a potential for improvement. Brief trial therapy is usually justified, and the program is likely to be carried out by caregivers trained by SLPs who prescribe the treatment. Educating caregivers may be reimbursable.

Memory and Problem-Solving

In conversation, people with DAT do not remember what was just said and do not remember a topical event that occurred the previous week. They may repeat a question over and over. **Spaced retrieval training** (SRT), introduced in Chapter 12, is adopted for memory practice. SRT requires recall of material at increasing intervals between presentation and test and, conversely, includes shortening the interval when there is recall failure (Brush & Camp, 1998; Camp, 2006). Let us suppose we tell an individual that lunch is going to be chicken salad and soup. We ask her to repeat it. Then a few seconds later, we ask her what is for lunch. If she is correct, we ask again a couple minutes later, stretching the interval out further. SRT has produced favorable results in naming therapy for aphasia (Fridriksson, Holland, Beeson, et al., 2005; see also Hopper, Mahendra, Kim, et al., 2005).

In articles and video presentations, Bayles alerted SLPs to the value of basic memory theory for providing comprehensive compensatory strategies (e.g., Hopper & Bayles, 2008). Her principles have been conveyed in various ways. Here we will consider a few of them.

One of Bayles's recommendations is to **reduce demands on episodic memory**. In conversation, this means avoiding requests to retrieve experiences from memory and, instead, stating the possibilities for easier recognition (e.g., yes/no response). Bayles recommended stimulating spared stores such as procedural memory (e.g., Zanetti et al., 2001). Also, *external memory aids*, like those used for traumatic brain injury, support long-term memory generally.

Bourgeois (1992, 2007) recommended a memory book or "memory wallet" as an external aid. It is a book of pictures and sentences pertaining to a person's common memory failures. Each page contains one sentence and a related picture or photograph. Nursing home residents were trained in three or four sessions to use wallets in conversations with nursing assistants. There was an increase in factual utterances by residents and a reduction of nonfacilitative behavior by nursing assistants. Additional training of the assistants reduced nonfacilitative behavior further, and turn-taking became more balanced (Hoerster, Hickey, & Bourgeois, 2001; Bourgeois, Camp, Rose, et al., 2003).

Another one of Bayles's recommendations is to **support working memory**. Limitations lead to forgetting utterances in an exchange, forgetting the topic of a conversation, and being susceptible to distraction. In principle, support comes from reducing distractions, writing down a topic or important information, and keeping statements short and simple.

A third suggestion from Bayles is **to provide stimulation and environments to evoke positive memory, emotion, and action**. This refers to programs of activity and environmental management in nursing homes and other facilities. On any day, we can visit one of these facilities and find residents being entertained with music or being involved in art, crafts, or gardening. The setting is sunlit and cheerful. A few nursing homes have created "50s environments" in which the décor is reminiscent of the time when residents were young adults. These will soon become "60s environments" and so on.

Field trips are common, and some are extensions of art therapy. Museums open their doors to people with Alzheimer's disease. For example, small groups with mild-to-moderate dementia pay weekly visits to New York's Museum of Modern Art and Boston's Museum of Fine Arts. Individuals are encouraged to say whatever comes to mind about the artworks, and caregivers have noticed increased energy and talkativeness after the visits.

Marshall, Capilouto, and McBride (2007) borrowed from a problem-solving test to create a task in which people with DAT would ask yes/no questions leading to identifying a target picture in an array of 32 pictures. The idea was to be efficient, asking as few questions as possible. Constraint questions, which efficiently eliminated more than one item, were good. Guesses were bad. After 12 sessions, participants increased constraint questioning and decreased guessing.

Caregivers

"Initially, I refused to believe my wife was suffering from dementia. Something was wrong, yes, but she was too perceptive, too alert for such an illness" (Wheeler, 2001, p. 3). A community-based program in Arizona is called Elder Rehab "because some participants and/or their families do not acknowledge an Alzheimer's disease (AD) diagnosis or prefer not to be publicly identified with AD" (Arkin, 2001, p. 273). Acceptance is a tough state to reach.

Caregivers struggle with what seems like a "36-hour day" (Mace & Rabins, 2011). Information is plentiful in print and online to support family and residential staff (e.g., Gruetzner, 2001; Schulz, 2000). Wheeler (2001) expressed his discomfort with the term *caregiver*. "It implies to me a constancy and stability . . . I wish I were capable of such behavior, but I'm not" (p. 1). He added, "Most mornings I crawl out of bed slowly. Not only slowly, but painfully. I'm in my mid-seventies" (p. 2).

The following is a sample of general recommendations:

- Educate yourself regarding DAT.
- Get appropriate medical care for your loved one.
- Make sure your loved one's legal documents are complete.
- Keep the impaired person active but not upset.
- Take care of yourself.
- Solve problems one at a time.
- Share the burden.
- Join a support group.

Some of these strategies are important for relieving the stress of adjusting to a new life. Support includes a "caregiver's bill of rights" and a caregiver stress test (Dean, 2004).

For SLPs, Danielle Ripich, president of the University of New England in Maine, developed a caregiver communication program called "FOCUSED." Each letter represents a strategy for successful communication: **F**ace to face, **O**rient to topic, **C**ontinuity of topic, **U**nstick blocks, **S**tructured questions, **E**xchange of turns, and **D**irect short sentences. The program is divided into modules with guidebooks to use in small-group training. Caregivers are encouraged to ask yes/no questions instead of open-ended questions, which has become a fairly consistent recommendation. In addition, Ripich developed a series of videotapes for independent learning by caregivers (Ripich, 1996; Ripich, Ziol, & Lee, 1998; see also Bourgeois, Schulz, Burgio, et al., 2002).

At the University of British Columbia, Jeff Small has been examining the interactions between caregivers and people with DAT. In one study, he compared what caregivers thought they were doing to support conversation with what they were actually doing and how successful they were. What should get our attention is that this study targeted 10 communication strategies frequently recommended by SLPs and others. In general, caregivers perceived themselves as following certain recommendations but were not actually employing them (Small, Gutman, Makela, et al., 2003).

In Small's study, simple sentences were the most effective strategy that caregivers thought they were using and were actually using. Also, encouraging the use of yes–no questions has been integral to some training programs. Most of the caregivers' questions were this type, and yes/no questions were relatively effective. Other successful strategies were to reduce distractions and avoid interrupting. Slowing the rate of speech and repeating verbatim were infrequently used and often ineffective for communication. Caregivers rarely encouraged circumlocution for conveying information.

Later, Small and Perry (2005) examined caregiver questions more closely. Semantic questions address conceptual information (e.g., What is this thing?). Episodic questions address experienced events that occurred recently (e.g., What did you eat for dinner yesterday?) or in the remotely distant past (e.g., Where did you go to college?). Conversations were between 18 caregivers and spouses with mild or moderate AD. Contrary to previous studies, caregivers asked open-ended questions as often as yes/no questions. Communication was more successful when the questions tapped into semantic memory than episodic memory, which is a result that is consistent with what we know about memory deficit in DAT. However, spouses asked many more episodic questions about recent information than about remote information. This result was somewhat surprising, considering the greater impairment of recent memory.

A variety of assistance is available for families (Table 13.6). The **Safe Return Program**, administered by the Alzheimer's Association, assists individuals who are at risk for wandering from home and getting lost. It provides identification bracelets or pendants with an identification number and a hotline number. It also maintains a national database in case a loved one is missing. The database includes a photograph and contact information.

TABLE 13.6   Resources on Alzheimer's disease for professionals and caregivers.

RESOURCE	WEB SITE	DESCRIPTION
Alzheimer's Association	alz.org	Main support and advocacy organization; provides updates on policies and legislation
Alzheimer's Information	alzinfo.org	Information source
ALZwell Caregiver Support	alzwell.com	Resource for caregivers
Geriatric Resources, Inc.	geriatric-resources.com	Company specializing in caregiving resources and services
theforgetting.com	randomhouse.com/features/forgetting	News about the disease, inspired by Shenk's (2002) book *The Forgetting*
Health Professions Press	healthpropress.com	Publisher specializing in gerontology and long-term care

Medical Treatments

A cautionary tale can be found in the development of drugs for Alzheimer's. The plot is driven by science, the pharmaceutical industry, the federal regulatory system, and the public. In the early 1970s, scientists discovered the deficiency in acetylcholine (ACH). In 1986, William Summers published a study extolling the effectiveness of a new drug, called tacrine, to boost the production of ACH. The scientific community was skeptical of the investigator's credentials and the study itself, which was completed on only 14 participants. The outcome measures were questioned, and the data appeared to be mainly anecdotal. The Food and Drug Administration (FDA) accused Summers of misrepresentation.

Nevertheless, word got out, and an anxious public was impressed with the possibility that a wonder drug could improve memory. They vilified the FDA "as heartlessly impeding the relief of suffering and demanded the immediate release of tacrine" (Gillick, 1998, p. 132). Hate mail sent to the director of the FDA illustrates the conflict between an "activist public" that wants any promising new drug immediately and a deliberate regulatory agency that seeks to protect the public.

The Tacrine Collaborative Study Group was formed. Their results, reported in 1992, were promising but also reinforced previous findings of damaging side effects. Another study of a stronger dose for a longer period prompted the FDA to approve tacrine in 1993. However, two of the authors were employees of the pharmaceutical company that made tacrine, and 70 percent of the participants had dropped out of the study because of the same side effects, namely liver toxicity or gastrointestinal problems of nausea, vomiting, and diarrhea. Tacrine also proved to be taxing on a patient and caregiver because it had to be taken four times per day.

Tacrine has been replaced by three FDA-approved drugs that have a similar mechanism of action on the brain. The goal of boosting ACH is achieved by inhibiting the action of cholinesterase, a chemical that breaks down ACH across the synapse. Thus, the drugs are classified as "cholinesterase inhibitors." The first, approved in 1996, goes by the increasingly familiar trade name **Aricept**® (donepezil). Its mechanism is the same as tacrine but without the liver toxicity side effect, and it is taken only once a day. An efficacy study, combined with cognitive stimulation, was described earlier (Chapman, et al., 2004).

According to the National Institute on Aging, other medications for early Alzheimer's may delay progression of symptoms. They include rivastigmine (e.g., Exelon®), or the Exelon Patch, and galantamine (e.g., Razadyne®, Reminyl®). Side effects include nausea, vomiting, and diarrhea. Memantine (e.g., Namenda®) is prescribed for moderate-to-severe Alzheimer's and also may delay progression of symptoms. Side effects include dizziness and headache (nia.nih.gov/alzheimers).

Soon after his diagnosis, DeBaggio (2002) used Aricept® and experienced its gastrointestinal side effect. His doctor also prescribed vitamin E soft gels and ibuprofen. Vitamin E is an "antioxidant," which combats toxic side effects. One study showed that a group taking a substantial amount of vitamin E had postponed institutionalization or death compared to a group taking a placebo. The American Academy of Neurologists has recommended its use. However, there has been no evidence that vitamin E slows intellectual deterioration. Scientists are still investigating the value of vitamins C and B, as well as vitamin E.

One can keep up with new possibilities by doing a Google search for "Alzheimer's news," where, for example, we can find "brain pacemakers" consisting of brain implants that deliver a constant electrical current to neural circuits. The implants have been around as *deep brain stimulation* for Parkinson's disease and other movement disorders. What is new is their application for Alzheimer's disease, and experiments take the shape of those reported for electrical stimulation and aphasia (Chapter 9). Also, a drug, called bexarotene, has been given to mice models of Alzheimer's disease with positive effects on their cognition (Cramer, Cirrito, Wesson, Lee, Karlo, 2012).

Primary Progressive Aphasia

A 60-year-old public speaker was having an unusual difficulty finding words and reading notes. He went to a neurologist, who diagnosed stroke and for 3 years treated him with medication. Yet instead of getting better, these difficulties got worse. The individual was referred to Marsel Mesulam at Northwestern University, who diagnosed primary progressive aphasia (Brody, 2011).

Chapter 2 introduced PPA as being caused by a mysterious atrophy of language areas of the left hemisphere. The history of this disorder reaches back to Arnold Pick in the late 1800s, and it has been associated from time to time with Pick's disease and *frontotemporal dementia*. The "early descriptions of PPA challenged widely held views about dementia" (Grossman & Ash, 2004, p. 4) until it became apparent that progressive disease causes a wider variety of disorders (Croot, 2009). Mesulam (1982, 2007) was the first to publicize PPA in the modern era.

PPA changes over time, and as the scenario for the public speaker suggests, diagnosis may not be confirmed until some time after onset. It usually starts as a difficulty with word-finding and then spreads to other language functions. Many have good auditory comprehension in the first 2 years. By the third year, cases are quite heterogeneous. Reading deficits are rarely seen before the fourth or fifth year. Thus, the classic multimodality feature of stroke-related aphasia may not factor into diagnosis in early stages. Some researchers suggest that isolated language deficit may last at least 2 years before other cognitive deficits and motor deficits begin to develop.

Variants of PPA

Like stroke-related aphasia, PPA takes different forms, basically nonfluent and fluent types. Adding a mixed variety, three types were recognized by an international group of PPA investigators (Gorno-Tempini, Hillis, Weintraub, et al., 2011; Mesulam, Grossman, Hillis, et al., 2003) with some variation in the United Kingdom (e.g., Sajjadi et al., 2012). The following types of PPA are discussed here:

- Progressive nonfluent aphasia (PNFA)
- Fluent semantic dementia (SD)
- Mixed or logopenic progressive aphasia (LPA)

There is some variation of labeling in this nascent area of research. Many researchers have based their diagnoses of PPA on criteria set forth by Mesulam (2001).

Progressive nonfluent aphasia (PNFA) is also called "agrammatic/nonfluent" progressive aphasia (PPA-G). Like Broca's aphasia, there is labored production and, of course, agrammatism. It is caused, in general terms, by left frontal lobe degeneration. Picture descriptions contain reduced words per minute, reduction of grammatical sentences, and impaired verb morphology and argument structure (Thompson, Cho, Hsu, et al., 2012). Similar to a group with stroke-related agrammatism, people with PNFA had more difficulty naming with verbs than nouns (Thompson, Lukic, King, et al., 2012). These results were substantiated by picture descriptions and structured interviews (Sajjadi et al., 2012).

A research team in the United Kingdom has pursued its own path in studies of aphasia. They have argued, without broad sourcing on aphasia, that PNFA is not the same as nonfluent aphasia. In one study, their group with stroke-related nonfluent aphasia was diagnosed based on effortful speech and phonological errors without mention of agrammatism (Patterson, Graham, Lambon Ralph, et al., 2006). In a quantitative analysis of picture description, the researchers found a reduction in quantity of words. Perhaps a slight difference from Thompson's findings, ratios pertaining to verbs and function words did not differ from controls (Graham, Patterson, & Hodges, 2004). The basic conclusion was that although one disorder is progressive and the other is not, the two nonfluent aphasias are not the same disorder.

The fluent version is **semantic dementia** (SD, or PPA-S), due to left temporal lobe degeneration including the hippocampus. People with SD talk like someone with anomic aphasia and experience increasing difficulty with noun comprehension but also, unlike stroke-related aphasia, a deterioration of object recognition (Harciarek & Kertesz, 2009). Also, sentence comprehension remains good "even as the disease progresses" (Ogar, Baldo, Wilson, et al., 2011).

Hillis and her colleagues (2006) uncovered a double dissociation regarding objects and actions (nouns and verbs) when comparing people in the main categories of progressive aphasia. People with PNFA had more impairment naming actions than objects, and people with SD had more impairment with objects than actions on a variety of semantic tasks. This reversal between types for nouns and verbs was repeated for comprehension as well as naming (Thompson et al., 2012).

Let us return to the priming paradigm that was mentioned earlier in studies of semantic memory and DAT. Again, Bénédicte Giffard's team in France compared coordinate and attribute relationships. This time, the coordinates were divided into close (e.g., tiger-lion) and distant (e.g., elephant-crocodile) relationships. The attribute pairs were divided into shared (e.g., duck-*feathers*) and distinctive (e.g., zebra-*stripes*) features. People with SD displayed hyperpriming for coordinates and extinction of priming first in distinctive attributes followed by shared attributes (Laisney, Giffard, Belliard, et al., 2011).

Extensive investigations of semantic dementia have been undertaken by the aforementioned team in the United Kingdom led by John Hodges and Karalyn Patterson of Cambridge and Matthew Lambon Ralph of Manchester. Early on, they considered SD to be progressive fluent aphasia (Hodges, Patterson, Oxbury, et al., 1992). Their studies have led them to the conclusion that the heart of SD is a *degraded semantic memory*, affecting all functions pertaining to objects, including recognizing and naming them. In a study of repetition priming, the investigators at Cambridge found slow recognition responses but also hyperpriming for repeated targets. The influence of degraded semantic memory was indicated by larger abnormal priming for predetermined "degraded" words (Cumming, Graham, & Patterson, 2006). In interviews, people with SD failed to retrieve intended content words and, somewhat surprisingly, made subtle grammatical errors (Meteyard & Patterson, 2009).

The third type, **logopenic** (or "logopaenic") **progressive aphasia** (LPA, PPA-L), is a mixture of the others (Gorno-Tempini, Dronkers, Rankin, et al., 2004). The area of atrophy is the posterior temporal and inferior parietal lobes. Speech is slow, and both syntactic comprehension and naming are impaired. In some of the research, there were no differences between nouns and verbs in naming (Thompson, Lukic, et al., 2012), and picture descriptions demonstrated a variability of fluency among individuals (Thompson, Cho, Hsu, et al., 2012).

Finally, remember the psycholinguistic study of naming with the picture-word interference task introduced in Chapter 3? This time, Thompson and her colleagues at Northwestern employed a semantic competitor in an attempt to induce semantic interference of object naming. They compared a group with agrammatic PNFA to a group with LPA. For both of these groups and a control group, a semantically related word interfered with object naming with short onset asynchronies between the word and the target object. This was indicative of a fairly normal spreading activation in semantic memory, except for the longest word-target interval in which both progressive aphasias displayed semantic interference. Thus, the groups with aphasia took longer to resolve semantic interference, consistent with cognitive slowing in progressive disease (Thompson, Cho, Price, et al., 2012).

Rehabilitation for PPA

Northwestern University became a "lifesaver" for our public speaker and his wife. The clinic helped with applying for disability insurance, and it provided the individual with alternative forms of communication and the family with emotional support and tips for communicating (Brody, 2011). In other words, we can help.

We maintain the same dual impairment-based and consequence-based approaches that we apply to the other disorders (Croot, Nickels, Laurence, et al., 2009). Also, medication has reduced the rate of decline in a few cases (Reed, Johnson, Thompson, et al., 2004). Repetitive transcranial magnetic stimulation (rTMS) for one person produced a temporary increase in action naming but not memory span (Finocchiaro, Maimone, Brighina, et al., 2006). Traditional therapy for impairment is based mostly on assumptions that semantic memory is degraded and that some relearning is necessary.

A computer-based naming therapy was provided to two people with nonfluent PPA (Jokel, Cupit, Rochon, et al., 2009). For fluent semantic dementia the goal was "to restore lost concepts" (Bier, Macoir, Gagnon, et al., 2009). The investigators instituted a semantic therapy in which the clinician responded to semantically related naming errors by showing a picture of the error and discussing how its attributes differ from attributes of the targeted object. This explanation of errors, aimed at meaning, differs from the simpler cueing restimulation provided in treatment for stroke-related aphasia.

A participant with SD and another with LPA received a cueing hierarchy naming therapy for about 9 weeks, roughly 3 days per week. The person with SD improved in treated items only. The person with LPA improved in naming treated and untreated items (Newhart, Davis, Kannan, et al., 2009; see also Dressel, Huber, Frings, et al., 2010). A home treatment restimulated naming failures with a printed word and evaluated progress with phonemic cueing (Mayberry, Sage, Ehsan, et al., 2011). For errorless learning, a clinician provided a printed word as prestimulation in naming practice (Robinson, Druks, Hodges, et al., 2009). One client stood out from less successful others by retaining relearned words for 6 months (Heredia, Sage, Lambon Ralph, et al., 2009).

More divergent semantic and word retrieval activities were instituted by Henry, Beeson, and Rapcsak (2008) for two individuals with fluent PPA. A brief intensive regimen consisted of twelve 90-minute sessions over 16 days. The treatment was called "guided lexical retrieval" in which participants produced exemplars of varied semantic categories. Considering the degradation of semantic memory, the SLPs wanted to provide "a boost to semantic representations" with cues and supplemental sorting tasks. One person with PPA demonstrated large treatment effects, whereas the other did not.

In general, rehabilitation for PPA emphasizes language and communication over memory and problem solving. SLPs draw from aphasia therapy with the main difference being expectations for PPA. Evidence indicates that therapies maintain performance for a while or slow the rate of functional decline, which now are sufficient outcomes for receiving Medicare benefits. Research has been limited to a few individuals, simple pre-post experimental designs, and small reaches of generalization (e.g., Jokel et al., 2009). It has become common practice to assess maintenance generalization of 1 to 6 months after concluding treatment.

Summary and Conclusions

This chapter maintained the logical (cause-effect) subtext of the first chapter. Alzheimer's disease (i.e., plaques and tangles) causes dementia of Alzheimer's type (i.e., disorientation, memory loss). Stories were told about discovering the nature of this disease and about developing drugs for improving memory. Research has been plentiful with respect to semantic memory, language comprehension, and word-finding for naming and discourse. Rehabilitation contains a heavy dose of linguistic and communicative activity. Language is often employed in compensatory strategies to support weakened memory systems. SLPs and other professionals provide training and support for caregivers who must cope with immense challenges that increase over time.

One problem in dealing with the literature and, thus, communicating with colleagues is that many researchers do not have a tightly wound psycholinguistic basis to steer conceptualizations of language impairments. Some think of language disorders as a broad contrast to motor disorders so that language exists vaguely in a conceptual realm. Some think of words as concepts so that something that happens with the lexicon is diagnosed as a semantic problem. This can be confusing for those who see connection and independence, like a marriage, between semantic and lexical representations. This helps to explain why, in *aphasia*, someone can clear mindedly know what he wants to say but just cannot find the words.

REFERENCES

Abel, S., Huber, W., & Dell, G. S. (2009). Connectionist diagnosis of lexical disorders in aphasia. *Aphasiology, 23,* 1353–1382.

Abel, S., Willmes, K., & Huber, W. (2007). Model-oriented naming therapy: Testing predictions of a connectionist model. *Aphasiology, 21,* 411–447.

Abutalebi, J., Della Rosa, P. A., Tettamanti, M., Green, D. W., & Cappa, S. F. (2009). Bilingual aphasia and language control: A follow-up fMRI and intrinsic connectivity study. *Brain and Language, 109,* 141–156.

Ackerman, D. (2011). *One hundred names for love: A stroke, a marriage, and the language of healing.* New York: W.W. Norton.

Adamovich, B. B., & Henderson, J. A. (1992). *Scales of Cognitive Ability for Traumatic Brain Injury* (SCATBI). Chicago: Riverside.

Adamovich, B. L. B. (2005). Traumatic brain injury. In L. L. LaPointe (Ed.), *Aphasia and related neurogenic language disorders* (3rd ed., pp. 225–236). New York: Thieme.

Adams, M. L., Reich, A. R., & Flowers, C. R. (1989). Verbal-fluency characteristics of normal and aphasic speakers. *Journal of Speech and Hearing Research, 32,* 871–879.

Agency for Healthcare Research and Quality. (2002). *Systems to rate the strength of scientific evidence: Summary.* [online] retrieved January 11, 2012 from http://archive.ahrq.gov/clinic/epcsums/strengthsum .htm

Aguirre, G. K., & D'Esposito, M. (1999). Topographical disorientation: A synthesis and taxonomy. *Brain, 122,* 1613–1628.

Ahlsén, E., Nespoulous, J.-L., Dordain, M., Stark, J., Jarema, G., et al. (1996). Noun phrase production by agrammatic patients: A cross-linguistic approach. *Aphasiology, 10,* 543–559.

Albert, M. L., & Obler, L. K. (1978). *The bilingual brain.* New York: Academic Press.

Albert, M. L., Sparks, R., & Helm, N. A. (1973). Melodic intonation therapy. *Archives of Neurology, 29,* 130–131.

Albright, E., & Purves, B. (2008). Exploring SentenceShaper™: Treatment and augmentative possibilities. *Aphasiology, 22,* 741–752.

Alcock, K. J., Wade, D., Anslow, P., & Passingham, R. E. (2000). Pitch and timing abilities in adult left-hemisphere-dysphasic and right-hemisphere-damaged subjects. *Brain and Language, 75,* 47–65.

Aleligay, A., Worrall, L. E., & Rose, T. A. (2008). Readability of written health information provided to people with aphasia. *Aphasiology, 22,* 383–407.

Alexander, M. P., Fischette, M. R., & Fischer, R. S. (1989). Crossed aphasias can be mirror image or anomalous: Case reports, review and hypothesis. *Brain, 112,* 953–973.

Alexander, M. P., Naeser, M. A., & Palumbo, C. L. (1987). Correlations of subcortical CT lesion sites and aphasia profiles. *Brain, 110,* 961–991.

Almor, A., Aronoff, J. M., MacDonald, M. C., Gonnerman, L. M., Kempler, D., Hintiryan, H., Hayes, U. L., Arunachalam, S., & Andersen, E. S. (2009). A common mechanism in verb and noun naming deficits in Alzheimer's patients. *Brain and Language, 111,* 8–19.

Amanzio, M., Geminiani, G., Leotta, D., & Cappa, S. (2008). Metaphor comprehension in Alzheimer disease: Novelty matters. *Brain and Language, 107,* 1–10.

American Psychiatric Association. (2013). *Diagnostic and statistical manual of mental disorders* (*DSM-5*). Arlington, VA: American Psychiatric Publishing.

Amunts, K., & Zilles, K. (2006). A multimodal analysis of structure and function in Broca's region. In Y. Grodzinsky & K. Amunts (Eds.), *Broca's region* (pp. 17–30). New York: Oxford University Press.

Andersen, G. (1997). Post-stroke depression and pathological crying: Clinical aspects and new pharmacological approaches. *Aphasiology, 11,* 651–664.

Anderson, J. M., Gilmore, R., Roper, S., Crosson, B., Bauer, M., et al. (1999). Conduction aphasia and the arcuate fasciculus: A reexamination of the Wernicke-Geschwind model. *Brain and Language, 70,* 1–12.

Anderson, J. R. (1983). *The architecture of cognition.* Cambridge, MA: Harvard University Press.

Anderson, S. W., Damasio, H., & Tranel, D. (1990). Neuropsychological impairments associated with lesions caused by tumor or stroke. *Archives of Neurology, 47,* 397–405.

Andrewes, D., (2001). *Neuropsychology: From theory to practice.* Hove, UK: Psychology Press.

Angeleri, R., Bosco, F. M., Zettin, M., Sacco, K., Colle, L., & Bara, B. G. (2008). Communicative impairment in traumatic brain injury: A complete pragmatic assessment. *Brain and Language, 107,* 229–245.

Ansaldo, A. I., Arguin, M., & Lecours, A. R. (2002). The contribution of the right cerebral hemisphere to the recovery from aphasia: A single longitudinal case study. *Brain and Language, 82,* 206–222.

Ansaldo, A. I., Saidi, L. G., & Ruiz, A. (2010). Model-driven intervention in bilingual aphasia: Evidence from a case of pathological language mixing. *Aphasiology, 24,* 309–324.

Ansell, B. J., & Flowers, C. R. (1982). Aphasic adults' use of heuristic and structural linguistic cues for sentence analysis. *Brain and Language, 16,* 61–72.

Antonucci, S. M. (2009). Use of semantic feature analysis in group aphasia treatment. *Aphasiology, 23,* 854–866.

Antonucci, S. M., Beeson, P. M., Labiner, D. M., & Rapcsak, S. Z. (2008). Lexical retrieval and semantic knowledge in patients with left inferior temporal lobe lesions. *Aphasiology, 22,* 281–304.

Appell, J., Kertesz, A., & Fisman, M. (1982). A study of language functioning in Alzheimer patients. *Brain and Language, 17,* 73–91.

Ardila, A. (2010). A proposed reinterpretation and reclassification of aphasic syndromes. *Aphasiology, 24,* 363–394.

Arguin, M., & Bub, D. (1993). Modulation of the directional attention deficit in visual neglect by hemispatial factors. *Brain and Cognition, 22,* 148–160.

Arguin, M., & Bub, D. (1997). Lexical constraints on reading accuracy in neglect dyslexia. *Cognitive Neuropsychology, 14,* 765–800.

Arkin, S. (2001). Alzheimer rehabilitation by students: Interventions and outcomes. *Neuropsychological Rehabilitation, 11,* 273–317.

Arkin, S., & Mahendra, N. (2001). Discourse analysis of Alzheimer's patients before and after intervention: Methodology and outcomes. *Aphasiology, 15,* 533–569.

Armstrong, E., Ciccone, N., Godecke, E., & Kok, B. (2011). Monologues and dialogues in aphasia: Some initial comparisons. *Aphasiology, 25,* 1347–1371.

Armstrong, L., Brady, M., Mackenzie, C., & Norrie, J. (2007). Transcription-less analysis of aphasic discourse: A clinician's dream or a possibility? *Aphasiology, 21,* 355–374.

Arrigoni, G., & DeRenzi, E. (1964). Constructional apraxia and hemispheric locus of lesion. *Cortex, 1,* 170–197.

Arvedson, J. C., McNeil, M. R., & West, T. L. (1985). Prediction of Revised Token Test overall, subtest, and linguistic unit scores by two shortened versions. In R. H. Brookshire (Ed.), *Clinical aphasiology* (Vol. 15, pp. 57–63). Minneapolis, MN: BRK.

Ashcraft, M. H. (1989). *Human memory and cognition.* Gleview, IL: Scott, Foresman.

Ashcraft, M. H., & Radvansky, G. A. (2010). *Cognition* (5th ed.). Boston: Prentice Hall.

Ashford J. W., Kumar, U., Barringer, M., Becker, M., Bice, J., et al. (1992). Assessing Alzheimer's severity with a global clinical scale. *International Psychogeriatrics, 4,* 55–74.

Ashton, C., Aziz, N. A., Barwood, C., French, R., Savina, E., et al. (2008). Communicatively accessible public transport for people with aphasia: A pilot study. *Aphasiology, 22,* 305–320.

Asp, E., Song, X., & Rockwood, K. (2006). Self-referential tags in the discourse of people with Alzheimer's disease. *Brain and Language, 97,* 41–52.

Astell, A. J., & Harley, T. A. (1996). Tip-of-the-tongue states and lexical access in dementia. *Brain and Language, 54,* 196–215.

Astell, A. J., & Harley, T. A. (1998). Naming problems in dementia: Semantic or lexical? *Aphasiology, 12,* 357–374.

Aten, J. L., & Lyon, J. G. (1978). Measures of PICA subtest variance: A preliminary assessment of their value as predictors of language recovery in aphasic patients. In R. H. Brookshire (Ed.), *Clinical aphasiology conference proceedings.* Minneapolis, MN: BRK.

Avent, J. R., Edwards, D. J., Franco, C. R., Lucero, C. J., & Pekowsky, J. I. (1995). A verbal and non-verbal treatment comparison study in aphasia. *Aphasiology, 9,* 295–303.

Babbitt, E. M., Heinemann, A. W., Semik, P., & Cherney, L. R. (2011). Psychometric properties of the Communication Confidence Rating Scale for Aphasia (CCRSA): Phase 2. *Aphasiology, 25,* 727–735.

Backus, O. (1947). The rehabilitation of persons with aphasia. In R. West, L. Kennedy, A. Carr, & O. Backus (Eds.), *The rehabilitation of speech* (2nd ed.). New York: Harper.

Baddeley, A. D. (1986). *Working memory.* London: Oxford University Press.

Baddeley, A. D. (1992). Implicit memory and errorless learning: A link between cognitive theory and neuropsychological rehabilitation? In L. R. Squire & N. Butters (Eds.), *Neuropsychology of memory* (2nd ed., pp. 309–314). New York: Guilford Press.

Baddeley, A. D. (1996). Exploring the central executive. *Quarterly Journal of Experimental Psychology, 49A,* 5–28.

Baddeley, A. D. (2004). *Your memory: A user's guide.* Buffalo, NY: Firefly Books.

Baddeley, A. D., Eysenck, M. W., & Anderson, M. C. (2009). *Memory.* New York: Psychology Press.

Baldo, J. V., Schwartz, S., Wilkins, D. P., & Dronkers, N. F. (2010). Double dissociation of letter and category fluency following left frontal and temporal lobe lesions. *Aphasiology, 24,* 1593–1604.

Ball, A. L., de Riesthal, M., Breeding, V. E., & Mendoza, D. E. (2011). Modified ACT and CART in severe aphasia. *Aphasiology, 25,* 836–848.

Ballard, C. (2000). Criteria for the diagnosis of dementia. In J. O'Brien, D. Ames, & A. Burns (Eds.), *Dementia* (2nd ed., pp. 29–40). London: Arnold.

Ballard, K. J., & Thompson, C. K. (1999). Treatment and generalization of complex sentence production in agrammatism. *Journal of Speech, Language, and Hearing Research, 42,* 690–707.

Bamber, L. (1980). *A retrospective study of language recovery in adult aphasics.* Unpublished thesis, Memphis State University.

Bara, B. G. (2005). *Cognitive pragmatics.* Cambridge, MA: MIT Press.

Barlow, D. H., Nock, M. K., & Hersen, M. (2008). *Single case experimental designs: Strategies for studying behavior change* (3rd ed.). Boston: Allyn & Bacon.

Barr, A., & Brandt, J. (1996). Word-list generation deficits in dementia. *Journal of Clinical and Experimental Neuropsychology, 18,* 810–822.

Barth, J. T., Broshek, D. K., & Freeman, J. R. (2006). Sports: A new frontier for neuropsychology. In R. J. Echemendía (Ed.), *Sports neuropsychology: Assessment and management of traumatic brain injury* (pp. 3–16). New York: Guilford Press.

Bartha, L., & Benke, T. (2003). Acute conduction aphasia: An analysis of 20 cases. *Brain and Language, 85,* 93–108.

Barthel, G., Meinzer, M., Djundja, D., & Rockstroh, B. (2008). Intensive language therapy in chronic aphasia: Which aspects contribute most? *Aphasiology, 22,* 408–421.

Bartlett, M. R., Fink, R. B., Schwartz, M. F., & Linebarger, M. (2007). Informativeness of messages created on an AAC processing prosthesis. *Aphasiology, 21,* 475–498.

Barton, M. I. (1971). Recall of generic properties of words in aphasic patients. *Cortex, 7,* 73–82.

Barwood, C. H. S., Murdoch, B. E., Whelan, B.-M., Lloyd, D., Riek, S., et al. (2011). Modulation of N400 in chronic non-fluent aphasia using low frequency Repetitive Transcranial Magnetic Stimulation (rTMS). *Brain and Language, 116,* 125–135.

Barwood, C. H. S., Murdoch, B. E., Whelan, B.-M., O'Sullivan, J. D., Wong, A., et al. (2012). Longitudinal modulation of N400 in chronic non-fluent aphasia using low-frequency rTMS: A randomised placebo controlled trial. *Aphasiology, 26,* 103–124.

Basso, A. (1992). Prognostic factors in aphasia. *Aphasiology, 6,* 337–348.

Basso, A. (1996). PALPA: An appreciation and a few criticisms. *Aphasiology, 10,* 190–193.

Basso, A. (2003). *Aphasia and its therapy.* New York: Oxford University Press.

Basso, A. (2005). How intensive/prolonged should an intensive/prolonged treatment be? *Aphasiology, 19,* 975–984.

Basso, A. (2008). Treatment for fluent aphasia from a cognitive-impairment perspective. In N. Martin, C. K. Thompson, & L. Worrall (Eds.). *Aphasia rehabilitation: The impairment and its consequences* (pp. 31–44). San Diego, CA: Plural Publishing.

Basso, A. (2010). "Natural" conversation: A treatment for severe aphasia. *Aphasiology, 24,* 466–479.

Basso, A., Capitani, E., & Moraschini, S. (1982). Sex differences in recovery from aphasia. *Cortex, 18,* 469–475.

Basso, A., Capitani, E., & Vignolo, L. A. (1979). Influence of rehabilitation on language skills in aphasic patients: A controlled study. *Archives of Neurology, 36,* 190–196.

Basso, A., Lecours, A. R., Moraschini, S., & Vanier, M. (1985). Anatomo-clinical correlations of aphasias as defined through computerized tomography: Exceptions. *Brain and Language, 26,* 201–229.

Basso, A., Razzano, C., Faglioni, P., & Zanobio, M. E. (1990). Confrontation naming, picture description and action naming in aphasic patients. *Aphasiology, 4,* 185–196.

Bastiaanse, R., Bosje, M., & Franssen, M. (1996). Deficit-oriented treatment of word-finding problems: Another replication. *Aphasiology, 10,* 363–383.

Bastiaanse, R., Edwards, S., & Kiss, K. (1996). Fluent aphasia in three languages: Aspects of spontaneous speech. *Aphasiology, 10,* 561–575.

Bastiaanse, R., Edwards, S., Maas, E., & Rispens, J. (2003). Assessing comprehension and production of verbs and sentences: The Verb and Sentence Test (VAST). *Aphasiology, 17,* 49–73.

Bastiaanse, R., Edwards, S., & Rispens, J. (2002). *Verb and Sentence Test* (VAST). New York: Pearson/PsychCorp.

Bastiaanse, R., Hurkmans, J., & Links, P. (2006). The training of verb production in Broca's aphasia: A multiple-baseline across-behaviors study. *Aphasiology, 20,* 298–311.

Bastiaanse, R., & Jonkers, R. (1998). Verb retrieval in action naming and spontaneous speech in agrammatism and anomic aphasia. *Aphasiology, 12,* 951–969.

Bastiaanse, R., & Thompson, C. K. (2003). Verb and auxiliary movement in agrammatic Broca's aphasia. *Brain and Language, 84,* 286–305.

Bates, E. A., Friederici, A. D., & Wulfeck, B. B. (1987a). Comprehension in aphasia: A cross-linguistic study. *Brain and Language, 32,* 19–67.

Bates, E. A., Friederici, A. D., & Wulfeck, B. B. (1987b). Grammatical morphology in aphasia: Evidence from three languages. *Cortex, 23,* 545–574.

Bates, E. A., Friederici, A. D., Wulfeck, B. B., & Juarez, L. A. (1988). On the preservation of word order in aphasia: Cross-linguistic evidence. *Brain and Language, 33,* 323–364.

Bates, E. A., Marchman, V., Harris, C., Wulfeck, B., & Kritchevsky, M. (1995). Production of complex syntax in normal ageing and Alzheimer's disease. *Language and Cognitive Processes, 10,* 487–539.

Bates, E. A., & Wulfeck, B. (1989). Comparative aphasiology: A cross-linguistic approach to language breakdown. *Aphasiology, 3,* 111–142.

Bauer, R. M., & Rubens, A. B. (1985). Agnosia. In K. M. Heilman & E. Valenstein (Eds.), *Clinical neuropsychology* (2nd ed., pp. 187–241). New York: Oxford University Press.

Baum, S. R. (1988). Syntactic processing in agrammatism: Evidence from lexical decision and grammaticality judgment tasks. *Aphasiology, 2,* 117–136.

Baum, S. R. (1989). On-line sensitivity to local and long-distance syntactic dependencies in Broca's aphasia. *Brain and Language, 37,* 327–338.

Baum, S. R. (1997). Phonological, semantic, and mediated priming in aphasia. *Brain and Language, 60,* 347–359.

Baum, S. R. (2001). Contextual influences on phonetic identification in aphasia: The effects of speaking rate and semantic bias. *Brain and Language, 76,* 266–281.

Baum, S. R., Daniloff, J., Daniloff, R., & Lewis, J. (1982). Sentence comprehension by Broca's aphasics: Effects of some suprasegmental variables. *Brain and Language, 17,* 261–271.

Baum, S. R., & Dwivedi, V. D. (2003). Sensitivity to prosodic structure in left- and right-hemisphere-damaged individuals. *Brain and Language, 87,* 278–289.

Baum, S. R., & Pell, M. D. (1997). Production of affective and linguistic prosody by brain-damaged patients. *Aphasiology, 11,* 177–198.

Baum, S. R., & Pell, M. D. (1999). The neural bases of prosody: Insights from lesion studies and neuroimaging. *Aphasiology, 13,* 581–608.

Bayles, K. A., & Tomoeda, C. K. (1993). *The Arizona Battery for Communication Disorders of Dementia.* Tucson, AZ: Canyonlands.

Bayles, K. A., & Tomoeda, C. K. (1994). *The Functional Linguistic Communication Inventory.* Tucson, AZ: Canyonlands.

Bayles, K. A., Tomoeda, C. K., & Rein, J. A. (1996). Phrase repetition in Alzheimer's disease: Effect of meaning and length. *Brain and Language, 54,* 246–261.

Beatty, W. W., Salmon, D. P., Bernstein, N., & Butters, N. (1987). Remote memory in a patient with amnesia due to hypoxia. *Psychological Medicine, 17,* 657–665.

Beauchamp, T. L., & Childress, J. F. (1994). *Principles of biomedical ethics* (4th ed.). New York: Oxford University Press.

Becker, B. (1975). Intellectual changes after closed head injury. *Journal of Clinical Psychology, 31,* 307–309.

Beeke, S., Wilkinson, R., & Maxim, J. (2007). Grammar without sentence structure: A conversation analytic investigation of agrammatism. *Aphasiology, 21,* 256–282.

Beeman, M. (1993). Semantic processing in the right hemisphere may contribute to drawing inferences from discourse. *Brain and Language, 44,* 80–120.

Beeson, P. M. (1999). Treating acquired writing impairment: Strengthening graphemic representations. *Aphasiology, 13,* 367–386.

Beeson, P. M., & Henry, M. L. (2008). Comprehension and production of written words. In R. Chapey (Ed.), *Language intervention strategies in aphasia and related neurogenic communication disorders* (5th ed., pp. 654–688). Philadelphia: Wolters Kluwer Health.

Beeson, P. M., Hirsch, F. M., & Rewega, M. A. (2002). Successful single-word writing treatment: Experimental analysis of four cases. *Aphasiology, 16,* 473–491.

Beeson, P. M., & Holland, A. L. (2007). Aphasia groups in a university setting. In R. J. Elman (Ed.), *Group treatment of neurogenic communication disorders: The expert clinician's approach* (2nd ed., pp. 145–158). San Diego, CA: Plural.

Beeson, P. M., Holland, A. L., & Murray, L. L. (1997). Naming famous people: An examination of tip-of-the-tongue phenomena in aphasia and Alzheimer's disease. *Aphasiology, 11,* 323–336.

Beeson, P. M., Rising, K., Kim, E. S., & Rapcsak, S. Z. (2008). A novel method for examining response to spelling treatment. *Aphasiology, 22,* 707–717.

Behrens, S. J. (1988). The role of the right hemisphere in the production of linguistic stress. *Brain and Language, 33,* 104–127.

Behrens, S. J. (1989). Characterizing sentence intonation in a right hemisphere-damaged population. *Brain and Language, 37,* 181–200.

Behrmann, M., & Byng, S. (1992). A cognitive approach to the neurorehabilitation of acquired language disorders. In D. I. Margolin (Ed.), *Cognitive neuropsychology in clinical practice* (pp. 327–350). New York: Oxford University Press.

Behrns, I., Hartelius, L., & Wengelin, Å. (2009). Aphasia and computerised writing aid supported treatment. *Aphasiology, 23,* 1276–1294.

Bélanger, N., Baum, S. R., & Titone, D. (2009). Use of prosodic cues in the production of idiomatic and literal sentences by individuals with right- and left-hemisphere damage. *Brain and Language, 110,* 38–42.

Bell, E. E., Chenery, H. J., & Ingram, J. C. L. (2001). Semantic priming in Alzheimer's dementia: Evidence for dissociation of automatic and attentional processes. *Brain and Language, 76,* 130–144.

Bellaire, K. J., Georges, J. B., & Thompson, C. K. (1991). Establishing functional communication board use for nonverbal aphasic subjects. In T. E. Prescott (Ed.), *Clinical aphasiology* (Vol. 19, pp. 219–228). Austin, TX: Pro-Ed.

Ben-Yishay, Y. (Ed.). (1980). *Working approaches to remediation of cognitive deficits in brain damaged persons.* New York: New York University Medical Center.

Berg, T. (2006). A structural account of phonological paraphasias. *Brain and Language, 96,* 331–356.

Berger, P. E., & Mensh, S. (2002). *How to conquer the world with one hand . . . and an attitude.* Merrifield, VA: Positive Power.

Bergner, M., Bobitt, R. A., Carter, W. B., & Gilson, B. S. (1981). The Sickness Impact Profile: Development and final revision of a health status measure. *Medical Care, 19,* 787–805.

Berman, M., & Peelle, L. M. (1967). Self-generated cues: A method for aiding aphasic and apractic patients. *Journal of Speech and Hearing Disorders, 32,* 372–376.

Berndt, R. S., Haendiges, A. N., Mitchum, C. C., & Sandson, J. (1997). Verb retrieval in aphasia. 2. Relationship to sentence processing. *Brain and Language, 56,* 107–137.

Berndt, R. S., Haendiges, A. N., Mitchum, C. C., & Wayland, S. C. (1996). An investigation of nonlexical reading impairments. *Cognitive Neuropsychology, 13,* 763–802.

Berndt, R. S., Mitchum, C. C., Haendiges, A. N., & Sandson, J. (1997). Verb retrieval in aphasia. Characterizing single word impairments. *Brain and Language, 56,* 68–106.

Berndt, R. S., Mitchum, C. C., & Wayland, S. (1997). Patterns of sentence comprehension in aphasia: A consideration of three hypotheses. *Brain and Language, 60,* 197–221.

Berndt, R. S., Wayland, S., Rochon, E., Saffran, E., & Schwartz, M. (2000). *Quantitative production analysis: A training manual for the analysis of aphasic sentence production.* Hove, UK: Psychology Press.

Bernstein-Ellis, E., & Elman, R. J. (2007). Aphasia group communication treatment: The Aphasia Center of California approach. In R. J. Elman (Ed.). *Group treatment of neurogenic communication disorders: The expert clinician's approach* (2nd ed., pp. 71–94). San Diego, CA: Plural.

Berthier, M. L. (1999). *Transcortical aphasias.* Hove, UK: Psychology Press.

Berthier, M. L., Hinojosa, J., Martin Mdel, C., & Fernandez, I. (2003). Open-label study of donepezil in chronic poststroke aphasia. *Neurology, 60,* 1218–1219.

Beukelman, D. R., Yorkston, K. M., & Garrett, K. L. (2007). An introduction to AAC services for adults with chronic medical conditions: Who, what, when, where, and why. In D. R. Beukelman, K. L. Garrett, & K. M. Yorkston (Eds.), *Augmentative communication strategies for adults with acute or chronic medical conditions* (pp. 1–16). Baltimore: Brookes.

Bhatnagar, S. C., Buckingham, H. W., Puglisi-Creegan, S., & Hacein-Bay, L. (2011). Crossed aphasia in a patient with congenital lesion in the right hemisphere. *Aphasiology, 25,* 27–42.

Bickel, C., Pantel, J., Eysenbach, K., & Schröder, J. (2000). Syntactic comprehension deficits in Alzheimer's disease. *Brain and Language, 71,* 432–448.

Bier, N., Macoir, J., Gagnon, L., Van der Linden, M., Louveaux, S., et al. (2009). Known, lost, and recovered: Efficacy of formal-semantic therapy and spaced retrieval method in a case of semantic dementia. *Aphasiology, 23,* 210–235.

Bihrle, A. M., Brownell, H. H., Powelson, J. A., & Gardner, H. (1986). Comprehension of humorous and nonhumorous materials by left and right brain damaged patients. *Brain and Cognition, 5,* 399–411.

Bilda, K. (2011). Video-based conversational script training for aphasia: A therapy study. *Aphasiology, 25,* 191–201.

Bisiach, E., Capitani, E., Luzzatti, C., & Perani, D. (1981). Brain and the conscious representation of outside reality. *Neuropsychologia, 19,* 543–551.

Bisiach, E., Vallar, G., Perani, D., Papagno, C., & Berti, A. (1986). Unawareness of disease following lesions of the right hemisphere: Anosognosia for hemiplegia and anosognosia for hemianopia. *Neuropsychologia, 24,* 471–482.

Blacker, D., Albert, M. S., Bassett, S. S., Go, R. C., Harrell, L. E., et al. (1994). Reliability and validity of NINCDS-ADRDA criteria for Alzheimer's disease. The National Institute of Mental Health Genetics Initiative. *Archives of Neurology, 51,* 1198–1204.

Blasi, V., Young, A. C., Tansy, A. P., Petersen, S. E., Snyder, A. Z., et al. (2002). Word retrieval learning modulates right frontal cortex in patients with left frontal damage. *Neuron, 36,* 159–170.

Blessed, G., Tomlinson, B. E., & Roth, M. (1968). The association between quantitative measures of dementia and of senile change in the cerebral gray matter of elderly subjects. *British Journal of Psychiatry, 114,* 797–811.

Blomert, L., Kean, M.-L., Koster, C., & Schokker, J. (1994). Amsterdam-Nijmegen Everyday Language Test: Construction, reliability and validity. *Aphasiology, 8,* 381–407.

Blonder, L. X., Bowers, D., & Heilman, K. M. (1991). The role of the right hemisphere in emotional communication. *Brain, 114,* 1115–1127.

Blonder, L. X., Burns, A. F., Bowers, D., Moore, R. W., & Heilman, K. M. (1993). Right hemisphere facial expressivity during natural conversation. *Brain and Cognition, 21,* 44–56.

Bloom, M., & Fischer, J. (1982). *Evaluating practice: Guidelines for the accountable professional.* Englewood Cliffs, NJ: Prentice-Hall.

Bloom, R. L., Borod, J. C., Obler, L. K., Santschi-Haywood, C., & Pick, L. (1995). An examination of coherence and cohesion in aphasia [abstract]. *Brain and Language, 51,* 206–209.

Blumenthal, A. L. (1970). *Language and psychology: Historical aspects of psycholinguistics.* New York: Wiley.

Blumstein, S. E. (1973). *A phonological investigation of aphasic speech.* The Hague, Netherlands: Mouton.

Blumstein, S. E., Cooper, W. E., Goodglass, H., Statlender, S., & Gottleib, J. (1980). Production deficits in aphasia: A voice-onset time analysis. *Brain and Language, 9,* 153–170.

Blumstein, S. E., Cooper, W. E., Zurif, E. B., & Caramazza, A. (1977). The perception and production of voice-onset time in aphasia. *Neuropsychologia, 15,* 371–383.

Blumstein, S. E., & Goodglass, H. (1972). The perception of stress as a semantic cue in aphasia. *Journal of Speech and Hearing Research, 15,* 800–806.

Blumstein, S. E., Katz, B., Goodglass, H., Shrier, R., & Dworetsky, B. (1985). The effects of slowed speech on auditory comprehension in aphasia. *Brain and Language, 24,* 246–265.

Blumstein, S. E., Milberg, W., Dworetzky, B., Rosen, A., & Gershberg, F. (1991). Syntactic priming effects in aphasia: An investigation of local syntactic dependencies. *Brain and Language, 40,* 393–421.

Boake, C., Millis, S. R., High, W. M., Jr., Delmonica, R. L., Kreutzer, J. S., et al. (2001). Using early neuropsychologic testing to predict long-term productivity outcome from traumatic brain injury. *Archives of Physical Medicine and Rehabilitation, 82,* 761–768.

Bock, K., & Levelt, W. (1994). Language production: Grammatical encoding. In M. A. Gernsbacher (Ed.), *Handbook of psycholinguistics* (pp. 945–984). San Diego, CA: Academic Press.

Boles, L. (1997). A comparison of naming errors in individuals with mild naming impairment following poststroke aphasia, Alzheimer's disease, and traumatic brain injury. *Aphasiology, 11,* 1043–1056.

Boller, F., & Vignolo, L. A. (1966). Latent sensory aphasia in hemisphere-damaged patients: An experimental study with the Token Test. *Brain, 89,* 815–830.

Bonakdarpour, B., Eftekharzadeh, A., & Ashayeri, H. (2003). Melodic intonation therapy in Persian aphasic patients. *Aphasiology, 17,* 75–95.

Bond, M. R., & Brooks, D. N. (1976). Understanding the process of recovery as a basis for the investigation of rehabilitation for the brain injured. *Scandinavian Journal of Rehabilitation Medicine, 8,* 127–133.

Boo, M., & Rose, M. L. (2011). The efficacy of repetition, semantic, and gesture treatments for verb retrieval and use in Broca's aphasia. *Aphasiology, 25,* 154–175.

Booth, S., & Perkins, L. (1999). The use of conversation analysis to guide individualized advice to carers and evaluate change in aphasia: A case study. *Aphasiology, 13,* 283–203.

Booth, S., & Swabey, D. (1999). Group training in communication skills for carers of adults with aphasia. *International Journal of Language and Communication Disorders, 34,* 291–309.

Borkowski, J. G., Benton, A. L., & Spreen, O. (1967). Word fluency and brain damage. *Neuropsychologia, 5,* 135–140.

Bormann, T., Fulke, F., Wallesch, C.-W., & Blanken, G. (2008). Omissions and semantic errors in aphasic naming: Is there a link? *Brain and Language, 104,* 24–32.

Borod, J. C., Andelman, F., Obler, L., Tweedy, J., & Welkowitz, J. (1992). Right hemisphere specialization for the identification of emotional words and sentences: Evidence from stroke patients. *Neuropsychologia, 30,* 827–844.

Borod, J. C., Carper, J. M., & Naeser, M. (1990). Long-term language recovery in left-handed aphasic patients. *Aphasiology, 4,* 561–572.

Borod, J. C., Fitzpatrick, P. M., Helm-Estabrooks, N., & Goodglass, H. (1989). The relationship between limb apraxia and the spontaneous use of communicative gesture in aphasia. *Brain and Cognition, 10,* 121–131.

Borod, J. C., Goodglass, H., & Kaplan, E. (1980). Normative data on the Boston Diagnostic Aphasia Examination, Parietal Lobe Battery, and the Boston Naming Test. *Journal of Clinical Neuropsychology, 2,* 209–215.

Borod, J. C., Koff, E., Perlman-Lorch, M., & Nicholas, M. (1986). The expression and perception of facial emotion in brain-damaged patients. *Neuropsychologia, 24,* 169–180.

Borson, S., Scanlan, J. M., Chen, P., & Ganguli, M. (2003). The Mini-Cog as a screen for dementia: Validation in a population-based sample. *Journal of the American Geriatrics Society, 51,* 1451–1454.

Bose, A., McHugh, T., Schollenberger, H., & Buchanan, L. (2009). Meaasuring quality of life in aphasia: Results from two scales. *Aphasiology, 23,* 797–808.

Botez, M. I., Botez, T., & Aube, M. (1980). Amusia: Clinical and computerized scanning (CT) correlations. *Neurology, 30,* 359.

Bottenberg, D. E., & Lemme, M. L. (1991). Effect of shared and unshared listener knowledge on narratives of normal and aphasic adults. In T. E. Prescott (Ed.), *Clinical aphasiology* (Vol. 19, pp. 109–116). Austin, TX: Pro-Ed.

Bottenberg, D. E., Lemme, M. L., & Hedberg, N. L. (1987). Effect of story content on narrative discourse of aphasic adults. In R. H. Brookshire (Ed.), *Clinical aphasiology* (Vol. 17, pp. 202–209). Minneapolis, MN: BRK.

Bourgeois, M. S. (1992). Evaluating memory wallets in conversations with patients with dementia. *Journal of Speech and Hearing Research, 35,* 1344–1357.

Bourgeois, M. S. (2007). *Memory books and other graphic cuing systems: Practical communication and memory aids for adults with dementia.* Bethesda, MD: Health Professions Press.

Bourgeois, M., Camp, C., Rose, M., Blanche, W., Malone, M., et al. (2003). A comparison of training strategies to enhance use of external aids by persons with dementia. *Journal of Communication Disorders, 36,* 361–378.

Bourgeois, M. S., & Hickey, E. (2009). *Dementia: From diagnosis to management—A functional approach.* New York: Psychology Press.

Bourgeois, M., Schulz, R., Burgio, L., & Beach, S. (2002). Skills training for spouses of patients with Alzheimer's disease: Outcomes of an intervention study. *Journal of Clinical Geropsychology, 8,* 53–73.

Bowers, D., Blonder, L. X., & Heilman, K. M. (1999). *Florida Affect Battery Manual.* Gainesville, FL: University of Florida. Retrieved from http://neurology.ufl.edu/research/memory-and-cognitive-disorders-research/behavioral-neurology-research

Bowes, K., & Martin, N. (2007). Longitudinal study of reading and writing rehabilitation using a bigraph-biphone correspondence approach. *Aphasiology, 21,* 687–701.

Bowling, A. (2004). *Measuring health: A review of quality of life measurement scales* (3rd ed.). Berkshire, UK: Open University Press.

Boyle, M. (1989). Reducing phonemic paraphasias in the connected speech of a conduction aphasic subject. In T. E. Prescott (Ed.), *Clinical aphasiology* (Vol. 18, pp. 379–393). Boston: College-Hill/Little, Brown.

Boyle, M. (2004). Semantic feature analysis treatment for anomia in two fluent aphasia syndromes. *American Journal of Speech-Language Pathology, 13,* 236–249.

Boyle, M. (2011). Discourse treatment for word retrieval impairment in aphasia: The story so far. *Aphasiology, 25,* 1308–1326.

Boyle, M., & Coelho, C. A. (1995). Application of semantic feature analysis as a treatment for aphasic dysnomia. *American Journal of Speech-Language Pathology, 4*(4), 94–98.

Boyle, M., Coelho, C. A., & Kimbarow, M. L. (1991). Word fluency tasks: A preliminary analysis of variability. *Aphasiology, 5,* 171–182.

Brady, M., Armstrong, L., & Mackenzie, C. (2005). Further evidence on topic use following right hemisphere brain damage: Procedural and descriptive discourse. *Aphasiology, 19,* 731–747.

Brady, M., Mackenzie, C., & Armstrong, L. (2003). Topic use following right hemisphere brain damage during three semi-structured conversational discourse samples. *Aphasiology, 17,* 881–904.

Brady, M. C., Kelly, H., Godwin, J., & Enderby, P. (2012). Speech and language therapy for aphasia following stroke. *Cochrane Database of Systematic Reviews,* Issue 5. Art. No.: CD000425. DOI: 10.1002/14651858.CD000425.pub3

Breese, E. L., & Hillis, A. E. (2004). Auditory comprehension: Is multiple choice really good enough? *Brain and Language, 89,* 3–8.

Brennan, A. D., Worrall, L. E., & McKenna, K. T. (2005). The relationship between specific features of aphasia-friendly written material and comprehension of written material for people with aphasia: An exploratory study. *Aphasiology, 19,* 693–711.

Brenneise-Sarshad, R., Nicholas, L. E., & Brookshire, R. H. (1991). Effects of apparent listener knowledge and picture stimuli on aphasic and non-brain-damaged speakers' narrative discourse. *Journal of Speech and Hearing Research, 34,* 168–176.

Brody, J. E. (2011). A thief that robs the brain of language. *New York Times,* May 3, D7.

Broida, H. (1977). Language therapy effects in long term aphasia. *Archives of Physical Medicine and Rehabilitation, 58,* 248–253.

Brooks, N., Campsie, L., Symington, C., Beattie, A., & McKinlay, W. (1986). The five year outcome of severe blunt head injury: A relative's view. *Journal of Neurology, Neurosurgery, and Psychiatry, 49,* 764–770.

Brooks, N., McKinlay, W., Symington, C., Beattie, A., & Campsie, L. (1987). Return to work within the first seven years of severe head injury. *Brain Injury, 1,* 5–19.

Brookshire, R. H. (1972). Effects of task difficulty on naming by aphasic subjects. *Journal of Speech and Hearing Research, 15,* 551–558.

Brookshire, R. H. (1983). Subject description and generality of results in experiments with aphasic adults. *Journal of Speech and Hearing Disorders, 48,* 342–346.

Brookshire, R. H. (1994). Group studies of treatment for adults with aphasia: Efficacy, effectiveness, and believability. *Special Interest Division 2 Newsletter, 4*(4), 5–14.

Brookshire, R. H. (2007). *Introduction to neurogenic communication disorders* (7th ed.). St. Louis, MO: Mosby Elsevier.

Brookshire, R. H., & Nicholas, L. E. (1978). Effects of clinician request and feedback behavior on responses of aphasic individuals in speech and language treatment sessions. In R. H. Brookshire (Ed.), *Clinical aphasiology conference proceedings* (pp. 40–48). Minneapolis, MN: BRK.

Brookshire, R. H., & Nicholas, L. E. (1984). Consistency of effects of slow rate and pauses on aphasic listeners' comprehension of spoken sentences. *Journal of Speech and Hearing Research, 27,* 323–328.

Brookshire, R. H., & Nicholas, L. E. (1993). *The Discourse Comprehension Test.* Tucson, AZ: Communication Skill Builders.

Brookshire, R. H., & Nicholas, L. E. (1994). Speech sample size and test-retest stability of connected speech measures for adults with aphasia. *Journal of Speech and Hearing Research, 37,* 399–407.

Brookshire, R. H., Nicholas, L. E., Krueger, K. M., & Redmond, K. J. (1978). The clinical interaction analysis system: A system for observational recording of aphasia treatment. *Journal of Speech and Hearing Disorders, 43,* 437–447.

Brown, J. R., & Schuell, H. M. (1950). A preliminary report of a diagnostic test for aphasia. *Journal of Speech and Hearing Disorders, 15,* 21–28.

Brown, K., Worrall, L., Davidson, B., & Howe, T. (2010). Snapshots of success: An insider perspective on living successfully with aphasia. *Aphasiology, 24,* 1267–1295.

Brownell, H. H. (1988). The neuropsychology of narrative comprehension. *Aphasiology, 2,* 247–250.

Brownell, H. H., Bihrle, A. M., & Michelow, D. (1986). Basic and subordinate level naming by agrammatic and fluent aphasic patients. *Brain and Language, 28,* 42–52.

Brownell, H. H., Griffin, R., Winner, E., Friedman, O., & Happé, F. (2000). Cerebral lateralization and theory of mind. In S. Baron-Cohen, H. Tager-Flusberg, & D. J. Cohen (Eds.), *Understanding other minds: Perspectives from autism and developmental cognitive neuroscience* (2nd ed., pp. 311–338). Oxford, UK: Oxford University Press.

Brownell, H. H., Michel, D., Powelson, J. A., & Gardner, H. (1983). Surprise but not coherence: sensitivity to verbal humor in right hemisphere patients. *Brain and Language, 18,* 20–27.

Brownell, H. H., Pincus, D., Blum, A., Rehak, A., & Winner, E. (1997). The effects of right-hemisphere brain-damage on patients' use of terms of personal reference. *Brain and Language, 57,* 60–79.

Brownell, H. H., Potter, H. H., Bihrle, A. M., & Gardner, H. (1986). Inference deficits in right brain-damaged patients. *Brain and Language, 27,* 310–321.

Bruce, C., & Edmundson, A. (2010). Letting the CAT out of the bag: A review of the Comprehensive Aphasia Test. Commentary on Howard, Swinburn, and Porter. *Aphasiology, 24,* 79–93.

Bruce, C., & Howard, D. (1988). Why don't Broca's aphasics cue themselves? An investigation of phonemic cueing and tip of the tongue information. *Neuropsychologia, 26,* 253–264.

Brumfitt, S. (1993). Losing your sense of self: What aphasia can do. *Aphasiology, 7,* 569–574.

Brush, J. A., & Camp, C. J. (1998). Using spaced retrieval as an intervention during speech-language therapy. *Clinical Gerontologist, 19,* 51–64.

Bryan, K. L. (1989). Language prosody and the right hemisphere. *Aphasiology, 3*(4), 285–300.

Bryan, K. L. (1995). *The Right Hemisphere Language Battery* (2nd ed.). London: Whurr.

Buchanan, L., McEwen, S., Westbury, C., & Libben, G. (2003). Semantics and semantic errors: Implicit access to semantic information from words and nonwords in deep dyslexia. *Brain and Language, 84,* 65–83.

Buchsbaum, B. R., Baldo, J., Okada, K., Berman, K. F., Dronkers, N., et al. (2011). Conduction aphasia, sensory-motor integration, and phonological short-term memory—An aggregate analysis of lesion and fMRI data. *Brain and Language, 119,* 119–128.

Buck, R., & Duffy, R. J. (1980). Nonverbal communication of affect in brain-damaged patients. *Cortex, 16,* 351–362.

Buckingham, H. W. (1981). Where do neologisms come from? In J. W. Brown (Ed.), *Jargonaphasia* (pp. 39–62). New York: Academic Press.

Buckingham, H. W. (1987). Phonemic paraphasias and psycholinguistic production models for neologistic jargon. *Aphasiology, 1,* 381–401.

Buckingham, H. W. (1989). Mechanisms underlying aphasic transformations. In A. Ardila & P. Ostrosky-Solis (Eds.), *Brain organization of language and cognitive processes* (pp. 123–145). New York: Plenum.

Buckingham, H. W., & Kertesz, A. (1976). *Neologistic jargon aphasia.* Amsterdam: Swets and Zeitlinger.

Bupp, H. (2012). Nine upsetting dilemmas: A look at the most commonly reported ethical quandaries in the professions. *ASHA Leader, 17*(14), 10–14.

Burchert, F., Meisner, N., & De Bleser, R. (2008). Production of non-canonical sentences in agrammatic aphasia: Limits in representation or rule application? *Brain and Language, 104,* 170–179.

Burke, H. L., Yeo, R. A., Delaney, H. D., & Conner, L. (1993). CT scan cerebral hemispheric asymmetries: Predictors of recovery from aphasia. *Journal of Clinical and Experimental Neuropsychology, 15,* 191–204.

Burkhardt, P., Piñango, M. M., & Wong, K. (2003). The role of the anterior left hemisphere in real-time sentence comprehension: Evidence from split intransivity. *Brain and Language, 86,* 9–22.

Busch, C. R. (1993). Functional outcome: Reimbursement issues. In M. L. Lemme (Ed.), *Clinical aphasiology* (Vol. 21, pp. 73–85). Austin, TX: Pro-Ed.

Busch, C. R. (2007). Reimbursement issues particular to group treatment. In R. J. Elman (Ed.), *Group treatment of neurogenic communication disorders: The expert clinician's approach* (2nd ed., pp. 63–70). San Diego, CA: Plural.

Busch, C. R., Brookshire, R. H., & Nicholas, L. E. (1988). Referential communication by aphasic and nonaphasic adults. *Journal of Speech and Hearing Disorders, 53,* 475–482.

Butfield, E., & Zangwill, O. L. (1946). Reeducation in aphasia: A review of 70 cases. *Journal of Neurology, Neurosurgery, and Psychiatry, 9,* 75–79.

Butler-Hinz, S., Caplan, D., & Waters, G. (1990). Characteristics of syntactic and semantic comprehension deficits following closed head injury versus left cerebrovascular accident. *Journal of Speech and Hearing Research, 33,* 269–280.

Byng, S. (1988). Sentence processing deficits: Theory and therapy. *Cognitive Neuropsychology, 5,* 629–676.

Byng, S., & Black, M. (1989). Some aspects of sentence production in aphasia. *Aphasiology, 3,* 241–263.

Byng, S., Kay, J., Edmundson, A., & Scott, C. (1990). Aphasia tests reconsidered. *Aphasiology, 4,* 67–92.

Byng, S., Nickels, L., & Black, M. (1994). Replicating therapy for mapping deficits in agrammatism: Remapping the deficit? *Aphasiology, 8,* 315–341.

Cahalan, S. (2012). *Brain on fire.* New York: Free Press.

Calvin, W. H., & Ojemann, G. A. (1980). *Inside the brain.* New York: Mentor.

Cameron, R. M., Wambaugh, J. L., & Mauszycki, S. C. (2010). Individual variability on discourse measures over repeated sampling times in persons with aphasia. *Aphasiology, 24,* 671–684.

Cameron, R. M., Wambaugh, J. L., Wright, S. M., & Nessler, C. L. (2006). Effects of a combined semantic/phonologic cueing treatment on word retrieval in discourse. *Aphasiology, 20,* 269–285.

Camp, C. J. (2006). Spaced retrieval: A model for dissemination of a cognitive intervention for persons with dementia. In D. K. Attix & K. A. Welsh-Bohmer (Eds.), *Geriatric neuropsychology: Assessment and intervention* (pp. 275–292). New York: Guilford Press.

Cannizzaro, M., & Coelho, C. (2012). Communication following executive dysfunction. In R. K. Peach & L. P. Shapiro (Eds.), *Cognition and acquired language disorders: An information processing approach* (pp. 227–240). St. Louis: Elsevier/Mosby.

Canter, G. J. (1988). Apraxia of speech and phonemic paraphasia. *Aphasiology, 2,* 251–254.

Canter, G. J., Trost, J. E., Burns, M. S. (1985). Contrasting speech patterns in apraxia of speech and phonemic paraphasia. *Brain and Language, 24,* 204–222.

Cao, Y., Vikingstad, E., George, K., Johnson, A., & Welch, K. (1999). Cortical language activation in stroke patients recovering from aphasia with functional MRI. *Stroke, 30,* 2331–2340.

Capilouto, G. J., Harris Wright, H., & Wagovich, S. A. (2006). Reliability of main event measurement in the discourse of individuals with aphasia. *Aphasiology, 20,* 205–216.

Capitani, E., Laiacona, M., Mahon, B., & Caramazza, A. (2003). What are the facts of semantic category-specific deficits? *Cognitive Neuropsychology, 20,* 213–262.

Caplan, D. (1985). Syntactic and semantic structures in agrammatism. In M.-L. Kean (Ed.), *Agrammatism* (pp. 125–151). Orlando, FL: Academic Press.

Caplan, D. (1987). *Neurolinguistics and linguistic aphasiology: An introduction.* Cambridge, UK: Cambridge University Press.

Caplan, D. (1991). Agrammatism is a theoretically coherent aphasic category. *Brain and Language, 40,* 274–281.

Caplan, D. (2002). The neural basis of syntactic processing: A critical look. In A. E. Hillis (Ed.), *The handbook of adult language disorders* (pp. 331–350). New York: Psychology Press.

Caplan, D., Baker, C., & Dehaut, F. (1985). Syntactic determinants of sentence comprehension in aphasia. *Cognition, 21,* 117–175.

Caplan, D., DeDe, G., & Brownell, H. (2006). Effects of syntactic features on sentence-picture matching in Broca's aphasics: A reply to Drai and Grodzinsky (2006). *Brain and Language, 96,* 129–134.

Caplan, D., DeDe, G., & Michaud, J. (2006). Task-independent and task-specific syntactic deficits in aphasic comprehension. *Aphasiology, 20,* 893–920.

Caplan, D., & Futter, C. (1986). Assignment of thematic roles to nouns in sentence comprehension by an agrammatic patient. *Brain and Language, 27,* 117–134.

Caplan, D., & Waters, G. (1996). Syntactic processing in sentence comprehension under dual-task conditions in aphasic patients. *Language and Cognitive Processes, 11,* 525–551.

Caplan, D., & Waters, G. (2003). On-line syntactic processing in aphasia: Studies with auditory moving window presentation. *Brain and Language, 84,* 222–249.

Caplan, D., Waters, G. S., & Hildebrandt, N. (1997). Determinants of sentence comprehension in aphasic patients in sentence-picture matching tasks. *Journal of Speech, Language, and Hearing Research, 40,* 542–555.

Caporali, A., & Basso, A. (2003). A survey of long-term outcome of aphasia and of chances of gainful employment. *Aphasiology, 17,* 815–834.

Cappa, S. F., Benke, T., Clarke, S., Rossi, B., Stemmer, B., et al. (2011). Cognitive rehabilitation. In N. E. Gilhus, M. P. Barnes, & M. Brainin (Eds.), *European handbook of neurological management: Volume 1* (2nd ed., pp. 545–562). Oxford, UK: Blackwell.

Cappa, S. F., Cavallotti, G., & Vignolo, L. (1981). Phonemic and lexical errors in fluent aphasia: Correlation with lesion site. *Neuropsychologia, 19,* 171–177.

Cappa, S. F., Papagno, C., & Vallar, G. (1990). Language and verbal memory after right hemispheric stroke: A clinical-CT scan study. *Neuropsychologia, 28,* 503–509.

Cappa, S. F., Perani, D., Grassi, F., Bressi, S., Alberoni, M., et al. (1997). A PET follow-up study of recovery after stroke in acute aphasics. *Brain and Language, 56,* 55–67.

Caramazza, A., & Badecker, W. (1991). Clinical syndromes are not God's gift to cognitive neuropsychology: A reply to a rebuttal to an answer to a response to the case against syndrome-based research. *Brain and Cognition, 16,* 211–227.

Caramazza, A., & Berndt, R. S. (1978). Semantic and syntactic processes in aphasia: A review of the literature. *Psychological Bulletin, 85,* 898–918.

Caramazza, A., & Berndt, R. S. (1985). A multicomponential deficit view of agrammatic Broca's aphasia. In M. L. Kean (Ed.), *Agrammatism* (pp. 27–63). Orlando, FL: Academic Press.

Caramazza, A., Capasso, R., Capitani, E., & Miceli, G. (2005). Patterns of comprehension performance in agrammatic Broca's aphasia: A test of the Trace Deletion Hypothesis. *Brain and Language, 94,* 43–53.

Caramazza, A., Papagno, C., & Ruml, W. (2000). The selective impairment of phonological processing in speech production. *Brain and Language, 75,* 428–450.

Caramazza, A., & Zurif, E. B. (1976). Dissociation of alogorithmic and heuristic processes in language comprehension: Evidence from aphasia. *Brain and Language, 3,* 572–582.

Carlesimo, G. A., Fadda, L., & Caltagirone, C. (1993). Basic mechanisms of constructional apraxia in unilateral brain-damaged patients: Role of visuoperceptual and executive disorders. *Journal of Clinical and Experimental Neuropsychology, 15,* 342–358.

Carlomagno, S., Losanno, N., Emanuelli, S., & Casadio, P. (1991). Expressive language recovery or improved communicative skills: Effects of P. A. C. E. therapy on aphasics' referential communication and story retelling. *Aphasiology, 5,* 419–424.

Carlomagno, S., Pandolfi, M., Labruna, L., Colombo, A., & Razzano, C. (2001). Recovery from moderate aphasia in the first year post-stroke: Effect of type of therapy. *Archives of Physical Medicine and Rehabilitation, 82,* 1073–1080.

Carney, N., Chestnut, R. M., Maynard, H., Mann, N. C., Patterson, P., et al. (1999). Effect of cognitive rehabilitation on outcomes for persons with traumatic brain injury. *Journal of Head Trauma Rehabilitation, 14,* 277–307.

Carr, C. (2011, June/July). The ABCs of aphasia. *Neurology Now,* 35–38.

Carr, T. H., & Hinckley, J. J. (2012). Attention: Architecture and process. In R. K. Peach & L. P. Shapiro (Eds.), *Cognition and acquired language disorders: An information processing approach* (pp. 61–93). St. Louis: Elsevier/Mosby.

Carragher, M., Conroy, P., Sage, K., & Wilkinson, R. (2012). Can impairment-focused therapy change the everyday conversations of people with aphasia? A review of the literature and future directions. *Aphasiology, 26,* 895–916.

Carreiras, M., and Clifton, Jr., C. (Eds.). (2004). *The online study of sentence comprehension: Eye-tracking, ERPs and beyond.* Brighton, UK: Psychology Press.

Centeno, J. G., & Ansaldo, A. I. (2013). Aphasia in multilingual populations. In I. Papathanasiou, P. Coppens, & C. Potages (Eds.), *Aphasia and related neurogenic communication disorders* (pp. 275–294). Burlington, MA: Jones & Bartlett Learning.

Chamberlain, M. A., Neumann, V., & Tennant, A. (Eds.). (1995). *Traumatic brain injury rehabilitation: Services, treatments and outcomes.* London: Chapman & Hall Medical.

Chan, A. S., Salmon, D. P., & De La Pena, J. (2001). Abnormal semantic network for "animals" but not "tools" in patients with Alzheimer's disease. *Cortex, 37,* 197–217.

Channon, S., Pellijeff, A., & Rule, A. (2005). Social cognition after head injury: Sarcasm and theory of mind. *Brain and Language, 93,* 123–134.

Chapey, R., Rigrodsky, S., & Morrison, E. B. (1977). Aphasia: A divergent semantic interpretation. *Journal of Speech and Hearing Disorders, 42,* 287–295.

Chapman, S. B., & Ulatowska, H. K. (1989). Discourse in aphasia: Integration deficits in processing reference. *Brain and Language, 36,* 651–668.

Chapman, S. B., Weiner, M. F., Rackley, A., Hynan, L. S., & Zientz, J. (2004). Effects of cognitive-communication stimulation for Alzheimer's disease patients treated with Donepezil. *Journal of Speech, Language, and Hearing Research, 47,* 1149–1163.

Chenery, H. J., Ingram, J. C. L., & Murdoch, B. B. (1990). Automatic and volitional semantic processing in aphasia. *Brain and Language, 38,* 215–232.

Cherney, L. R. (2010). Oral Reading for Language in Aphasia (ORLA): Impact of aphasia severity on cross-modal outcomes in chronic nonfluent aphasia. *Seminars in Speech-Language Pathology, 31,* 42–51.

Cherney, L. R., Erickson, R. K., & Small, S. L. (2010). Epidural cortical stimulation as adjunctive treatment for non-fluent aphasia: Preliminary findings. *Journal of Neurology, Neurosurgery and Psychiatry, 81,* 1014–1021.

Cherney, L. R., & Halper, A. S. (2007). Group treatment for patients with right hemisphere damage. In R. J. Elman (Ed.), *Group treatment of neurogenic communication disorders: The expert clinician's approach* (2nd ed., pp. 269–296). San Diego, CA: Plural.

Cherney, L. R., Halper, A., Holland, A., & Cole, R. (2008). Computerized script training in aphasia: Preliminary results. *American Journal of Speech and Language Pathology, 17,* 19–34.

Cherney, L. R., Halper, A. S., Kwasnica, C. M., Harvey, R. L., & Zhang, M. (2001). Recovery of functional status after right hemisphere stroke: Relationship with unilateral neglect. *Archives of Physical Medicine and Rehabilitation, 82,* 322–328.

Cherney, L. R., Harvery, R. L., Babbitt, E. M., Hurwitz, R., Kaye, R. C., et al. (2012). Epidural cortical stimulation and aphasia therapy. *Aphasiology, 26,* 1192–1217.

Cherney, L. R., Patterson, J. P., Raymer, A., Frymark, T., & Schooling, T. (2008). Evidence-based systematic review: Effects of intensity of treatment and constraint-induced language therapy for individuals with stroke-induced aphasia. *Journal of Speech, Language, and Hearing Research, 51,* 1282–1299.

Chertkow, H., Bub, D., Deaudon, C., & Whitehead, V. (1997). On the status of object concepts in aphasia. *Brain and Language, 58,* 203–232.

Chertkow, H., Bub, D., & Seidenberg, M. (1989). Priming and semantic memory loss in Alzheimer's disease. *Brain and Language, 36,* 420–446.

Chialant, D., Costa, A., & Caramazza, A. (2002). Models of naming. In A. E. Hillis (Ed.), *The handbook of adult language disorders: Integrating cognitive neuropsychology, neurology, and rehabilitation* (pp. 123–142). New York: Psychology Press.

Cho, S., & Thompson, C. K. (2010). What goes wrong during passive sentence production in agrammatic aphasia: An eyetracking study. *Aphasiology, 24,* 1576–1592.

Cho-Reyes, S., & Thompson, C. K. (2012). Verb and sentence production and comprehension in aphasia: Northwestern Assessment of Verbs and Sentences (NAVS). *Aphasiology, 26,* 1250–1277.

Chomsky, N. (1957). Syntactic structures. The Hague: Mouton.

Choy, J. J., & Thompson, C. K. (2010). Binding in agrammatic aphasia: Processing to comprehension. *Aphasiology, 24,* 551–579.

Christiansen, J. A. (1995a). Coherence violations and propositional usage in the narratives of fluent aphasics. *Brain and Language, 51,* 291–317.

Christiansen, J. A. (1995b). Getting to the point: Relevance in story production and comprehension by aphasic patients [abstract]. *Brain and Language, 51,* 201–204.

Chue, W. L., Rose, M. L., & Swinburn, K. (2010). The reliability of the Communication Disability Profile: A patient-reported outcome measure for aphasia. *Aphasiology, 24,* 940–956.

Ciaghi, M., Pancheri, E., & Miceli, G. (2010). Semantic paralexias: A group-case study on the underlying functional mechanisms, incidence and clinical features in a consecutive series of 340 Italian aphasics. *Brain and Language, 115,* 121–132.

Cicerone, K. D., Dahlberg, C., Malec, J. F., Langenbahn, D. M., Felicetti, T., et al. (2005). Evidence-based cognitive rehabilitation: Updated review of the literature from 1998 through 2002. *Archives of Physical Medicine and Rehabilitation, 86,* 1681–1692.

Cicerone, K. D., & Giacino, J. T. (1992). Remediation of executive function deficits after traumatic brain injury. *Neuropsychological Rehabilitation, 2,* 12–22.

Cimino-Knight, A. M., Hollingsworth, A. L., & Gonzalez Rothi, L. J. (2005). The transcortical aphasias. In L. L. LaPointe (Ed.), *Aphasia and related neurogenic language disorders* (3rd ed., pp. 169–185). New York: Thieme.

Clare, L., Wilson, B. A., Carter, G., Hodges, J. R., & Adams, M. (2001). Long-term maintenance of treatment gains following a cognitive rehabilitation intervention in early dementia of Alzheimer type: A single case study. *Neuropsychological Rehabilitation, 11,* 477–494.

Clark, C. M., & Ryan, L. (1993). Implications of statistical tests of variance and means. *Journal of Clinical and Experimental Neuropsychology, 15,* 619–622.

Clark, L. W., & Witte, K. (1995). Nature and efficacy of communication management in Alzheimer's disease. In R. Lubinski (Ed.), *Dementia and communication* (pp. 238–256). San Diego, CA: Singular.

Clements, A. M., Rimrodt, S. L., Abel, J. R., Blankner, J. G., Mostofsky, S. H., et al. (2006). Sex differences in cerebral laterality of language and visuospatial processing. *Brain and Language, 98,* 150–158.

Clérébaut, N., Coyette, F., Feyereisen, P., & Seron, X. (1984). Une method de rééducation fonctionelle des aphasiques: La P.A.C.E. *Rééducation Orthophonique, 22,* 329–345.

Cocks, N., Hird, K., & Kirsner, K. (2007). The relationship between right hemisphere damage and gesture in spontaneous discourse. *Aphasiology, 21,* 299–319.

Code, C. (2004). Ten years of PALPAring in aphasia. *Aphasiology, 18,* 75–76.

Coelho, C. A. (1990). Acquisition and generalization of simple manual sign grammars by aphasic subjects. *Journal of Communication Disorders, 23,* 383–400.

Coelho, C. A. (1991). Manual sign acquisition and use in two aphasic subjects. In T. E. Prescott (Ed.), *Clinical aphasiology* (Vol. 19, pp. 209–218). Austin, TX: Pro-Ed.

Coelho, C. A. (2002). Story narratives of adults with closed head injury and non-brain-injured adults: Influence of socioeconomic status, elicitation task, and executive functioning. *Journal of Speech, Language, and Hearing Research, 45,* 1232–1248.

Coelho, C. A., DeRuyter, F., & Stein, M. (1996). Treatment efficacy: Cognitive-communicative disorders resulting from traumatic brain injury in adults. *Journal of Speech and Hearing Research, 39,* S5–S17.

Coelho, C. A., Liles, B. Z., & Duffy, R. J. (1991). Discourse analyses with closed head injured adults: Evidence for differing patterns of deficits. *Archives of Physical Medicine and Rehabilitation, 72,* 465–468.

Coelho, C. A., Liles, B. Z., Duffy, R. J., & Clarkson, J. V. (1993). Conversational patterns of aphasic, closed-head-injured, and normal speakers. In M. L. Lemme (Ed.), *Clinical aphasiology* (Vol. 21, pp. 183–192). Austin, TX: Pro-Ed.

Coelho, C. A., McHugh, R. E., & Boyle, M. (2000). Semantic feature analysis as a treatment for aphasic dysnomia: A replication. *Aphasiology, 14,* 133–142.

Coelho, C. A., Sinotte, M. P., & Duffy, J. R. (2008). Schuell's stimulation approach to rehabilitation. In R. Chapey (Ed.), *Language intervention strategies in aphasia and related neurogenic communication disorders* (5th ed., pp. 403–449). Philadelphia: Wolters Kluwer Health.

Coelho, C. A., Youse, K. M., & Lê, K. N. (2002). Conversational discourse in closed-head-injured and nonbrain-injured adults. *Aphasiology, 16,* 659–671.

Coelho, C. A., Youse, K. M., Lê, K. N, & Feinn, R. (2003). Narrative and conversational discourse of adults with closed head injuries and non-brain-injured adults: A discriminant analysis. *Aphasiology, 17,* 499–510.

Coelho, C., Lê, K., Mozeiko, J., Hamilton, M., Tyler, E., et al. (2013). Characterizing discourse deficits following penetrating head injury: A preliminary model. *American Journal of Speech-Language Pathology* (Supplement), *22,* S438–S448.

Cohen, R. Kelter, S. & Woll, G. (1980). Analytical competence and language impairment in aphasia. *Brain and Language, 10,* 331–347.

Cole-Virtue, J., & Nickels, L. (2004). Spoken word to picture matching from PALPA: A critique and some new matched sets. *Aphasiology, 18,* 77–101.

Collette, F., & Van der Linden, M. (2002). Brain imaging of the central executive component of working memory. *Neuroscience & Neurobehavioral Reviews, 26,* 105–125.

Collie, A., Maruff, P., Darby, D., Makdissi, M., McCrory, P., et al. (2006). CogSport. In R. J. Echemendía (Ed.), *Sports neuropsychology: Assessment and management of traumatic brain injury* (pp. 240–262). New York: Guilford Press.

Collins, M. (2005). Global aphasia. In L. L. LaPointe (Ed.), *Aphasia and related neurogenic language disorders* (3rd ed., pp. 186–198). New York: Thieme.

Collins, M. J. (1986). *Diagnosis and treatment of global aphasia.* San Diego: Singular.

Collins, M. J., McNeil, M. R., Lentz, S., Shubitowski, Y., & Rosenbek, J. C. (1984). Word fluency and aphasia: Some linguistic and not-so-linguistic considerations. In R. H. Brookshire (Ed.), *Clinical aphasiology conference proceedings* (pp. 78–84). Minneapolis, MN: BRK.

Conner, L. T., Obler, L. K., Tocco, M., Fitzpatrick, P. M., & Albert, M. L. (2001). Effect of socioeconomic status on aphasia severity and recovery. *Brain and Language, 78,* 254–257.

Conroy, P., Sage, K., & Lambon Ralph, M. A. (2006). Towards theory-driven therapies for aphasic verb impairments: A review of current theory and practice. *Aphasiology, 20,* 1159–1185.

Conroy, P., Sage, K., & Lambon Ralph, M. A. (2009a). A comparison of word versus sentence cues as therapy for verb naming in aphasia. *Aphasiology, 23,* 462–483.

Conroy, P., Sage, K., & Lambon Ralph, M. A. (2009b). Errorless and errorful therapy for verb and noun naming in aphasia. *Aphasiology, 23,* 1311–1337.

Cook, L., Smith, D. S., & Truman, G. (1994). Using Functional Independence Measure profiles as an index of outcome in the rehabilitation of brain-injured patients. *Archives of Physical Medicine and Rehabilitation, 75,* 390–393.

Cooper, W. E., Soares, C., Nicol, J., Michelow, D., & Goloskie, S. (1984). Clausal intonation after unilateral brain damage. *Language and Speech, 27,* 17–24.

Coppens, P., Hungerford, S., Yamaguchi, S., & Yamadori, A. (2002). Crossed aphasia: An analysis of the symptoms, their frequency, and a comparison with left-hemisphere aphasia symptomatology. *Brain and Language, 83,* 425–463.

Corbett, F., Jefferies, E., & Lambon Ralph, M. A. (2008). The use of cueing to alleviate recurrent verbal perseverations: Evidence from transcortical sensory aphasia. *Aphasiology, 22,* 363–382.

Corina, D., Kritchevsky, M., & Bellugi, U. (1996). Visual language processing and unilateral neglect: Evidence from American Sign Language. *Cognitive Neuropsychology, 13,* 321–356.

Correll, A., van Steenbrugge, W., & Scholten, I. (2010). Judging conversation: How much is enough? *Aphasiology, 24,* 612–622.

Corrigan, J. D., Selassie, A. W., & Orman, J. A. (2010). The epidemiology of traumatic brain injury. *Journal of Head Trauma Rehabilitation, 25,* 72–80.

Corsten, S., Mende, M., Cholewa, J., & Huber, W. (2007). Treatment of input and output phonology in aphasia: A single case study. *Aphasiology, 21,* 587–603.

Coughlan, A. K., & Warrington, E. K. (1978). Word comprehension and word retrieval in patients with localized cerebral lesions. *Brain, 101,* 163–185.

Craig, H. K., Hinckley, J. J., Winkelseth, M., Carry, L., Walley, J., et al. (1993). Quantifying connected speech samples of adults with chronic aphasia. *Aphasiology, 7,* 155–164.

Cramer, P. E., Cirrito, J. R., Wesson, D. W., Lee, C. Y. D., Karlo, J. C., et al. (2012). ApoE-directed therapeutics rapidly clear ?-amyloid and reverse deficits in AD mouse models. *Science, 335,* 1503–1506.

Cranfill, T. B., & Harris Wright, H. (2010). Importance of health-related quality of life for persons with aphasia, their significant others, and SLPs. *Aphasiology, 24,* 957–970.

Crary, M. A., Haak, N. J., & Malinsky, A. E. (1989). Preliminary psychometric evaluation of an acute aphasia screening protocol. *Aphasiology, 3,* 611–618.

Crary, M. A., Wertz, R. T., & Deal, J. L. (1992). Classifying aphasias: Cluster analysis of Western Aphasia Battery and Boston Diagnostic Aphasia Examination results. *Aphasiology, 6,* 29–36.

Crawford, J. R., Johnson, D. A., Mychalkiw, B., & Moore, J. W. (1997). WAIS-R performance following closed-head injury: A comparison of the clinical utility of summary IQs, factor scores, and subtest scatter indices. *Clinical Neuropsychologist, 11,* 345–355.

Crawford, J. R., Parker, D. M., Stewart, L. E., Besson, J. A. O., & DeLacey, E. (1989). Prediction of WAIS IQ with the National Adult Reading Test: Cross-validation and extension. *British Journal of Clinical Psychology, 28,* 267–273.

Crepaldi, D., Berlingeri, M., Paulesu, E., & Luzzatti, C. (2011). A place for nouns and a place for verbs? A critical review of neurocognitive data on grammatical-class effects. *Brain and Language, 116,* 33–49.

Crepeau, F., & Scherzer, P. (1993). Predictors and indicators of work status after traumatic brain injury: A meta-analysis. *Neuropsychological Rehabilitation, 3,* 5–35.

Crimmins, C. (2000). *Where is the Mango Princess?* New York: Vintage Books.

Cripe, L. I. (1987). The neuropsychological assessment and management of closed head injury: General guidelines. *Cognitive Rehabilitation, 5,* 18–22.

Critchley, M. (1960). Jacksonian ideas and the future, with special reference to aphasia. *British Medical Journal, 6,* 6–11.

Croisile, B., Ska, B., Brabant, M. J., Duchene, A., Lepage, Y., Aimard, G., et al. (1996). Comparative study of oral and written picture description in patients with Alzheimer's disease. *Brain and Language, 53,* 1–19.

Croot, K. (2009). Progressive language impairments: Definitions, diagnoses, and prognoses. *Aphasiology, 23,* 302–330.

Croot, K., Nickels, L., Laurence, F., & Manning, M. (2009). Impairment- and activity/participation-directed interventions in progressive language impairment: Clinical and theoretical issues. *Aphasiology, 23,* 125–160.

Crossley, M., D'Arcy, C., & Rawson, N. (1997). Letter and category fluency in community-dwelling Canadian seniors: A comparison of normal participants to those with dementia of the Alzheimer or vascular type. *Journal of Clinical and Experimental Neuropsychology, 19,* 52–62.

Croteau, C., & Le Dorze, G. (2006). Overprotection, "speaking for," and conversational participation: A study of couples with aphasia. *Aphasiology, 20,* 327–336.

Croteau, C., Le Dorze, G., & Morin, C. (2008). The influence of aphasia severity on how both members of a couple participate in an interview situation. *Aphasiology, 22,* 802–812.

Crowe, S. F. (1992). Dissociation of two frontal lobe syndromes by a test of verbal fluency. *Journal of Clinical and Experimental Neuropsychology, 14,* 327–339.

Cruice, M. (2007). Issues of access and inclusion with aphasia. *Aphasiology, 21,* 3–8.

Cruice, M., Hill, R., Worrall, L., & Hickson, L. (2010). Conceptualising quality of life for older people with aphasia. *Aphasiology, 24,* 327–347.

Cruice, M., Worrall, L., & Hickson, L. (2006). Quantifying aphasic people's social lives in the context of non-aphasic peers. *Aphasiology, 20,* 1210–1225.

Cruice, M., Worrall, L., Hickson, L., & Murison, R. (2003). Finding a focus for quality of life with aphasia: Social and emotional health, and psychological well-being. *Aphasiology, 17,* 333–353.

Cruice, M., Worrall, L., Hickson, L., & Murison, R. (2005). Measuring quality of life: Comparing family members' and friends' ratings with those of their aphasic partners. *Aphasiology, 19,* 111–129.

Cubelli, R., Foresti, A., & Consolini, T. (1988). Reeducation strategies in conduction aphasia. *Journal of Communication Disorders, 21,* 239–249.

Cuetos, F., Gonzalez-Nosti, M., & Martinez, C. (2005). The picture-naming task in the analysis of cognitive deterioration in Alzheimer's disease. *Aphasiology, 19,* 545–557.

Cullum, C. M., & Bigler, E. D. (1986). Ventricle size, cortical atrophy and the relationship with neuropsychological status in closed-head injury: A quantitative analysis. *Journal of Clinical and Experimental Neuropsychology, 8,* 437–452.

Cullum, C. M., Weiner, M. F., & Saine, K. C. (2009). *Texas Functional Living Scale* (TFLS). San Antonio, TX: Pearson.

Cumming, T. B., Graham, K. S., & Patterson, K. (2006). Repetition priming and hyperpriming in semantic dementia. *Brain and Language, 98,* 221–234.

Cunningham, R., & Ward, C. (2003). Evaluation of a training program to facilitate conversation between people with aphasia and their partners. *Aphasiology, 17,* 687–707.

Cupit, J., Rochon, E., Leonard, C., & Laird, L. (2010). Social validation as a measure of improvement after aphasia treatment: Its usefulness and influencing factors. *Aphasiology, 24,* 1486–1500.

Cutica, H., Bucciarelli, M., & Bara, B. G. (2006). Neuropragmatics: Extralinguistic pragmatic ability is better preserved in left-hemisphere-damaged patients than in right-hemisphere-damaged patients. *Brain and Language, 98,* 12–25.

Cutting, L. (1978). Study of anosognosia. *Journal of Neurology, Neurosurgery, and Psychiatry, 41,* 548–555.

Cycyk, L. M., & Harris Wright, H. (2008). Frontotemporal dementia: Its definition, differential diagnosis, and management. *Aphasiology, 22,* 422–446.

Cyr-Stafford, C. (1993). The dynamics of speech therapy in aphasia. In D. Lafond, Y. Joanette, J. Ponzio, R. Degiovani, & M. T. Sarno (Eds.), *Living with aphasia: Psychosocial issues* (pp. 103–116). San Diego, CA: Singular.

Dahlberg, C. C., & Jaffe, J. (1977). *Stroke: A doctor's personal story of his recovery.* New York: Norton.

Dalemans, R. J. P., De Witte, L. P., Wade, D. T., & Van den Heuvel, W. J. A. (2008). A description of social participation in working-age persons with aphasia: A review of the literature. *Aphasiology, 22,* 1071–1091.

Damasio, A. R. (2007). How the brain creates the mind. In F. E. Bloom (Ed.), *Best of the brain from Scientific American.* New York: Dana Press.

Damasio, H. (2008). Neural basis of language disorders. In R. Chapey (Ed.), *Language intervention strategies in aphasia and related neurogenic communication disorders* (5th ed., pp. 20–41). Philadelphia: Wolters Kluwer Health.

Damasio, H. D., & Damasio, A. R. (1980). The anatomical basis of conduction aphasia. *Brain, 103,* 337–350.

Damasio, H., Grabowski, T., Frank, R., Galaburda, A. M., & Damasio, A. R. (1994). The return of Phineas Gage: Clues about the brain from the skull of a famous patient. *Science, 264,* 1102–1105.

Damico, J. S., & Simmons-Mackie, N. N. (2003). Qualitative research and speech-language pathology: A tutorial for the clinical realm. *American Journal of Speech-Language Pathology, 12,* 131–143.

Daniloff, J. K., Fritelli, G., Buckingham, H. W., Hoffman, P. R., & Daniloff, R. G. (1986). Amer-Ind versus ASL: Recognition and imitation in aphasic subjects. *Brain and Language, 28,* 95–113.

Daniloff, J. K., Lloyd, L., & Fristoe, M. (1983). Amer-Ind transparency. *Journal of Speech and Hearing Disorders, 48,* 103–110.

Daniloff, J. K., Noll, J. D., Fristoe, M., & Lloyd, L. L. (1982). Gesture recognition in patients with aphasia. *Journal of Speech and Hearing Disorders, 47,* 43–49.

Darley, F. L. (1982). *Aphasia.* Philadelphia: W. B. Saunders.

Darley, F. L., Aronson, A. E., & Brown, J. R. (1975). *Motor speech disorders* (audio seminar). Philadelphia: W. B. Saunders.

Dash, P., & Villemarette-Pittman, N. (2005). *Alzheimer's disease.* New York: American Academy of Neurology Press.

Daum, I., Riesch, G., Sartori, G., & Birbaumer, N. (1996). Semantic memory impairment in Alzheimer's disease. *Journal of Clinical and Experimental Neuropsychology, 18,* 648–665.

Davidson, B., & Worrall, L. (2013). Living with aphasia: A client-centered approach. In I. Papathanasiou, P. Coppens, & C. Potages (Eds.), *Aphasia and related neurogenic communication disorders* (pp. 255–274). Burlington, MA: Jones & Bartlett Learning.

Davidson, B., Worrall, L., & Hickson, L. (2003). Identifying the communication activities of older people with aphasia: Evidence from naturalistic observation. *Aphasiology, 17,* 243–264.

Davidson, B., Worrall, L., & Hickson, L. (2008). Exploring the interactional dimension of social communication: A collective case study of older people with aphasia. *Aphasiology, 22,* 235–257.

Davie, G. L., Hutcheson, K. A., Barringer, D. A., Weinberg, J. S., & Lewin, J. S. (2009). Aphasia in patients after brain tumour resection. *Aphasiology, 23,* 1196–1206.

Davies, R., Cuetos, F., & Rodriguez-Ferreiro, J. (2010). Recovery in reading: A treatment study of acquired deep dyslexia in Spanish. *Aphasiology, 24,* 1115–1131.

Davis, C., Farias, D., & Baynes, K. (2009). Implicit phoneme manipulation for the treatment of apraxia of speech and co-occurring aphasia. *Aphasiology, 23,* 503–530.

Davis, C., Kleinman, J. T., Newhart, M., Gingis, L., Pawlak, M., et al. (2008). Speech and language functions that require a functioning Broca's area. *Brain and Language, 105,* 50–58.

Davis, C. H., Harrington, G., & Baynes, K. (2006). Intensive semantic intervention in fluent aphasia: A pilot study with fMRI. *Aphasiology, 20,* 59–83.

Davis, G. A. (1973). Linguistics and language therapy: The sentence construction board. *Journal of Speech and Hearing Disorders, 38,* 205–214.

Davis, G. A. (1983). *A survey of adult aphasia.* Englewood Cliffs, NJ: Prentice-Hall.

Davis, G. A. (1994). Theory as the base on which to build treatment of aphasia. *American Journal of Speech-Language Pathology, 3*(1), 8–10.

Davis, G. A. (2005). PACE revisited. *Aphasiology, 19,* 21–38.

Davis, G. A. (2007a). *Aphasiology: Disorders and clinical practice* (2nd ed.). Boston: Allyn & Bacon/Longman.

Davis, G. A. (2007b). Cognitive pragmatics of language disorders in adults. *Seminars in Speech and Language, 28,* 111–121.

Davis, G. A. (2012). The cognition of language and communication. In R. K. Peach & L. P. Shapiro (Eds.), *Cognition and acquired language disorders: An information processing approach* (pp. 1–12). St. Louis, MO: Elsevier.

Davis, G. A., & Coelho, C. A. (2004). Referential cohesion and logical coherence of narration after closed head injury. *Brain and Language, 89,* 508–523.

Davis, G. A., & Holland, A. L. (1981). Age in understanding and treating aphasia. In D. S. Beasley & G. A. Davis (Eds.), *Aging: Communication processes and disorders* (pp. 207–228). New York: Grune & Stratton.

Davis, G. A., O'Neil-Pirozzi, T. M., & Coon, M. (1997). Referential cohesion and logical coherence of narration after right hemisphere stroke. *Brain and Language, 56,* 183–210.

Davis, G. A., & Wilcox, M. J. (1985). *Adult aphasia rehabilitation: Applied pragmatics.* San Diego: Singular.

Davis, K. L., Price, C. C., Moore, P., Campea, S., & Grossman, M. (2001). Evaluating the clinical diagnosis of frontotemporal degeneration: A re-examination of Neary et al., 1998. *Neurology, 56,* A144–A145.

Dawson, D. R., & Chipman, M. (1995). The disablement experienced by traumatically brain-injured adults living in the community. *Brain Injury, 9,* 339–353.

Deal, J. L., & Deal, L. A. (1978). Efficacy of aphasia rehabilitation: Preliminary results. In R. H. Brookshire (Ed.), *Clinical aphasiology conference proceedings* (pp. 66–77). Minneapolis, MN: BRK.

Dean, C. (2004). *The everything Alzheimer's book.* Avon, MA: Adams Media.

DeBaggio, T. (2002). *Losing my mind: An intimate look at life with Alzheimer's.* New York: Free Press.

De Bleser, R., Schwarz, W., & Burchert, F. (2006). Quantitative neurosyntactic analyses: The final word? *Brain and Language, 96,* 143–146.

De Boissezon, X., Peran, P., de Boysson, C., & Demonet, J.-F. (2007). Pharmacotherapy of aphasia: Myth or reality? *Brain and Language, 102,* 114–125.

de Jong-Hagelstein, M., van de Sandt-Koenderman, W. M. E., Prins, N. D., Dippel, D. W. J., Koudstaal, P. J., & Visch-Brink, E. G. (2011). Efficacy of early cognitive-linguistic treatment and communicative treatment in aphasia after stroke: A randomised controlled trial (RATS-2). *Journal of Neurology, Neurosurgery and Psychiatry, 82,* 399–404.

Dekoskey, S., Heilman, K. M., Bowers, D., & Valenstein, E. (1980). Recognition and discrimination of emotional faces and pictures. *Brain and Language, 9,* 206–214.

Delis, D. C., Kaplan, E., & Kramer, J. H. (2001). *Delis-Kaplan Executive Function System* (D-KEFS). New York: Pearson.

Delis, D. C., Wapner, W., Gardner, H., & Moses, J. A., Jr. (1983). The contribution of the right hemisphere to the organization of paragraphs. *Cortex, 19,* 43–50.

Dell, G. S., Lawler, E. N., Harris, H. D., & Gordon, J. K. (2004). Models of errors of omission in aphasic naming. *Cognitive Neuropsychology, 21,* 125–146.

Dell, G. S., & O'Seaghdha, P. G. (1992). Stages of lexical access in language production. *Cognition, 42,* 287–314.

Dell, G. S., Schwartz, M. F., Martin, N., Saffran, E. M., & Gagnon, D. A. (1997). Lexical access in aphasic and nonaphasic speakers. *Psychological Review, 104,* 801–838.

Deloche, G., Hannequin, D., Dordain, M., Perrier, D., Cardebat, D., et al. (1997). Picture written naming: Performance parallels and divergencies between aphasic patients and normal subjects. *Aphasiology, 11,* 219–234.

del Toro, C. M., Altmann, L. J. P., Raymer, A. M., Leon, S., Blonder, L. X., et al. (2008). Changes in aphasic discourse after contrasting treatments for anomia. *Aphasiology, 22,* 881–892.

Denes, G., Perazzolo, C., Piani, A., & Piccione, F. (1996). Intensive versus regular speech therapy in global aphasia: A controlled study. *Aphasiology, 10,* 385–394.

de Partz, M.-P. (1986). Re-education of a deep dyslexic patient: Rationale of the methods and results. *Cognitive Neuropsychology, 3,* 149–177.

DeRenzi, E., & Faglioni, P. (1978). Normative data and screening power of a shortened version of the Token Test. *Cortex, 14,* 41–49.

DeRenzi, E., Faglioni, P., & Scotti, G. (1969). Impairment of memory for position following brain damage. *Cortex, 5,* 274–284.

DeRenzi, E., & Lucchelli, F. (1988). Ideational apraxia. *Brain, 111,* 1173–1188.

DeRenzi, E., Motti, F., & Nichelli, P. (1980). Imitating gestures: A quantitative approach to ideomotor apraxia. *Archives of Neurology, 37,* 6–10.

DeRenzi, E., & Vignolo, L. A. (1962). The Token Test: A sensitive test to detect receptive disturbances in aphasics. *Brain, 85,* 665–678.

de Riesthal, M., & Wertz, R. T. (2004). Prognosis for aphasia: Relationship between selected biographical and behavioural variables and outcome and improvement. *Aphasiology, 18,* 899–915.

de Roo, E., Kolk, H., & Hofstede, B. (2003). Structural properties of syntactically reduced speech: A comparison of normal speakers and Broca's aphasics. *Brain and Language, 86,* 99–115.

Devescovi, A., Bates, E., D'Amico, S., Hernandez, A., Marangolo, P., et al. (1997). An on-line study of grammaticality judgments in normal and aphasic speakers of Italian. *Aphasiology, 11,* 543–579.

Diaz, M., Sailor, K., Cheung, D., & Kuslansky, (2004). Category size effects in semantic and letter fluency in Alzheimer's patients. *Brain and Language, 89,* 108–114.

Dickey, M. W., Choy, J. J., & Thompson, C. K. (2007). Real-time comprehension of Wh-movement in aphasia: Evidence from eye-tracking while listening. *Brain and Language, 100,* 1–22.

Dickey, M. W., & Thompson, C. K. (2004). The resolution and recovery of filler-gap dependencies in aphasia: Evidence from on-line anomaly detection. *Brain and Language, 88,* 108–127.

Dickey, M. W., & Thompson, C. K. (2007). The relation between syntactic and morphological recovery in agrammatic aphasia: A case study. *Aphasiology, 21,* 604–616.

Dickey, M. W., & Thompson, C. K. (2009). Automatic processing of wh- and NP-movement in agrammatic aphasia: Evidence from eye-tracking. *Journal of Neurolinguistics, 22,* 563–583.

Dickey, M. W., & Yoo, H. (2010). Predicting outcomes for linguistically specific sentence treatment protocols. *Aphasiology, 24,* 787–801.

Difrancesco, S., Pulvermüller, F., & Mohr, B. (2012). Intensive language-action therapy (ILAT): The methods. *Aphasiology, 26,* 1317–1351.

DiSimoni, F., Keith, R. L., Holt, D. L., & Darley, F. L. (1975). Practicality of shortening the Porch Index of Communicative Ability. *Journal of Speech and Hearing Research, 18,* 491–497.

Doesborgh, S. J. C., van de Sandt-Koenderman, M. W. E., Dippel, D. W. J., van Harskamp, F., Koudstaal, P. J., et al. (2004). Effects of semantic treatment on verbal communication and linguistic processing in aphasia after stroke: A randomized controlled trial. *Stroke, 35,* 141–146.

Doidge, N. (2007). *The brain that changes itself.* New York: Penguin.

Dollaghan, C. A. (2007). *The handbook for evidence-based practice in communication disorders.* Baltimore: Brookes.

Donovan, N. J., Rosenbek, J. C., Kerrerson, T. U., & Velozo, C. A. (2006). Adding meaning to measurement: Initial Rasch analysis of the ASHA FACS Social Communication Subtest. *Aphasiology, 20,* 362–373.

Dotson, V. M., Singletary, F., Fuller, R., Koehler, S., Bacon Moore, A., et al. (2008). Treatment of word-finding deficits in fluent aphasia through the manipulation of spatial attention: Preliminary findings. *Aphasiology, 22,* 103–118.

Douglas, J. M., Bracy, C. A., & Snow, P. C. (2007). Exploring the factor structure of the La Trobe Communication Questionnaire: Insights into the nature of communication deficits following traumatic brain injury. *Aphasiology, 21,* 1181–1194.

Douglas, J. M., O'Flaherty, C. A., & Snow, P. (2000). Measuring perception of communicative ability: The development and evaluation of the La Trobe Communication Questionnaire. *Aphasiology, 14,* 251–268.

Douglas, K. (2002). *My stroke of luck.* New York: William Morrow.

Doyle, P. J., & Goldstein, H. (1985). Experimental analysis of acquisition and generalization of syntax in Broca's aphasia. In R. H. Brookshire (Ed.), *Clinical aphasiology* (Vol. 15, pp. 205–213). Minneapolis, MN: BRK.

Doyle, P. J., Goldstein, H., & Bourgeois, M. S. (1987). Experimental analysis of syntax training in Broca's aphasia: A generalization and social validation study. *Journal of Speech and Hearing Disorders, 52,* 143–155.

Doyle, P. J., Hula, W. D., McNeil, M. R., Mikolic, J. M., & Matthews, C. (2005). An application of Rasch Analysis to the measurement of communicative functioning. *Journal of Speech, Language, and Hearing Research, 48,* 1412–1428.

Doyle, P. J., McNeil, M. R., Hula, W. D., & Mikolic, J. M. (2003). The Burdon of Stroke Scale (BOSS): Validating patient-reported communication difficulty and associated psychological distress in stroke survivors. *Aphasiology, 17,* 291–304.

Doyle, P. J., McNeil, M. R., Le, K., Hula, W. D., & Ventura, M. B. (2008). Measuring communicative functioning in community-dwelling stroke survivors: Conceptual foundation and item development. *Aphasiology, 22,* 718–728.

Doyle, P. J., McNeil, M. R., Park, G., Goda, A., Rubenstein, E., et al. (2000). Linguistic validation of four parallel forms of a story retelling procedure. *Aphasiology, 15,* 537–549.

Doyle, P. J., Thompson, C. K., Oleyar, K., Wambaugh, J., & Jackson, A. (1994). The effects of setting variables on conversational discourse in normal and aphasic adults. In M. L. Lemme (Ed.), *Clinical aphasiology* (Vol. 22, pp. 135–144). Austin, TX: Pro-Ed.

Doyle, P. J., Tsironas, D., Goda, A. J., & Kalinyak, M. (1996). The relationship between objective measures and listeners' judgments of the communicative informativeness of the connected discourse of adults with aphasia. *American Journal of Speech-Language Pathology, 5*(3), 53–60.

Dragoy, O., & Bastiaanse, R. (2010). Verb production and word order in Russian agrammatic speakers. *Aphasiology, 24,* 28–55.

Drai, D., & Grodzinsky, Y. (2006). A new empirical angle on the variability debate: Quantitative neurosyntactic analyses of a large data set from Broca's aphasia. *Brain and Language, 96,* 117–128.

Drake, C. T., & Iadecola, C. (2007). The role of neuronal signaling in controlling cerebral blood flow. *Brain and Language, 102,* 141–152.

Dressel, K., Huber, W., Frings, L., Kümmerer, D., Saur, D., Mader, I., Hüll, M., Weiller, C., & Abel, S. (2010). Model-oriented naming therapy in semantic dementia: A single-case fMRI study. *Aphasiology, 24,* 1537–1558.

Dressler, R. A., Buder, E. H., & Cannito, M. P. (2009). Rhythmic patterns during conversational repairs in speakers with aphasia. *Aphasiology, 23,* 731–748.

Drew, R., & Thompson, C. K. (1999). Model-based semantic treatment for naming deficits in aphasia. *Journal of Speech, Language, and Hearing Research, 42,* 972–989.

Druks, J., & Masterson, J. (2000). *An Object and Action Naming Battery.* Philadelphia: Taylor & Francis.

Druks, J., Masterson, J., Kopelman, M., Clare, L., Rose, A., et al. (2006). Is action naming better preserved (than object naming) in Alzheimer's disease and why should we ask? *Brain and Language, 98,* 332–340.

DuBay, M. F., Laures-Gore, J. S., Matheny, K., & Romski, M. A. (2011). Coping resourses in individuals with aphasia. *Aphasiology, 25,* 1016–1029.

Dubois, B., Feldman, H. H., Jacova, C., Dekosky, S. T., Barberger-Gateau, P., et al. (2007). Research criteria for the diagnosis of Alzheimer's disease: Revising the NINCDS-ADRDA criteria. *Lancet Neurology, 6,* 734–746.

Dudas, R. B., Berrios, G. E., & Hodges, J. R. (2005). The Addenbrooke's Cognitive Examination (ACE) in the differential diagnosis of early dementias versus affective disorder. *American Journal of Geriatric Psychiatry, 13,* 218–226.

Duff, M. C., Hengst, J. A., Tranel, D., & Cohen, N. J. (2008). Collaborative discourse facilitates efficient communication and new learning in amnesia. *Brain and Language, 106,* 41–54.

Duff, M. C., Hengst, J. A., Tranel, D., & Cohen, N. J. (2009). Hippocampal amnesia disrupts verbal play and creative use of language in social interaction. *Aphasiology, 23,* 926–939.

Duffy, J. R. (2012). *Motor speech disorders: Substrates, differential diagnosis, and management* (3rd ed.). St. Louis, MO: Mosby.

Duffy, J. R., & Duffy, R. J. (1989). The limb apraxia test: An imitative measure of upper limb apraxia. In T. E. Prescott (Ed.), *Clinical aphasiology* (Vol. 18, pp. 145–160). Boston: College-Hill/Little, Brown.

Duffy, J. R., Keith, R. L., Shane, H., & Podraza, B. L. (1976). Performance of normal (non-brain-injured) adults on the Porch Index of Communicative Ability. In R. H. Brookshire (Ed.). *Clinical aphasiology conference proceedings* (pp. 32–42). Minneapolis, MN: BRK.

Duffy, J. R., & Myers, P. S. (1991). Group comparisons across neurologic communication disorders: Some methodological issues. In T. E. Prescott (Ed.), *Clinical aphasiology* (Vol. 19, pp. 1–14). Austin, TX: Pro-Ed.

Duffy, R. J., & Duffy, J. R. (1981). Three studies of deficits in pantomimic expression and pantomimic recognition in aphasia. *Journal of Speech and Hearing Research, 24,* 70–84.

Duffy, R. J., & Duffy, J. R. (1984). *Assessment of Nonverbal Communication.* Tigard, OR: C. C. Publications.

Duffy, R. J., Duffy, J. R., & Mercaitis, P. A. (1984). Comparison of the performance of a fluent and a nonfluent aphasic on a pantomimic referential task. *Brain and Language, 21,* 260–273.

Duffy, R. J., Duffy, J. R., & Pearson, K. (1975). Pantomime recognition in aphasia. *Journal of Speech and Hearing Research, 18,* 115–132.

Duffy, R. J., Watt, J. H., & Duffy, J. R. (1994). Testing causal theories of pantomimic deficits in aphasia using path analysis. *Aphasiology, 8,* 361–379.

Duncan, J. (1986). Disorganisation of behaviour after frontal lobe damage. *Cognitive Neuropsychology, 3,* 271–290.

Duncan, P. W., Wallace, D., Lai, S. M., Johnson, D., Embretson, S., et al. (1999). The stroke impact scale version 2.0: Evaluation of reliability, validity, and sensitivity to change. *Stroke, 30,* 2131–2140.

Eaton, E., Marshall, J., & Pring, T. (2011). Mechanisms of change in the evolution of jargon aphasia. *Aphasiology, 25,* 1543–1561.

Edelman, G. (1987). Global aphasia: The case for treatment. *Aphasiology, 1,* 75–80.

Edmonds, L. A., Nadeau, S. E., & Kiran, S. (2009). Effect of Verb Network Strengthening Treatment (VNeST) on lexical retrieval of content words in sentences in persons with aphasia. *Aphasiology, 23,* 402–426.

Edwards, S., & Tucker, K. (2006). Verb retrieval in fluent aphasia: A clinical study. *Aphasiology, 20,* 644–675.

Ehrlich, J. S. (1988). Selective characteristics of narrative discourse in head-injured and normal adults. *Journal of Communication Disorders, 21,* 1–9.

Eisenson, J. (1954). *Examining for aphasia.* New York: The Psychological Corporation.

Eisenson, J. (1962). Language and intellectual findings associated with right cerebral damage. *Language and Speech, 5,* 49–53.

Eisenson, J. (1984). *Adult aphasia* (2nd ed.). Englewood Cliffs, NJ: Prentice-Hall.

Ellis, A. W., Flude, B. M., & Young, A. W. (1987). "Neglect dyslexia" and the early visual processing of letters in words and nonwords. *Cognitive Neuropsychology, 4,* 439–464.

Ellis, A. W., Kay, J., & Franklin, S. (1992). Anomia: Differentiating between semantic and phonological deficits. In D. I. Margolin (Ed.), *Cognitive neuropsychology in clinical practice* (pp. 207–228). New York: Oxford University Press.

Ellis, A. W., & Young, A. W. (1988). *Human cognitive neuropsychology.* London: Erlbaum.

Elman, R. J. (2005). Social and life participation approaches to aphasia intervention. In L. L. LaPointe (Ed.), *Aphasia and related neurogenic language disorders* (3rd ed., pp. 39–50). New York: Thieme.

Elman, R. J. (Ed.). (2007). *Group treatment of neurogenic communication disorders: The expert clinician's approach* (2nd ed.). San Diego, CA: Plural.

Elman, R. J., & Bernstein-Ellis, E. (1999). The efficacy of group communication treatment in adults with chronic aphasia. *Journal of Speech, Language, and Hearing Research, 42,* 411–419.

Emmorey, K. D. (1987). The neurological substrates for prosodic aspects of speech. *Brain and Language, 30,* 305–320.

Enderby, P. M., John, A., & Petheram, B. (2006). *Therapy outcome measures for rehabilitation* (2nd ed.). Chichester, UK: Wiley.

Enderby, P. M., Wood, V., & Wade, D. (2006). *Frenchay Aphasia Screening Test* (2nd Ed.). London: Whurr.

Engell, B., Hütter, B.-O., Willmes, K., & Huber, W. (2003). Quality of life in aphasia: Validation of a pictorial self-rating procedure. *Aphasiology, 17,* 383–396.

England, J. E., O'Neill, J. J., & Simpson, R. K. (1996). Pragmatic assessment of communication in dementia (PAC-D). *American Journal of Alzheimer's Disease, 11,* 7–10.

Erez, A. B., Katz, N., Ring, H., & Soroker, N. (2009). Assessment of spatial neglect using computerised feature and conjunction visual search tasks. *Neuropsychological Rehabilitation, 19,* 677–695.

Erickson, R. J., Goldinger, S. D., & LaPointe, L. L. (1996). Auditory vigilance in aphasic individuals: Detecting nonlinguistic stimuli with full or divided attention. *Brain and Cognition, 30,* 244–253.

Eriksen, B. A., & Eriksen, C. W. (1974). Effects of noise letters upon the identification of a target letter in a nonsearch task. *Perception & Psychophysics, 16,* 143–149.

Eriksson, P. S., Perfilieva, E., Björk-Eriksson, T., Alborn, A.-M., Nordborg, C., et al. (1998). Neurogenesis in the adult human hippocampus. *Nature Medicine, 4,* 1313–1317.

Estes, C., & Bloom, R. L. (2011). Using voice recognition software to treat dysgraphia in a patient with conduction aphasia. *Aphasiology, 25,* 366–385.

Estevis, E., Basso, M. R., & Combs, D. (2012). Effects of practice on the Wechsler Adult Intelligence Scale-IV across 3- and 6-month intervals. *Clinical Neuropsychology, 26,* 239–254.

Eysenck, M. W. (2006). *Fundamentals of cognition.* New York: Psychology Press.

Fabbro, F. (2001). The bilingual brain: Bilingual aphasia. *Brain and Language, 79,* 201–210

Faglioni, P., Spinnler, H., & Vignolo, L. (1969). Contrasting behavior of right and left hemisphere-damaged patients on a discriminative and a semantic task of auditory recognition. *Cortex, 5,* 366–389.

Falconer, C., & Antonucci, S. M. (2012). Use of semantic feature analysis in group discourse treatment for aphasia: Extension and expansion. *Aphasiology, 26,* 64–82.

Farias, D., Davis, C., & Harrington, G. (2006). Drawing: Its contribution to naming in aphasia. *Brain and Language, 97,* 53–63.

Faroqi-Shah, Y., & Dickey, M. W. (2009). On-line processing of tense and temporality in agrammatic aphasia. *Brain and Language, 108,* 97–111.

Faroqi-Shah, Y., & Thompson, C. K. (2003). Effect of lexical cues on the production of active and passive sentences in Broca's and Wernicke's aphasia. *Brain and Language, 85,* 409–426.

Faroqi-Shah, Y., & Virion, C. R. (2009). Constraint-induced language therapy for agrammatism: Role of grammaticality constraints. *Aphasiology, 23,* 977–988.

Fasold, R. W., & Connor-Linton, J. (2006). (Eds.). *An introduction to language and linguistics.* Cambridge, UK: Cambridge University Press.

Fassbinder, W., & Tompkins, C. A. (2001). Slowed lexical-semantic activation in individuals with right hemisphere brain damage? *Aphasiology, 15,* 1079–1090.

Ferguson, A. (1994). The influence of aphasia, familiarity and activity on conversational repair. *Aphasiology, 8,* 143–157.

Ferguson, A., & Armstrong, E. (1996). The PALPA: A valid investigation of language? *Aphasiology, 10,* 193–197.

Ferguson, A., & Harper, A. (2010). Contributions to the talk of individuals with aphasia in multiparty interactions. *Aphasiology, 24,* 1605–1620.

Ferguson, A., Worrall, L., McPhee, J., Buskell, R., Armstrong, E., et al. (2003). Testamentary capacity and aphasia: A descriptive case report with implications for clinical practice. *Aphasiology, 17,* 965–980.

Fernandez, B., Cardebat, D., Demonet, J. F., Joseph, P. A., Mazaux, J. M., et al. (2004). Functional MRI follow-up study of language processes in healthy subjects and during recovery in a case of aphasia. *Stroke, 35,* 2171–2176.

Ferro, J. M. (1992). The influence of infarct location on recovery from global aphasia. *Aphasiology, 6,* 415–430.

Ferro, J. M., & Kertesz, A. (1987). Comparative classification of aphasic disorders. *Journal of Clinical and Experimental Neuropsychology, 9,* 365–375.

Ferro, J. M., Santos, M. E., Castro-Caldas, A., & Mariano, G. (1980). Gesture recognition in aphasia. *Journal of Clinical Neuropsychology, 2,* 277–292.

Feyereisen, P., Barter, D., Goosens, M., & Clarebaut, N. (1988). Gestures and speech referential communication by aphasic subjects: Channel use and efficiency. *Aphasiology, 2,* 21–32.

Feyereisen, P., & Seron, X. (1982). Nonverbal communication and aphasia: A review. I. Comprehension. *Brain and Language, 16,* 191–212.

Fields, R. B. (1998). The dementias. In P. J. Snyder & P. D. Nussbaum (Eds.), *Clinical neuropsychology: A pocket handbook for assessment* (pp. 211–239). Washington, DC: American Psychological Association.

Fink, M., Churan, J., & Wittman, M. (2006). Temporal processing and context dependency of phoneme discrimination in patients with aphasia. *Brain and Language, 98,* 1–11.

Fink, R. B., Bartlett, M. R., Lowery, J. S., Linebarger, M. C., & Schwartz, M. F. (2008). Aphasic speech with and without SentenceShaper: Two methods for assessing informativeness. *Aphasiology, 22,* 679–690.

Fink, R. B., Brecher, A., Schwartz, M. F., & Robey, R. R. (2002). A computer-implemented protocol for treatment of naming disorders: Evaluation of clinician-guided and partially self-guided instruction. *Aphasiology, 16,* 1061–1086.

Fink, R. B., Schwartz, M. F., & Myers, J. L. (1997). Effects of multilevel training on verb retrieval: Is more always better? (abstract). *Brain and Language, 60,* 444.

Fink, R. B., Schwartz, M. F., Rochon, E., Myers, J. L., Socolof, G. S., et al. (1995). Syntax stimulation revisited: An analysis of generalization of treatment effects. *American Journal of Speech-Language Pathology, 4*(4), 99–104.

Finocchiaro, C., Maimone, M., Brighina, F., Piccoli, T., Giglia, G., et al. (2006). A case study of primary progressive aphasia: Improvement on verbs after rTMS treatment. *Neurocase, 12,* 317–321.

Fisher, C. A., Wilshire, C. E., & Ponsford, J. L. (2009). Word discrimination therapy: A new technique for the treatment of a phonologically based word-finding impairment. *Aphasiology, 23,* 676–693.

Fishman, S. (1988). *A bomb in the brain.* New York: Avon.

Fitch West, J., Sands, E. S., & Ross-Swain, D. (1998). *Bedside Evaluation Screening Test* (2nd ed.). Austin, TX: Pro-Ed.

Fleming, V. B., & Harris, J. L. (2009). Test-retest discourse performance of individuals with mild cognitive impairment. *Aphasiology, 23,* 940–950.

Flowers, C. R., & Wyse, M. (1985). Assessing gestural intelligibility of normal and aphasic subjects. In R. H. Brookshire (Ed.), *Clinical aphasiology* (Vol. 15, pp. 64–71). Minneapolis, MN: BRK.

Flynn, L., Cumberland, A., & Marshall, J. (2009). Public knowledge about aphasia: A survey with comparative data. *Aphasiology, 23,* 393–401.

Foldi, N. S. (1987). Appreciation of pragmatic interpretations of indirect commands: Comparison of right and left hemisphere brain-damaged patients. *Brain and Language, 31,* 88–108.

Folstein, M. F., Folstein, S. E., & McHugh, P. R. (1975). Mini-mental state. *Journal of Psychiatric Research, 12,* 189–198.

Fotopoulou, A., Rudd, A., Holmes, P., and Kopelman, M. (2009). Self-observation reinstates motor awareness in anosognosia for hemiplegia. *Neuropsychologia, 47,* 1256–1260.

Fox, S., Armstrong, E., & Boles, L. (2009). Conversational treatment in mild aphasia: A case study. *Aphasiology, 23,* 951–964.

Foygel, D., & Dell, G. S. (2000). Models of impaired lexical access in speech production. *Journal of Memory and Language, 43,* 182–216.

Francis, D. R., Clark, N., & Humphreys, G. W. (2002). Circumlocution-induced naming (CIN): A treatment for affecting generalization in anomia? *Aphasiology, 16,* 243–260.

Francis, D. R., Clark, N., & Humphreys, C. W. (2003). The treatment of an auditory working memory deficit and the implications for sentence comprehension abilities in mild "receptive" aphasia. *Aphasiology, 17,* 723–750.

Frankel, T., & Penn, C. (2007). Perseveration and conversation in TBI: Response to pharmacological intervention. *Aphasiology, 21,* 1039–1078.

Frankel, T., Penn, C., & Ormond-Brown, D. (2007). Executive dysfunction as an explanatory basis for conversation symptoms of aphasia: A pilot study. *Aphasiology, 21,* 814–828.

Franklin, R. D., Allison, D. B., & Gorman, B. S. (1996). *Design and analysis of single-case research.* Mahwah, NJ: Erlbaum.

Franklin, S. (1989). Dissociations in auditory word comprehension: Evidence from nine fluent aphasic patients. *Aphasiology, 3,* 189–207.

Franklin, S. E., Buerk, F., & Howard, D. (2002). Generalised improvement in speech production for a subject with reproduction conduction aphasia. *Aphasiology, 16,* 1087–1114.

Frattali, C. M., Thompson, C. M., Holland, A. L., Wohl, C. B., & Ferketic, M. M. (1995). The FACS of life: ASHA FACS—A functional outcome measure for adults. *Asha, 37*(4), 40–46.

Freed, D. (2009). A short history of the Veterans Administration's influence on aphasia assessment tools. *Aphasiology, 23,* 1146–1157.

Freed, D., Celery, K., & Marshall, R. C. (2004). Effectiveness of personalized and phonological cueing in long-term naming performance by aphasic subjects: A clinical investigation. *Aphasiology, 18,* 743–757.

Freedman, M., & Cermak, L. S. (1986). Semantic encoding deficits in frontal lobe disease and amnesia. *Brain and Cognition, 5,* 108–114.

Fridriksson, J. (2010). Preservation and modulation of specific left hemisphere regions is vital for treated recovery from anomia in stroke. *Journal of Neuroscience, 30,* 11558–11564.

Fridriksson, J., Bonilha, L., Baker, J. M., Moser, D., & Rorden, C. (2010). Activity in preserved left hemisphere regions predicts anomia severity in aphasia. *Cerebral Cortex, 20,* 1013–1019.

Fridriksson, J., Holland, A. L. Beeson, P., & Morrow, L. (2005). Spaced retrieval treatment of anomia. *Aphasiology, 19,* 99–109.

Fridriksson, J., Holland, A. L., Coull, B. M., Plante, E., Trouard, T. P., et al. (2002). Aphasia severity: Association with cerebral perfusion and diffusion. *Aphasiology, 16,* 859–871.

Fridriksson, J., Kjartansson, O., Morgan, P., Hjaltason, H., Magnusdottir, S., et al. (2010). Impaired speech repetition and left parietal lobe damage. *Journal of Neuroscience, 30,* 11057–11061.

Fridriksson, J., Richardson, J. D., Baker, J. M., & Rorden, C. (2011). Transcranial direct current stimulation improves naming reaction time in fluent aphasia: A double-blind, sham-controlled study. *Stroke, 42,* 819–821.

Friederici, A. D., Wessels, J. M. I., Emmorey, K., & Bellugi, U. (1992). Sensitivity to inflectional morphology in aphasia: A real-time processing perspective. *Brain and Language, 43,* 747–763.

Friedmann, N. (2006). Speech production in Broca's agrammatic aphasia: Syntactic tree pruning. In Y. Grodzinsky & K. Amunts (Eds.), *Broca's region* (pp. 63–82). New York: Oxford University Press.

Friedmann, N., & Grodzinsky, Y. (1997). Tense and agreement in agrammatic production: Pruning the syntactic tree. *Brain and Language, 56,* 397–425.

Friedmann, N., & Gvion, A. (2003). Sentence comprehension and working memory limitation in aphasia: A dissociation between semantic-syntactic and phonological reactivation. *Brain and Language, 86,* 23–39.

Friedmann, N., & Gvion, A. (2007). As far as individuals with conduction aphasia understood these sentences were ungrammatical: Garden path in conduction aphasia. *Aphasiology, 21,* 570–586.

Fromm, D., Holland, A., Armstrong, E., Forbes, M., MacWhinney, B., et al. (2011). "Better but no cigar": Persons with aphasia speak about their research. *Aphasiology, 25,* 1431–1447.

Fryer, L. J., & Haffey, W. J. (1987). Cognitive rehabilitation and community readaptation: Outcomes from two program models. *Journal of Head Trauma Rehabilitation, 2,* 51–63.

Gaddie, A., Naeser, M. A., Palumbo, C. L., & Stiassny-Eder, D. (1989). Recovery of auditory comprehension after one year: A computed tomography scan study. In T. E. Prescott (Ed.), *Clinical aphasiology* (Vol. 18, pp. 463–478). Boston: College-Hill/Little, Brown.

Gainotti, G. (1972). Emotional behavior and hemispheric side of lesion. *Cortex, 8,* 41–55.

Gainotti, G., Caltagirone, C., & Ibba, A. (1975). Semantic and phonemic aspects of auditory language comprehension in aphasia. *Linguistics, 154/5,* 15–29.

Gainotti, G., Caltagirone, C., & Miceli, G. (1983). Selective impairment of semantic-lexical discrimination in right-brain-damaged patients. In E. Perecman (Ed.). *Cognitive processing in the right hemisphere* (pp. 149–167). New York: Academic Press.

Gainotti, G., Caltagirone, C., Miceli, G., & Masullo, C. (1981). Selective semantic-lexical impairment of language comprehension in right brain-damaged patients. *Brain and Language, 13,* 201–211.

Gainotti, G., Carlomagno, S., Craca, A., & Silveri, M. C. (1986). Disorders of classificatory activity in aphasia. *Brain and Language, 28,* 181–195.

Gainotti, G., & Lemmo, M. A. (1976). Comprehension of symbolic gestures in aphasia. *Brain and Language, 3,* 451–460.

Gainotti, G., & Tiacci, C. (1970). Patterns of drawing disability in right and left hemispheric patients. *Neuropsychologia, 8,* 379–384.

Gallagher, T. M. (1998). National initiatives in outcomes measurement. In C. M. Frattali (Ed.), *Measuring outcomes in speech-language pathology* (pp. 527–557). New York: Thieme.

Gallaher, A. J. (1979). Temporal reliability of aphasic performance on the Token Test. *Brain and Language, 7,* 34–41.

Gallaher, A. J., & Canter, G. J. (1982). Reading and listening comprehension in Broca's aphasia: Lexical versus syntactical errors. *Brain and Language, 17,* 183–192.

Gandour, J., Marshall, R. C., Kim, S. Y., & Neuburger, S. (1991). On the nature of conduction aphasia: A longitudinal case study. *Aphasiology, 5,* 291–306.

Gansler, D. A., Covall, S., McGrath, N., & Oscar-Berman, M. (1996). Measures of prefrontal dysfunction after closed head injury. *Brain and Cognition, 30,* 194–204.

Garcia, L. J., Barrette, J., & Laroche, C. (2000). Perceptions of the obstacles to work reintegration for persons with aphasia. *Aphasiology, 14,* 269–290.

Gardner, H. (1974). *The shattered mind.* New York: Vintage Books.

Gardner, H. (1982). Missing the point: Language and the right hemisphere. In H. Gardner, *Art, mind, and brain: A cognitive approach to creativity* (pp. 309–317). New York: Basic Books.

Gardner, H., & Brownell, H. H. (1986). *Right hemisphere communication battery.* Boston: Psychology Service, Veterans Administration Medical Center.

Gardner, H., Brownell, H. H., Wapner, W., & Michelow, D. (1983). Missing the point: The role of the right hemisphere in the processing of complex linguistic materials. In E. Perecman (Ed.), *Cognitive processing in the right hemisphere* (pp. 169–191). New York: Academic Press.

Gardner, H., & Denes, G. (1973). Connotative judgements by aphasic patients on a pictorial adaptation of the semantic differential. *Cortex, 9,* 183–196.

Gardner, H., Denes, G., & Weintraub, S. (1975). Comprehending a word: The influence of speed and redundancy on auditory comprehension in aphasia. *Cortex, 11,* 155–162.

Gardner, H., Ling, P. K., Flamm, L., & Silverman, J. (1975). Comprehension and appreciation of humorous material following brain damage. *Brain, 98,* 399–412.

Gardner, H., Zurif, E. B., Berry, T., & Baker, E. (1976). Visual communication in aphasia. *Neuropsychologia, 14,* 275–292.

Garrett, K. L., Staltari, C. F., & Moir, L. J. (2007). Contextual group communication therapy for persons with aphasia: A scaffolded discourse approach. In R. J. Elman (Ed.), *Group treatment of neurogenic communication disorders* (pp. 159–192). San Diego, CA: Plural Publishing.

Garrett, M. F. (1984). The organization of processing structure for language production: Applications to aphasic speech. In D. Caplan, A. R. Lecours, &

A. Smith (Eds.), *Biological perspectives on language* (pp. 172–193). Cambridge, MA: MIT Press.

Gazzaniga, M. S., Ivry, R. B., & Mangun, G. R. (2008). *Cognitive neuroscience: The biology of the mind* (3rd ed.). Norton.

Geigenberger, A., & Ziegler, W. (2001). Receptive prosodic processing in aphasia. *Aphasiology, 15,* 1169–1187.

Germani, M. J., & Pierce, R. S. (1995). Semantic attribute knowledge in adults with right and left hemisphere damage. *Aphasiology, 9,* 1–21.

Gerratt, B., & Jones, D. (1987). Aphasic performance on a lexical decision task: Multiple meanings and word frequency. *Brain and Language, 30,* 106–115.

Geschwind, N. (1965). Disconnexion syndromes in animals and man. *Brain, 88,* 237–294, 585–644.

Geschwind, N. (1967). The varieties of naming errors. *Cortex, 3,* 96–112.

Gianico, J. L., & Altarriba, J. (2008). The psycholinguistics of bilingualism. In J. Altarriba, & R. R. Heredia (Eds.), *An introduction to bilingualism: Principles and processes* (pp. 71–103). New York: Erlbaum.

Gibbs, R. W., Jr. (2006). Figurative language. In M. J. Traxler & M. A. Gernsbacher (Eds.), *Handbook of psycholinguistics* (2nd ed., pp. 835–861). London: Elsevier.

Giffard, B., Desgranges, B., & Eustache, F. (2005). Semantic memory disorders in Alzheimer's disease: Clues from semantic priming effects. *Current Alzheimer's Research, 2,* 425–434.

Giffard, B., Desgranges, B., Nore-Mary, F., Lalevée, C., de la Sayette, V., et al. (2001). The nature of semantic memory deficits in Alzheimer's disease: New insights from hyperpriming effects. *Brain, 124,* 1522–1532.

Giffords, G., & Kelly, M. (2011). *Gabby: A story of courage and hope.* New York: Scribner.

Giles, E., Patterson, K., & Hodges, J. R. (1996). Performance on the Boston Cookie Theft picture description task in patients with early dementia of the Alzheimer's type: Missing information. *Aphasiology, 10,* 395–408.

Gillespie, A., Murphy, J., & Place, M. (2010). Divergences of perspective between people with aphasia and their family caregivers. *Aphasiology, 24,* 1559–1575.

Gillick, M. R. (1998). *Tangled minds: Understanding Alzheimer's disease and other dementias.* New York: Plume.

Gillis, R. J. (Ed.). (1996). *Traumatic brain injury rehabilitation for speech-language pathologists.* Boston: Butterworth-Heinemann.

Gillis, R. J. (2007a). Community-oriented group treatment for traumatic brain injury. In R. J. Elman (Ed.), *Group treatment of neurogenic communication disorders* (pp. 317–339). San Diego, CA: Plural Publishing.

Gillis, R. J. (2007b). Traumatic brain injury: Early intervention. In R. J. Elman (Ed.), *Group treatment of*

neurogenic communication disorders (pp. 297–316). San Diego, CA: Plural Publishing.

Glass, A. V., Gazzaniga, M. S., & Premack, D. (1973). Artificial language training in global aphasia. *Neuropsychologia, 11,* 95–103.

Glasser, M. F., & Rilling, J. K. (2008). DTI tractography of the human brain's language pathways. *Cerebral Cortex, 18,* 2471–2482.

Gleason, J. B., Goodglass, H., Green, E., Ackerman, N., & Hyde, M. R. (1975). The retrieval of syntax in Broca's aphasia. *Brain and Language, 2,* 451–471.

Gleason, J. B., Goodglass, H., Obler, L., Green, E., Hyde, M. R., et al. (1980). Narrative strategies of aphasic and normal-speaking subjects. *Journal of Speech and Hearing Research, 23,* 370–382.

Glindemann, R., & Springer, L. (1995). An assessment of PACE therapy. In C. Code & D. J. Müller (Eds.), *The treatment of aphasia: From theory to practice* (pp. 90–107). San Diego, CA: Singular.

Glindemann, R., Willmes, K., Huber, W., & Springer, L. (1991). The efficacy of modeling in PACE-therapy. *Aphasiology, 5,* 425–430.

Glosser, G., & Deser, T. (1991). Patterns of discourse production among neurological patients with fluent language disorders. *Brain and Language, 40,* 67–88.

Glosser, G., Friedman, R. B., Grugan, P. K., Lee, J. H., & Grossman, M. (1998). Lexical semantic and associative priming in Alzheimer's disease. *Neuropsychology, 12,* 218–224.

Glosser, G., Wiener, M., & Kaplan, E. (1986). Communicative gestures in aphasia. *Brain and Language, 27,* 345–359.

Godfrey, C. M., & Douglass, E. (1959). The recovery process in aphasia. *Canadian Medical Association Journal, 80,* 618–624.

Godfrey, H. P. D., Partridge, F. M., Knight, R. G., & Bishara, S. (1993). Course of insight disorder and emotional dysfunction following closed-head injury: A controlled cross-sectional follow-up study. *Journal of Clinical and Experimental Neuropsychology, 15,* 503–515.

Gold, B. T., & Kertesz, A. (2000). Right hemisphere semantic processing of visual words in an aphasic patient: An fMRI study. *Brain and Language, 73,* 456–465.

Gold, B. T., & Kertesz, A. (2001). Phonologically related lexical repetition disorder: A case study. *Brain and Language, 77,* 241–265.

Goldblum, G., & Alant, E. (2009). Sales assistants serving customers with traumatic brain injury. *Aphasiology, 23,* 87–109.

Goldenberg, G., & Spatt, J. (1994). Influence of size and site of cerebral lesions on spontaneous recovery of aphasia and on success of language therapy. *Brain and Language, 47,* 684–698.

Goldstein, K. (1942). *Aftereffects of brain injuries in war.* New York: Grune & Stratton.

Goodenough, C., Zurif, E. B., Weintraub, S., & Von Stockert, T. (1977). Aphasics' attention to grammatical morphemes. *Language and Speech, 20,* 11–19.

Goodglass, H., Blumstein, S. E., Gleason, J. B., Hyde, M. R., Green, E., et al. (1979). The effect of syntactic encoding on sentence comprehension in aphasia. *Brain and Language, 7,* 201–209.

Goodglass, H., Kaplan, E., & Barresi, B. (2001). *The assessment of aphasia and related disorders* (3rd ed.). Philadelphia: Lippincott, Williams & Wilkins.

Goodglass, H., Kaplan, E., Weintraub, S., & Ackerman, N. (1976). The "tip-of-the-tongue" phenomenon in aphasia. *Cortex, 12,* 145–153.

Goodglass, H., & Mayer, J. (1958). Agrammatism in aphasia. *Journal of Speech and Hearing Disorders, 23,* 99–111.

Goodglass, H., & Stuss, D. T. (1979). Naming to picture versus description in three aphasic subgroups. *Cortex, 15,* 199–211.

Goodglass, H., Wingfield, A., & Ward, S. E. (1997). Judgments of concept similarity by normal and aphasic subjects: Relation to naming and comprehension. *Brain and Language, 56,* 138–158.

Goral, M., & Kempler, D. (2009). Training verb production in communicative context: Evidence from a person with chronic non-fluent aphasia. *Aphasiology, 23,* 1383–1397.

Goral, M., Levy, E. S., & Kastl, R. (2010). Cross-language treatment generalization: A case of trilingual aphasia. *Aphasiology, 24,* 170–187.

Gordon, J. K. (2006). A quantitative production analysis of picture description. *Aphasiology, 20,* 188–204.

Gordon, J. K. (2007). A contextual approach to facilitating word retrieval in agrammatic aphasia. *Aphasiology, 21,* 643–657.

Gorno-Tempini, M. L., Dronkers, N. F., Rankin, K. P., Ogar, J. M., Phrengrasamy, L., et al. (2004). Cognition and anatomy in three variants of primary progressive aphasia. *Annals of Neurology, 55,* 335–346.

Gorno-Tempini, M. L., Hillis, A. E., Weintraub, S., Kertesz, A., Mendez, M., et al. (2011). Recommendations for the classification of primary progressive aphasia and its variants. *Neurology, 76,* 1006–1014.

Gould, E., & Gross, C. G. (2002). Adult neurogenesis: Some progress and problems. *Journal of Neuroscience, 22,* 619–623.

Gould, E., Reeve, A. J., Graziano, M. S. A., & Gross, C. G. (1999). Neurogenesis in the neocortex of adult primates. *Science, 286,* 548–552.

Graham, N., Patterson, K., & Hodges, J. (2004). When more yields less: Speaking and writing deficits in nonfluent progressive aphasia. *Neurocase, 10,* 141–155.

Grandmaison, E., & Simard, M. (2003). A critical review of memory stimulation programs in Alzheimer's disease. *Journal of Neuropsychiatry and Clinical Neurosciences, 15,* 13–144.

Granger, C. V., Cotter, A. C., Hamilton, B. B., & Fiedler, R. C. (1993). Functional assessment scales: A study of persons after stroke. *Archives of Physical Medicine and Rehabilitation, 74,* 133–138.

Grant, D. A., & Berg, E. A. (1948). A behavioral analysis of degree of reinforcement and ease of shifting to new responses in a Weigl-type card-sorting problem. *Journal of Experimental Psychology, 38,* 404–411.

Green, D. W., Grogan, A., Crinion, J., Ali, N., Sutton, C., et al. (2010). Language control and parallel recovery of language in individuals with aphasia. *Aphasiology, 24,* 188–209.

Green, E., & Boller, F. (1974). Features of auditory comprehension in severely impaired aphasics. *Cortex, 10,* 133–145.

Greenwood, A., Grassly, J., Hickin, J., & Best, W. (2010). Phonological and orthographic cueing therapy: A case of generalised improvement. *Aphasiology, 24,* 991–1016.

Gregory, C., Lough, S., Stone, V., Erzinclioglu, S., Marton, L., et al. (2002). Theory of mind in patients with frontal variant frontotemporal dementia and Alzheimer's disease: Theoretical and practical implications. *Brain, 125,* 752–764.

Greitemann, G., & Wolf, E. (1991). *Making dynamic use of different modes of expression: The efficacy of the PACE-approach.* Paper presented to the Academy of Aphasia, Rome.

Grice, L. P. (1975). Logic and conversation. In P. Cole & J. L. Morgan (Ed.), *Syntax and semantics: Speech acts* (Vol. 3, pp. 41–58). New York: Academic Press.

Grindrod, C. M. (2012). Effects of left and right hemisphere damage on sensitivity to global context during lexical ambiguity resolution. *Aphasiology, 26,* 933–952.

Grindrod, C. M., & Baum, S. R. (2003). Sensitivity to local sentence context information in lexical ambiguity resolution: Evidence from left- and right-hemisphere-damaged individuals. *Brain and Language, 85,* 503–523.

Grober, E., & Sliwinski, M. (1991). Development and validation of a model for estimating premorbid verbal intelligence in the elderly. *Journal of Clinical and Experimental Neuropsychology, 13,* 933–949.

Grodzinsky, Y. (1989). Agrammatic comprehension of relative clauses. *Brain and Language, 37,* 480–499.

Grodzinsky, Y. (1991). There is an entity called agrammatic aphasia. *Brain and Language, 41,* 555–564.

Grodzinsky, Y., & Amunts, K. (Eds.). (2006). *Broca's region.* New York: Oxford University Press.

Grosjean, F. (1989). Neurolinguists, beware! The bilingual is not two monolinguals in one person. *Brain and Language, 36,* 3–15.

Gross, R. A., & Johnston, K. C. (2008). Levels of evidence: Taking *Neurology*® to the next level. *Neurology, 72,* 8–10.

Grossman, M. (1981). A bird is a bird is a bird: Making reference within and without superordinate categories. *Brain and Language, 12,* 313–331.

Grossman, M. (1988). Drawing deficits in brain-damaged patients' freehand pictures. *Brain and Cognition, 8,* 189–205.

Grossman, M., & Ash, S. (2004). Primary progressive aphasia: A review. *Neurocase, 10,* 3–18.

Grossman, M., & Haberman, S. (1982). Aphasics' selective deficits in appreciating grammatical agreements. *Brain and Language, 16,* 109–120.

Grossman, M., & Wilson, M. (1987). Stimulus categorization by brain-damaged patients. *Brain and Cognition, 6,* 55–71.

Gruen, A. K., Frankle, B. C., & Schwartz, R. (1990). Word fluency generation skills of head-injured patients in an acute trauma center. *Journal of Communication Disorders, 23,* 163–170.

Gruetzner, H. (2001). *Alzheimer's: A caregiver's guide and sourcebook* (3rd ed.). New York: Wiley.

Guendouzi, J., & Müller, N. (2006). *Approaches to discourse in dementia.* Mahwah, NJ: Erlbaum.

Güngör, L., Terzi, M., & Onar, M. K. (2011). Does long term use of piracetam improve speech disturbances due to ischemic cerebrovascular diseases? *Brain and Language, 117,* 23–27.

Guns, B. (2008). *Rewire your brain, rewire your life: A handbook for stroke survivors & their caregivers.* Livermore, CA: Wingspan Press.

Gupta, S. R., Mlcoch, A. G., Scolaro, C., & Moritz, T. (1995). Bromocriptine treatment for nonfluent aphasia. *Neurology, 45,* 2170–2173.

Haaland, K. Y., & Flaherty, D. (1984). The different types of limb apraxia errors made by patients with left vs. right hemisphere damage. *Brain and Cognition, 3,* 370–384.

Haarmann, H. J., Just, M. A., & Carpenter, P. A. (1997). Aphasic sentence comprehension as a resource deficit: A computational approach. *Brain and Language, 59,* 76–120.

Haarmann, H. J., & Kolk, H. H. J. (1991). Syntactic priming in Broca's aphasics: Evidence for slow activation. *Aphasiology, 5,* 247–264.

Hadar, U., Wenkert-Olenik, D., Krauss, R., & Soroker, N. (1998). Gesture and processing of speech: Neuropsychological evidence. *Brain and Language, 62,* 107–126.

Hageman, C. F., & Folkestad, A. (1986). Performance of aphasic listeners on an expanded Revised Token Test subtest presented verbally and nonverbally. In R. H. Brookshire (Ed.), *Clinical aphasiology* (Vol. 16, pp. 227–233). Minneapolis, MN: BRK.

Hagen, C. (1981). Language disorders secondary to closed head injury: Diagnosis and treatment. *Topics in Language Disorders, 1,* 73–87.

Hagiwara, H., & Caplan, D. (1990). Syntactic comprehension in Japanese aphasics: Effects of category and thematic role order. *Brain and Language, 38,* 159–170.

Hagoort, P. (1997). Semantic priming in Broca's aphasics at a short SOA: No support for an automatic access deficit. *Brain and Language, 56,* 287–300.

Hagoort, P., Brown, C., & Swaab, T. (1995). Semantic deficits in right hemisphere patients (abstract). *Brain and Language, 51,* 161–163.

Hale, S. (2003). *The man who lost his language.* London: Penguin.

Hall, K. M., & Cope, D. N. (1995). The benefit of rehabilitation in traumatic brain injury: A literature review. *Journal of Head Trauma Rehabilitation, 10,* 1–13.

Hall, K. M., Cope, D. N., & Rappaport, M. (1985). Glasgow Outcome Scale and Disability Rating Scale: Comparative usefulness in following recovery in traumatic brain injury. *Archives of Physical Medicine and Rehabilitation, 66,* 35–37.

Hall, K. M., Hamilton, B. B., & Keith, R. A. (1993). Characteristics and comparisons of functional assessment indices: Disability Rating Scale, Functional Independence Measure, and Functional Assessment Measure. *Journal of Head Trauma Rehabilitation, 8,* 60–74.

Halper, A. S., Cherney, L. R., & Burns, M. S. (1996). *Clinical management of right hemisphere dysfunction: Procedural manual* (2nd ed.). Gaithersburg, MD: Aspen.

Halpern, H., & Goldfarb, R. (2013). *Language and motor speech disorders in adults* (3rd ed.). Burlington, MA: Jones & Bartlett Learning.

Halstead, W. C., & Wepman, J. M. (1949). The Halstead-Wepman aphasia screening test. *Journal of Speech and Hearing Disorders, 14,* 9–15.

Hamilton, B. B., Laughlin, J. A., Granger, C. V., & Kayton, R. M. (1991). Interrater agreement of the seven-level Functional Independence Measure (FIM) [abstract]. *Archives of Physical Medicine and Rehabilitation, 72,* 790.

Hanlon, R. E., Brown, J. W., & Gerstman, L. J. (1990). Enhancement of naming in nonfluent aphasia through gesture. *Brain and Language, 38,* 298–314.

Hannay, H. J., & Levin, H. S. (1989). Visual continuous recognition memory in normal and closed head-injured adolescents. *Journal of Clinical and Experimental Neuropsychology, 11,* 444–460.

Hanne, S., Sekerina, I. A., Vasishth, S., Burchert, F., & De Bleser, R. (2011). Chance in agrammatic sentence comprehension: What does it really mean? Evidence from eye movements of German agrammatic aphasic patients. *Aphasiology, 25,* 221–244.

Hanson, W. R., & Cicciarelli, A. W. (1978). The time, amount, and pattern of language improvement in adult aphasics. *British Journal of Disorders of Communication, 13,* 59–63.

Hanson, W. R., Metter, E. J., & Riege, W. H. (1989). The course of chronic aphasia. *Aphasiology, 3,* 19–30.

Haravon, A., Obler, L. K., & Sarno, M. T. (1994). A method for microanalysis of discourse in brain-damaged patients. In R. L. Bloom, L. K. Obler, S. De Santi, & J. S. Ehrlich (Eds.), *Discourse analysis and applications: Studies in adult clinical populations* (pp. 47–80). Hillsdale, NJ: Erlbaum.

Harciarek, M., & Kertesz, A. (2009). Longitudinal study of single-word comprehension in semantic dementia: A comparison with primary progressive aphasia and Alzheimer's disease. *Aphasiology, 23,* 606–626.

Harding, D., & Pound, C. (1999). Needs, function, and measurement: Juggling with multiple language impairment. In S. Byng, K. Swinburn, & C. Pound (Eds.), *The aphasia therapy file* (pp. 13–39). Hove, UK: Psychology Press.

Harley, T. A., Jessiman, L. J., MacAndrew, S. B. G., & Astell, A. (2008). I don't know what I know: Evidence of preserved semantic knowledge but impaired metalinguistic knowledge in adults with probable Alzheimer's disease. *Aphasiology, 22,* 321–335.

Harris, J. L. (1997). Reminiscence: A culturally and developmentally appropriate language intervention for older adults. *American Journal of Speech-Language Pathology, 6,* 19–26.

Harris, L., Olson, A., & Humphreys, G. (2012). Rehabilitation of past tense verb production and non-canonical sentence production in left inferior frontal non-fluent aphasia. *Aphasiology, 26,* 143–161.

Harris Wright, H., & Capilouto, G. J. (2009). Manipulating task instructions to change narrative discourse performance. *Aphasiology, 23,* 1295–1310.

Harris Wright, H., Capilouto, G. J., Wagovich, S. A., Cranfill, T., & Davis, J. (2005). Development and reliability of a quantitative measure of adults' narratives. *Aphasiology, 19,* 263–273.

Harris Wright, H., Marshall, R. C., Wilson, K. B., & Page, J. L. (2008). Using a written cueing hierarchy to improve verbal naming in aphasia. *Aphasiology, 22,* 522–536.

Harris Wright, H., & Newhoff, M. (2004). Inference revision processing in adults with and without aphasia. *Brain and Language, 89,* 450–463.

Hartje, W., Kerschensteiner, M., Poeck, K., & Orgass, B. (1973). A cross-validation study on the Token Test. *Neuropsychologia, 11,* 119–121.

Hartley, L. L. (1995). *Cognitive-communicative abilities following brain injury: A functional approach.* San Diego, CA: Singular.

Hartley, L. L., & Levin, H. S. (1990). Linguistic deficits after closed head injury: A current appraisal. *Aphasiology, 4,* 353–370.

Harvey, M., Milner, A. D., & Roberts, R. C. (1995). An investigation of hemispatial neglect using the Landmark Task. *Brain and Cognition, 27,* 59–78.

Hashimoto, N., & Thompson, C. K. (2010). The use of the picture-word interference paradigm to examine naming abilities in aphasic individuals. *Aphasiology, 24,* 580–611.

Haut, M. W., Petros, T. V., Frank, R. G., & Haut, J. S. (1991). Speed of processing within semantic memory following severe closed head injury. *Brain and Cognition, 17,* 31–41.

Hawkins, K. A., & Bender, S. (2002). Norms and the relationship of Boston Naming Test performance to vocabulary and education: A review. *Aphasiology, 16,* 1143–1153.

Hawley, C. A., Taylor, R., Hellawell, D. J., & Pentland, B. (1999). Use of the Functional Assessment Measure (FIM+FAM) in head injury rehabilitation: A psychometric analysis. *Journal of Neurology, Neurosurgery, and Psychiatry, 67,* 749–754.

Haynes, W. O., & Oratio, A. R. (1978). A study of clients' perceptions of therapeutic effectiveness. *Journal of Speech and Hearing Disorders, 43,* 21–33.

Head, H. (1920). Aphasia and kindred disorders of speech. *Brain, 43,* 87–165.

Heath, R. L., & Blonder, L. X. (2005). Spontaneous humor among right hemisphere stroke survivors. *Brain and Language, 93,* 267–276.

Heeschen, C. (1980). Strategies of decoding actor-object relations by aphasic patients. *Cortex, 16,* 5–19.

Heeschen, C., & Schegloff, E. A. (1999). Agrammatism, adaptation theory, conversation analysis: On the role of so-called telegraphic style in talk-in-interaction. *Aphasiology, 13,* 365–405.

Heilman, K. M., Bowers, D., Speedie, L., & Coslett, H. B. (1984). Comprehension of affective and non-affective prosody. *Neurology, 34,* 917–921.

Heilman, K. M., Safran, A., & Geschwind, N. (1971). Closed head trauma and aphasia. *Journal of Neurology, Neurosurgery, and Psychiatry, 34,* 265–269.

Heilman, K. M., & Scholes, R. J. (1976). The nature of comprehension errors in Broca's, conduction and Wernicke's aphasics. *Cortex, 12,* 258–265.

Heilman, K. M., Schwartz, H. D., & Watson, R. T. (1978). Hypoarousal in patients with the neglect syndrome and emotional indifference. *Neurology, 28,* 229–232.

Heiss, W.-D., & Thiel, A. (2006). A proposed regional hierarchy in recovery of post-stroke aphasia. *Brain and Language, 98,* 118–123.

Helm, N. A., & Barresi, B. (1980). Voluntary control of involuntary utterances: A treatment approach for severe aphasia. In R. H. Brookshire (Ed.), *Clinical aphasiology conference proceedings* (pp. 308–315). Minneapolis, MN: BRK.

Helm-Estabrooks, N. (1981). *Helm Elicited Language Program for Syntax Stimulation (HELPSS)*. Chicago: Riverside.

Helm-Estabrooks, N. (1991). *Test of Oral and Limb Apraxia (TOLA)*. Austin, TX: Pro-Ed.

Helm-Estabrooks, N. (1992). *Aphasia Diagnostic Profiles*. Austin, TX: Pro-Ed.

Helm-Estabrooks, N., & Albert, M. L. (2004). *Manual of aphasia and aphasia therapy* (2nd ed.). Austin, TX: Pro-Ed.

Helm-Estabrooks, N., Fitzpatrick, P. M., & Barresi, B. N. (1981). Response of an agrammatic patient to a syntax stimulation program for aphasia. *Journal of Speech Hearing Disorders, 46*, 422–427.

Helm-Estabrooks, N., Fitzpatrick, P. M., & Barresi, B. N. (1982). Visual action therapy for global aphasia. *Journal of Speech and Hearing Disorders, 47*, 385–389.

Helm-Estabrooks, N., & Hotz, G. (1990). *Brief Test of Head Injury (BTHI)*. Austin, TX: Pro-Ed.

Helm-Estabrooks, N., & Nicholas, M. (1999). *Sentence production program for aphasia*. Austin, TX: Pro-Ed.

Helm-Estabrooks, N., Nicholas, M., & Morgan, A. (1989). *Melodic intonation therapy program*. Austin, TX: Pro-Ed.

Helm-Estabrooks, N., & Ramsberger, G. (1986). Treatment of agrammatism in long-term Broca's aphasia. *British Journal of Disorders of Communication, 21*, 39–45.

Helm-Estabrooks, N., Ramsberger, G., Morgan, A. R., & Nicholas, M. (1989). *Boston Assessment of Severe Aphasia (BASA)*. Austin, TX: Pro-Ed.

Henderson, L. W., Frank, E. M., Pigatt, T., Abramson, R. K., & Houston, M. (1998). Race, gender, and educational level effects on Boston Naming Test scores. *Aphasiology, 12*, 901–911.

Hengst, J. A., (2003). Collaborative referencing between individuals with aphasia and routine communication partners. *Journal of Speech, Language, and Hearing Research, 46*, 831–848.

Hengst, J. A. (2006). "That mea::n dog": Linguistic mischief and verbal play as a communicative resource in aphasia. *Aphasiology, 20*, 312–326.

Hengst, J. A., Duff, M. C., & Dettmer, A. (2010). Rethinking repetition in therapy: Repeated engagement as the social ground of learning. *Aphasiology, 24*, 887–901.

Hengst, J. A., Frame, S. R., Neuman-Stritzel, T., & Gannaway, R. (2005). Using others' words: Conversational use of reported speech by individuals with aphasia and their communication partners. *Journal of Speech, Language, and Hearing Research, 48*, 137–156.

Henley, S., Pettit, S., Todd-Pokropek, A., & Tupper, A. (1985). Who goes home? Predictive factors in stroke recovery. *Journal of Neurology, Neurosurgery, and Psychiatry, 48*, 1–6.

Henry, M. L., Beeson, P. M., & Rapcsak, S. Z. (2008). Treatment for lexical retrieval in progressive aphasia. *Aphasiology, 22*, 826–838.

Herbert, R., Hickin, J., Howard, D., Osborne, F., & Best, W. (2008). Do picture-naming tests provide a valid assessment of lexical retrieval in conversation in aphasia? *Aphasiology, 22*, 184–203.

Heredia, C. G., Sage, K., Lambon Ralph, M. A., & Berthier, M. L. (2009). Relearning and retention of verbal labels in a case of semantic dementia. *Aphasiology, 23*, 192–209.

Hernández, M., Costa, A., Juncadella, M., Sebastián-Gallés, N., & Reñé, R. (2008). Category-specific semantic deficits in Alzheimer's disease: A semantic priming study. *Neuropsychologia, 46*, 935–946.

Herrmann, M., Johannsen-Horbach, H., & Wallesch, C. W. (1993). Empathy and aphasia rehabilitation—Are there contradictory requirements of treatment and psychological support? *Aphasiology, 7*, 575–579.

Herrmann, M., Koch, U., Johannsen-Horbach, H., & Wallesch, C.-W. (1989). Communicative skills in chronic and severe nonfluent aphasia. *Brain and Language, 37*, 339–352.

Herrmann, M., & Wallesch, C. W. (1989). Psychosocial changes and psychosocial adjustment with chronic and severe nonfluent aphasia. *Aphasiology, 3*, 513–526.

Hersh, D. (2009). How do people with aphasia view their discharge from therapy. *Aphasiology, 23*, 331–350.

Hersh, D., Worrall, L., Howe, T., Sherratt, S., & Davidson, B. (2012). SMARTER goal setting in aphasia rehabilitation. *Aphasiology, 26*, 220–233.

Hersh, N. A., & Treadgold, L. G. (1994). Neuropage: The rehabilitation of memory dysfunction by prosthetic memory and cuing. *Neurorehabilitation, 4*, 187–197.

Hesketh, A., Long, A., & Bowen, A. (2011). Agreement on outcome: Speaker, carer, and therapist perspectives on functional communication after stroke. *Aphasiology, 25*, 291–308.

Hesketh, A., Long, A., Patchick, E., Lee, J., & Bowen, A. (2008). The reliability of rating conversation as a measure of functional communication following stroke. *Aphasiology, 22*, 970–984.

Hickin, J., Best, W., Herbert, R., Howard, D., & Osborne, F. (2002). Phonological therapy for word-finding difficulties: A re-evaluation. *Aphasiology, 16*, 981–1000.

Hickok, G., Love-Geffen, T., & Klima, E. S. (2002). Role of the left hemisphere in sign language comprehension. *Brain and Language, 82*, 167–178.

Hilari, K., Byng, S., Lamping, D. L., & Smith, S. C. (2003). Stroke and aphasia quality of life scale-39 (SAQOL-39): Evaluation of acceptability, reliability, and validity. *Stroke, 34,* 1944–1950.

Hilari, K., & Cruice, M. (2013). Quality-of-life approach to aphasia. In I. Papathanasiou, P. Coppens, & C. Potages (Eds.), *Aphasia and related neurogenic communication disorders* (pp. 233–254). Burlington, MA: Jones & Bartlett Learning.

Hilari, K., & Northcott, S. (2006). Social support in people with chronic aphasia. *Aphasiology, 20,* 17–36.

Hill, A. J., Theodoros, D. G., Russell, T. G., Ward, E. C., & Wootton, R. (2009). The effects of aphasia severity on the ability to assess language disorders via telerehabilitation. *Aphasiology, 23,* 627–642.

Hillis, A. E. (2001). The organization of the lexical system. In B. Rapp (Ed.), *The handbook of cognitive neuropsychology* (pp. 185–210). Philadelphia: Psychology Press.

Hillis, A. E. (2007). Magnetic resonance perfusion imaging in the study of language. *Brain and Language, 102,* 165–175.

Hillis, A. E., Barker, P. B., Wityk, R. J., Aldrich, E. M., Restrepo, L., et al. (2004). Variability in subcortical aphasia is due to variable sites of cortical hypoperfusion. *Brain and Language, 89,* 524–530.

Hillis, A. E., & Caramazza, A. (1991). Category-specific naming and comprehension impairment: A double dissociation. *Brain, 114,* 2081–2094.

Hillis, A. E., & Caramazza, A. (1992). The reading process and its disorders. In D. I. Margolin (Ed.), *Cognitive neuropsychology in clinical practice* (pp. 229–261). New York: Oxford University Press.

Hillis, A. E., & Heidler, J. (2002). Mechanisms of early aphasia recovery. *Aphasiology, 16,* 885–895.

Hillis, A. E., & Heidler, J. (2005). Contributions and limitations of the cognitive neuropsychological approach to treatment: Illustrations from studies of reading and spelling therapy. *Aphasiology, 19,* 985–993.

Hillis, A. E., Heidler-Gary, J., Newhart, M., Chang, S., Ken, L., & Bak, T. H. (2006). Naming and comprehension in primary progressive aphasia: The influence of grammatical word class. *Aphasiology, 20,* 246–256.

Hillis, A. E., Kane, A., Tuffiash, E., Ulatowski, J. A., Barker, P. B., et al. (2001). Reperfusion of specific brain regions by raising blood pressure restores selective language functions in subacute stroke. *Brain and Language, 79,* 495–510.

Hillis, A. E., Newhart, M., Heidler, J., Marsh, E. B., Barker, P., et al. (2005). The neglected role of the right hemisphere in spatial representation of words for meaning. *Aphasiology, 19,* 225–238.

Hillis, A. E., Ulatowska, J. A., Barker, P. B., Torbey, M., Ziai, W., et al. (2003). A pilot randomized trial of induced blood pressure elevation: Effects on function and focal perfusion in acute and subacute stroke. *Cerebrovascular Diseases, 16,* 236–246.

Hinckley, J. J. (2002). Vocational and social outcomes of adults with chronic aphasia. *Journal of Communication Disorders, 35,* 543–560.

Hinckley, J. J., & Carr, T. H. (2005). Comparing the outcomes of intensive and non-intensive context-based aphasia treatment. *Aphasiology, 19,* 965–974.

Hinckley, J. J., & Douglas, N. F. (2013). Treatment fidelity: Its importance and reported frequency in aphasia treatment studies. *American Journal of Speech-Language Pathology* (Supplement), 22, S279–S284.

Hinckley, J. J., Patterson, J. P., & Carr, T. H. (2001). Differential effects of context- and skill-based treatment approaches: Preliminary findings. *Aphasiology, 15,* 463–476.

Hirsch, F. M., & Holland, A. L. (2000). Beyond activity: Measuring participation in society and quality of life. In L. E. Worrall & C. M. Frattali (Eds.), *Neurogenic communication disorders: A functional approach* (pp. 35–54). New York: Thieme.

Hodges, J. R., & McCarthy, R. A. (1993). Autobiographical amnesia resulting from bilateral paramedian thalamic infarction. *Brain, 116,* 921–940.

Hodges, J. R., Patterson, K., Oxbury, S., & Funnell, E. (1992). Semantic dementia: Progressive fluent aphasia with temporal lobe atrophy. *Brain, 115,* 1783–1806.

Hoen, B., Thelander, M., & Worsley, J. (1997). Improvement in psychological well-being of people with aphasia and their families: Evaluation of a community-based programme. *Aphasiology, 11,* 681–691.

Hoerster, L., Hickey, E., & Bourgeois, M. (2001). Effects of memory aids on conversations between nursing home residents with dementia and nursing assistants. *Neuropsychological Rehabilitation, 11,* 399–427.

Holland, A. L. (1970). Case studies in aphasia rehabilitation using programmed instruction. *Journal of Speech and Hearing Disorders, 35,* 377–390.

Holland, A. L. (1975). *Aphasics as communicators: A model and its implications.* Paper presented to the American Speech and Hearing Association, November, Washington, D.C.

Holland, A. L. (1978). Functional communication in the treatment of aphasia. In L. J. Branford (Ed.), *Communicative disorders: An audio journal for continuing education.* New York: Grune & Stratton.

Holland, A. L. (1982). When is aphasia aphasia? The problem of closed head injury. In R. H. Brookshire (Ed.), *Clinical aphasiology conference proceedings* (pp. 345–349). Minneapolis, MN: BRK.

Holland, A. L. (1991). Pragmatic aspects of intervention in aphasia. *Journal of Neurolinguistics, 6,* 197–211.

Holland, A. L. (1995). Patient inputs to increasing understanding of communicative drawing. *Aphasiology, 9,* 57–59.

Holland, A. L. (1998). Why can't clinicians talk to aphasic adults? Comments on supported conversation for adults with aphasia: Methods and resources for training conversational partners. *Aphasiology, 12,* 844–846.

Holland, A. L. (2007). *Counseling in communication disorders: A wellness perspective.* San Diego, CA: Plural.

Holland, A. L., & Beeson, P. M. (1993). Finding a new sense of self: What the clinician can do to help. *Aphasiology, 7,* 581–584.

Holland, A. L., Frattali, C. M., & Fromm, D. (1999). *Communication activities of daily living* (2nd ed.). Austin, TX: Pro-Ed.

Holland, A. L., & Fridriksson, J. (2001). Aphasia management during the early phases of recovery following stroke. *American Journal of Speech-Language Pathology, 10,* 19–28.

Holland, A. L., Fromm, D. S., DeRuyter, F., & Stein, M. (1996). Treatment efficacy: Aphasia. *Journal of Speech and Hearing Research, 39,* S27–S36.

Holland, A. L., Greenhouse, J., Fromm, D., & Swindell, C. S. (1989). Predictors of language restitution following stroke: A multivariate analysis. *Journal of Speech and Hearing Research, 32,* 232–238.

Holland, A. L., Halper, A. S., & Cherney, L. R. (2010). Tell me your story: Analysis of script topics selected by persons with aphasia. *American Journal of Speech-Language Pathology, 19,* 198–203.

Holland, A. L., Swindell, C. S., & Forbes, M. M. (1985). The evolution of initial global aphasia: Implications for prognosis. In R. H. Brookshire (Ed.), *Clinical aphasiology* (Vol. 15, pp. 169–175). Minneapolis, MN: BRK.

Holland, R., & Crinion, J. (2012). Can tDCS enhance treatment of aphasia after stroke? *Aphasiology, 26,* 1169–1191.

Holtzapple, P., Pohlman, K., LaPointe, L. L., & Graham, L. F. (1989). Does SPICA mean PICA? In T. E. Prescott (Ed.), *Clinical aphasiology* (Vol. 18, pp. 131–144). Boston: College-Hill/Little, Brown.

Hom, J., & Reitan, R. M. (1990). Generalized cognitive function after stroke. *Journal of Clinical and Experimental Neuropsychology, 12,* 644–654.

Hopper, T. (2007). Group treatment for people with dementia. In R. J. Elman (Ed.), *Group treatment of neurogenic communication disorders* (pp. 341–354). San Diego, CA: Plural Publishing.

Hopper, T., & Bayles, K. A. (2008). Management of neurogenic communication disorders associated with dementia. In R. Chapey (Ed.), *Language intervention strategies in aphasia and related neurogenic communication disorders* (5th ed., pp. 988–1008). Philadelphia: Wolters Kluwer Health.

Hopper, T., & Holland, A. L. (1998). Situation-specific training for adults with aphasia: An example. *Aphasiology, 12,* 933–944.

Hopper, T., Holland, A., & Rewega, M. (2002). Conversational coaching: Treatment outcomes and future directions. *Aphasiology, 16,* 745–762.

Hopper, T., Mahendra, N., Kim, E., Azuma, T., Bayles, K. A., et al. (2005). Evidence-based practice recommendations for working with individuals with dementia: Spaced-retrieval training. *Journal of Medical Speech-Language Pathology, 13,* xxvii–xxxiv.

Horner, J., Dawson, D., Heyman, A., & Fish, A. M. (1992). The usefulness of the Western Aphasia Battery for differential diagnosis of Alzheimer dementia and focal stroke syndromes: Preliminary evidence. *Brain and Language, 42,* 77–88.

Horner, J., & Wheeler, M. (2005, November 8). HIPAA: Impact on research practices. *The ASHA Leader,* 8–9, 26–27.

Horton, S. (2006). A framework for description and analysis of therapy for language impairment in aphasia. *Aphasiology, 20,* 528–564.

Horton, S. (2008). Learning-in-interaction: Resourceful work by people with aphasia and therapists in the course of language impairment therapy. *Aphasiology, 22,* 985–1014.

Hosomi, A., Nagakane, Y., Yamada, K., Kuriyama, N., Mizuno, T., et al. (2009). Assessment of arcuate fasciculus with diffusion-tensor tractography may predict the prognosis of aphasia in patients with left middle cerebral artery infarcts. *Neuroradiology, 51,* 549–555.

Hough, M. S. (1989). Category concept generation in aphasia: The influence of context. *Aphasiology, 3,* 553–568.

Hough, M. S. (1990). Narrative comprehension in adults with right and left hemisphere brain-damage: Theme organization. *Brain and Language, 38,* 253–277.

Hough, M. S. (1993). Treatment of Wernicke's aphasia with jargon: A case study. *Journal of Communication Disorders, 26,* 101–111.

Hough, M. S. (2008). Word retrieval failure episodes after traumatic brain injury. *Aphasiology, 22,* 644–654.

Hough, M. S. (2010). Melodic Intonation Therapy and aphasia: Another variation on a theme. *Aphasiology, 24,* 775–786.

Hough, M. S., & Barrow, I. (2003). Descriptive discourse abilities of traumatic brain-injured adults. *Aphasiology, 17,* 183–191.

Hough, M. S., & Givens, G. D. (2004). Word fluency skills in dementia of the Alzheimer's type for common and goal-directed categories. *Aphasiology, 18,* 357–371.

Hough, M. S., & Johnson, R. K. (2009). Use of AAC to enhance linguistic communication skills in an adult with chronic severe aphasia. *Aphasiology, 23,* 965–976.

Howard, D., & Gatehouse, C. (2006). Distinguishing semantic and lexical word retrieval deficits in people with aphasia. *Aphasiology, 20,* 921–951.

Howard, D., & Patterson, K. (1992). *Pyramids and palm trees.* San Antonio, TX: Harcourt Assessment.

Howard, D., Patterson, K., Franklin, S., Orchard-Lisle, V., & Morton, J. (1985). Treatment of word retrieval deficits in aphasia. *Brain, 108,* 817–829.

Howard, D., Swinburn, K., & Porter, G. (2010). Putting the CAT out: What the Comprehensive Aphasia Test has to offer. *Aphasiology, 24,* 56–74.

Howe, T. J., Worrall, L. E., & Hickson, L. M. H. (2004). What is an aphasia-friendly environment? *Aphasiology, 18,* 1015–1037.

Howe, T. J., Worrall, L. E., & Hickson, L. M. H. (2008). Interviews with people with aphasia: Environmental factors that influence their community participation. *Aphasiology, 22,*1092–1122.

Huber, M. (1946). Linguistic problems of brain-injured servicemen. *Journal of Speech and Hearing Disorders, 11,* 143–147.

Huber, W., & Gleber, J. (1982). Linguistic and nonlinguistic processing of narratives in aphasia. *Brain and Language, 16,* 1–18.

Huber, W., Poeck, K., & Willmes, K. (1984). The Aachen Aphasia Test. In F. C. Rose (Ed.), *Progress in aphasiology* (pp. 291–303). New York: Raven Press.

Huff, F. J., Collins, C., Corkin, S., & Rosen, J. T. (1986). Equivalent forms of the Boston Naming Test. *Journal of Clinical and Experimental Neuropsychology, 8,* 556–562.

Hula, W., Donovan, N. J., Kendall, D. L., & Gonzalez-Rothi, L. J. (2010). Item response theory analysis of the Western Aphasia Battery. *Aphasiology, 24,* 1326–1341.

Hunt, J. (1999). Drawing on the semantic system: The use of drawing as a therapy medium. In S. Byng, K. Swinburn, & C. Pound (Eds.), *The aphasia therapy file* (pp. 41–60). Hove, UK: Psychology Press.

Hurkmans, J., de Bruijn, M., Boonstra, A. M., Jonkers, R., Bastiaanse, R., et al. (2012). Music in the treatment of neurological language and speech disorders: A systematic review. *Aphasiology, 26,* 1–19.

Hutton, C. (2005). *After a stroke: 300 tips for making life easier.* New York: Demos Medical Publishing.

Hux, K., Buechter, M., Wallace, S., & Weissling, K. (2010). Using visual scene displays to create a shared communication space for a person with aphasia. *Aphasiology, 24,* 643–660.

Hux, K., Weissling, K., & Wallace, S. (2008). Communication-based interventions: Augmented and alternative communication for people with aphasia. In R. Chapey (Ed.), *Language intervention strategies in aphasia and related neurogenic communication disorders* (5th ed., pp. 814–836). Philadelphia: Wolters Kluwer Health.

Hye, A., Lynham, S., Thambisetty, M., Causevic, M., Campbell, J., et al. (2006). Proteome-based plasma biomarkers for Alzheimer's disease. *Brain, 129,* 3042–3050.

Illes, J., Metter, E. J., Dennings, R., Jackson, C., Kempler, D., et al. (1989). Spontaneous language production in mild aphasia: Relationship to left prefrontal glucose hypometabolism. *Aphasiology, 3,* 527–537.

Ip, R. Y., Dornan, J., & Schentag, C. (1995). Traumatic brain injury: Factors predicting return to work or school. *Brain Injury, 9,* 517–532.

Irwin, W. H., Wertz, R. T., & Avent, J. R. (2002). Relationships among language impairment, functional communication, and pragmatic performance in aphasia. *Aphasiology, 16,* 823–835.

Itoh, M., Sasanuma, S., Hirose, H., Yoshioka, H., & Sawashima, M. (1983). Velar movements during speech in two Wernicke aphasic patients. *Brain and Language, 19,* 283–292.

Itoh, M., Sasanuma, S., Tatsumi, I. F., Murakami, S., Fukusako, Y., et al. (1982). Voice onset time characteristics in apraxia of speech. *Brain and Language, 17,* 193–210.

Ivanova, M. V., & Hallowell, B. (2009). Short form of the Bilingual Aphasia Test in Russian: Psychometric data of persons with aphasia. *Aphasiology, 23,* 544–556.

Iverson, G. L., Lovell, M. R., & Collins, M. W. (2003). Interpreting change on ImPACT following sport concussion. *The Clinical Neuropsychologist, 17,* 460–467.

Jacobs, B. J., & Thompson, C. K. (2000). Cross-modal generalization effects of training noncanonical sentence comprehension and production in agrammatic aphasia. *Journal of Speech, Language, and Hearing Research, 43,* 5–20.

Jakobson, R. (1955). Aphasia as a linguistic problem. In H. Werner (Ed.), *On expressive language.* Worcester, MA: Clark University Press.

Janse, E. (2010). Spoken word processing and the effect of phonemic mismatch in aphasia. *Aphasiology, 24,* 3–27.

Jennett, B., & Bond, M. (1975). Assessment of outcome after severe brain damage. *Lancet, 1,* 480–484.

Jennett, B., & Teasdale, G. (1981). *Management of head injuries.* Philadelphia: F. A. Davis.

Jinguji, T. M., Bompadre, V., Harmon, K. G., Satchell, E. K., Gilbert, K., et al. (2012). Sport Concussion Assessment Tool-2: Baseline values for high school athletes. *British Journal of Sports Medicine, 46,* 365–370.

Joanette, Y., Goulet, P., & Le Dorze, G. (1988). Impaired word naming in right-brain-damaged right-handers: Error types and time-course analyses. *Brain and Language, 34,* 54–64.

Joanette, Y., Goulet, P., Ska, B., & Nespoulous, J.-L. (1986). Informative content of narrative discourse in right-brain-damaged right-handers. *Brain and Language, 29,* 81–105.

Johnson, R. (1998). How do people get back to work after severe head injury? A 10 year follow-up study. *Neuropsychological Rehabilitation, 8,* 61–79.

Johnson-Laird, P. N. (1983). *Mental models.* Cambridge, UK: Cambridge University Press.

Johnstone, B., & Stonnington, H. H. (Eds.). (2001). *Rehabilitation of neuropsychological disorders: A practical guide for rehabilitation professionals.* Philadelphia: Psychology Press.

Jokel, R., Cupit, J., Rochon, E., & Leonard, C. (2009). Relearning lost vocabulary in nonfluent progressive aphasia with MossTalk Words®. *Aphasiology, 23,* 175–191.

Jones, D., Pierce, R. S., Mahoney, M., & Smeach, K. (2007). Effect of familiar content on paragraph comprehension in aphasia. *Aphasiology, 21,* 1218–1229.

Jonkers, R., & Bastiannse, R. (1998). How selective are selective word class deficits. Two case studies of action and object naming. *Aphasiology, 12,* 245–256.

Jordan, B. D. (2000). Cognitive rehabilitation following traumatic brain injury. *Journal of the American Medical Association, 283,* 3123–3124.

Junque, C., Vendrell, P., Vendrell-Brucet, J. M., & Tobena, A., (1989). Differential recovery in naming in bilingual aphasics. *Brain and Language, 36,* 16–22.

Kaan, E., & Swaab, T. Y. (2003). Electrophysiological evidence for serial sentence processing: A comparison between non-preferred and ungrammatical continuations. *Cognitive Brain Research, 17,* 621–635.

Kagan, A. (1998). Supported conversation for adults with aphasia: Methods and resources for training conversation partners. *Aphasiology, 12,* 816–830.

Kagan, A., Black, S. E., Duchan, J. F., Simmons-Mackie, N., & Square, P. (2001). Training volunteers as conversation partners using "Supported Conversation for Adults with Aphasia" (SCA): A controlled trial. *Journal of Speech, Language, and Hearing Research, 44,* 624–638.

Kagan, A., Cohen-Schneider, R., Sherman, C., & Podolsky, L. (2007). Groups in the Aphasia Institute's *Introductory Program*: Preparing to live successfully with aphasia. In R. J. Elman (Ed.), *Group treatment of neurogenic communication disorders: The expert clinician's approach* (2nd ed., pp. 211–232). San Diego, CA: Plural.

Kagan, A., & Simmons-Mackie, N. (2007). Beginning with the end: Outcome driven assessment and intervention with life participation in mind. *Topics in Language Disorders,* 27, 309–317.

Kagan, A., Simmons-Mackie, N., Rowland, A., Huijbregts, M., Shumway, W., et al. (2008). Counting what counts: A framework for capturing real-life outcomes of aphasia intervention. *Aphasiology, 22,* 258–280.

Kagan, A., Winckel, J., Black, S., Duchan, J. F., Simmons-Mackie, N., et al. (2004). A set of observational measures for rating support and participation in conversation between adults with aphasia and their conversation partners. *Topics in Stroke Rehabilitation, 11,* 67–83.

Kahn, H. J., Joanette, Y., Ska, B., & Goulet, P. (1990). Discourse analysis in neuropsychology: Comment on Chapman and Ulatowska. *Brain and Language, 38,* 454–461.

Kalinyak-Fliszar, M., Kohen, F., & Martin, N. (2011). Remediation of language processing in aphasia: Improving activation and maintenance of linguistic representations in (verbal) short-term memory. *Aphasiology, 25,* 1095–1131.

Kaplan, E., Goodglass, H., & Weintraub, (1983). *The Boston Naming Test.* Philadelphia: Lea & Febiger.

Kaplan, J. A., Brownell, H. H., Jacobs, J. R., & Gardner, H. (1990). The effects of right hemisphere damage on the pragmatic interpretation of conversational remarks. *Brain and Language, 38,* 315–333.

Kapur, N. (1994). Remembering Norman Schwarzkopf: Evidence for two distinct long-term fact learning mechanisms. *Cognitive Neuropsychology, 11,* 661–670.

Karbe, H., Thiel, A., Weber-Luxenburger, G., Herholz, K., Kessler, J., et al. (1998). Brain plasticity in poststroke aphasia: What is the contribution of the right hemisphere? *Brain and Language, 64,* 215–230.

Karow, C. M., Marquardt, T. P., & Marshall, R. C. (2001). Affective processing in left and right hemisphere brain-damaged subjects with and without subcortical involvement. *Aphasiology, 15,* 715–729.

Karr, M. (1995). *The liars' club.* New York: Penguin.

Karzmark, P., Heaton, R. K., Lehman, R. A. W., & Crouch, J. (1985). Utility of the Seashore Tonal Memory Test in neuropsychological assessment. *Journal of Clinical and Experimental Neuropsychology, 7,* 367–374.

Kashiwagi, T., Kashiwagi, A., Kunimori, Y., Yamadori, A., Tanabe, H., et al. (1994). Preserved capacity to copy drawings in severe aphasics with little premorbid experience. *Aphasiology, 8,* 427–442.

Katz, R. C. (2008). Computer applications in aphasia treatment. In R. Chapey (Ed.), *Language intervention strategies in aphasia and related neurogenic communication disorders* (5th ed., pp. 852–876). Philadelphia: Wolters Kluwer Health.

Katz, W. F. (1988). An investigation of lexical ambiguity in Broca's aphasics using an auditory lexical priming technique. *Neuropsychologia, 26,* 747–752.

Kay, J., Lesser, R., & Coltheart, M. (1992). *PALPA: Psycholinguistic Assessments of Language Processing in Aphasia.* Hove, UK: Erlbaum.

Kay, J., Lesser, R., & Coltheart, M. (1996a). Psycholinguistic Assessments of Language Processing in Aphasia (PALPA): An introduction. *Aphasiology, 10,* 159–180.

Kay, J., Lesser, R., & Coltheart, M. (1996b). PALPA: The proof of the pudding is in the eating. *Aphasiology, 10,* 202–215.

Kay, J., & Terry, R. (2004). Ten years on: Lessons learned from published studies that cite the PALPA. *Aphasiology, 18,* 127–151.

Kazdin, A. E. (1982). *Single-case research designs: Methods for clinical and applied settings.* New York: Oxford University Press.

Kazdin, A. E. (2010). *Single-case research designs: Methods for clinical and applied settings* (2nd ed.). New York: Oxford University Press.

Kearns, K. P. (1985). Response elaboration training for patient initiated utterances. In R. H. Brookshire (Ed.), *Clinical aphasiology* (Vol. 15, pp. 196–204). Minneapolis, MN: BRK.

Kearns, K. P. (1986a). Flexibility of single-subject experimental designs. Part II: Design selection and arrangement of experimental phases. *Journal of Speech and Hearing Disorders, 51,* 204–214.

Kearns, K. P. (1986b). Systematic programming of verbal elaboration skills in chronic Broca's aphasia. In R. C. Marshall (Ed.), *Case studies in aphasia rehabilitation: For clinicians by clinicians* (pp. 225–244). Austin, TX: Pro-Ed.

Kearns, K. P. (1989). Methodologies for studying generalization. In L. V. McReynolds & J. Spradlin (Eds.). *Generalization strategies in the treatment of communication disorders* (pp. 13–30). Lewiston, NY: BC Decker.

Kearns, K. P. (2005). Broca's aphasia. In L. L. LaPointe (Ed.), *Aphasia and related neurogenic language disorders* (3rd ed., pp. 117–141). New York: Thieme.

Kearns, K. P., & Elman, R. J. (2008). Group therapy for aphasia: Theoretical and practical considerations. In R. Chapey (Ed.), *Language intervention strategies in aphasia and related neurogenic communication disorders* (5th ed., pp. 376–400). Philadelphia: Wolters Kluwer Health.

Kearns, K. P., & Salmon, S. J. (1984). An experimental analysis of auxiliary and copula verb generalization in aphasia. *Journal of Speech and Hearing Disorders, 49,* 152–163.

Kearns, K. P., & Scher, G. P. (1989). The generalization of response elaboration training effects. In T. E. Prescott (Ed.), *Clinical aphasiology* (Vol. 18, pp. 223–246). Boston: College-Hill.

Kearns, K. P., & Yedor, K. (1991). An alternating treatments comparison of loose training and a convergent treatment strategy. In T. E. Prescott (Ed.), *Clinical aphasiology* (Vol. 20, pp. 223–238). Austin, TX: Pro-Ed.

Keefe, K. A. (1995). Applying basic neuroscience to aphasia therapy: What the animals are telling us. *American Journal of Speech-Language Pathology, 4*(4), 88–93.

Keenan, J. S., & Brassell, E. G. (1974). A study of factors related to prognosis for individual aphasic patients. *Journal of Speech and Hearing Disorders, 39,* 257–269.

Keenan, J. S., & Brassell, E. G. (1975). *Aphasia language performance scales.* Murfreesboro, TN: Pinnacle Press.

Kemmerer, D., & Tranel, D. (2000a). Verb retrieval in brain-damaged subjects: 1. Analysis of stimulus, lexical, and conceptual factors. *Brain and Language, 73,* 347–392.

Kemmerer, D., & Tranel, D. (2000b). Verb retrieval in brain-damaged subjects: 2. Analysis of errors. *Brain and Language, 73,* 393–420.

Kempermann, G., Kuhn, H. G., & Gage, F. H. (1997). More hippocampal neurons in adult mice living in an enriched environment. *Nature, 386,* 493–495.

Kempler, D., Curtiss, S., & Jackson, C. (1987). Syntactic preservation in Alzheimer's disease. *Journal of Speech and Hearing Research, 30,* 343–350.

Kempler, D., & Goral, M. (2011). A comparison of drill- and communication-based treatment for aphasia. *Aphasiology, 25,* 1327–1346.

Kendall, D. L., McNeil, M. R., & Small, S. L. (1998). Rule-based treatment for acquired phonological dyslexia. *Aphasiology, 12,* 587–600.

Kenin, M., & Swisher, L. P. (1972). A study of pattern of recovery in aphasia. *Cortex, 8,* 56–68.

Kennedy, C., Coelho, C., Ylvisaker, M., Turkstra, L., Sohlberg, M. M., et al. (2008). Intervention for executive functions after traumatic brain injury: A systematic review, meta-analysis and clinical recommendations. *Neuropsychological Rehabilitation, 18,* 257–299.

Kennedy, M., & Murdoch, B. E. (1991). Patterns of speech and language recovery following left striato-capsular hemorrhage. *Aphasiology, 5,* 489–510.

Kennedy, M., & Murdoch, B. E. (1994). Thalamic aphasia and striato-capsular aphasia as independent aphasic syndromes. *Aphasiology, 8,* 303–313.

Kennedy, M. R. T. (2000). Topic scenes in conversations with adults with right-hemisphere brain damage. *American Journal of Speech-Language Pathology, 9,* 72–86.

Kennedy, M. R. T., & Nawrocki, M. D. (2003). Delayed predictive accuracy of narrative recall after traumatic brain injury: Salience and explicitness. *Journal of Speech, Language, and Hearing Research, 46,* 98–112.

Kerr, J., Hilari, K., & Litosseliti, L. (2010). Information needs after stroke: What to include and how to structure it on a website. A qualitative study using focus groups and card sorting. *Aphasiology, 24,* 1170–1196.

Kertesz, A. (1979). *Aphasia and associated disorders: Taxonomy, localization, and recovery.* New York: Grune & Stratton.

Kertesz, A. (1985). Recovery and treatment. In K. M. Heilman & E. Valenstein (Eds.), *Clinical neuro psychology* (2nd ed., pp. 481–505). New York: Oxford University Press.

Kertesz, A. (2007). *Western Aphasia Battery-Revised*. New York: Pearson/PsychCorp.

Kertesz, A. (2010). Ardila's attempt to alter aphasiology. *Aphasiology, 24*, 404–407

Kertesz, A., & Benson, D. F. (1970). Neologistic jargon—A clinicopatholgical study. *Cortex, 6*, 362–386.

Kertesz, A., Ferro, J. M., & Shewan, C. M. (1984). Apraxia and aphasia: The functional-anatomical basis for their dissociation. *Neurology, 34*, 40–47.

Kertesz, A., Harlock, W., & Coates, R. (1979). Computer topographic localization, lesion size and prognosis in aphasia. *Brain and Language, 8*, 34–50.

Kertesz, A., Lau, W. K., & Polk, M. (1993). The structural determinants of recovery in Wernicke's aphasia. *Brain and Language, 44*, 153–165.

Kertesz, A., Lesk, D., & McCabe, P. (1977). Isotope localization of infarcts in aphasia. *Archives of Neurology, 34*, 590–601.

Kertesz, A., & McCabe, P. (1975). Intelligence and aphasia: Performance of aphasics on Raven's Coloured Progressive Matrices (RCPM). *Brain and Language, 2*, 387–395.

Kertesz, A., & McCabe, P. (1977). Recovery patterns and prognosis in aphasia. *Brain, 100*, 1–18.

Kertesz, A., & Phipps, J. B. (1977). Numerical taxonomy of aphasia. *Brain and Language, 4*, 1–10.

Kertesz, A., & Poole, E. (1974). The aphasia quotient: The taxonomic approach to measurement of aphasic disability. *Canadian Journal of Neurological Sciences, 1*, 7–16.

Kessler, J., Thiel, A., Karbe, H., & Heiss, W. D. (2000). Piracetam improves activated blood flow and facilitates rehabilitation of poststroke aphasic patients. *Stroke, 31*, 2112–2116.

Kiernan, R. J., Mueller, J., Langston, J. W., & Van Dyke, C. (1987). The Neurobehavioral Cognitive Status Examination: A brief but quantitative approach to cognitive assessment. *Annals of Internal Medicine, 107*, 481–485.

Kilov, A. M., Togher, L., & Grant, S. (2009). Problem solving with friends: Discourse participation and performance of individuals with and without traumatic brain injury. *Aphasiology, 23*, 584–605.

Kim, M., & Thompson, C. K. (2000). Patterns of comprehension and production of nouns and verbs in agrammatism: Implications for lexical organization. *Brain and Language, 74*, 1–25.

Kim, M., & Thompson, C. K. (2004). Verb deficits in Alzheimer's disease and agrammatism: Implications for lexical organization. *Brain and Language, 88*, 10–20.

Kimbarow, M. L. (Ed.). (2011). *Cognitive communication disorders*. San Diego, CA: Plural.

Kimmel, D. C. (1974). *Adulthood and aging*. New York: Wiley.

King, J. T., Carlier, P. M., & Marion, D. W. (2005). Early Glasgow Outcome Scale scores predict long-term functional outcome in patients with severe traumatic brain injury. *Journal of Neurotrauma, 22*, 947–954.

King, K. A., Hough, M. S., Vos, P., Walker, M. M., & Givens, G. (2006). Word retrieval following mild TBI: Implications for categorical deficits. *Aphasiology, 20*, 233–245.

Kintsch, W. (1998). *Comprehension: A paradigm for cognition*. Cambridge, UK: Cambridge University Press.

Kiran, S., & Roberts, P. M. (2010). Semantic feature analysis treatment in Spanish-English and French-English bilingual aphasia. *Aphasiology, 24*, 231–261.

Kiran, S., Sandberg, C., & Abbott, K. (2009). Treatment for lexical retrieval using abstract and concrete words in persons with aphasia: Effect of complexity. *Aphasiology, 23*, 835–853.

Kiran, S., & Thompson, C. K. (2003a). Effect of typicality on online category verification of animate category exemplars in aphasia. *Brain and Language, 85*, 441–450.

Kiran, S., & Thompson, C. K. (2003b). The role of semantic complexity in treatment of naming deficits: Training semantic categories in fluent aphasia by controlling exemplar typicality. *Journal of Speech, Language, and Hearing Research, 46*, 773–787.

Kirk, A., & Kertesz, A. (1994). Cortical and subcortical aphasias compared. *Aphasiology, 8*, 65–82.

Kirmess, M., & Lind, M. (2011). Spoken language production as outcome measurement following constraint induced language therapy. *Aphasiology, 25*, 1207–1238.

Kirmess, M., & Maher, L. M. (2010). Constraint induced language therapy in early aphasia rehabilitation. *Aphasiology, 24*, 725–736.

Kirshner, H. S., Casey, P. F., Henson, J., & Heinrich, J. J. (1989). Behavioural features and lesion localization in Wernicke's aphasia. *Aphasiology, 3*, 169–176.

Kirshner, H. S., Webb, W. G., & Duncan, G. W. (1981). Word deafness in Wernicke's aphasia. *Journal of Neurology, Neurosurgery, and Psychiatry, 45*, 197–201.

Klepousniotou, E., & Baum, S. R. (2005). Unilateral brain damage effects on processing homonymous and polysemous words. *Brain and Language, 93*, 308–326.

Klima, E. S., Bellugi, U., & Poizner, H. (1988). Grammar and space in sign aphasiology. *Aphasiology, 2*, 319–328.

Knopman, D. S., Selnes, O. A., Niccum, N., & Rubens, A. B. (1984). Recovery of naming in aphasia: Relationship to fluency, comprehension and CT findings. *Neurology, 34*, 1461–1471.

Koemeda-Lutz, M., Cohen, R., & Meier, E. (1987). Organization of and access to semantic memory in aphasia. *Brain and Language, 30*, 321–337.

Koenig-Bruhin, M., & Studer-Eichenberger, F. (2007). Therapy of verbal short-term memory disorders in fluent aphasia: A single case study. *Aphasiology, 21,* 448–458.

Kohn, S. E., & Goodglass, H. (1985). Picture-naming in aphasia. *Brain and Language, 24,* 266–283.

Kohn, S. E., & Smith, K. L. (1995). Serial effects of phonemic planning during word production. *Aphasiology, 9,* 209–222.

Kohn, S. E., Smith, K. L., & Arsenault, J. (1990). The remediation of conduction aphasia via sentence repetition: A case study. *British Journal of Disorders of Communication, 25,* 45.

Kohnert, K. (2008). Primary language impairments in bilingual children and adults. In J. Altarriba, & R. R. Heredia (Eds.), *An introduction to bilingualism: Principles and processes* (pp. 295–320). New York: Erlbaum.

Kok, P., van Doorn, A., & Kolk, H. (2007). Inflection and computational load in agrammatic speech. *Brain and Language, 102,* 273–283.

Kolb, B., Morshead, C., Gonzalez, C., Kim, M., Gregg, C., et al. (2006). Growth factor-stimulated generation of new cortical tissue and functional recovery after stroke damage to the motor cortex of rats. *Journal of Cerebral Blood Flow & Metabolism,* 1–15.

Kolk, H. H. J., & Heeschen, C. (1990). Adaptation symptoms and impairment symptoms in Broca's aphasia. *Aphasiology, 4,* 221–232.

Kolk, H. H. J., & Heeschen, C. (1992). Agrammatism, paragrammatism and the management of language. *Language and Cognitive Processes, 7,* 89–130.

Kolk, H. H. J., & van Grunsven, M. M. (1985). Agrammatism as a variable phenomenon. *Cognitive Neuropsychology, 2,* 347–384.

Kopelman, M. D., Wilson, B. A., and Baddeley, A. D. (1989). The Autobiographical Memory Interview: A new assessment of personal and autobiographical semantic memory in amnesic patients. *Journal of Clinical and Experimental Neuropsychology, 11,* 724–744.

Kortte, K., & Hillis, A. E. (2009). Recent advances in the understanding of neglect and anosognosia following right hemisphere stroke. *Current Neurology and Neuroscience Reports, 9,* 459–465.

Kumar, V. P., & Humphreys, G. W. (2008). The role of semantic knowledge in relearning spellings: Evidence from deep dysgraphia. *Aphasiology, 22,* 489–504.

Kurland, J., Baldwin, K., & Tauer, C. (2010). Treatment-induced neuroplasticity following intensive naming therapy in a case of chronic Wernicke's aphasia. *Aphasiology, 24,* 737–751.

Kurland, J., Pulvermüller, F., Silva, N., Burke, K., & Andrianopoulos, M. (2012). Constrained versus unconstrained intensive language therapy in two individuals with *chronic,* moderate-to-severe aphasia and apraxia of speech: Behavioral and fMRI outcomes.

American Journal of Speech-Language Pathology, 21, 565–587.

Labourel, D., & Martin, M.-M. (1993). The person with aphasia and the family. In D. Lafond, Y. Joanette, J. Ponzio, R. Degiovani, & M. T. Sarno (Eds.), *Living with aphasia: Psychosocial issues* (pp. 151–172). San Diego, CA: Singular.

Laiacona, M., & Caramazza, A. (2004). The noun/verb dissociation in language production: Varieties of causes. *Cognitive Neuropsychology, 21,* 103–124.

Laine, M., Goodglass, H., Niemi, J., Kolvuselkä-Sallinen, P., Tuomainen, J., et al. (1993). Adaptation of the Boston Diagnostic Aphasia Examination and the Boston Naming Test into Finnish. *Scandanavian Journal of Logopedics and Phoniatrics, 18,* 83–92.

Laine, M., & Martin, N. (2012). Cognitive neuropsychology has been, is, and will be significant to aphasiology. *Aphasiology, 26,* 1362–1375.

Laisney, M., Giffard, B., Belliard, S., de la Sayette, V., Desgranges, B., et al. (2011). When the zebra loses its stripes: Semantic priming in early Alzheimer's disease and semantic dementia. *Cortex, 47,* 35–46.

Langlois, J. A., Rutland-Brown, W., & Wald, M. M. (2006). The epidemiology and impact of traumatic brain injury: A brief overview. *Journal of Head Trauma Rehabilitation, 21,* 375–378.

Lanyon, L., & Rose, M. L. (2009). Do the hands have it? The facilitation effects of arm and hand gesture on word retrieval in aphasia. *Aphasiology, 23,* 809–822.

LaPointe, L. L. (1985). Aphasia therapy: Some principles and strategies for treatment. In D. F. Johns (Ed.), *Clinical management of neurogenic communicative disorders* (pp. 179–241). Boston: Little, Brown.

LaPointe, L. L., & Eisenson, J. (2008). *Examining for aphasia* (4th ed.). Austin, TX: Pro-Ed.

LaPointe, L. L., & Horner, J. (1998). *Reading Comprehension Battery for Aphasia* (rev. ed.). Austin, TX: Pro-Ed.

Lasker, J. P., & Garrett, K. L. (2006). Using the *Multimodal Communication Screening Test for Persons with Aphasia* (MCST-A) to guide the selection of alternative communication strategies for people with aphasia. *Aphasiology, 20,* 217–232.

Lasker, J. P., Garrett, K. L., & Fox, L. E. (2007). Severe aphasia. In D. R. Beukelman, K. L. Garrett, & K. M. Yorkston (Eds.), *Augmentative communication strategies for adults with acute or chronic medical conditions* (pp. 163–206). Baltimore: Brookes.

Lasprilla, J. C. A., Iglesias, J., & Lopera, F. (2003). Neuropsychological study of familial Alzheimer's disease caused by mutation E280A in the presenilin 1 gene. *American Journal of Alzheimer's Disease and Other Dementias, 18,* 137–146.

Laures-Gore, J., Shisler Marshall, R., & Verner, E. (2011). Performance of individuals with left hemisphere stroke and aphasia and individuals with right brain damage on forward and backward digit span tasks. *Aphasiology, 25,* 43–57.

Law, B. M. (2012a). Getting in tune with clients with aphasia. *ASHA Leader, 17*(7), 12–13.

Law, B. M. (2012b). If I can talk, you can talk. *ASHA Leader, 17*(7), 14–16.

Lawton, M. P., & Brody, E. M. (1969). Assessment of older people: Self-maintaining and instrumental activities of daily living. *Gerontologist, 9,* 179–186.

Lawton, M. P., & Rubinstein, R. L. (Eds.). (2000). *Interventions in dementia care: Toward improving quality of life.* New York: Springer.

Lê, K., Coelho, C., Mozeiko, J., & Grafman, J. (2011). Measuring goodness of story narratives. *Journal of Speech, Language, and Hearing Research, 54,* 118–126.

Lê, K., Coelho, C., Mozeiko, J., Krueger, F., & Grafman, J. (2011). Measuring goodness of story narratives: Implications for traumatic brain injury. *Aphasiology, 25,* 748–750.

Le Dorze, G., Boulay, N., Gaudreau, J., & Brassard, C. (1994). The contrasting effects of a semantic versus a formal-semantic technique for the facilitation of naming in a case of anomia. *Aphasiology, 8,* 127–141.

Le Dorze, G., & Brassard, C. (1995). A description of the consequences of aphasia on aphasic persons and their relatives and friends, based on the WHO model of chronic diseases. *Aphasiology, 9,* 239–255.

Le Dorze, G., Tremblay, V., & Croteau, C. (2009). A qualitative longitudinal case study of a daughter's adaptation process to her father's aphasia and stroke. *Aphasiology, 23,* 483–502.

Lee, B. H., Suh, M. K., Kim, E. J., Seo, S. W., Choi, K. M, et al. (2009). Neglect dyslexia: Frequency, association with other hemispatial neglects, and lesion localization. *Neuropsychologia, 47,* 704–710.

Lee, C., Grossman, M., Morris, J., Stern, M. B., & Hurtig, H. I. (2003). Attentional resource and processing speed limitations during sentence processing in Parkinson's disease. *Brain and Language, 85,* 347–356.

Lee, J., Fowler, R., Rodney, D., Cherney, L., & Small, S. L. (2010). IMITATE: An intensive computer-based treatment of aphasia based on action observation and imitation. *Aphasiology, 24,* 449–465.

Lee, J., Milman, L. H., & Thompson, C. K. (2008). Functional category production in English agrammatism. *Aphasiology, 22,* 893–905.

Lee, J., & Thompson, C. K. (2011). Real-time production of unergative and unaccusative sentences in normal and agrammatic speakers: An eyetracking study. *Aphasiology, 25,* 813–825.

Lee, J. B., & Sohlberg, M. M. (2013). Evaluation of attention training and metacognitive facilitation to improve reading comprehension in aphasia.

American Journal of Speech-Language Pathology (Supplement), *22,* S318–S333.

Lee, J. B., Kaye, R. C., & Cherney, L. R. (2009). Conversational script performance in adults with non-fluent aphasia: Treatment intensity and aphasia severity. *Aphasiology, 23,* 885–897.

Lee, S. W., Clemenson, G. D., & Gage, F. H. (2012). New neurons in an aged brain. *Behavior and Brain Research, 227,* 497–507.

Legg, C., Young, L., & Bryer, A. (2003). Training sixth-year medical students in obtaining case-history information from adults with aphasia. *Aphasiology, 19,* 559–575.

Lehman Blake, M. T. (2005). Right hemisphere syndrome. In L. L. LaPointe (Ed.), *Aphasia and related neurogenic language disorders* (3rd ed., pp. 213–224). New York: Thieme.

Lehman Blake, M. T. (2007). Perspectives on treatment for communication deficits associated with right hemisphere brain damage. *American Journal of Speech-Language Pathology, 16,* 331–342.

Lehman Blake, M. T., Duffy, J. R., Myers, P. S., & Tompkins, C. A. (2002). Prevalence and patterns of right hemisphere cognitive/communicative deficits: Retrospective data from an inpatient rehabilitation unit. *Aphasiology, 16,* 537–548.

Lehman Blake, M. T., Duffy, J. R., Tompkins, C. A., & Myers, P. A. (2003). Right hemisphere syndrome is in the eye of the beholder. *Aphasiology, 17,* 423–432.

Lehman Blake, M. T., & Lesniewicz, K. S. (2005). Contextual bias and predictive inferencing in adults with and without right hemisphere brain damage. *Aphasiology, 19,* 423–434.

Leker, R. R., Soldner, F., Velasco, I., Gavin, D. K., Androutsellis-Theotokis, A., et al. (2007). Long-lasting regeneration after ischemia in the cerebral cortex. *Stroke, 28,* 153–161.

Le May, A., David, R., & Thomas, A. P. (1988). The use of spontaneous gesture by aphasic patients. *Aphasiology, 2,* 137–146.

Lemme, M. L., Hedberg, N. L., & Bottenberg, D. E. (1984). Cohesion in narratives of aphasic adults. In R. H. Brookshire (Ed.), *Clinical aphasiology conference proceedings* (pp. 215–222). Minneapolis, MN: BRK.

Lendrem, W., & Lincoln, N. B. (1985). Spontaneous recovery of language in patients with aphasia between 4 and 34 weeks after stroke. *Journal of Neurology, Neurosurgery, and Psychiatry, 48,* 743–748.

Leonard, C., Rochon, E., & Laird, L. (2008). Treating naming impairments in aphasia: Findings from a phonological components analysis treatment. *Aphasiology, 22,* 923–947.

Leonard, L. L. (1998). *Children with specific language impairment.* Cambridge, MA: MIT Press.

Lesser, R., & Perkins, L. (1999). *Cognitive neuropsychology and conversation analysis in aphasia: An introductory casebook.* London: Whurr.

Levin, H. S., Goldstein, F. C., High, W. M., & Williams, D. (1988). Automatic and effortful processing after severe closed head injury. *Brain and Cognition, 7,* 283–297.

Levin, H. S., Grossman, R. G., & Kelly, P. J. (1976). Aphasic disorders in patients with closed head injury. *Journal of Neurology, Neurosurgery, and Psychiatry, 39,* 1062–1070.

Levin, H. S., Grossman, R. G., Sarwar, M., & Meyers, C. A. (1981). Linguistic recovery after closed head injury. *Brain and Language, 12,* 360–374.

Levin, H. S., O'Donnell, V. M., & Grossman, R. G. (1979). The Galveston orientation and amnesia test: A practical scale to assess cognition after head injury. *Journal of Nervous and Mental Disease, 167,* 675–684.

Lezak, M. D., Howleson, D. B., Bigler, E. D., & Tranel, D. (2012). *Neuropsychological assessment* (6th ed.). New York: Oxford University Press.

Lezak, M. D., & O'Brien, K. P. (1988). Longitudinal study of emotional, social, and physical changes after traumatic brain injury. *Journal of Learning Disability, 21,* 456–465.

Li, E. C., Kitselman, K., Dusatko, D., & Spinelli, C. (1988). The efficacy of PACE in the remediation of naming deficits. *Journal of Communication Disorders, 21,* 491–503.

Li, E. C., & Williams, S. E. (1989). The efficacy of two types of cues in aphasic patients. *Aphasiology, 3,* 619–626.

Li, E. C., & Williams, S. E. (1990). The effects of grammatic class and cue type on cueing responsiveness in aphasia. *Brain and Language, 38,* 48–60.

Liles, B. Z., Coelho, C. A., Duffy, R. J., & Zalagens, M. R. (1989). Effects of elicitation procedures on the narratives of normal and closed head-injured adults. *Journal of Speech and Hearing Disorders, 54,* 356–366.

Lilienfeld, S. O., Lynn, S. J., & Lohr, J. M. (Eds.). (2003). *Science and pseudoscience in clinical psychology.* New York: Guilford.

Lincoln, N. B., & Ells, P. (1980). A shortened version of the PICA. *British Journal of Disorders of Communication, 15,* 183–187.

Lincoln, N. B., McGuirk, E., Mully, G. P., Lendrem, W., Jones, A. C., & Mitchell, J. R. A. (1984). The effectiveness of speech therapy for aphasic stroke patients: A randomized controlled trial. *Lancet, 1,* 1197–1200.

Lindenberg, R., Fangerau, H., & Seitz, R. J. (2007). "Broca's area" as a collective term? *Brain and Language, 102,* 22–29.

Linebarger, M. C. (1990). Neuropsychology of sentence parsing. In A. Caramazza (Ed.), *Cognitive neuropsychology and neurolinguistics: Advances in models of cognitive function and impairment* (pp. 55–122). Hillsdale, NJ: Erlbaum.

Linebarger, M. C., McCall, D., Virata, T., & Berndt, R. S. (2007). Widening the temporal window: Processing support in the treatment of aphasic language production. *Brain and Language, 100,* 53–68.

Linebarger, M. C., Romania, J. F., Fink, R. B., Bartlett, M. R., & Schwartz, M. F. (2008). Building on residual speech: A portable processing prosthesis for aphasia. *Journal of Rehabilitation Research & Development, 45,* 1401–1414.

Linebarger, M. C., Schwartz, M. F., Romania, J. R., Kohn, S. E., & Stephens, D. L. (2000). Grammatical encoding in aphasia: Evidence from a "processing prosthesis." *Brain and Language, 75,* 416–427.

Linebarger, M. C., Schwartz, M. F., & Saffran, E. M. (1983). Sensitivity to grammatical structure in so-called agrammatic aphasics. *Cognition, 13,* 361–392.

Linebaugh, C. W. (1983). Treatment of anomic aphasia. In W. H. Perkins (Ed.), *Language handicaps in adults* (pp. 35–44). New York: Thieme-Stratton.

Linebaugh, C. W., Margulies, C. P., & Mackisack-Morin, E. L. (1984). The effectiveness of comprehension-enhancing strategies employed by spouses of aphasic patients. In R. H. Brookshire (Ed.), *Clinical aphasiology conference proceedings* (pp. 188–197). Minneapolis, MN: BRK.

Links, P., Hurkmans, J., & Bastiaanse, R. (2010). Training verb and sentence production in agrammatic Broca's aphasia. *Aphasiology, 24,* 1303–1325.

Lock, S., Wilkinson, R., & Bryan, K. (2001). *SPPARC: Supporting partners of people with aphasia in relationships and conversation.* Bicester, UK: Speechmark.

Lohman, T., Ziggas, D., & Pierce, R. S. (1989). Word fluency performance on common categories by subjects with closed head injuries. *Aphasiology, 3,* 685–694.

Lomas, J., & Kertesz, A. (1978). Patterns of spontaneous recovery in aphasic groups: A study of adult stroke patients. *Brain and Language, 5,* 388–401.

Lomas, J., Pickard, L., Bester, S., Elbard, H., Finlayson, A., et al. (1989). The Communicative Effectiveness Index: Development and psychometric evaluation of a functional communication measure for adult aphasia. *Journal of Speech and Hearing Disorders, 54,* 113–124.

Lorenz, A., & Nickels, L. (2007). Orthographic cueing in anomic aphasia: How does it work? *Aphasiology, 21,* 670–686.

Lott, S. N., Carney, A. S., Glezer, L. S., & Friedman, R. B. (2010). Overt use of a tactile/kinesthetic strategy shifts to covert processing in rehabilitation of letter-by-letter reading. *Aphasiology, 24,* 1424–1442.

Lott, S. N., Sperling, A. J., Watson, N. L., & Friedman, R. B. (2009). Repetition priming in oral text reading: A therapeutic strategy for phonologic text alexia. *Aphasiology, 23,* 659–675.

Love, R. J., & Webb, W. J. (1977). The efficacy of cueing techniques in Broca's aphasia. *Journal of Speech and Hearing Disorders, 42,* 170–178.

Love, T., & Brumm, K. (2012). Language processing disorders. In R. K. Peach & L. P. Shapiro (Eds.), *Cognition and acquired language disorders: An information processing approach* (pp. 202–226). St. Louis, MO: Elsevier.

Love, T., & Oster, E. (2002). On the categorization of aphasic typologies: The S.O.A.P., a test of syntactic complexity. *Journal of Psycholinguistic Research, 31,* 503–529.

Love, T., Swinney, D., Walenski, M., & Zurif, E. (2008). How left inferior frontal cortex participates in syntactic processing: Evidence from aphasia. *Brain and Language, 107,* 203–219.

Love, T., Swinney, D., Wong, E., & Buxton, R. (2002). Perfusion imaging and stroke: A more sensitive measure of the brain bases of cognitive deficits. *Aphasiology, 16,* 873–883.

Lovell, M. R. (2006). Neuropsychological assessment of the professional athlete. In R. J. Echemendía (Ed.), *Sports neuropsychology: Assessment and management of traumatic brain injury* (pp. 176–192). New York: Guilford Press.

Loverso, F. L., Prescott, T. E., & Selinger, M. (1988). Cueing verbs: A treatment strategy for aphasic adults. *Journal of Rehabilitation Research, 25,* 47–60.

Lowell, S., Beeson, P. M., & Holland, A. L. (1995). The efficacy of a semantic cueing procedure on naming performance of adults with aphasia. *American Journal of Speech-Language Pathology, 4*(4), 109–114.

Lubinski, R. (2008). Environmental approach to adult aphasia. In R. Chapey (Ed.), *Language intervention strategies in aphasia and related neurogenic communication disorders* (5th ed., pp. 319–348). Philadelphia: Wolters Kluwer Health.

Lubinski, R., Duchan, J., & Weitzner-Lin, B. (1980). Analysis of breakdowns and repairs in aphasic adult communication. In R. H. Brookshire (Ed.), *Clinical aphasiology conference proceedings* (pp. 111–116). Minneapolis: BRK.

Luck, A. M., & Rose, M. L. (2007). Inverviewing people with aphasia: Insights into method adjustments from a pilot study. *Aphasiology, 21,* 208–224.

Lundgren, K., Brownell, H., Cayer-Meade, C., Milione, J., & Kearns, K. (2011). Treating metaphor interpretation deficits subsequent to right hemisphere brain damage: Preliminary results. *Aphasiology, 25,* 456–474.

Luria, A. R. (1966). *Higher cortical functions in man.* New York: Basic Books.

Luria, A. R. (1970). *Traumatic aphasia.* The Hague, Netherlands: Mouton.

Luzzatti, C., Willmes, K., Taricco, M., Colombo, C., & Chiesa, G. (1989). Language disturbances after severe head injury: Do neurological or other associated cognitive disorders influence type, severity and evolution of the verbal impairment? A preliminary report. *Aphasiology, 3,* 643–654.

Lyon, J. G. (1992). Communication use and participation in life for adults with aphasia in natural settings: The scope of the problem. *American Journal of Speech-Language Pathology, 1*(3), 7–14.

Lyon, J. G. (1995). Communicative drawing: An augmentative mode of interaction. *Aphasiology, 9,* 84–94.

Lyon, J. G. (1998). *Coping with aphasia.* San Diego, CA: Singular.

Lyon, J. G. (2001). Treating life consequences of aphasia's chronicity. In R. Chapey (Ed.), *Language intervention strategies in adult aphasia and related neurogenic communication disorders* (4th ed., pp. 297–315). Philadelphia: Lippincott Williams & Wilkins.

Lyon, J. G., Cariski, D., Keisler, L., Rosenbek, J., Levine, R., et al. (1997). Communication partners: Enhancing participation in life and communication for adults with aphasia in natural settings. *Aphasiology, 11,* 693–708.

Lyon, J. G., & Sims, E. (1989). Drawing: Its use as a communicative aid with aphasic and normal adults. In T. E. Prescott (Ed.), *Clinical aphasiology* (Vol. 18, pp. 339–355). Boston: College-Hill/Little, Brown.

MacDonald, S. (1998). *Functional assessment of verbal reasoning and executive strategies* (FAVRES). Guelph, ON: CCD Publishing.

MacDonald, M. C., Almor, A., Henderson, V. W., Kempler, D., & Andersen, E. S. (2001). Assessing working memory and language comprehension in Alzheimer's disease. *Brain and Language, 78,* 17–42.

Mace, N. L., & Rabins, P. V. (2011). *The 36-hour day* (5th ed.). Baltimore: Johns Hopkins University Press.

MacGinitie, W. H., MacGinitie, R. K., Maria, K., & Dreyer, L. G. (2006). *Gates-MacGinitie Reading Tests* (4th ed.). Chicago: Riverside.

Mackenzie, C., Brady, M., Norrie, J., & Poedjianto, N. (2007). Picture description in neurologically normal adults: Concepts and topic coherence. *Aphasiology, 21,* 340–354.

Mackenzie, C., & Paton, G. (2003). Resumption of driving with aphasia following stroke. *Aphasiology, 17,* 107–121.

MacWhinney, B., Fromm, D., Forbes, M., & Holland, A. (2011). AphasiaBank: Methods for studying discourse. *Aphasiology, 25,* 1286–1307.

MacWhinney, B., Fromm, D., Holland, A., Forbes, M., & Wright, H. H. (2010). Automated analysis of the Cinderella story. *Aphasiology, 24,* 856–868.

Mahendra, N. (2004). *Modifying the Communicative Abilities of Daily Living (CADL-2) for use with illiterate persons with aphasia: Preliminary results.* Retrieved October 21, 2005, from http://speechpathology.com/ articles/pf_arc_disp.asp?id=242

Mahendra, N., Arkin, S. M., & Kim, E. S. (2007). Individuals with Alzheimer's disease achieve implicit and explicit learning: Previous success replicated with different stimuli. *Aphasiology, 21*, 187–207.

Maher, L. M., Kendall, D. L., Swearengin, J. A., Rodriguez, A., Leon, S. A., Pingel, K., et al. (2006). A pilot study of use-dependent learning in the context of constraint induced language therapy. *Journal of the International Neuropsychological Society, 12*, 843–852.

Mahoney, F. I., & Barthel, D. (1965). Functional evaluation: The Barthel Index. *Maryland Medical Journal, 14*, 56–61.

Majerus, S., Van der Kaa, M. A., Renard, C., Van der Linden, M., & Poncelet, P. (2005). Treating verbal short-term memory deficits by increasing the duration of temporary phonological representations: A case study. *Brain and Language, 95*, 174–175.

Mandleberg, I. A., & Brooks, D. N. (1975). Cognitive recovery after severe head injury: 1. Serial testing on the Wechsler Adult Intelligence Scale. *Journal of Neurology, Neurosurgery, and Psychiatry, 38*, 1121–1126.

Mannheim, L. M., Halper, A. S., & Cherney, L. R. (2009). Patient-reported changes in communication after computer-based script training for aphasia. *Archives of Physical Medicine and Rehabilitation, 90*, 623–627.

Mariner, W. K. (1994). Outcomes assessment in health care reform: Promise and limitations. *American Journal of Law & Medicine, 20*, 36–57.

Marini, A., Carlomagno, S., Caltagirone, C., & Nocentini, U. (2005). The role played by the right hemisphere in the organization of complex textual structures. *Brain and Language, 93*, 46–54.

Marini, A., Caltagirone, C., Pasqualetti, P., & Carlomagno, S. (2007). Patterns of language improvement in adults with non-chronic non-fluent aphasia after specific therapies. *Aphasiology, 21*, 164–186.

Marks, M. M., Taylor, M., & Rusk, H. A. (1957). Rehabilitation of the aphasic patient: A survey of three years' experience in a rehabilitation setting. *Neurology, 7*, 837–843.

Markwardt, F. C., Jr. (1989). *The Peabody Individual Achievement Test-Rrevised*. Circle Pines, MN: American Guidance Service.

Marler, J. R. (2005). *Stroke for dummies*. Indianapolis, IN: Wiley.

Marshall, J. (1996). The PALPA: A commentary and consideration of the clinical implications. *Aphasiology, 10*, 197–202.

Marshall, J. (1999a). Doing something about a verb impairment: Two therapy approaches. In S. Byng, K. Swinburn, & C. Pound (Eds.), *The aphasia therapy file* (pp. 111–130). Hove, UK: Psychology Press.

Marshall, J. (1999b). "Who ends up with the fiver?"—A sentence production therapy. In S. Byng, K. Swinburn, & C. Pound (Eds.). *The aphasia therapy file* (pp. 143–149). Hove, UK: Psychology Press.

Marshall, J. (2006). Jargon aphasia: What have we learned? *Aphasiology, 20*, 387–410.

Marshall, J. (2009). Framing ideas in aphasia: The need for thinking therapy. *International Journal of Language and Communication Disorders*, 44, 1–14.

Marshall, J., Atkinson, J., Woll, B., & Thacker, A. (2005). Aphasia in a bilingual user of British Sign Language and English: Effects of cross-linguistic cues. *Cognitive Neuropsychology, 22*, 719–736.

Marshall, J., & Cairns, D. (2005). Therapy for sentence processing problems in aphasia: Working on thinking for speaking. *Aphasiology, 19*, 1009–1020.

Marshall, J., Pound, C., White-Thomson, M., & Pring, T. (1990). The use of picture/word matching tasks to assist word retrieval in aphasic patients. *Aphasiology, 4*, 167–184.

Marshall, J., Pring, T., & Chiat, S. (1993). Sentence processing therapy: Working at the level of the event. *Aphasiology, 7*, 177–199.

Marshall, J., Pring, T., & Chiat, S. (1998). Verb retrieval and sentence production in aphasia. *Brain and Language, 63*, 159–183.

Marshall, J., Robson, J., Pring, T., & Chiat, S. (1998). Why does monitoring fail in jargon aphasia? Comprehension, judgment, and therapy evidence. *Brain and Language, 63*, 79–107.

Marshall, R. C. (1976). Word retrieval behavior of aphasic adults. *Journal of Speech and Hearing Disorders, 41*, 444–451.

Marshall, R. C., Capilouto, G. J., & McBride, J. M. (2007). Treatment of problem solving in Alzheimer's disease: A short report. *Aphasiology, 21*, 235–249.

Marshall, R. C., McGurk, S. R., Karow, C. M., & Kairy, T. J. (2007). Problem-solving abilities of participants with and without diffuse neurologic involvement. *Aphasiology, 21*, 750–762.

Marshall, R. C., & Tompkins, C. A. (1982). Verbal self-correction behaviors of fluent and nonfluent aphasic subjects. *Brain and Language, 15*, 292–306.

Martin, I., & McDonald, S. (2003). Weak coherence, no theory of mind, or executive dysfunction: Solving the puzzle of pragmatic language disorders. *Brain and Language, 85*, 451–466.

Martin, I., & McDonald, S. (2005). Evaluating the causes of impaired irony comprehension following traumatic brain injury. *Aphasiology, 19*, 712–730.

Martin, N. (2012). Management of communication deficits associated with memory impairments. In R. K. Peach & L. P. Shapiro (Eds.), *Cognition and acquired language disorders: An information processing approach* (pp. 275–297). St. Louis: Elsevier/Mosby.

Martin, N., & Ayala, J. (2004). Measurements of auditory-verbal STM span in aphasia: Effects of item, task, and lexical impairment. *Brain and Language, 89*, 464–498.

Martin, N., Thompson, C. K., & Worrall, L. (Eds.). (2008). *Aphasia rehabilitation: The impairment and its consequences*. San Diego, CA: Plural Publishing.

Martin, N., Fink, R., Laine, M., & Ayala, J. (2004). Immediate and short-term effects of contextual priming. *Aphasiology, 18,* 867–898.

Martin, R. C., & Miller, M. (2002). Sentence comprehension deficits: Independence and interaction of syntax, semantics, and working memory. In A. E. Hillis (Ed.), *The handbook of adult language disorders* (pp. 295–310). New York: Psychology Press.

Martin, R. C., Shelton, J. R., & Yaffee, L. S. (1994). Language processing and working memory: Neuropsychological evidence for separate phonological and semantic capacities. *Journal of Memory and Language, 33,* 83–111.

Mason, R. A., Just, M. A., Keller, T. A., & Carpenter, P. A. (2003). Ambiguity in the brain: What brain imaging reveals about the processing of syntactically ambiguous sentences. *Journal of Experimental Psychology: Learning, Memory, and Cognition, 29,* 1319–1338.

Mathuranath, P. S., Nestor, P. J., Berrios, G. E., Rakowicz, W., & Hodges, J. R. (2000). A brief cognitive test battery to differentiate Alzheimer's disease and frontotemporal dementia. *Neurology, 55,* 1613–1620.

Matlin, M. W. (2009). *Cognition* (7th ed.). Hoboken, NJ: Wiley.

Mattis, S. (1988). *Dementia Rating Scale* (DRS). Odessa, FL: Psychological Assessment Resources.

Mauthe, R. W., Haaf, D. C., Hayn, P., & Krall, J. M. (1996). Predicting discharge destination of stroke patients using a mathematical model based on six items from the Functional Independence Measure. *Archives of Physical Medicine and Rehabilitation, 77,* 10–13.

Mavis, I., Colay, K., Topbas, S., & Tanrıdağ, O. (2007). Standardization, validity and reliability study of Gülhane Aphasia Test-2 (GAT-2). *Turkish Journal of Neurology, 13,* 89–98.

Mayberry, E. J., Sage, K., Ehsan, S., & Lambon Ralph, M. A. (2011). An emergent effect of phonemic cueing following relearning in semantic dementia. *Aphasiology, 25,* 1069–1077.

Mayer, J. F., & Murray, L. L. (2003). Functional measures of naming in aphasia: Word retrieval in confrontation naming versus connected speech. *Aphasiology, 17,* 481–497.

Mazzocchi, F., & Vignolo, L. A. (1979). Localization of lesions in aphasia: Clinical-CT scan correlations in stroke patients. *Cortex, 15,* 627–654.

Mazzoni, M., Vista, M., Pardossi, L., Avila, L., Bianchi, F., et al. (1992). Spontaneous evolution of aphasia after ischaemic stroke. *Aphasiology, 6,* 387–396.

McCarthy, R. A., & Warrington, E. K. (1990). *Cognitive neuropsychology: A clinical introduction*. San Diego, CA: Academic Press.

McCleary, C. (1988). The semantic organization and classification of fourteen words by aphasic patients. *Brain and Language, 34,* 183–202.

McCleary, C., & Hirst, W. (1986). Semantic classification in aphasia: A study of basic, superordinate, and function relations. *Brain and Language, 27,* 199–209.

McCrae, K., Jared, D., & Seidenberg, M. S. (1990). On the roles of frequency and lexical access in word naming. *Journal of Memory and Language, 29,* 43–65.

McCrum, R. (1998). *My year off: Recovering life after a stroke*. New York: W.W. Norton.

McDermott, F. B., Horner, J., & DeLong, E. R. (1996). Evolution of acute aphasia as measured by the Western Aphasia Battery. In M. L. Lemme (Ed.), *Clinical aphasiology* (Vol. 24, pp. 159–172). Austin, TX: Pro-Ed.

McDonald, S. (1993). Viewing the brain sideways? Frontal versus right hemisphere explanations of non-aphasic language disorders. *Aphasiology, 7,* 535–549.

McDonald, S., Bornhofen, C., Shum, D., Long, E., Saunders, C., et al. (2006). Reliability and validity of The Awareness of Social Inference Test (TASIT): A clinical test of social perception. *Disability Rehabilitation, 30,* 1529–1542.

McDonald, S., Flanagan, S., & Rollins, J. (2011). *Awareness of Social Inference Test–Revised (TASIT-R)*. New York: Pearson.

McDonald, S., & Pearce, S. (1996). Clinical insights into pragmatic theory: Frontal lobe deficits and sarcasm. *Brain and Language, 53,* 81–104.

McDonald, S., & Pearce, S. (1998). Requests that overcome listener reluctance: Impairment associated with executive dysfunction in brain injury. *Brain and Language, 61,* 88–104.

McDonald, S., Tate, R. L., & Rigby, J. (1994). Error types in ideomotor apraxia: A qualitative analysis. *Brain and Cognition, 25,* 250–270.

McDonald, S., Tate, R., Togher, L., Perdices, M., Moseley, A., et al. (2006). Improving evidence-based practice in rehabilitation: Introducing PsycBITE™. *Aphasiology, 20,* 676–683.

McDonald, S., & van Sommers, P. (1993). Pragmatic language skills after closed head injury: Ability to negotiate requests. *Cognitive Neuropsychology, 10,* 297–315.

McDonald, S., & Wales, R. (1986). An investigation of the ability to process inferences in language following right hemisphere brain damage. *Brain and Language, 29,* 68–80.

McGlinchey-Berroth, R., Milberg, W. P., Verfaellie, M., Alexander, M., & Kilduff, P. T. (1993). Semantic processing in the neglected visual field: Evidence from a lexical decision task. *Cognitive Neuropsychology, 10,* 79–108.

McGlynn, S. M., & Schacter, D. L. (1989). Unawareness of deficits in neuropsychological syndromes. *Journal of Clinical and Experimental Neuropsychology, 11,* 143–205.

McGurk, R., Kneebone, I. I., & Pit ten Cate, I. M. (2011). "Sometimes we get it wrong but we keep on trying": A cross-sectional study of coping with communication problems by informal carers of stroke survivors with aphasia. *Aphasiology, 25,* 1507–1522.

McIntosh, K. W., Ramsberger, G., & Prescott, T. E. (1996). Relationships between and among language impairment, communication disability and quality of life outcome assessments in aphasic patients [abstract]. *Brain and Language, 55,* 23–26.

McKee, A. C., Cantu, R. C., Nowinski, C. J., Hedley-White, E. T., Gavett, B. E., et al. (2009). Chronic traumatic encephalopathy in athletes: Progressive tauopathy following repetitive head injury. *Journal of Neuropathology and Experimental Neurology, 68,* 709–735.

McKeith, J. G., Fairbarn, A. F., Perry, R. H., & Thompson, P. (1994). The clinical diagnosis of senile dementia of Lewy body type (SDLT). *British Journal of Psychiatry, 165,* 324–332.

McKenna, P., & Warrington, E. K. (1980). Testing for nominal dysphasia. *Journal of Neurology, Neurosurgery, and Psychiatry, 43,* 781–788.

McKhann, G., Drachman, D., Folstein, M., Katzman, R., Price, D., et al. (1984). Clinical diagnosis of Alzheimer's disease: Report of the NINCDS-ADRDA work group under the auspices of the Department of Health and Human Services Task Force on Alzheimer's disease. *Neurology, 34,* 939–944.

McNamara, T. P. (2005). *Semantic priming: Perspectives from memory and word recognition.* New York: Psychology Press.

McNeil, M. R., Doyle, P. J., Fossett, T. R. D., Park, G. H., & Goda, A. J. (2001). Reliability and concurrent validity of the information unit scoring metric for the Story Retell Procedure. *Aphasiology, 10/11,* 991–1006.

McNeil, M. R., Doyle, P. J., Park, G. H., Fossett, T. R. D., & Brodsky, M. B. (2002). Increasing the sensitivity of the Story Retell Procedure for the discrimination of normal elderly subjects from persons with aphasia. *Aphasiology, 16,* 815–822.

McNeil, M. R., Hula, W. D., Matthews, C. T., & Doyle, P. J. (2004). Resource theory and aphasia: A fugacious theoretical dismissal. *Aphasiology, 18,* 836–839.

McNeil, M. R., Hula, W. D., & Sung, J. E. (2011). The role of memory and attention in aphasic language performance. In J. Guendouzi, F. Lonke, & M. J. Williams (Eds.), *The handbook of psycholinguistic and cognitive processes: Perspectives on communication disorders* (pp. 551–578). New York: Psychology Press.

McNeil, M. R., Matthews, C. T., Hula, W. D., Doyle, P. J., & Fossett, T. R. D. (2006). Effects of visual-

manual tracking under dual-task conditions on auditory language comprehension and story retelling in persons with aphasia. *Aphasiology, 20,* 167–174.

McNeil, M. R., & Prescott, T. E. (1978). *Revised Token Test.* Baltimore, MD: University Park Press.

McNeil, M. R., Sung, J. E., Yang, D., Pratt, S. R., Fossett, T. R., et al. (2007). Comparing connected language elicitation procedures in persons with aphasia: Concurrent validation of the Story Retell Procedure. *Aphasiology, 21,* 775–790.

McVicker, S., Parr, S., Pound, C., & Duchan, J. (2009). The Communication Partner Scheme: A project to develop long-term, low-cost access to conversation for people living with aphasia. *Aphasiology, 23,* 52–71.

Medina, J., Norise, C., Faseyitan, O., Coslett, H. B., Turkeltaub, P. E., et al. (2012). Finding the right words: Transcranial magnetic stimulation improves discourse productivity in non-fluent aphasia after stroke. *Aphasiology, 26,* 1153–1168.

Meinzer, M., & Breitenstein, C. (2008). Functional imaging studies of treatment-induced recovery in chronic aphasia. *Aphasiology, 22,* 1251–1268.

Meinzer, M., Flaisch, T., Breitnestein, C., Wienbruch, C., Elbert, T., et al. (2008). Functional re-recruitment of dysfunctional brain areas predicts language recovery in chronic aphasia. *Neuroimage, 39,* 2038–2046.

Meinzer, M., Harnish, S., Conway, T., & Crosson, B. (2011). Recent developments in functional and structural imaging of aphasia recovery after stroke. *Aphasiology, 25,* 271–290.

Mentis, M., & Prutting, C. A. (1987). Cohesion in the discourse of normal and head-injured adults. *Journal of Speech and Hearing Research, 30,* 88–98.

Mesulam, M.-M. (1982). Slowly progressive aphasia without generalized dementia. *Annals of Neurology, 11,* 592–598.

Mesulam, M.-M. (2001). Primary progressive aphasia. *Annals of Neurology, 49,* 425–432.

Mesulam, M.-M. (2007). Primary progressive aphasia: A 25-year retrospective. *Alzheimer Disease & Associated Disorders, 21,* S8–Sll.

Mesulam, M.-M., Grossman, M., Hillis, A. E., Kertesz, A., & Weintraub, S. (2003). The core and halo of primary progressive aphasia and semantic dementia. *Annals of Neurology, 54,* S11–S14.

Meteyard, L., & Patterson, K. (2009). The relation between content and structure in language production: An analysis of speech errors in semantic dementia. *Brain and Language, 110,* 121–134.

Metter, E. J. (1985). Feature: Letter. *Asha, 27,* 43.

Mey, J. L. (2001). *Pragmatics: An introduction* (2nd ed.). Malden, MA: Blackwell.

Miceli, G., Amitrano, A., Capasso, R., & Caramazza, A. (1996). The treatment of anomia resulting from output lexical damage: Analysis of two cases. *Brain and Language, 52,* 150–174.

Miceli, G., Gainotti, G., Caltagirone, C., & Masulo, C. (1980). Some aspects of phonological impairment in aphasia. *Brain and Language, 11,* 159–170.

Miceli, G., Silveri, M. C., Romani, C., & Caramazza, A. (1989). Variation in the pattern of omissions and substitutions of grammatical morphemes in the spontaneous speech of so-called agrammatic patients. *Brain and Language, 36,* 447–492.

Miceli, G., Silveri, M. C., Villa, G., & Caramazza, A. (1984). On the basis for the agrammatic's difficulty in producing main verbs. *Cortex, 20,* 207–220.

Milberg, W., & Blumstein, S. (1981). Lexical decision and aphasia: Evidence for semantic processing. *Brain and Language, 14,* 371–385.

Milberg, W., Blumstein, S. E., & Dworetzky, B. (1987). Processing of lexical ambiguities in aphasia. *Brain and Language, 31,* 151–170.

Miller, J., & Iglesias, A. (2008). *Systematic analysis of language transcripts* (SALT) [computer software]. Madison, WI: University of Wisconsin, Waisman Research Center, Language Analysis Laboratory.

Miller, N. (2010). Ruby McDonough allowed to testify in Sudbury sexual assault case. *MetroWest Daily News.* Retrieved November, 29, 2010, from http://www .metrowestdailynews.com/features/x298229494/ Ruby-McDonough-allowed-to-testify-in-Sudbury-sexual-assault-case

Mills, H. (2004). *A mind of my own: Memoir of recovery from aphasia.* Bloomington, IN: AuthorHouse.

Milner, B., Corkin, S., & Teuber, H.-L. (1968). Further analysis of the hippocampal amnesic syndrome: 14-year follow-up of H. M. *Neuropsychologia, 6,* 215–234.

Miozzo, M., Costa, A., Hernández, M., & Rapp, B. (2010). Lexical processing in the bilingual brain: Evidence from grammatical/morphological deficits. *Aphasiology, 24,* 262–287.

Milton, S. B., Wertz, R. T., Katz, R. C., & Prutting, C. A. (1981). Stimulus saliency in the sorting behavior of aphasic adults. In R. H. Brookshire (Ed.), *Clinical aphasiology conference proceedings* (pp. 46–54). Minneapolis, MN: BRK.

Mitchum, C. C., Haendiges, A. N., & Berndt, R. S. (1995). Treatment of thematic mapping in sentence comprehension: Implications for normal processing. *Cognitive Neuropsychology, 12,* 503–547.

Mitchum, C. C., Haendiges, A. N., & Berndt, R. S. (2004). Response strategies in aphasic sentence comprehension: An analysis of two cases. *Aphasiology, 18,* 675–691.

Mitchum, C. C., Ritgert, B., Sandson, J., & Berndt, R. S. (1990). The use of response analysis in confrontation naming. *Aphasiology, 4,* 261–279.

Mlcoch, A. G., & Metter, E. J. (2008). Medical aspects of stroke rehabilitation. In R. Chapey (Ed.), *Language intervention strategies in aphasia and related neurogenic communication disorders* (5th ed., pp. 42–63). Philadelphia: Wolters Kluwer Health.

Mohr, J. P., Pessin, M., Finkelstein, S., Funkenstein, H., Duncan, G., et al. (1978). Broca's aphasia: pathologic and clinical. *Neurology, 28,* 311–324.

Mohr, J. P., Weiss, G., Caveness, W. F., Dillon, J. D., Kistler, et al. (1980). Language and motor deficits following penetrating head injury in Vietnam. *Neurology, 30,* 1273–1279.

Molrine, C. J., & Pierce, R. S. (2002). Black and white adults' expressive language performance on three tests of aphasia. *American Journal of Speech-Language Pathology, 11,* 139–150.

Monoi, H., Fukusako, Y., Itoh, M., & Sasanuma, S. (1983). Speech sound errors in patients with conduction and Broca's aphasia. *Brain and Language, 20,* 175–194.

Montanes, P., Goldblum, M. C., & Boller, F. (1996). Classification deficits in Alzheimer's disease with special reference to living and nonliving things. *Brain and Language, 54,* 335–358.

Moore, S., Sandman, C. A., McGrady, K., & Kesslak, J. P. (2001). Memory training improves cognitive ability in patients with dementia. *Neuropsychological Rehabilitation, 11,* 245–261.

Moore, W. H. (1989). Language recovery in aphasia: A right hemisphere perspective. *Aphasiology, 3,* 101–110.

Moreaud, O., David, D., Charnallet, A., & Pellat, J. (2001). Are semantic errors actually semantic?: Evidence from Alzheimer's disease. *Brain and Language, 77,* 176–186.

Moreno-Martinez, F. J., & Montoro, P. R. (2010). Longitudinal patterns of fluency impairment in dementia: The role of domain and "nuisance variables." *Aphasiology, 24,* 1389–1399.

Morgan, A. L. R., & Helm-Estabrooks, N. (1987). Back to the drawing board: A treatment program for nonverbal aphasic patients. In R. H. Brookshire (Ed.), *Clinical aphasiology* (Vol. 17, pp. 64–72). Minneapolis, MN: BRK.

Morgan, G. A., Gliner, J. A., & Harmon, R. J. (2006). *Understanding and evaluating research in applied and clinical settings.* Mahwah, NJ: Erlbaum.

Morganstein, S., & Certner-Smith, M. (2008). Thematic language-stimulation therapy. In R. Chapey (Ed.), *Language intervention strategies in aphasia and related neurogenic communication disorders* (5th ed., pp. 450–468). Philadelphia: Wolters Kluwer Health.

Morley, G. K., Lundgren, S., & Haxby, J. (1979). Comparison and clinical applicability of auditory comprehension scores on the Behavioral Neurology

Deficit Examination, Boston Diagnostic Aphasia Examination, Porch Index of Communicative Ability and Token Test. *Journal of Clinical Neuropsychology, 1,* 249–258.

Morris, J., Franklin, S., Menger, F., & GD (2011). Returning to work with aphasia: A case study. *Aphasiology, 25,* 890–907.

Morrow, L., Vrtunski, P. B., Kim, Y., & Boller, F. (1981). Arousal responses to emotional stimuli and laterality of lesion. *Neuropsychologia, 19,* 65–71.

Mortley, J., Wade, J., & Enderby, P. (2004). Superhighway to promoting a client-therapist partnership? Using the Internet to deliver word-retrieval computer therapy, monitored remotely with minimal speech and language therapy input. *Aphasiology, 18,* 193–212.

Mowrer, D. E. (1982). *Methods of modifying speech behaviors: Learning theory in speech pathology* (2nd ed.). Prospect Heights, IL: Waveland Press.

Mozeiko, J., Lê, K., Coelho, C., Krueger, F., & Grafman, J. (2011). The relationship of story grammar and executive function following TBI. *Aphasiology, 25,* 826–835.

Mullen, R. (2003, August 8). National outcomes measurement system (NOMS): 2003. Retrieved December 7, 2005, from www.speechpathology.com/articles/pf_arc_disp.asp?id=17

Muñoz, M. L., & Marquardt, T. P. (2008). The performance of neurologically normal bilingual speakers of Spanish and English on the short version of the Bilingual Aphasia Test. *Aphasiology, 22,* 3–19.

Muñoz, M. L., Marquardt, T. P., & Copeland, G. (1999). A comparison of the code-switching patterns of aphasic and neurologically normal bilingual speakers of English and Spanish. *Brain and Language, 66,* 249–274.

Murray, L., Timberlake, A., & Eberle, R. (2007). Treatment of underlying forms in a discourse context. *Aphasiology, 21,* 139–163.

Murray, L. L. (2002). Attention deficits in aphasia: Presence, nature, and assessment and treatment. *Seminars in Speech and Language, 23,* 107–116.

Murray, L. L., & Clark, H. M. (2006). *Neurogenic disorders of language: Theory driven clinical practice.* Clifton Park, NY: Thomson Delmar.

Murray, L. L., Holland, A. L., & Beeson, P. M. (1998). Spoken language of individuals with mild fluent aphasia under focused and divided-attention conditions. *Journal of Speech Language and Hearing Research, 41,* 213–227.

Myers, P. S. (1979). Profiles of communication deficits in patients with right cerebral hemisphere damage. In R. H. Brookshire (Ed.), *Clinical aphasiology conference proceedings* (pp. 38–46). Minneapolis, MN: BRK.

Myers, P. S. (1999). *Right hemisphere damage.* San Diego, CA: Singular.

Myers, P. S., & Brookshire, R. H. (1994). The effects of visual and inferential complexity on the picture descriptions of non-brain-damaged and right-hemisphere-damaged adults. In M. L. Lemme (Ed.), *Clinical aphasiology* (Vol. 22, pp. 25–34). Austin, TX: Pro-Ed.

Myers, P. S., & Lehman Blake, M. (2008). Communication disorders associated with right-hemisphere damage. In R. Chapey (Ed.), *Language intervention strategies in aphasia and related neurogenic communication disorders* (5th ed., pp. 963–987). Philadelphia: Wolters Kluwer Health.

Myers, P. S., Linebaugh, C. W., & Mackisack-Morin, L. (1985). Extracting implicit meaning: Right versus left hemisphere damage. In R. H. Brookshire (Ed.), *Clinical aphasiology* (Vol. 15, pp. 72–82). Minneapolis, MN: BRK.

Nabors, N., Millis, S., & Rosenthal, M. (1997). Use of the Neurobehavioral Cognitive Status Examination (Cognistat) in traumatic brain injury. *Journal of Head Trauma Rehabilitation, 12,* 79–84.

Nadeau, S. E., & Crosson, B. (1997). Subcortical aphasia. *Brain and Language, 58,* 355–402.

Naeser, M. A. (1988). Some effects of subcortical white matter lesions on language behavior in aphasia. *Aphasiology, 2,* 363–368.

Naeser, M. A. (1994). Neuroimaging and recovery of auditory comprehension and spontaneous speech in aphasia with some implications for treatment of severe aphasia. In A. Kertesz (Ed.), *Localization and neuroimaging in neuropsychology* (pp. 245–296). San Diego, CA: Academic Press.

Naeser, M. A., & Hayward, R. W. (1978). Lesion localization in aphasia with cranial computed tomography and the Boston Diagnostic Aphasia Exam. *Neurology, 28,* 545–551.

Naeser, M. A., Martin, P. I., Theoret, H., Kobayashi, M., Fregni, F., et al. (2011). TMS suppression of right pars triangularis, but not pars opercularis, improves naming in aphasia. *Brain and Language, 119,* 206–213.

Naeser, M. A., Palumbo, C. L., Prete, M. N., Fitzpatrick, P. M., Mimura, M., et al. (1998). Visible changes in lesion borders on CT scan after five years poststroke, and long-term recovery in aphasia. *Brain and Language, 62,* 1–28.

Nagata, K., Yunoki, K., Kabe, S., Suzuki, A., & Araki, G. (1986). Regional cerebral blood flow correlates of aphasia outcome in cerebral hemorrhage and cerebral infarction. *Stroke, 17,* 417–423.

Nasreddine, Z. S., Phillips, N. A., Bedirian, V., Charbonneau, S., Whitehead, V., et al. (2005). The Montreal Cognitive Assessment, MoCA: A brief screening tool for mild cognitive impairment. *Journal of the American Geriatric Society, 53,* 695–699.

Nebes, R. D., Brady, C. B., & Huff, F. J. (1989). Automatic and attentional mechanisms of semantic priming in Alzheimer's disease. *Journal of Clinical and Experimental Neuropsychology, 11,* 219–230.

Needham, L. S., & Swisher, L. P. (1972). A comparison of three tests of auditory comprehension for adult aphasics. *Journal of Speech and Hearing Disorders, 37,* 123–131.

Nelson, E., Wasson, J., Kirk, J., Keller, A., Clark, D., et al. (1987). Assessment of function in routine clinical practice: Description of the COOP Chart method and preliminary findings. *Journal of Chronic Disease, 40,* 55S–63S.

Nelson, H. E., & O'Connell, A. (1978). Dementia: The estimation of premorbid intelligence levels using the New Adult Reading Test. *Cortex, 14,* 234–244.

Nespoulous, J., Dordain, M., Perron, C., Ska, B., Bub, D., et al. (1988). Agrammatism in sentence production without comprehension deficits: Reduced availability of syntactic structures and/or of grammatical morphemes? A case study. *Brain and Language, 33,* 273–295.

Neumann, M. A., & Cohn, R. (1953). Incidence of Alzheimer's disease in a large mental hospital. *Archives of Neurology and Psychiatry, 69,* 615–636.

Newcombe, F. (1969). *Missile wounds to the brain: A study of psychological deficits.* Oxford: Clarendon Press.

Newhart, M., Davis, C., Kannan, V., Heidler-Gary, J., Cloutman, L., et al. (2009). Therapy for naming deficits in two variants of primary progressive aphasia. *Aphasiology, 23,* 823–834.

Ni, W., Shankweiler, D., Harris, K. S., & Fulbright, R. K. (1997). Production and comprehension of relative clause syntax in nonfluent aphasia: A coordinated study [abstract]. *Brain and Language, 60,* 93–95.

Nicholas, L. E., & Brookshire, R. H. (1987). Error analysis and passage dependency of test items from a standardized test of multiple-sentence reading comprehension for aphasic and non-brain-damaged adults. *Journal of Speech and Hearing Disorders, 52,* 358–366.

Nicholas, L. E., & Brookshire, R. H. (1993). A system for quantifying the informativeness and efficiency of the connected speech of adults with aphasia. *Journal of Speech and Hearing Research, 36,* 338–350.

Nicholas, L. E., & Brookshire, R. H. (1995a). Comprehension of spoken narrative discourse by adults with aphasia, right-hemisphere brain damage, or traumatic brain injury. *American Journal of Speech-Language Pathology, 4*(3), 69–81.

Nicholas, L. E., & Brookshire, R. H. (1995b). Presence, completeness, and accuracy of main concepts in the connected speech of non-brain-damaged adults and adults with aphasia. *Journal of Speech and Hearing Research, 38,* 145–156.

Nicholas, L. E., MacLennan, D. L., & Brookshire, R. H. (1986). Validity of multiple-sentence reading comprehension tests for aphasic adults. *Journal of Speech and Hearing Disorders, 51,* 82–87.

Nicholas, M., Obler, L. K., Au, R., & Albert, M. L. (1996). On the nature of naming errors in aging and dementia: A study of semantic relatedness. *Brain and Language, 54,* 184–195.

Nicholas, M., Sinotte, M. P., & Helm-Estabrooks, N. (2005). Using a computer to communicate: Effect of executive function impairments in people with severe aphasia. *Aphasiology, 19,* 1052–1065.

Nicholas, M. L., Helm-Estabrooks, N., Ward-Lonergan, J., & Morgan, A. R. (1993). Evolution of severe aphasia in first two years post onset. *Archives of Physical Medicine and Rehabilitation, 74,* 830–836.

Nickels, L. (1995). Getting it right? Using aphasic naming errors to evaluate theoretical models of spoken word production. *Language and Cognitive Processes, 10,* 13–45.

Nickels, L. (2001). Spoken word production. In B. Rapp (Ed.), *The handbook of cognitive neuropsychology* (pp. 291–320). Philadelphia: Psychology Press.

Nickels, L. (2002). Therapy for naming disorders: Revisiting, revising, and reviewing. *Aphasiology, 16,* 935–979.

Nickels, L., & Best, W. (1996). Therapy for naming deficits (part II): Specifics, surprises and suggestions. *Aphasiology, 10,* 109–136.

Noll, J. D., & Randolf, S. R. (1978). Auditory semantic, syntactic, and retention errors made by aphasic subjects on the Token Test. *Journal of Communication Disorders, 11,* 543–553.

Norman, D. A., & Shallice, T. (1986). Attention to action: Willed and automatic control of behavior. In R. J. Davidson, G. E. Schwarts, & D. Shapiro (Eds.). *Consciousness and self-regulation: Advances in research and therapy* (pp. 1–18). New York: Plenum.

Nowicki, S., Jr., & Carton, J. S. (1993). The measurement of emotional intensity from facial expressions. *Journal of Social Psychology, 133,* 749–750.

Obler, L. K., & Albert, M. L. (1977). Influence of aging on recovery from aphasia in polyglots. *Brain and Language, 4,* 460–463.

Oczkowski, W. J., & Barreca, S. (1993). The Functional Independence Measure: Its use to identify rehabilitation needs in stroke survivors. *Archives of Physical Medicine and Rehabilitation, 74,* 1291–1294.

Odell, K. H., Wollack, J. A., & Flynn, M. (2005). Functional outcomes in patients with right hemisphere brain damage. *Aphasiology, 19,* 807–830.

Oelschlaeger, M. L., & Damico, J. S. (1998). Spontaneous verbal repetition: A social strategy in aphasic conversation. *Aphasiology, 12,* 971–988.

Oelschlaeger, M. L., & Thorne, J. C. (1999). Application of the correct information unit analysis to the naturally occurring conversation of a person with aphasia. *Journal of Speech, Language, and Hearing Research, 42,* 636–648.

Ogar, J. M., Baldo, J. V., Wilson, S. M., Brambati, S. M., Miller, B. L., et al. (2011). Semantic dementia and persisting Wernicke's aphasia: Linguistic and anatomical profiles. *Brain and Language, 117,* 28–33.

Oleyar, K. S., Doyle, P. J., Keefe, K., & Goldstein, H. (1991). The effects of a time-delay procedure on comprehension of verb-noun commands in severe aphasia. In T. E. Prescott (Ed.), *Clinical aphasiology* (Vol. 20, pp. 271–284). Austin, TX: Pro-Ed.

Olness, G. S. (2006). Genre, verb, and coherence in picture-elicited discourse of adults with aphasia. *Aphasiology, 20,* 175–187.

Olness, G. S., Matteson, S. E., & Stewart, C. T. (2010). "Let me tell you the point": How speakers with aphasia assign prominence to information in narratives. *Aphasiology, 24,* 697–708.

Olsen, E., Freed, D. B., & Marshall, R. C. (2012). Generalization of personalized cueing to enhance word finding in natural settings. *Aphasiology, 26,* 618–631.

Orfei, M. D., Robinson, R. G., Prigatano, G. P., Starkstein, S., Rüsch, N., et al. (2007). Anosognosia for hemiplegia after stroke is a multifaceted phenomenon: A systematic review of the literature. *Brain, 130,* 3075–3090.

Osborn, C. L. (1998). *Over my head: A doctor's own story of head injury from the inside looking out.* Kansas City, MO: Andrews McMeel.

Osgood, C. E., & Sebeok, T. A. (eds.). (1965). *Psycholinguistics: A survey of theory and research problems.* Bloomington: Indiana University Press.

Ostrin, R. K., & Schwartz, M. F. (1986). Reconstructing from a degraded trace: A study of sentence repetition in agrammatism. *Brain and Language, 28,* 328–345.

Ousset, P. J., Viallard, G., Puel, M., Celsis, P., Démonet, J. F., et al. (2002). Lexical therapy and episodic word learning in dementia of the Alzheimer type. *Brain and Language, 80,* 14–20.

Panton, A., & Marshall, J. (2008). Improving spelling and everyday writing after a CVA: A single-case therapy study. *Aphasiology, 22,* 164–183.

Papathanasiou, I., Coppens, P., & Ansaldo, A. (2013). Plasticity and recovery in aphasia. In I. Papathanasiou, P. Coppens, & C. Potages (Eds.), *Aphasia and related neurogenic communication disorders* (pp. 49–66). Burlington, MA: Jones & Bartlett Learning.

Paradis, M. (1977). Bilingualism and aphasia. In H. Whitaker & H. A. Whitaker (Eds.), *Studies in neurolinguistics* (Vol. 3, pp. 65–122). New York: Academic Press.

Paradis, M. (1998). Aphasia in bilinguals: How atypical is it? In P. Coppens, Y. Lebrun, & A. Basso (Eds.), *Aphasia in atypical populations* (pp. 35–66). Mahwah, NJ: Erlbaum.

Paradis, M., Goldblum, M-C., & Abidi, R. (1982). Alternate antagonism with paradoxical translation behavior in two bilingual aphasic patients. *Brain and Language, 15,* 55–69.

Paradis, M., & Libben, G. (1997). *The assessment of bilingual aphasia.* Hillsdale, NJ: Erlbaum.

Park, G. H., McNeil, M. R., & Tompkins, C. A. (2000). Reliability of the five-item Revised Token Test for individuals with aphasia. *Aphasiology, 14,* 527–535.

Parr, S. (1994). Coping with aphasia: Conversations with 20 aphasic people. *Aphasiology, 8,* 457–466.

Parr, S. (2007). Living with severe aphasia: Tracking social interaction. *Aphasiology, 21,* 98–123.

Pashek, G. V., & Holland, A. L. (1988). Evolution of aphasia in the first year post-stroke. *Cortex, 24,* 411–423.

Pashek, G. V., & Tompkins, C. A. (2002). Context and word class influences on lexical retrieval in aphasia. *Aphasiology, 16,* 261–286.

Patricaou, A., Psallida, E., Pring, T., & Dipper, L. (2007). The Boston Naming Test in Greek: Normative data and the effects of age and education on naming. *Aphasiology, 21,* 1157–1170.

Patronas, N. J., Deveikis, J. P., & Schellinger, D. (1987). The use of computed tomography in studying the brain. In H. G. Mueller & V. C. Geoffrey (Eds.), *Communication disorders in aging: Assessment and management* (pp. 107–134). Washington, DC: Gallaudet University Press.

Patterson, K., Graham, N. L., Lambon Ralph, M. A., & Hodges, J. R. (2006). Progressive non-fluent aphasia is not a progressive form of non-fluent (post-stroke) aphasia. *Aphasiology, 20,* 1018–1034.

Patterson, K. E., & Wilson, B. (1990). A ROSE is a ROSE or a NOSE: A deficit in initial letter identification. *Cognitive Neuropsychology, 7,* 447–478.

Paul, D. R., Frattali, C. M., Holland, A. L., Thompson, C. K., Caperton, C. J., et al. (2004). *Quality of Communication Life Scale* (ASHA QCL). Rockville, MD: American Speech-Language-Hearing Association.

Paul, N. A., & Sanders, G. F. (2010). Applying an ecological framework to education needs of communication partners of individuals with aphasia. *Aphasiology, 24,* 1095–1114.

Peach, R. K. (1987). A short-term memory treatment approach to the repetition deficit in conduction aphasia. In R. H. Brookshire (Ed.), *Clinical aphasiology* (Vol. 17, pp. 35–45). Minneapolis, MN: BRK.

Peach, R. K. (1996). Treatment for aphasic phonological output planning deficits. In M. L. Lemme (Ed.), *Clinical aphasiology* (Vol. 24, pp. 109–120). Austin, TX: Pro-Ed.

Peach, R. K. (2008). Global aphasia: Identification and management. In R. Chapey (Ed.), *Language intervention strategies in aphasia and related neurogenic communication disorders* (5th ed., pp. 565–594). Philadelphia: Wolters Kluwer Health.

Peach, R. K. (2012). Better a diamond with a flaw than a pebble without one: What cognitive neuropsychology can't do, what it can, and what it should: Commentary on Laine and Martin, "Cognitive neuropsychology has been, is, and will be significant to aphasiology." *Aphasiology, 26,* 1376–1380.

Peach, R. K., Canter, G. J., & Gallaher, A. J. (1988). Comprehension of sentence structure in anomic and conduction aphasia. *Brain and Language, 35,* 119–137.

Peach, R. K., & Reuter, K. A. (2010). A discourse-based approach to semantic feature analysis for the treatment of aphasic word retrieval failures. *Aphasiology, 24,* 971–990.

Peach, R. K., Rubin, S. S., & Newhoff, M. (1994). A topographic event-related potential analysis of the attention deficit for auditory processing in aphasia. In M. L. Lemme (Ed.), *Clinical aphasiology* (Vol. 22, pp. 81–96). Austin, TX: Pro-Ed.

Peach, R. K., & Shapiro, L. P. (eds.). (2012). *Cognition and acquired language disorders: An information processing approach.* St. Louis, MO: Elsevier.

Pease, D. M., & Goodglass, H. (1978). The effects of cuing on picture naming in aphasia. *Cortex, 14,* 178–189.

Pell, M. D. (2006). Cerebral mechanisms for understanding emotional prosody in speech. *Brain and Language, 96,* 221–234.

Pell, M. D. (2007). Reduced sensitivity to prosodic attitudes in adults with focal right hemisphere brain damage. *Brain and Language, 101,* 64–79.

Pell, M. D., & Baum, S. R. (1997). Unilateral brain damage, prosodic comprehension deficits, and the acoustic cues to prosody. *Brain and Language, 57,* 195–214.

Penfield, W., & Perot, P. (1963). The brain's record of visual and auditory experience: A final summary and discussion. *Brain, 86,* 595–696.

Penn, C., Frankel, T., Watermeyer, J., & Russell, N. (2010). Executive function and conversational strategies in bilingual aphasia. *Aphasiology, 24,* 288–308.

Penn, C., & Jones, D. (2000). Functional communication and the workplace: A neglected domain. In L. E. Worrall & C. M. Frattali (Eds.). *Neurogenic communication disorders: A functional approach* (pp. 103–124), New York: Thieme.

Perecman, E. (1984). Spontaneous translation and language mixing in a polyglot aphasic. *Brain and Language, 23,* 43–63.

Peretz, I. (2001). Music perception and recognition. In B. Rapp (Ed.), *The handbook of cognitive neuropsychology* (pp. 519–540). Philadelphia: Psychology Press.

Peretz, I., Champod, A. S., & Hyde, K. (2003, November). Varieties of musical disorders. The Montreal Battery of Evaluation of Amusia. *Annals of the New York Academy of Sciences, 999,* 58–75.

Perkins, L., Whitworth, A., & Lesser, R. (1997). *Conversation analysis profile for people with cognitive impairment.* Chichester, UK: Whurr Publishers.

Perri, R., Zannino, G. D., Caltagirone, C., & Carlesimo, G. A. (2011). Semantic priming for coordinate distant concepts in Alzheimer's disease patients. *Neuropsychologia, 49,* 839–847.

Petersen, R. (2002). *Mayo Clinic on Alzheimer's disease.* Rochester, MN: Mayo Clinic Health Information.

Petersen, R. C., Smith, G. E., Tangalos, E. G., Kokmen, E., & Ivnik, R. J. (1993). Longitudinal outcome of patients with a mild cognitive impairment. *Annals of Neurology, 34,* 294–295.

Peterson, L. N., & Kirshner, H. S. (1981). Gestural impairment and gestural ability in aphasia: A review. *Brain and Language, 14,* 333–348.

Phillips, P. P., & Halpin, G. (1978). Language impairment evaluation in aphasic patients. *Archives of Physical Medicine and Rehabilitation, 59,* 327–329.

Pickard, R., McAllister, J., & Horton, S. (2010). Spontaneous recovery of writing after stroke: A case study of the first 100 days. *Aphasiology, 24,* 1223–1242.

Pickersgill, M. J., & Lincoln, N. B. (1983). Prognostic indicators and the pattern of recovery of communication in aphasic stroke patients. *Journal of Neurology, Neurosurgery, and Psychiatry, 46,* 130–139.

Pierce, R. S., & Wagner, C. M. (1985). The role of context in facilitating syntactic decoding in aphasia. *Journal of Communication Disorders, 18,* 203–219.

Pimental, P. A., & Knight, J. A. (2000). *The Mini Inventory of Right Brain Injury* (MIRBI-2). Austin, TX: Pro-Ed.

Pizzamiglio, L., Mammucari, A., & Razzano, C. (1985). Evidence for sex differences in brain organization in recovery in aphasia. *Brain and Language, 25,* 213–223.

Poeck, K., Huber, W., & Willmes, K. (1989). Outcome of intensive language treatment in aphasia. *Journal of Speech and Hearing Disorders, 54,* 471–478.

Poirier, J., & Shapiro, L. P. (2012). Linguistic and psycholinguistic foundations. In R. K. Peach & L. P. Shapiro (Eds.). *Cognition and acquired language disorders: An information processing approach* (pp. 121–146). St. Louis, MO: Elsevier.

Poizner, H., Klima, E. S., & Bellugi, U. (1987). *What the hands reveal about the brain.* Cambridge, MA: MIT Press.

Polovoy, C. (2012, February 14). Baltimore's "aphasia-friendly" businesses. *ASHA Leader,* 24–25.

Ponsford, J., & Kinsella, G. (1992). Attentional deficits following closed-head injury. *Journal of Clinical and Experimental Neuropsychology, 14,* 822–838.

Ponsford, J., Olver, J., Nelms, R., Curran, C., & Ponsford, M. (1999). Outcome measurement in an inpatient and outpatient traumatic brain injury rehabilitation program. *Neuropsychological Rehabilitation, 9,* 517–534.

Ponsford, J., Sloan, S., & Snow, P. (1995). *Traumatic brain injury: Rehabilitation for everyday adaptive living.* Hove, UK: Psychology Press.

Ponzio, J., & Degiovani, R. (1993). Typical behavior of persons with aphasia and their families. In D. Lafond, Y. Joanette, J. Ponzio, R. Degiovani, & M. T. Sarno (Eds.), *Living with aphasia: Psychosocial issues* (pp. 117–128). San Diego, CA: Singular.

Porch, B. E. (1967). *Porch Index of Communicative Ability, Volume I: Theory and development.* Palo Alto, CA: Consulting Psychologists Press.

Porch, B. E. (1981). *Porch Index of Communicative Ability, Volume II: Administration, scoring, and interpretation* (3rd ed.). Palo Alto, CA: Consulting Psychologists Press.

Porch, B. E., Collins, M., Wertz, R. T., & Friden, T. P. (1980). Statistical prediction of change in aphasia. *Journal of Speech and Hearing Research, 23,* 312–321.

Porch, B. E., & Palmer, P. M. (1986). Right hemisphere PICA percentiles revised. In R. H. Brookshire (Ed.), *Clinical aphasiology* (Vol 16, pp. 275–280). Minneapolis, MN: BRK.

Porter, J. L., & Dabul, B. (1977). The application of transactional analysis to therapy with wives of adult aphasic patients. *Asha, 19,* 244–248.

Posner, M. I., Walker, J. A., Friedrich, F. J., & Rafal, R. D. (1987). How do the parietal lobes direct covert attention. *Neuropsychologia, 25,* 135–146.

Pound, C., Duchan, J., Penman, T., Hewitt, A., & Parr, S. (2007). Communication access to organizations: Inclusionary practices for people with aphasia. *Aphasiology, 22,* 23–38.

Prather, P. A., Love, T., Finkel, L., & Zurif, E. B. (1994). Effects of slowed processing on lexical activation: Automaticity without encapsulation [abstract]. *Brain and Language, 47,* 326–329.

Price, C. C., & Grossman, M. (2005). Verb agreements during on-line sentence processing in Alzheimer's disease and frontotemporal dementia. *Brain and Language, 94,* 217–232.

Price, C. J., Seghier, M. L., & Leff, A. P. (2010). Predicting language outcome and recovery after stroke: The PLORAS system. *Nature Reviews Neurology, 6,* 202–210.

Prigatano, G. P. (1999). *Principles of neuropsychological rehabilitation.* New York: Oxford University Press.

Prigatano, G. P., & Klonoff, P. S. (1998). A clinician's rating scale for evaluating impaired self-awareness and denial of disability after brain injury. *Clinical Neuropsychologist, 12,* 56–67.

Pring, T., Hamilton, A., Harwood, A., & Macbride, L. (1993). Generalization of naming after picture/word

matching tasks: Only items appearing in therapy benefit. *Aphasiology, 7,* 383–394.

Prins, R. S., Snow, C. E., & Wagenaar, E. (1978). Recovery from aphasia: Spontaneous speech versus language comprehension. *Brain and Language, 6,* 192–211.

Prior, M., Kinsella, G., & Giese, J. (1990). Assessment of musical processing in brain-damaged patients: Implications for laterality of music. *Journal of Clinical and Experimental Neuropsychology, 12,* 301–312.

Pulvermüller, F., & Berthier, M. L. (2008). Aphasia therapy on a neuroscience basis. *Aphasiology, 22,* 563–599.

Pulvermüller, F., Neininger, B., Elbert, T., Mohr, B., Rockstroh, B., et al. (2001). Constraint-induced therapy of chronic aphasia after stroke. *Stroke, 32,* 1621–1626.

Punt, T. D., Kitadono, K., Hulleman, J., Humphreys, G. W., & Riddoch, M. J. (2008). From both sides now: Crossover effects influence navigation in patients with unilateral neglect. *Journal of Neurology, Neurosurgery and Psychiatry, 79,* 464–466.

Purdy, M., & Hindenlang, J. (2005). Educating and training caregivers of persons with aphasia. *Aphasiology, 19,* 377–387.

Purdy, M., & Koch, A. (2006). Prediction of strategy usage by adults with aphasia. *Aphasiology, 20,* 337–348.

Purdy, M. H., Duffy, R. J., & Coelho, C. A. (1994). An investigation of the communicative use of trained symbols following multimodality training. In M. L. Lemme (Ed.), *Clinical aphasiology* (Vol. 22, pp. 345–356). Austin, TX: Pro-Ed.

Purves, B. A. (2009). The complexities of speaking for another. *Aphasiology, 23,* 914–925.

Quinn, D. A. (1998). *Conquering the darkness: One woman's story of recovering from brain injury.* St. Paul, MN: Paragon House.

Raboyeau, G., De Boissezon, X., Marie, N., Balduyck, S., Puel, M., et al. (2008). Right hemisphere activation in recovery from aphasia: Lesion effect or function recruitment? *Neurology, 70,* 290–298.

Radanovic, M., & Mansur, L. L. (2002). Performance of a Brazilian population sample in the Boston Diagnostic Aphasia Examination: A pilot study. *Brazilian Journal of Medical and Biological Research, 35,* 305–317.

Radanovic, M., & Scaff, M. (2003). Speech and language disturbances due to subcortical lesions. *Brain and Language, 84,* 337–352.

Radin, L., & Radin, G. (2003). *What if it's not Alzheimer's?* Amherst, NY: Prometheus.

Rao, P. R. (1995). Drawing conclusions on the efficacy of 'drawing' as a treatment for persons with severe aphasia. *Aphasiology, 9,* 59–62.

Rapp, B. (Ed.). (2001). *The handbook of cognitive neuropsychology.* Philadelphia: Psychology Press.

Rapp, B., Folk, J. R., & Tainturier, M.-J. (2001). Word reading. In B. Rapp (Ed.), *The handbook of cognitive neuropsychology* (pp. 233–262). Philadelphia: Psychology Press.

Rappaport, M., Herrero-Backe, C., Rappaport, M. L., & Winterfield, K. M. (1989). Head injury outcome up to ten years later. *Archives of Physical Medicine and Rehabilitation, 70,* 885–892.

Raskin, S. A., & Sohlberg, M. M. (1996). The efficacy of prospective memory training in two adults with brain injury. *Journal of Head Trauma Rehabilitation, 11,* 32–51.

Rastle, K., Tyler, L. K., & Marslen-Wilson, W. (2006). New evidence for morphological errors in deep dyslexia. *Brain and Language, 97,* 189–199.

Rautakoski, P., Korpijaakko-Huuhka, A.-M., & Klippi, A. (2008). People with severe and moderate aphasia and their partners are estimators of communicative skills: A client-centered evaluation. *Aphasiology, 22,* 1269–1293.

Raven, J. C. (1938/1965). *Progressive Matrices.* New York: Psychological Corporation.

Raymer, A. M. (2005). Naming and word-retrieval problems. In L. L. LaPointe (Ed.), *Aphasia and related neurogenic language disorders* (3rd ed., pp. 68–82). New York: Thieme

Raymer, A. M., Ciampitti, M., Holliway, B., Singletary, F., Blonder, L. H., et al. (2007). Semantic-phonologic treatment for noun and verb retrieval impairments in aphasia. *Neuropsychological Rehabilitation, 17,* 244–270.

Raymer, A. M., & Ellsworth, T. A. (2002). Response to contrasting verb retrieval treatments: A case study. *Aphasiology, 16,* 1031–1045.

Raymer, A. M., & Gonzalez Rothi, L. J. (2008). Impairments of word comprehension and production. In R. Chapey (Ed.), *Language intervention strategies in aphasia and related neurogenic communication disorders* (5th ed., pp. 607–631). Philadelphia: Wolters Kluwer Health.

Raymer, A. M., Kohen, F. P., & Saffell, D. (2006). Computerized training for impairments of word comprehension and retrieval in aphasia. *Aphasiology, 20,* 257–268.

Raymer, A. M., Maher, L. M., Foundas, A. L., Heilman, K. M., & Rothi, L. J. G. (1997). The significance of body part as tool errors in limb apraxia. *Brain and Cognition, 34,* 287–292.

Raymer, A. M., Moberg, P., Crosson, B., Nadeau, S., & Rothi, L. J. (1997). Lexical-semantic deficits in two patients with dominant thalamic infarction. *Neuropsychologia, 35,* 211–219.

Raymer, A. M., Rowland, L., Haley, M., & Crosson, B. (2002). Nonsymbolic movement training to improve sentence generation in transcortical motor aphasia: A case study. *Aphasiology, 16,* 493–506.

Raymer, A. M., Thompson, C. K., Jacobs, B., & Le Grand, H. R. (1993). Phonological treatment of naming deficits in aphasia: Model-based generalization analysis. *Aphasiology, 7,* 27–53.

Recinto, R. (2012). Crash survivor preaches dangers of texting while driving. Retrieved August 3, 2012, from http://news.yahoo.com/ blogs/lookout/crash-survivor-preaches-dangers-texting-while-driving

Reed, D. A., Johnson, N. A., Thompson, C., Weintraub, S., & Mesulam, M.-M. (2004). A clinical trial of bromocriptine for treatment of primary progressive aphasia. *Annals of Neurology, 56,* 750.

Reisberg, B., Ferris, S. H., de Leon, M. J., & Crook, T. (1982). The Global Deterioration Scale for assessment of primary degenerative dementia. *American Journal of Psychiatry, 139,* 1136–1139.

Reisberg, B., Ferris, S. H., & Franssen, E. (1985). An ordinal functional assessment tool for Alzheimer's type dementia. *Hospital and Community Psychiatry, 36,* 939–944.

Reitan, R. M., & Wolfson, D. (1993). *The Halstead-Reitan Neuropsychological Test Battery: Theory and clinical interpretation.* Tucson, AZ: Neuropsychology Press.

Reitan, R. M., & Wolfson, D. (1995). Category Test and Trail Making Test as measures of frontal lobe functions. *Clinical Neuropsychologist, 9,* 50–55.

Renvall, K., Laine, M., & Martin, N. (2007). Treatment of anomia with contextual priming: Exploration of a modified procedure with additional semantic and phonological tasks. *Aphasiology, 21,* 499–527.

Richardson, J. T. E. (2000). *Clinical and neuropsychological aspects of closed head injury* (2nd ed.). Hove, UK: Psychology Press.

Riddoch, M. J., Humphreys, G. W., Cleton, P., & Ferry, P. (1990). Interaction of attentional and lexical processes in neglect dyslexia. *Cognitive Neuropsychology, 7,* 479–518.

Riege, W. H., Metter, E. J., & Hanson, W. R. (1980). Verbal and nonverbal recognition memory in aphasic and nonaphasic stroke patients. *Brain and Language, 10,* 60–70.

Riley, E. A., & Thompson, C. K. (2010). Semantic typicality effects in acquired dyslexia: Evidence for semantic impairment in deep dyslexia. *Aphasiology, 24,* 802–813.

Rimel, R. W., & Jane, J. A. (1983). Characteristics of the head-injured patient. In M. Rosenthal, E. R. Griffith, M. R. Bond, & J. D. Miller (Eds.), *Rehabilitation of the head injured adult* (pp. 9–22). Philadelphia: F. A. Davis.

Rinnert, C., & Whitaker, H. A. (1973). Semantic confusions by aphasic patients. *Cortex, 9,* 56–81.

Ripich, D. N. (1996). *Alzheimer's disease communication guide: The FOCUSED program for caregivers.* San Antonio, TX: The Psychological Corporation.

Ripich, D. N., Ziol, E., & Lee, M. M. (1998). Longitudinal effects of communication training on caregivers of persons with Alzheimer's disease. *Clinical Gerontologist, 19,* 37–55.

Rivers, D. L., & Love, R. J. (1980). Language performance on visual processing tasks in right hemisphere lesion cases. *Brain and Language, 10,* 348–366.

Roach, A., Schwartz, M. F., Martin, N., Grewal, R. S., & Brecher, A. (1996). The Philadelphia Naming Test: Scoring and rationale. In M. L. Lemme (Ed.), *Clinical aphasiology* (Vol. 24, pp. 121–134). Austin, TX: Pro-Ed.

Roberts, J. A., & Wertz, R. T. (1989). Comparison of spontaneous and elicited oral-expressive language in aphasia. In T. E. Prescott (Ed)., *Clinical aphasiology* (Vol. 18, pp. 479–488). Boston: College-Hill/Little, Brown.

Roberts, P. M. (2008). Issues in assessment and treatment for bilingual and culturally diverse patients. In R. Chapey (Ed.), *Language intervention strategies in aphasia and related neurogenic communication disorders* (5th ed., pp. 245–275). Philadelphia: Wolters Kluwer Health.

Roberts, P. M., Code, C., & McNeil, M. R. (2003). Describing participants in aphasia research: Part 1. Audit of current practice. *Aphasiology, 17,* 911–932.

Roberts, P. M., & Kiran, S. (2009). Assessment and treatment of bilingual aphasia and bilingual anomia. In G. Ibanescu & S. Pescariu (Eds.), *Aphasia: Symptoms, diagnosis and treatment* (pp. 133–156). New York: Nova Biomedical.

Robertson, I. H., Ward, T., Ridgeway, V., & Nimmo-Smith, I. (1996). The structure of normal human attention: The Test of Everyday Attention. *Journal of the International Neuropsychological Society, 2,* 525–534.

Robey, R. R. (1998). A meta-analysis of clinical outcomes in the treatment of aphasia. *Journal of Speech, Language, and Hearing Research, 41,* 172–187.

Robey, R. R., & Dalebout, S. D. (1998). A tutorial on conducting meta-analyses of clinical outcome research. *Journal of Speech Language and Hearing Research, 41,* 1227–1241.

Robey, R. R., Schultz, M. C., Crawford, A. B., & Sinner, C. A. (1999). Single-subject clinical-outcome research: Designs, data, effect sizes, and analyses. *Aphasiology, 13,* 445–473.

Robinson, R. G., Kubos, K. L., Starr, L. B., Rao, K., & Price, T. R. (1984). Mood disorders in stroke patients: Importance of location of lesion. *Brain, 107,* 81–93.

Robinson, S., Druks, J., Hodges, J., & Garrard, P. (2009). The treatment of object naming, definition, and object use in semantic dementia: The effectiveness of errorless learning. *Aphasiology, 23,* 749–780.

Robson, J., Marshall, J., Pring, T., Montagu, A., & Chiat, S. (2004). Processing proper nouns in aphasia: Evidence from assessment and therapy. *Aphasiology, 18,* 917–935.

Rochon, E., Leonard, C., Burianova, H., Laird, L., Soros, P., Graham, S., & Grady, C. (2010). Neural changes after phonological treatment for anomia: An fMRI study. *Brain & Language, 114,* 164–179.

Rochon, E., Saffran, E. M., Berndt, R. S., & Schwartz, M. F. (2000). Quantitative analysis of aphasic sentence production: Further development and new data. *Brain and Language, 72,* 193–218.

Rochon, E., Waters, G. S., & Caplan, D. (1994). Sentence comprehension in patients with Alzheimer's disease. *Brain and Language, 46,* 329–349.

Rodriguez, A. D., Raymer, A. M., & Gonzalez Rothi, L. J. (2006). Effects of gesture+verbal and semantic-phonologic treatments for verb retrieval in aphasia. *Aphasiology, 20,* 286–297.

Rogalsky, C., Pitz, E., Hillis, A. E., & Hickok, G. (2008). Auditory word comprehension impairment in acute stroke: Relative contribution of phonemic versus semantic factors. *Brain and Language, 107,* 167–169.

Rogers, C. R. (1951). *Client-centered therapy.* Boston: Houghton Mifflin.

Rohde, A., Townley-O'Neill, K., Trendall, K., Worrall, L., & Cornwell, P. (2012). A comparison of client and therapist goals for people with aphasia: A qualitative exploratory study. *Aphasiology, 26,* 1298–1315.

Rohling, M. L., Faust, M. E., Beverly, B., & Demakis, G. (2009). Effectiveness of cognitive rehabilitation following acquired brain injury: A meta-analytic re-examination of Cicerone et al.'s (2000, 2005) systematic reviews. *Neuropsychology, 23,* 20–39.

Rolak, L. A. (Ed.). (1993). *Neurology secrets.* Philadelphia: Hanley & Belfus.

Roman, M., Brownell, H. H., Potter, H. H., Seibold, M. S., & Gardner, H. (1987). Script knowledge in right hemisphere-damaged and in normal elderly adults. *Brain and Language, 31,* 151–170.

Rose, M. (2006). The utility of arm and hand gestures in the treatment of aphasia. *Advances in Speech-Language Pathology, 8,* 92–109.

Rose, M. L. (2013). Releasing the constraints on aphasia therapy: The positive impact of gesture and multimodality treatments. *American Journal of Speech-Language Pathology* (Supplement), *22,* S227–S239.

Rose, M., & Douglas, J. (2008). Treating a semantic word production deficit in aphasia with verbal and gestural methods. *Aphasiology, 22,* 20–41.

Rose, S. (1989). *The conscious brain* (rev. ed.). New York: Paragon.

Rose, T. A., Worrall, L. E., Hickson, L. M., & Hoffman, T. C. (2011). Exploring the use of graphics in written health information for people with aphasia. *Aphasiology, 25,* 1579–1599.

Rosen, W. G., Mohs, R. C., & Davis, K. L. (1984). A new rating scale for Alzheimer's disease. *American Journal of Psychiatry, 141,* 1356–1364.

Rosenbek, J. C., LaPointe, L. L., & Wertz, R. T. (1989). *Aphasia: A clinical approach.* San Diego: Singular.

Rosenbek, J. C., Rodreiguez, A. D., Hieber, B., Leon, S. A., Crusian, G. P., et al. (2006). Effects of two treatments for aprosodia secondary to acquired brain injury. *Journal of Rehabilitation Research & Development, 43,* 379–390.

Rosenberg, B., Zurif, E., Brownell, H., Garrett, M., & Bradley, D. (1985). Grammatical class effects in relation to normal and aphasic sentence processing. *Brain and Language, 26,* 287–303.

Ross, A., Winslow, I., Marchant, P., & Brumfitt, S. (2006). Evaluation of communication, life participation and psychological well-being in chronic aphasia: The influence of group intervention. *Aphasiology, 20,* 427–448.

Ross, E. D. (1981). The aprosodias: Functional-anatomic organization of the affective components of language in the right hemisphere. *Archives of Neurology, 38,* 561–569.

Ross, E. D., & Mesulam, M. (1979). Dominant language functions of the right hemisphere? Prosody and emotional gesturing. *Archives of Neurology, 36,* 144–148.

Ross, E. D., & Monnot, M. (2008). Neurology of affective prosody and its functional-anatomic organization in right hemisphere. *Brain and Language, 104,* 51–74.

Ross, E. D., & Monnot, M. (2011). Affective prosody: What do comprehension errors tell us about hemispheric lateralization of emotions, sex and aging effects, and the role of cognitive appraisal. *Neuropsychologia, 49,* 866–877.

Ross, E. D., Thompson, R. D., & Yenkosky, J. (1997). Lateralization of affective prosody in brain and the collosal integration of hemispheric language functions. *Brain and Language, 56,* 27–54.

Ross, K. B., & Wertz, R. T. (1999). Comparison of impairment and disability measures for assessing severity of, and improvement in, aphasia. *Aphasiology, 13,* 113–124.

Ross, K. B., & Wertz, R. T. (2002). Relationships between language-based disability and quality of life in chronically aphasic adults. *Aphasiology, 16,* 791–800.

Ross, K. B., & Wertz, R. T. (2003). Quality of life with and without aphasia. *Aphasiology, 17,* 355–364.

Ross, K. B., & Wertz, R. T. (2004). Accuracy of formal tests for diagnosing mild aphasia: An application of evidence-based medicine. *Aphasiology, 18,* 337–355.

Ross, K. B., & Wertz, R. T. (2005). Advancing appraisal: Aphasia and the WHO. *Aphasiology, 19,* 860–870.

Rossi, E., & Bastiaanse, R. (2008). Spontaneous speech in Italian agrammatic aphasia: A focus on verb production. *Aphasiology, 22,* 347–362.

Rothi, L. J. G., Mack, L., Verfaellie, M., Brown, P., & Heilman, K. M. (1988). Ideomotor apraxia: Error pattern analysis. *Aphasiology, 2,* 381–388.

Rubens, A. B. (1977a). The role of changes within the central nervous system during recovery from aphasia. In M. Sullivan & M. S. Kommers (Eds.), *Rationale for adult aphasia therapy* (pp. 28–43). Omaha: University of Nebraska Medical Center.

Rubens, A. B. (1977b). What neurologists expect of clinical aphasiologists. In R. H. Brookshire (Ed.), *Clinical aphasiology conference proceedings* (pp. 1–4). Minneapolis, MN: BRK.

Ruff, R. M., Marshall, L. F., Crouch, J., & Klauber, M. R. (1993). Predictors of outcome following severe head trauma: Follow-up data from the Traumatic Coma Data Bank. *Brain Injury, 7,* 101–111.

Ruiter, M. B., Kolk, H. H. J., Rietveld, T. C. M., Dijkstra, N., & Lotgering, E. (2011). Towards a quantitative measure of verbal effectiveness and efficiency in the Amsterdam-Nijmegen Everyday Language Test (ANELT). *Aphasiology, 25,* 961–975.

Russell, W. R., & Espir, M. L. E. (1961). *Traumatic aphasia.* London: Oxford University Press.

Ryff, C. D. (1989). Happiness is everything, or is it? Explorations on the meaning of well-being. *Journal of Personality and Social Psychology, 57,* 1069–1081.

Sabbagh, M. A. (1999). Communicative intentions and language: Evidence from right-hemisphere damage and autism. *Brain and Language, 70,* 29–69.

Sabe, L., Salvarezza, F., Garcia Cuerva, A., Leiguarda, R., & Starkstein, S. (1995). A randomized, double-blind, placebo-controlled study of bromocriptine in nonfluent aphasia. *Neurology, 45,* 2272–2274.

Sacchett, C., & Black, M. (2011). Drawing as a window to event conceptualisation: Evidence from two people with aphasia. *Aphasiology, 25,* 3–26.

Sacks, O. (1985). *The man who mistook his wife for a hat and other clinical tales.* New York: Summit.

Saffran, E. M., Schwartz, M. F., & Linebarger, M. C. (1998). Semantic influences on thematic role assignment: Evidence from normals and aphasics. *Brain and Language, 62,* 255–297.

Sagar, H. J., Sullivan, E. V., & Corkin, S. (1991). Autobiographical memory in normal ageing and dementia. *Behavioural Neurology, 4,* 235–248.

Sage, K., & Ellis, A. W. (2006). Using orthographic neighbours to treat a case of graphemic buffer disorder. *Aphasiology, 20,* 851–870.

Sahraoui, H., & Nespoulous, J.-L. (2012). Across-task variability in agrammatic performance. *Aphasiology, 26,* 785–810.

Sajjadi, S. A., Patterson, K., Tomek, M., & Nestor, P. J. (2012). Abnormalities of connected speech in the non-semantic variants of primary progressive aphasia. *Aphasiology, 26,* 1219–1237.

Salvatore, A. P. (1985). Experimental analysis of acquisition and generalization of syntax in Broca's aphasia. In R. H. Brookshire (Ed.), *Clinical aphasiology* (Vol. 15, pp. 214–221). Minneapolis, MN: BRK.

Salvatore, A. P., & Sirmon Fjordbak, B. (2011). Concussion management: The speech-language pathologist's role. *Medical Speech-Language Pathology, 19,* 1–12.

Samples, J. M., & Lane, V. W. (1980). Language gains in global aphasia over a three-year period: Case study. *Journal of Communication Disorders, 13,* 49–57.

Sampson, M., & Faroqi-Shah, Y. (2011). Investigation of self-monitoring in fluent aphasia with jargon. *Aphasiology, 25,* 505–528.

Sanders, S. B., & Davis, G. A. (1978). A comparison of the Porch Index of Communicative Ability and the Western Aphasia Battery. In R. H. Brookshire (Ed.), *Clinical aphasiology conference proceedings* (pp. 117–126). Minneapolis, MN: BRK.

Sands, E., Sarno, M. T., & Shankweiler, D. (1969). Long-term assessment of language function in aphasia due to stroke. *Archives of Physical Medicine and Rehabilitation, 50,* 202–207.

Santo Pietro, M. J., & Boczko, F. (1998). The Breakfast Club: Results of a study examining the effectiveness of a multi-modality group communication treatment. *American Journal of Alzheimer's Disease, 13,* 146–158.

Saporta S. (Ed.). (1961). *Psycholinguistics: A book of readings.* New York: Holt, Rinehart and Winston.

Sarno, J. E., Sarno, M. T., & Levita, E. (1971). Evaluating language improvement after completed stroke. *Archives of Physical Medicine and Rehabilitation, 52,* 73–78.

Sarno, M. T. (1969). *The functional communication profile manual of directions.* Rehabilitation Monograph *42,* New York University Medical Center.

Sarno, M. T. (1980). The nature of verbal impairment after closed head injury. *Journal of Nervous and Mental Disease, 168,* 685–692.

Sarno, M. T. (1993). Aphasia rehabilitation: Psychosocial and ethical considerations. *Aphasiology, 7,* 321–334.

Sarno, M. T., Buonaguro, A., & Levita, E. (1987). Aphasia in closed head injury and stroke. *Aphasiology, 1,* 331–338.

Sarno, M. T., & Levita, E. (1971). Natural course of recovery in severe aphasia. *Archives of Physical Medicine and Rehabilitation, 52,* 175–178.

Sarno, M. T., & Levita, E. (1979). Recovery in treated aphasia during the first year post-stroke. *Stroke, 10,* 663–670.

Sarno, M. T., & Levita, E. (1981). Some observations on the nature of recovery in global aphasia after stroke. *Brain and Language, 13,* 1–12.

Sarno, M. T., Silverman, M., & Sands, E. (1970). Speech therapy and language recovery in severe aphasia. *Journal of Speech and Hearing Research, 13,* 607–623.

Saur, D., Lange, R., Baumgaertner, A., Schraknepper, V., Willmes, K., et al. (2006). Dynamics of language reorganization after stroke. *Brain, 129,* 1371–1384.

Saur, D., Ronneberger, O., Kümmerer, D., Mader, I., Weiller, C., et al. (2010). Early functional magnetic resonance imaging activations predict language outcome after stroke. *Brain, 133,* 1252–1264.

Schacter, D. L. (1996). *Searching for memory: The brain, the mind, and the past.* New York: BasicBooks.

Schacter, D. L., & Graf, P. (1986). Preserved learning in amnesic patients: Perspectives from research on direct priming. *Journal of Clinical and Experimental Neuropsychology, 8,* 727–743.

Scharp, V. L., & Tompkins, C. A. (2013) Suppression and narrative time shifts in adults with right-hemisphere brain damage. *American Journal of Speech-Language Pathology* (Supplement), *22,* S256–S267

Scharp, V. L., Tompkins, C. A., & Iverson, J. M. (2007). Gesture and aphasia: Helping hands? *Aphasiology, 21,* 717–725.

Scheinberg, S., & Holland, A. (1980). Conversational turn-taking in Wernicke's aphasia. In R. Brookshire (Ed.), *Clinical aphasiology conference proceedings* (pp. 106–110). Minneapolis, MN: BRK.

Scherzer, E. (1992). Functional assessment: A clinical perspective. *Aphasiology, 6,* 101–104.

Schiffrin, D. (2006). Discourse. In R. W. Fasold, & J. Connor-Linton (Eds.). *An introduction to language and linguistics* (pp. 169–203). Cambridge, UK: Cambridge University Press.

Schlanger, B. B., Schlanger, P., & Gerstman, L. J. (1976). The perception of emotionally toned sentences by right hemisphere-damaged and aphasic subjects. *Brain and Language, 3,* 396–403.

Schlanger, P. H., & Schlanger, B. B. (1970). Adapting role playing activities with aphasic patients. *Journal of Speech and Hearing Disorders, 35,* 229–235.

Schlaug, G., Renga, V., & Nair, D. (2008). Transcranial direct current stimulation in stroke recovery. *Archives of Neurology, 65,* 1571–1576.

Schmidt, P. A., & Dark, V. J. (1998). Attentional processing of "unattended" flankers: Evidence for a failure of selective attention. *Perception & Psychophysics, 60,* 227–238.

Schmitter-Edgecombe, M. E., Marks, W., Fahy, J. F., & Long, C. J. (1992). Effects of severe closed-head injury on three stages of information processing. *Journal of Clinical and Experimental Neuropsychology, 14,* 717–737.

Schneider, S. L., & Thompson, C. K. (2003). Verb production in agrammatic aphasia: The influence of semantic class and argument structure properties on generalization. *Aphasiology, 17,* 213–241.

Schnitzer, M. L. (1978). Toward a neurolinguistic theory of language. *Brain and Language, 6,* 342–361.

Schretlin, D., Bobholz, J. H., & Brandt, J. (1996). Development and psychometric properties of the Brief Test of Attention. *Clinical Neuropsychologist, 10,* 80–89.

Schriefers, H., Meyer, A. S., & Levelt, W. J. M. (1990). Exploring the time course of lexical access in language production: Picture-word interference studies. *Journal of Memory and Language, 29,* 86–102.

Schuell, H. M. (1965). *Minnesota Test for Differential Diagnosis of Aphasia.* Minneapolis: University of Minnesota Press.

Schuell, H. M. (1966). A re-evaluation of the short examination for aphasia. *Journal of Speech and Hearing Disorders, 31,* 137–147.

Schuell, H. M. (1969). *Aphasia in adults.* In *Human communication and its disorders—an overview.* Bethesda, MD: U.S. Department of Health, Education, and Welfare.

Schuell, H. M. (1973). *Differential diagnosis of aphasia with the Minnesota test* (2nd ed., revised by Sefer, J. W.). Minneapolis: University of Minnesota Press.

Schuell, H. M., & Jenkins, J. J. (1961). Reduction of vocabulary in aphasia. *Brain, 84,* 243–261.

Schuell, H. M., Jenkins, J. J., & Jimenez-Pabon, E. (1964). *Aphasia in adults.* New York: Harper and Row.

Schulz, R. (2000). *Handbook on dementia caregiving.* New York: Springer.

Schwartz, M. F. (1987). Patterns of speech production deficit within and across aphasia syndromes: Application of a psycholinguistic model. In M. Coltheart, G. Sartori, & R. Job (Eds.). *The cognitive neuropsychology of language* (pp. 163–199). London: Erlbaum.

Schwartz, M. F., Dell, G. S., Martin, N., Gahl, S., & Sobel, P. (2006). A case-series test of the interactive two-step model of lexical access: Evidence from picture naming. *Journal of Memory and Language, 54,* 223–264.

Schwartz, M. F., Linebarger, M. C., & Saffran, E. M. (1985). The status of the syntactic deficit theory of agrammatism. In M.-L. Kean (Ed.), *Agrammatism* (pp. 83–124). Orlando, FL: Academic Press.

Schwartz, M. F., Linebarger, M. C., Saffran, E. M., & Pate, D. S. (1987). Syntactic transparency and sentence interpretation in aphasia. *Language and Cognitive Processes, 2,* 85–114.

Schwartz, M. F., Saffran, E. M., Fink, R., Myers, J., & Martin, N. (1994). Mapping therapy: A treatment programme for agrammatism. *Aphasiology, 8,* 19–54.

Schwartz, M. F., Saffran, E. M., & Marin, O. S. M. (1980). The word order problem in agrammatism. I. Comprehension. *Brain and Language, 10,* 249–262.

Schwartz, M. F., Wilshire, C. E., Gagnon, D. A., & Polansky, M. (2004). Origins of nonword phonological errors in aphasic picture naming. *Cognitive Neuropsychology, 21,* 159–186.

Schwartz, R. G. (2009). (Ed.). *Handbook of child language disorders.* New York: Psychology Press.

Schwartz-Cowley, R., & Stepanik, M. J. (1989). Communication disorders and treatment in the acute trauma center setting. *Topics in Language Disorders, 9,* 1–14.

Schweinberger, S. R. (1995). Personal name recognition and associative priming in patients with unilateral brain damage. *Brain and Cognition, 29,* 23–35.

Scott, C., & Byng, S. (1989). Computer assisted remediation of a homophone comprehension disorder in surface dyslexia. *Aphasiology, 3,* 301–320.

Scoville, W. B., & Milner, B. (1957). Loss of recent memory after bilateral hippocampal lesions. *Journal of Neurology, Neurosurgery and Psychiatry, 20,* 11–21.

Searle, J. R. (1969). *Speech acts.* London: Cambridge University Press.

Sebastian, R., & Kiran, S. (2011). Task-modulated neural activation patterns in chronic stroke patients with aphasia. *Aphasiology, 25,* 927–951.

Seddoh, S. A. (2002). How discrete or independent are "affective prosody" and "linguistic prosody"? *Aphasiology, 16,* 683–692.

Seddoh, S. A. (2008). Conceptualisation of deviations in intonation production in aphasia. *Aphasiology, 22,* 1294–1312.

Seddoh, S. A., Robin, D., Sim, H., Hageman, C., Moon, J., et al. (1996). Speech timing in apraxia of speech versus conduction aphasia. *Journal of Speech, Language, and Hearing Research, 39,* 590–603.

Seel, R. T., Kreutzer, J. S., Rosenthal, M., Hammond, F. M., Corrigan, J. S., et al. (2003). Depression after traumatic brain injury: A National Institute on Disability and Rehabilitation Model Systems multicenter investigation. *Archives of Physical Medicine and Rehabilitation, 84,* 177–184.

Seidenberg, M. S., Tanenhaus, M. K., Leiman, J. M., & Bienkowski, M. (1982). Automatic access of the meanings of ambiguous words in context: Some limitations of knowledge-based processing. *Cognitive Psychology, 14,* 489–537.

Senelick, R. C. (2010). *Living with stroke: A guide for families* (4th ed.). Birmingham, AL: Healthsouth Press.

Seron, X., & de Partz, M.-P. (1993). The re-education of aphasics: Between theory and practice. In A. L. Holland & M. M. Forbes (Eds.), *Aphasia treatment: World perspectives* (pp. 131–144). San Diego, CA: Singular.

Seron, X., Van Der Kaa, M., Remitz, A., & Van Der Linden, M. (1979). Pantomime interpretation and aphasia. *Neuropsychologia, 17,* 661–668.

Shadden, B. B. (2007). Rebuilding identity through stroke support groups: Embracing the person with aphasia and significant others. In R. J. Elman (Ed.), *Group treatment of neurogenic communication disorders* (pp. 111–126). San Diego, CA: Plural Publishing.

Shah, A. P., Baum, S. R., & Dwivedi, V. D. (2006). Neural substrates of linguistic prosody: Evidence from syntactic disambiguation in the production of brain-damaged patients. *Brain and Language, 96,* 78–89.

Shahripour, R. B., Shamsaei, G., Pakdamen, H., Majdinasab, N., Nejad, E. M, et al. (2011). The effect of NeuroAiD™ (MLC601) on cerebral blood flow velocity in subjects' post brain infarct in the middle cerebral artery territory. *European Journal of Internal Medicine, 22,* 509–513.

Shallice, T., & Warrington, E. K. (1977). Auditory-verbal short-term memory impairment and spontaneous speech. *Brain and Language, 4,* 479–491.

Shapiro, B. E., & Danly, M. (1985). The role of the right hemisphere in the control of speech prosody in propositional and affective contexts. *Brain and Language, 25,* 19–36.

Shapiro, B. E., Grossman, M., & Gardner, H. (1981). Selective musical processing deficits in brain damaged populations. *Neuropsychologia, 19,* 161–169.

Shapiro, L. P., Gordon, B., Hack, N., & Killackey, J. (1993). Verb-argument structure processing in complex sentences in Broca's and Wernicke's aphasia. *Brain and Language, 45,* 423–447.

Shapiro, L. P., & Levine, B. A. (1990). Verb processing during sentence comprehension in aphasia. *Brain and Language, 38,* 21–47.

Shapiro, L. P., Swinney, D., & Borsky, S. (1998). Online examination of language performance in normal and neurologically impaired adults. *American Journal of Speech-Language Pathology, 7,* 49–60.

Shapiro, L. P., & Thompson, C. K. (2006). Treating language deficits in Broca's aphasia. In Y. Grodzinsky & K. Amunts (Eds.), *Broca's region* (pp. 119–134). New York: Oxford University Press.

Sheehan, V. M. (1946). Rehabilitation of aphasics in an army hospital. *Journal of Speech and Hearing Disorders, 11,* 149–157.

Sheehy, L. M., & Haines, M. E. (2004). Crossed Wernicke's aphasia: A case report. *Brain and Language, 89,* 203–206.

Shelton, J. R., & Caramazza, A. (2001). The organization of semantic memory. In B. Rapp (Ed.), *The handbook of cognitive neuropsychology* (pp. 423–443). Philadelphia: Psychology Press.

Shelton, J. R., Weinrich, M., McCall, D., & Cox, D. M. (1996). Differentiating globally aphasic patients: Data from in-depth language assessments and production training using C-VIC. *Aphasiology, 10,* 319–342.

Shenaut, G. K., & Ober, B. A. (1996). Methodological control of semantic priming in Alzheimer's disease. *Psychology and Aging, 11,* 443–448.

Shenk, D. (2002). *The forgetting: Alzheimer's: Portrait of an epidemic.* New York: Anchor Books.

Shephard, J. M., & Kosslyn, S. M. (2005). The Minicog Rapid Assessment Battery: Developing a "blood pressure cuff for the mind." *Aviation, Space & Environmental Medicine, 76,* B192–197.

Sherer, M., Parsons, O. A., Nixon, S. J., & Adams, R. L. (1991). Clinical validity of the Speech-Sounds Perception Test and the Seashore Rhythm Test. *Journal of Clinical and Experimental Neuropsychology, 13,* 741–751.

Sherer, M., Sander, A. M., Nick, T. G., High, W. M., Jr., Males, J. F., et al. (2002). Early cognitive status and productivity outcome after traumatic brain injury: Findings from the TBI Model Systems. *Archives of Physical Medicine and Rehabilitation, 83,* 183–192.

Sherratt, S. (2007). Right brain damage and the verbal expression of emotion: A preliminary investigation. *Aphasiology, 21,* 320–339.

Shewan, C. M. (1979). *Auditory Comprehension Test for Sentences.* Chicago: Biolinguistics Clinical Institutes.

Shewan, C. M. (1982). To hear is not to understand: Auditory processing deficits and factors influencing performance in aphasic individuals. In N. J. Lass (Ed.), *Speech and language: Advances in basic research and practice* (Vol. 7, pp. 1–70). New York: Academic Press.

Shewan, C. M., & Bandur, D. L. (1986). *Treatment of aphasia: A language-oriented approach.* San Diego, CA: Singular.

Shewan, C. M., & Canter, G. J. (1971). Effects of vocabulary, syntax, and sentence length on auditory comprehension in aphasic patients. *Cortex, 7,* 209–226.

Shewan, C. M., & Kertesz, A. (1980). Reliability and validity characteristics of the Western Aphasia Battery (WAB). *Journal of Speech and Hearing Disorders, 45,* 308–324.

Shewan, C. M., & Kertesz, A. (1984). Effects of speech and language treatment on recovery from aphasia. *Brain and Language, 23,* 272–299.

Shuster, L. I. (2004). Resource theory and aphasia reconsidered: Why alternative theories can better guide our research. *Aphasiology, 18,* 811–830.

Shuster, L. I., & Thompson, J. C. (2004). Resource theory: Here, there, and everywhere. *Aphasiology, 18,* 850–854.

SI.com. (2002). Teenager struck by puck dies. Retrieved September 5, 2012, from http://www.sportsillustrated.cnn.com/hockey/news/2002/03/19/puck_death_ap/

Sidtis, J. J. (2007). Some problems for representations of brain organization based on activation in functional imaging. *Brain and Language, 102,* 130–140.

Sidtis, J. J., & Volpe, B. T. (1988). Selective loss of complex-pitch or speech discrimination after unilateral lesion. *Brain and Language, 34,* 235–245.

Sies, L. F. (Ed.). (1974). *Aphasia theory and therapy: Selected lectures and papers of Hildred Schuell.* Baltimore: University Park Press.

Silberman, E. K., & Weingartner, H. (1986). Hemispheric lateralization of functions related to emotion. *Brain and Cognition, 5,* 322–354.

Simmons, N. N., Kearns, K. P., & Potechin, G. (1987). Treatment of aphasia through family member training. In R. H. Brookshire (Ed.), *Clinical aphasiology* (Vol. 17, pp. 106–116). Minneapolis, MN: BRK.

Simmons-Mackie, N. (2005). Conduction aphasia. In L. L. LaPointe (Ed.), *Aphasia and related neurogenic language disorders* (3rd ed., pp. 155–168). New York: Thieme.

Simmons-Mackie, N. (2008). Social approaches to aphasia intervention. In R. Chapey (Ed.), *Language intervention strategies in aphasia and related neurogenic communication disorders* (5th ed., pp. 290–318). Philadelphia: Wolters Kluwer Health.

Simmons-Mackie, N., Code, C., Armstrong, E., Stiegler, L., & Elman, R. (2002). What is aphasia? Results of an international survey. *Aphasiology, 16,* 837–848.

Simmons-Mackie, N. N., & Damico, J. S. (1996). The contribution of discourse markers to communicative competence in aphasia. *American Journal of Speech-Language Pathology, 5,* 37–43.

Simmons-Mackie, N. N., & Damico, J. S. (1997). Reformulating the definition of compensatory strategies in aphasia. *Aphasiology, 11,* 761–781.

Simmons-Mackie, N., & Damico, J. S. (2007). Access and social inclusion in aphasia: Interactional principles and applications. *Aphasiology, 21,* 81–97.

Simmons-Mackie, N., Elman, R. J., Holland, A. L., & Damico, J. S. (2007). Management of discourse in group therapy for aphasia. *Topics in Language Disorders, 27,* 5–23.

Simmons-Mackie, N. N., & Kagan, A. (1999). Communication strategies used by 'good' versus 'poor' speaking partners of individuals with aphasia. *Aphasiology, 13,* 807–820.

Simmons-Mackie, N., Kagan, A., O'Neill Christie, C., Huijbregts, M., McEwen, S., et al. (2007). Communicative access and decision making for people with aphasia: Implementing sustainable healthcare systems change. *Aphasiology, 22,* 39–66.

Simmons-Mackie, N., Kingston, D., & Schultz, M. (2004). Speaking for another: The management of participant frames in aphasia. *American Journal of Speech Language Pathology, 13,* 114–127.

Simon, A. (2012). No "aphasia" for Giffords? *ASHA Leader, 17*(4), 4.

Simpson, G. B., & Burgess, C. (1985). Activation and selection processes in the recognition of ambiguous words. *Journal of Experimental Psychology: Human Perception and Performance, 11,* 28–39.

Skelly, M. (1975). Aphasic patients talk back. *American Journal of Nursing, 75,* 1140–1142.

Skelly, M. (1979). *Amer-Ind gestural code based on universal American Indian hand talk.* New York: Elsevier.

Skilbeck, C. E., Wade, D. T., Hewer, R. L., & Wood, V. A. (1983). Recovery after stroke. *Journal of Neurology, Neurosurgery, and Psychiatry, 46,* 5–8.

Skotko, B. G., Andrews, E., & Einstein, G. (2005). Language and the medial temporal lobe: Evidence from H. M.'s spontaneous discourse. *Journal of Memory and Language, 53,* 397–415.

Small, J. A., Gutman, G., Makela, S., & Hillhouse, B. (2003). Effectiveness of communication strategies used by caregivers of persons with Alzheimer's disease during activities of daily living. *Journal of Speech, Language, and Hearing Research, 46,* 353–367.

Small, J. A., & Perry, J. (2005). Do you remember? How caregivers question their spouses who have Alzheimer's disease and the impact on communication. *Journal of Speech, Language, and Hearing Research, 48,* 125–136.

Small, J. A., & Sandhu, N. (2008). Episodic and semantic memory influences on picture naming in Alzheimer's disease. *Brain and Language, 104,* 1–9.

Small, S. L. (2002). Biological approaches to the treatment of aphasia. In A. E. Hillis (Ed.), *The handbook of adult language disorders* (pp. 397–411). New York: Psychology Press.

Small, S. L. (2004). A biological model of aphasia rehabilitation: Pharmacological perspectives. *Aphasiology, 18,* 476–491.

Smith, F. (1982). *Understanding reading: A psycholinguistic analysis of reading and learning to read* (3rd ed.). New York: Holt, Rinehart and Winston.

Smith, T., Gildeh, N., & Holmes, C. (2007). The Montreal Cognitive Assessment: Validity and utility in a memory clinic setting. *Canadian Journal of Psychiatry, 52,* 329–332.

Snyder, P. J., Nussbaum, P. D., & Robins, D. L. (2006). *Clinical neuropsychology: A pocket handbook for assessment* (2nd ed.). Washington, DC: American Psychological Association.

Sohlberg, M. M., Avery, J., Kennedy, M., Ylvisaker, M., Coelho, C., et al. (2003). Practice guidelines for direct attention training. *Journal of Medical Speech-Language Pathology, 11,* xix–xxxix.

Sohlberg, M. M., & Mateer, C. A. (1987). Effectiveness of an attention training program. *Journal of Clinical and Experimental Neuropsychology, 9,* 117–130.

Sohlberg, M. M., & Mateer, C. A. (1989). Training use of compensatory memory books: A three-stage behavioral approach. *Journal of Clinical and Experimental Neuropsychology, 11,* 871–891.

Sohlberg, M. M., & Mateer, C. A. (2001). *Cognitive rehabilitation: An integrative neuropsychological approach.* New York: Guilford Press.

Sohlberg, M. M., & Mateer, C. (2011). *Attention Process Training APT-3: Direct Attention Training Program for Persons with Acquired Brain Injury*. Youngsville, NC: Lash & Associates.

Sohlberg, M. M., McLaughlin, K., Pavese, A., Heidrich, A., & Posner, M. (2000). Evaluation of attention process training and brain injury education in persons with acquired brain injury. *Journal of Clinical and Experimental Neuropsychology, 22*, 656–676.

Sohlberg, M. M., Turkstra, L. S., & Wilson, B. A. (2011). *Optimizing cognitive rehabilitation: Effective instructional methods*. New York: Guilford Press.

Sohlberg, M. M., White, O., Evans, E., & Mateer, C. A. (1992). An investigation into the effects of prospective memory training. *Brain Injury, 6*, 139–154.

Sohrabi, H. R., Weinborn, M., Badcock, J., Bates, K. A., Clarnette, R., et al. (2011). New lexicon and criteria for the diagnosis of Alzheimer's disease. *Lancet Neurology, 10*, 299–300.

Sokoloff, L. (1989). Circulation and energy metabolism of the brain. In G. Segal, B. Agranoff, R. W. Albers, & P. Molinoff (Eds.), *Basic neurochemistry* (pp. 565–590). New York: Raven Press.

Solin, D. (1989). The systematic misrepresentation of bilingual-crossed aphasia data and its consequences. *Brain and Language, 36*, 92–116.

Solso, R. L. (1988). *Cognitive psychology* (2nd ed.). Boston: Allyn & Bacon.

Song, A. W., Huettel, S. A., & McCarthy, G. (2006). Functional neuroimaging: Basic principles of functional MRI. In R. Cabeza, & A. Kingstone (Eds.). *Handbook of functional neuroimaging of cognition* (2nd ed., pp. 21–52). Cambridge, MA: MIT Press.

Soni, M., Lambon Ralph, M. A., & Woollams, A. M. (2012). Repetition priming of picture naming in semantic aphasia: The impact of intervening items. *Aphasiology, 26*, 44–63.

Sorin-Peters, R., McGilton, K. S., & Rochon, E. (2010). The development and evaluation of a training programme for nurses working with persons with communication disorders in a complex continuing care facility. *Aphasiology, 24*, 1511–1536.

Sparks, R. W. (1978). Parastandardized examination guidelines for adult aphasia. *British Journal of Disorders of Communication, 13*, 135–146.

Sparks, R. W., Helm, N. A., & Albert, M. L. (1974). Aphasia rehabilitation resulting from melodic intonation therapy. *Cortex, 10*, 303–316.

Sparks, R. W., & Holland, A. L. (1976). Method: Melodic intonation therapy for aphasia. *Journal of Speech and Hearing Disorders, 41*, 287–297.

Spector, A., Orrell, M., Davies, S., & Woods, B. (2001). Can reality orientation be rehabilitated? Development and piloting of an evidence-based programme of cognition-based therapies for people with dementia. *Neuropsychological Rehabilitation, 11*, 377–397.

Spellacy, F. J., & Spreen, O. (1969). A short form of the Token Test. *Cortex, 5*, 390–397.

Sperber, D., & Wilson, D. (1986). *Relevance: Communication and cognition*. Cambridge, MA: Harvard University Press.

Spreen, O., & Benton, A. L. (1977). *Neurosensory center comprehensive examination for aphasia* (NCCEA) (Revised). Victoria, British Columbia: Neuropsychology Laboratory, University of Victoria.

Springer, L., Glindemann, R., Huber, W., & Willmes, K. (1991). How efficacious is PACE-therapy when "Language Systematic Training" is incorporated? *Aphasiology, 5*, 391–399.

Springer, L., Huber, W., Schlenck, K.-J., & Schlenck, C. (2000). Agrammatism: Deficit or compensation? Consequences for aphasia therapy. *Neuropsychological Rehabilitation, 10*, 279–309.

Springer, S. P., & Deutsch, G. (1998). *Left brain, right brain* (5th ed.). New York: W. H. Freeman.

Squire, L. R. (1987). *Memory and brain*. New York: Oxford University Press.

Stadie, N., Schröder, A., Postler, J., Lorenz, A., Swoboda-Moll, M., et al. (2008). Unambiguous generalization effects after treatment of non-canonical sentence production in German agrammatism. *Brain and Language, 104*, 211–229.

Stambrook, M., Moore, A. D., Peters, L. C., Zubek, E., McBeath, S., et al. (1991). Head injury and spinal cord injury: Differential effects on psychosocial functioning. *Journal of Clinical and Experimental Neuropsychology, 13*, 521–530.

Stanczak, L., Waters, G., & Caplan, D. (2006). Typicality-based learning and generalisation in aphasia: Two case studies of anomia treatment. *Aphasiology, 20*, 374–383.

Stanovich, K. E. (2007). *How to think straight about psychology* (8th ed.). Boston: Allyn and Bacon.

Starch, S., & Falltrick, E. (1990). The importance of a home evaluation for brain injured clients: A team approach. *Cognitive Rehabilitation, 8*(6), 28–32.

Starkstein, S. E., & Robinson, R. G. (1988). Aphasia and depression. *Aphasiology, 2*, 1–20.

State University of New York at Buffalo. (1990). *Guide for use of the uniform data set for medical rehabilitation*. Buffalo, NY: Research Foundation.

Stein, J. (2004). *Stroke and the family: A new guide*. Cambridge, MA: Harvard University Press.

Stein, N. L., & Glenn, C. G. (1979). An analysis of story comprehension in elementary school children. In R. O. Freedle (Ed.), *New directions in discourse processes* (pp. 53–120). Norwood, NJ: Ablex.

Stemmer, B., Giroux, F., & Joanette, Y. (1994). Production and evaluation of requests by right hemisphere brain-damaged individuals. *Brain and Language, 47,* 1–31.

Stenneken, P., Hofmann, M. J., & Jacobs, A. M. (2008). Sublexical units in aphasic jargon and in the standard language: Comparative analyses of neologisms in connected speech. *Aphasiology, 22,* 1142–1156.

Sternberg, S. (1975). Memory scanning: New findings and current controversies. In D. Deutsch & J. A. Deutsch (Eds.), *Short-term memory.* New York: Academic Press.

Stimley, M. A., & Noll, J. D. (1991). The effects of semantic and phonemic prestimulation cues on picture naming in aphasia. *Brain and Language, 41,* 496–509.

Stimley, M. A., & Noll, J. D. (1994). The effects of communication partner familiarity on the verbal abilities of aphasic adults. *Aphasiology, 8,* 173–180.

Stokes, T. F., & Baer, D. M. (1977). An implied technology of generalization. *Journal of Applied Behavior Analysis, 10,* 349–357.

Stoler, D. R., & Hill, B. A. (1998). *Coping with mild traumatic brain injury: A guide to living with the challenges associated with concussion/brain injury.* New York: Avery.

Strand, E. A. (1995). Ethical issues related to progressive disease. *Special Interest Division 2 Newsletter, 5*(3), 3–8.

Stubbs, M. (1983). *Discourse analysis: The sociolinguistic analysis of natural language.* Chicago: University of Chicago Press.

Sunderland, A., Harris, J. E., & Baddeley, A. D. (1983). Do laboratory tests predict everyday memory? A neuropsychological study. *Journal of Verbal Learning and Verbal Behavior, 22,* 341–357.

Sundet, K. (1986). Sex differences in cognitive impairment following unilateral brain damage. *Journal of Clinical and Experimental Neuropsychology, 8,* 51–61.

Sung, J. E., McNeil, M. R., Pratt, S. R., Dickey, M. W., Fassbinder, W., et al. (2011). Real-time processing in reading sentence comprehension for normal adult individuals and persons with aphasia. *Aphasiology, 25,* 57–70.

Sung, J. E., McNeil, M. R., Pratt, S. R., Dickey, M. W., Hula, W. D., et al. (2009). Verbal working memory and its relationship to sentence-level reading and listening comprehension in persons with aphasia. *Aphasiology, 23,* 1040–1052.

Sutton, M. (2012). APP-titude: Apps for brain injury rehab. Retrieved September 9, 2012, from http://www.asha.org/Publications/Leader/2012/120703

Swaab, T. Y., Brown, C., & Hagoort, P. (1998). Understanding ambiguous words in sentence contexts: Electrophysiological evidence for delayed contextual selection in Broca's aphasia. *Neuropsychologia, 36,* 737–761.

Swet, P. (1998). *Cracking up: Nice day for a brain hemorrhage.* Center City, MN: Hazelden.

Swinburn, K., Porter, G., & Howard, D. (2005). *The Comprehensive Aphasia Test.* Hove, UK: Psychology Press.

Swindell, C. S., Holland, A. L., & Fromm, D. (1984). Classification of aphasia: WAB type versus clinical impression. In R. H. Brookshire (Ed.), *Clinical aphasiology conference proceedings* (pp. 48–54). Minneapolis, MN: BRK.

Swindell, C. S., Holland, A. L., Fromm, D., & Greenhouse, J. B. (1988). Characteristics of recovery of drawing ability in left and right brain-damaged subjects. *Brain and Cognition, 7,* 16–30.

Swinney, D. A. (1979). Lexical access during sentence comprehension: (Re)consideration of context effects. *Journal of Verbal Learning and Verbal Behavior, 20,* 645–660.

Swinney, D. A., & Zurif, E. (1995). Syntactic processing in aphasia. *Brain and Language, 50,* 225–239.

Swinney, D. A., Zurif, E., & Cutler, A. (1980). Effects of sentential stress and word class upon comprehension in Broca's aphasics. *Brain and Language, 10,* 132–144.

Swinney, D. A., Zurif, E., & Nicol, J. (1989). The effects of focal brain damage on sentence processing: An examination of the neurological organization of a mental module. *Journal of Cognitive Neuroscience, 1,* 25–37.

Swisher, L. P., & Sarno, M. T. (1969). Token Test scores of three matched patient groups: Left brain-damaged with aphasia; right brain-damaged without aphasia, non-brain damaged. *Cortex, 5,* 264–273.

Taber, K. H., Warden, D. L., & Hurley, R. A. (2006). Blast-related traumatic brain injury: What is known? *Journal of Neuropsychiatry & Clinical Neurosciences.* Retrieved September 8, 2012, from http://neuro.psychiatryonline.org/article.aspx?articleid=102725

Tanner, D. C., & Gerstenberger, D. L. (1988). The grief response in neuropathologies of speech and language. *Aphasiology, 2,* 79–84.

Tanridag, O., Kirshner, H. S., & Casey, P. F. (1987). Memory functions in aphasic and non-aphasic stroke patients. *Aphasiology, 1,* 201–214.

Taub, E., Crago, J. E., Burgio, L. D., Groomes, T. E., Cook, E. W., et al. (1994). An operant approach to rehabilitation medicine: Overcoming learned nonuse by shaping. *Journal of Experimental Analysis of Behavior, 61,* 281–293.

Taylor, J. B. (2006). *My stroke of insight: A brain scientist's personal journey.* New York: Viking.

Taylor, M. L., & Marks, M. M. (1959). *Aphasia rehabilitation manual and therapy kit.* New York: McGraw-Hill.

Teng, E. L., & Chui, H. C. (1987). The modified minimental state (3MS) examination. *Journal of Clinical Psychiatry, 48,* 314–318.

Tesak, J., & Niemi, J. (1997). Telegraphese and agrammatism: A cross-linguistic study. *Aphasiology, 11,* 145–155.

Thiel, A., Habedank, B., Herholz, K., Kessler, J., Winhuisen, L., et al. (2006). From the left to the right: How the brain compensates progressive loss of language function. *Brain and Language, 98,* 57–65.

Thompson, C. K. (1989). Generalization research in aphasia: A review of the literature. In T. E. Prescott (Ed). *Clinical aphasiology* (Vol. 18, pp. 195–222). Austin, TX: Pro-Ed.

Thompson, C. K. (2005). Functional neuroimaging: Applications for studying aphasia. In L. L. LaPointe (Ed.), *Aphasia and related neurogenic language disorders* (3rd ed., pp. 19–38). New York: Thieme.

Thompson, C. K. (2008). Treatment of syntactic and morphologic deficits in agrammatic aphasia: Treatment of underlying forms. In R. Chapey (Ed.), *Language intervention strategies in aphasia and related neurogenic communication disorders* (5th ed., pp. 735–755). Philadelphia: Wolters Kluwer Health.

Thompson, C. K. and Byrne, M. E. (1984). Across setting generalization of social conventions in aphasia: An experimental analysis of "loose training." In R. H. Brookshire (Ed.), *Clinical aphasiology conference proceedings* (pp. 132–144). Minneapolis, MN: BRK.

Thompson, C. K., Cho, S., Hsu, C.-J., Wieneke, C., Rademaker, A., et al. (2012). Dissociations between fluency and agrammatism in primary progressive aphasia. *Aphasiology, 26,* 20–43.

Thompson, C. K., Cho, S., Price, C., Wieneke, C., Bonakdarpour, B., et al. (2012). Semantic interference during object naming in agrammatic and logopenic primary progressive aphasia. *Brain and Language, 120,* 237–250.

Thompson, C. K., Choy, J. J., Holland, A., & Cole, R. (2010). Sentactics®: Computer-automated treatment of underlying forms. *Aphasiology, 24,* 1242–1266.

Thompson, C. K., den Ouden, D.-B., Bonakdarpour, B., Garibaldi, K., & Parrish, T. B. (2010). Neural plasticity and treatment-induced recovery of sentence processing in agrammatism. *Neuropsychologia, 48,* 3211–3227.

Thompson, C. K., & Johnson, N. (2006). Language interventions in dementia. In D. K. Attix & K. A. Welsh-Bohmer (Eds.), *Geriatric neuropsychology: Assessment and intervention* (pp. 315–332). New York: Guilford Press.

Thompson, C. K., & Kearns, K. P. (1981). An experimental analysis of acquisition, generalization, and maintenance of naming behavior in a patient with anomia. In R. H. Brookshire (Ed.), *Clinical aphasiology conference proceedings* (pp. 35–45). Minneapolis, MN: BRK.

Thompson, C. K., Lange, K. L., Schneider, S. L., & Shapiro, L. P. (1997). Agrammatic and non-brain-damaged subjects' verb and verb argument structure production. *Aphasiology, 11,* 473–490.

Thompson, C. K., Lukic, S., King, M. C., Mesulam, M. M., & Weintraub, S. (2012). Verb and noun deficits in stroke-induced and primary progressive aphasia: The Northwestern Naming Battery. *Aphasiology, 26,* 632–655.

Thompson, C. K., & McReynolds, L. V. (1986). *Wh* interrogative production in agrammatic aphasia: An experimental analysis of auditory-visual stimulation and direct-production treatment. *Journal of Speech and Hearing Research, 29,* 193–206.

Thompson, C. K., & Shapiro, L. P. (2005). Treating agrammatic aphasia within a linguistic framework: Treatment of underlying forms. *Aphasiology, 19,* 1021–1036.

Thompson, C. K., Shapiro, L. P., Ballard, K. J., Jacobs, B. J., Schneider, S. S., et al. (1997). Training and generalized production of wh- and NP-movement structures in agrammatic aphasia. *Journal of Speech, Language, and Hearing Research, 40,* 228–244.

Thompson, C. K., Shapiro, L. P., Kiran, S., & Sobecks, J. (2003). The role of syntactic complexity in treatment of sentence deficits in agrammatic aphasia: The complexity account of treatment efficacy (CATE). *Journal of Speech, Language, and Hearing Research, 46,* 591–607.

Thompson, C. K., Shapiro, L. P., Tait, M. E., Jacobs, B. J., & Schneider, S. L. (1996). Training Wh-question production in agrammatic aphasia: Analysis of argument and adjunct movement. *Brain and Language, 52,* 175–228.

Thompson, J., & Enderby, P. (1979). Is all your Schuell really necessary? *British Journal of Disorders of Communication, 14,* 195–201.

Thomson, A. M., Taylor, R., Fraser, D., & Whittle, I. R. (1997a). Stereotactic biopsy of nonpolar tumors in the dominant hemisphere: A prospective study of effects on language functions. *Journal of Neurosurgery, 86,* 923–926.

Thomson, A. M., Taylor, R., Fraser, D., & Whittle, I. R. (1997b). The utility of the Right Hemisphere Language Battery in patients with brain tumours. *European Journal of Disorders of Communication, 32,* 325–332.

Thorndyke, P. W. (1977). Cognitive structures in comprehension and memory of narrative discourse. *Cognitive Psychology, 9,* 77–110.

Threats, T. (2007). Access for persons with neurogenic communication disorders: Influence of Personal and Environmental Factors of the ICF. *Aphasiology, 21,* 67–80.

Thurlborn, K. R., Carpenter, P., & Just, M. A. (1999). Plasticity of language-related brain function during recovery from stroke. *Stroke, 30,* 749–754.

Tirassa, M. (1999). Communicative competence and the architecture of the mind/brain. *Brain and Language, 68,* 419–441.

Tissen, A., Weber, S., Grande, M., & Gunther, T. (2007). The "tree pruning hypothesis" in bilingualism. *Aphasiology, 21*, 548–557.

Togher, L. (2012). Clinical approaches to communication impairments due to executive dysfunction. In R. K. Peach & L. P. Shapiro (Eds.), *Cognition and acquired language disorders: An information processing approach* (pp. 326–345). St. Louis: Elsevier/Mosby.

Togher, L., Hand, L., & Code, C. (1997). Measuring service encounters with the traumatic brain injury population. *Aphasiology, 11*, 491–504.

Togher, L., McDonald, S., Code, C., & Grant, S. (2004). Training communication partners of people with traumatic brain injury: A randomized controlled trial. *Aphasiology, 18*, 313–335.

Togher, L., Power, E., Tate, R., McDonald, S., & Rietdijk, R. (2010). Measuring the social interactions of people with traumatic brain injury and their communication partners: The adapted Kagan scales. *Aphasiology, 24*, 914–927.

Togher, L., Schultz, R., Tate, R., McDonald, S., Perdices, M., et al. (2009). The methodological quality of aphasia therapy research: An investigation of group studies using the PsycBITE™ evidence-based practice database. *Aphasiology, 23*, 694–706.

Tombaugh, T. N., & Hubley, A. M. (1997). The 60-item Boston Naming Test: Norms for cognitively intact adults aged 26 to 88 years. *Journal of Clinical and Experimental Neuropsychology, 19*, 922–932.

Tompkins, C. A. (1990). Knowledge and strategies for processing lexical metaphor after right or left hemisphere brain damage. *Journal of Speech and Hearing Research, 33*, 307–316.

Tompkins, C. A. (1995). *Right hemisphere communication disorders: Theory and management*. San Diego, CA: Singular.

Tompkins, C. A., Baumgaertner, A., Lehman Blake, M. T., & Fassbinder, W. (2000). Mechanisms of discourse comprehension impairment after right hemisphere brain damage: Suppression and enhancement in lexical ambiguity resolution. *Journal of Speech, Language, and Hearing Research, 43*, 62–78.

Tompkins, C. A., Blake, M. T., Wambaugh, J., & Meigh, K. (2011). A novel, implicit treatment for language comprehension processes in right hemisphere brain damage: Phase I data. *Aphasiology, 25*, 789–799.

Tompkins, C. A., Bloise, C. G. R., Timko, M. L., & Baumgaertner, A. (1994). Working memory and inference revision in brain-damaged and normally aging adults. *Journal of Speech and Hearing Research, 37*, 896–912.

Tompkins, C. A., Boada, R., & McGarry, K. (1992). The access and processing of familiar idioms by brain-damaged and normally aging adults. *Journal of Speech and Hearing Research, 35*, 626–637.

Tompkins, C. A., Fassbinder, W., Lehman Blake, M., Baumgaertner, A., & Jayaram, N. (2004). Inference generation during text comprehension by adults with right hemisphere brain damage: Activation failure versus multiple activation. *Journal of Speech, Language, and Hearing Research, 47*, 1380–1395.

Tompkins, C. A., Fassbinder, W., Scharp, V. L., & Meigh, K. M. (2008). Activation and maintenance of peripheral semantic features of unambiguous words after right hemisphere brain damage in adults. *Aphasiology, 22*, 119–138.

Tompkins, C. A., Jackson, S. T., & Schulz, R. (1990). On prognostic research in adult neurologic disorders. *Journal of Speech and Hearing Research, 33*, 398–401.

Tompkins, C. A., Lehman Blake, M. T., Baumgaertner, A., & Fassbinder, W. (2002). Characterising comprehension difficulties after right brain damage: Attention demands of suppression function. *Aphasiology, 16*, 559–572.

Tompkins, C. A., Meigh, K., Gibbs Scott, A., & Guttentag Lederer, L. (2009). Can high-level inferencing be predicted by Discourse Comprehension Test performance in adults with right hemisphere brain damage? *Aphasiology, 23*, 1016–1027.

Tompkins, C. A., Scharp, V. L., Fassbinder, W., Meigh, K. M., & Armstrong, E. M. (2008). A different story on "Theory of Mind" deficit in adults with right hemisphere brain damage. *Aphasiology, 22*, 42–61.

Tompkins, C. A., Scharp, V. L., & Marshall, R. C. (2006). Communicative value of self cues in aphasia: A re-evaluation. *Aphasiology, 20*, 684–704.

Tompkins, C. A., Scharp, V. L., Meigh, K. M., & Fassbinder, W. (2008). Coarse coding and discourse comprehension in adults with right hemisphere damage. *Aphasiology, 22*, 204–223.

Tompkins, C. A., Scharp, V. L., Meigh, K. M., Lehman Blake, M., & Wambaugh, J. (2012). Generalization of a novel implicit treatment for coarse coding deficit in right hemisphere brain damage: A single-participant experiment. *Aphasiology, 26*, 689–708.

Tonkovich, J. D., & Loverso, F. (1982). A training matrix approach for gestural acquisition by the agrammatic patient. In R.H. Brookshire (Ed.), *Clinical aphasiology conference proceedings* (pp. 283–288). Minneapolis, MN: BRK.

Traxler, M. J., & Gernsbacher, M. A. (Eds.). (2006). *Handbook of psycholinguistics* (2nd ed.). London: Elsevier.

Tree, J. J., Kay, J., & Perfect, T. J. (2005). "Deep" language disorders in nonfluent progressive aphasia: An evaluation of the "summation" account of semantic errors across language production tasks. *Cognitive Neuropsychology, 22*, 643–660.

True, G., Bartlett, M. R., Fink, R. B., Linebarger, M. C., & Schwartz, M. (2010). Perspectives of persons with aphasia toward SentenceShaper To Go: A qualitative study. *Aphasiology, 24,* 1032–1050.

Trupe, E. H. (1984). Reliability of rating spontaneous speech in the Western Aphasia Battery: Implications for classification. In R. H. Brookshire (Ed.), *Clinical aphasiology conference proceedings* (pp. 55–69). Minneapolis, MN: BRK.

Trupe, E. H., & Hillis, A. (1985). Paucity vs. verbosity: Another analysis of right hemisphere communication deficits. In R. H. Brookshire (Ed.), *Clinical Aphasiology* (Vol. 15, pp. 83–96). Minneapolis, MN: BRK.

Tschirren, M., Laganaro, M., Michel, P., Martory, M.-D., Di Pietro, M., et al. (2011). Language and syntactic impairment following stroke in late bilingual aphasics. *Brain and Language,* 119, 238–242.

Tseng, C.-H., McNeil, M. R., & Milenkovic, P. (1993). An investigation of attention allocation deficits in aphasia. *Brain and Language, 45,* 276–296.

Tulving, E. (1972). Episodic and semantic memory. In E. Tulving & W. Donaldson (Eds.), *Organization of memory* (pp. 382–403). New York: Academic Press.

Turner, S., & Whitworth, A. (2006). Conversational partner training programmes in aphasia: A review of key themes and participants' roles. *Aphasiology, 20,* 483–510.

Turton, A. J., Dewar, S. J., Lievesley, A., O'Leary, K., Gabb, J., et al. (2009). Walking and wheelchair navigation in patients with left visual neglect. *Neuropsychological Rehabilitation, 19,* 274–290.

Tyler, L. K. (1987). Spoken language comprehension in aphasia: A real-time processing perspective. In M. Coltheart, G. Sartori, & R. Job (Eds.), *The cognitive neuropsychology of language* (pp. 145–162). London: Erlbaum.

Tyler, L. K., & Moss, H. E. (1997). Imageability and category-specificity. *Cognitive Neuropsychology, 14,* 293–318.

Tyler, L. K., Ostrin, R. K., Cooke, M., & Moss, E. (1995). Automatic access of lexical information in Broca's aphasics: Against the automaticity hypothesis. *Brain and Language, 48,* 131–162.

Udell, R., Sullivan, R. A., & Schlanger, P. H. (1980). Legal competency of aphasic patients: Role of speech-language pathologists. *Archives of Physical Medicine and Rehabilitation, 61,* 374–375.

Ulatowska, H. K., Freedman-Stern, R., Doyel, A. W., Macaluso-Haynes, S., & North, A. J. (1983). Production of narrative discourse in aphasia. *Brain and Language, 19,* 317–334.

Ulatowska, H. K., Reyes, B. A., Santos, T. O., & Worle, C. (2011). Stroke narratives in aphasia: The role of reported speech. *Aphasiology, 25,* 93–105.

Uryase, D., Duffy, R. J., & Liles, B. Z. (1990). Analysis and description of narrative discourse in right-hemisphere-damaged adults: A comparison to neurologically normal and left-hemisphere-damaged aphasic adults. In T. E. Prescott (Ed.), *Clinical aphasiology* (Vol. 19). Austin, TX: Pro-Ed.

U.S. National Institutes of Health. (n.d.). An investigation of constraint induced language therapy for aphasia. Retrieved March 30, 2006, from www .clinicaltrials.gov/ct/show/NCT00223847

Van Demark, A. A., Lemmer, E. C., & Drake, M. L. (1982). Measurement of reading comprehension in aphasia with the RCBA. *Journal of Speech and Hearing Disorders, 47,* 288–291.

Van der Linden, M., Brédart, S., Depoorter, N., & Coyette, F. (1996). Semantic memory and amnesia: A case study. *Cognitive Neuropsychology, 13,* 391–414.

van de Sandt-Koenderman, W. M. E., Wiegers, J., Wielaert, S. M., Duivenvoorden, H. J., & Ribbers, G. M. (2007). High-tech AAC and severe aphasia: Candidacy for TouchSpeak (TS). *Aphasiology, 21,* 459–474.

van Gompel, R. P. G., Pickering, M. J., Pearson, J., & Liversedge, S. P. (2005). Evidence against competition during syntactic ambiguity resolution. *Journal of Memory and Language, 52,* 284–307.

Van Gorp, W., Satz, P., Klersch, M. E., & Henry, R. (1986). Normative data on the Boston Naming Test for a group of normal older adults. *Journal of Clinical and Experimental Neuropsychology, 8,* 702–705.

Van Lancker, D. R., & Kempler, D. (1987). Comprehension of familiar phrases by left- but not by right-hemisphere damaged patients. *Brain and Language, 32,* 265–277.

Van Lancker, D. R., Kreiman, J., & Cummings, J. (1989). Voice perception deficits: Neuroanatomical correlates of phonagnosia. *Journal of Clinical and Experimental Neuropsychology, 11,* 665–674.

Van Lancker Sidtis, D., & Postman, W. A. (2006). Formulaic expressions in spontaneous speech of left- and right-hemisphere-damaged subjects. *Aphasiology, 20,* 411–426.

Varney, N. R. (1980). Sound recognition in relation to aural language comprehension in aphasia. *Journal of Neurology, Neurosurgery, and Psychiatry, 43,* 71–75.

Varney, N. R. (1982). Pantomime recognition defect in aphasia: Implications for the concept of asymbolia. *Brain and Language, 15,* 32–39.

Vergun, D. (2012). Army, NFL team up to fight traumatic brain injury. Retrieved September 7, 2012, from http://www.defense.gov/ news/newsarticle.aspx?id =117721

Vickers, C. P. (2010). Social networks after the onset of aphasia: The impact of aphasia group attendance. *Aphasiology, 24,* 902–913.

Vignolo, L. A., Boccardi, E., & Caverni, L. (1986). Unexpected CT-scan findings in global aphasia. *Cortex, 22,* 55–69.

Visch-Brink, E. G., van Harskamp, F., Van Amerongen, N. M., Wielaert, S. M., & van de Sandt-Koenderman, M. E. (1993). A multidisciplinary approach to aphasia therapy. In A. L. Holland & M. M. Forbes (Eds.), *Aphasia treatment: World perspectives* (pp. 227–262). San Diego, CA: Singular.

Vocat, R., Staub, F., Stroppini, T., & Vuilleumier, P. (2010). Anosognosia for hemiplegia: A clinical-anatomical prospective study. *Brain, 133,* 3578–3597.

Vogel, D., & Costello, R. M. (1986). Bilingual aphasic adults: Measures of word retrieval. In R. H. Brookshire (Ed.). *Clinical aphasiology* (Vol. 16, pp. 80–86). Minneapolis, MN: BRK.

Vukovic, M., Vuksanovic, J., & Vokovic, I. (2008). Comparison of the recovery patterns of language and cognitive functions in patients with post-traumatic language processing deficits and in patients with aphasia following a stroke. *Journal of Communication Disorders, 41,* 531–552.

Wade, D. T. (2009). Goal-setting in rehabilitation: An overview of what, why, and how. *Clinical Rehabilitation, 23,* 291–295.

Waldron, H., Whitworth, A., & Howard, D. (2011). Comparing monitoring and production based approaches to the treatment of phonological assembly difficulties in aphasia. *Aphasiology, 25,* 1153–1173.

Walker, J. P., Daigle, T., & Buzzard, M. (2002). Hemispheric specialization in processing prosodic structures: Revisited. *Aphasiology, 16,* 1155–1172.

Walker-Batson, D., Barton, M. M., Wendt, J. S., & Reynolds, S. (1987). Symbolic and affective non-verbal deficits in left- and right-hemisphere injured adults. *Aphasiology, 1,* 257–262.

Walker-Batson, D., Curtis, S., Natarajan, R., Ford, J., Dronkers, N., et al. (2001). A double-blind, placebo-controlled study of the use of amphetamine in the treatment of aphasia. *Stroke, 32,* 2093–2098.

Wallace, G. L., & Canter, G. J. (1985). Effects of personally relevant language materials on the performance of severely aphasic individuals. *Journal of Speech and Hearing Disorders, 50,* 385–390.

Wallander, J. L., Conger, A. J., & Conger, J. C. (1985). Development and evaluation of a behaviorally referenced rating system for heterosocial skills. *Behavioral Assessment, 7,* 137–153.

Wallesch, C.-W., Bak, T., & Schulte-Mönting, J. (1992). Acute aphasia—Patterns and prognosis. *Aphasiology, 6,* 373–385.

Wambaugh, J. L., Cameron, R., Kalinyak-Fliszar, M., Nessler, C., & Wright, S. (2004). Retrieval of action names in aphasia: Effects of two cueing treatments. *Aphasiology, 18,* 979–1004.

Wambaugh, J. L., & Ferguson, M. (2007). Application of semantic feature analysis to retrieval of action names in aphasia. *Journal of Rehabilitation Research and Development, 44,* 381–394.

Wambaugh, J. L., Martinez, A. L., & Alegre, M. N. (2001). Qualitative changes following application of modified response elaboration training with apraxic-aphasic speakers. *Aphasiology, 15,* 965–976.

Wambaugh, J. L., Nessler, C., & Wright, S. (2013). Modified response elaboration training: Application to procedural discourse and personal recounts. *American Journal of Speech-Language Pathology* (Supplement), *22,* S409–S425.

Wambaugh, J. L., & Wright, S. (2007). Improved effects of word-retrieval treatments subsequent to addition of the orthographic form. *Aphasiology, 21,* 632–642.

Wang, L., & Goodglass, H. (1992). Pantomime, praxis, and aphasia. *Brain and Language, 42,* 402–418.

Ward, J. (2010). *The student's guide to cognitive neuroscience* (2nd ed.). Hove, UK: Psychology Press.

Warden, D. (2006). Military TBI during the Iraq and Afghanistan wars. *Journal of Head Trauma Rehabilitation, 21,* 398–402.

Warrington, E. K. (1991). Right neglect dyslexia: A single case study. *Cognitive Neuropsychology, 8,* 193–212.

Warrington, E. K. (1997). The Graded Naming Test: A restandardization. *Neuropsychological Rehabilitation, 7,* 143–146.

Warrington, E. K., & Shallice, T. (1984). Category-specific semantic impairments. *Brain, 107,* 829–854.

Waters, G. S., & Caplan, D. (1996). The capacity theory of sentence comprehension: Critique of Just and Carpenter (1992). *Psychological Review, 103,* 761–772.

Waters, G. S., Caplan, D., & Hildebrandt, N. (1991). On the structure of verbal short-term memory and its functional role in sentence comprehension: Evidence from neuropsychology. *Cognitive Neuropsychology, 8,* 81–126.

Waters, G. S., Caplan, D., & Rochon, E. (1995). Processing capacity and sentence comprehension in patients with Alzheimer's disease. *Cognitive Neuropsychology, 12,* 1–30.

Waters, G. S., Rochon, E., & Caplan, D. (1998). Task demands and sentence comprehension in patients with dementia of Alzheimer's type. *Brain and Language, 62,* 361–397.

Watson, C. M., Chenery, H. J., & Carter, M. S. (1999). An analysis of trouble and repair in the natural conversations of people with dementia of the Alzheimer's type. *Aphasiology, 13,* 195–218.

Watts, A. J., & Douglas, J. M. (2006). Interpreting facial expression and communication competence following traumatic brain injury. *Aphasiology, 20,* 707–722.

Webster, J., Franklin, S., & Howard, D. (2001). An investigation of the interaction between thematic and phrasal structure in nonfluent agrammatic subjects. *Brain and Language, 78,* 197–211.

Webster, J., Morris, J., & Franklin, S. (2005). Effects of therapy targeted at verb retrieval and the realization of the predicate argument structure: A case study. *Aphasiology, 19,* 748–764

Webster, J. S., Cottam, G., Gouvier, W. D., Blanton, P., Beissel, G. F., et al. (1988). Wheelchair obstacle course performance in right cerebral vascular accident victims. *Journal of Clinical and Experimental Neuropsychology, 11,* 295–310.

Wechsler, D. (2008). *Wechsler Adult Intelligence Scale-Fourth Edition (WAIS-IV).* New York: Pearson.

Wechsler, D. (2009). *Wechsler Memory Scale-Fourth Edition (WMS-IV).* New York: Pearson.

Weed, E., McGregor, W., Nielsen, J. F., Roepstorff, A., & Frith, U. (2010). Theory of mind in adults with right hemisphere damage: What's the story? *Brain & Language, 113,* 65–72.

Weekes, B. S. (2010). Issues in bilingual aphasia: An introduction. *Aphasiology, 24,* 123–125.

Weekes, B., & Coltheart, M. (1996). Surface dyslexia and surface dysgraphia: Treatment studies and their theoretical implications. *Cognitive Neuropsychology, 13,* 277–315.

Wehman, P., Bricout, J., & Targett, P. (1999). Supported employment for persons with traumatic brain injury. In R. T. Fraiser & D. C. Clemmons (Eds.), *Traumatic brain injury rehabilitation: Practical vocational, neuropsychological, and psychotherapy interventions.* London: CRC Press.

Weiller, C., Isensee, C., Rijntjes, M., Huber, W., Muller, S., et al. (1995). Recovery from Wernicke's aphasia: A positron emission tomographic study. *Annals of Neurology, 37,* 723–732.

Weinrich, M., Shelton., J. R., Cox, D. M., & McCall, D. (1997). Remediating production of tense morphology improves verb retrieval in chronic aphasia. *Brain and Language, 58,* 23–45.

Welch, L. W., Doineau, D., Johnson, S., & King, D. (1996). Educational and gender normative data for the Boston Naming Test in a group of older adults. *Brain and Language, 53,* 260–266.

Welland, R. J., Lubinski, R., & Higginbotham, D. J. (2002). Discourse Comprehension Test performance of elders with dementia of Alzheimer type. *Journal of Speech, Language, and Hearing Research, 45,* 1175–1187.

Wepman, J. M. (1951). *Recovery from aphasia.* New York: Ronald Press.

Wepman, J. M. (1968). Aphasia therapy: Some "relative" comments and some purely personal prejudices. In J. W. Black & E. G. Jancosek (Eds.), *Proceedings of the conference on language retraining for aphasics* (pp. 95–107). Columbus, OH: Ohio State University.

Wepman, J. M. (1972). Aphasia therapy: A new look. *Journal of Speech and Hearing Disorders, 37,* 203–214.

Wepman, J. M., & Jones, L. V. (1961). *Studies in aphasia: An approach to testing.* Chicago: Education-Industry Service.

Wepman, J. M., & Van Pelt, D. (1955). A theory of cerebral language disorders based on therapy. *Folia Phoniatrica, 7,* 223–235.

Wertz, R. T. (1983). Classifying the aphasias: Commodious or chimerical? In R. H. Brookshire (Ed.), *Clinical aphasiology conference proceedings* (pp. 296–303). Minneapolis, MN: BRK.

Wertz, R. T. (1985). Neuropathologies of speech and language: An introduction to patient management. In D. F. Johns (Ed.), *Clinical management of neurogenic communicative disorders* (2nd ed., pp. 1–96). Boston: Little, Brown.

Wertz, R. T. (1996). The PALPA's proof is in the predicting. *Aphasiology, 10,* 180–190.

Wertz, R. T., Auther, L. L., & Ross, K. B. (1997). Aphasia in African-Americans and Caucasians: Severity, improvement, and rate of improvement. *Aphasiology, 11,* 533–542.

Wertz, R. T., Collins, M. J., Weiss, D. G., Kurtzke, J. F., Friden, T., et al. (1981). Veterans Administration cooperative study on aphasia: A comparison of individual and group treatment. *Journal of Speech and Hearing Research, 24,* 580–594.

Wertz, R. T., Deal, J. L., Holland, A. L., Kurtzke, J. F., & Weiss, D. G. (1986). Comments on an uncontrolled aphasia no treatment trial. *Asha, 28,* 31.

Wertz, R. T., Deal, J. L., & Robinson, A. J. (1984). Classifying the aphasias: A comparison of the Boston Diagnostic Aphasia Examination and the Western Aphasia Battery. In R. H. Brookshire (Ed.), *Clinical aphasiology conference proceedings* (pp. 40–47). Minneapolis, MN: BRK.

Wertz, R. T., Deal, L. M., & Deal, J. L. (1980). Prognosis in aphasia: Investigation of the High-Overall Prediction (HOAP) method and the Short-Direct or HOAP-Slope method to predict change in PICA performance. In R. H. Brookshire (Ed.), *Clinical aphasiology conference proceeding* (pp. 164–173). Minneapolis, MN: BRK.

Wertz, R. T., Deal, L. M., & Deal, J. L. (1981). Clinical significance of the PICA high-low gap. In R. H. Brookshire (Ed.), *Clinical aphasiology conference proceedings.* Minneapolis, MN: BRK.

Wertz, R. T., & Dronkers, N. F. (1994). PICA performance following left or right hemisphere brain damage: Influence of side and severity. M. L. Lemme (Ed.), *Clinical aphasiology* (Vol. 22, pp. 157–164).

Wertz, R. T., Dronkers, N. F., & Shubitowski, Y. (1986). Discriminant function analysis of performance by normals and left hemisphere, right hemisphere, and bilaterally brain damaged patients on a word fluency measure. In R. H. Brookshire (Ed.), *Clinical aphasiology* (Vol. 16, pp. 257–266). Minneapolis, MN: BRK.

Wertz, R. T., & Katz, R. C. (2004). Outcomes of computer-provided treatment for aphasia. *Aphasiology, 18,* 229–244.

Wertz, R. T., Weiss, D. G., Aten, J. L., Brookshire, R. H., Garcia-Bunuel, L., et al. (1986). Comparison of clinic, home, and deferred language treatment for aphasia: A Veterans Administration cooperative study. *Archives of Neurology, 43,* 653–658.

Westmacott, R., Freedman, M., Black, S. E., Stokes, K. A., & Moscovitch, M. (2004). Temporally graded semantic memory loss in Alzheimer's disease: Cross-sectional and longitudinal studies. *Cognitive Neuropsychology, 21,* 353–378.

Weylman, S. T., Brownell, H. H., Roman, M., & Gardner, H. (1989). Appreciation of indirect requests by left- and right-brain-damaged patients: The effects of verbal context and conventionality of wording. *Brain and Language, 36,* 580–591.

Whatmough, C., Chertkow, H., Murtha, S., Templeman, D., Babins, L., et al. (2003). The semantic category effect increases with worsening anomia in Alzheimer's type dementia. *Brain and Language, 84,* 134–147.

Wheeler, B. M. (2001). *Close to me, but far away: Living with Alzheimer's.* Columbia, MO: University of Missouri Press.

Whittle, I. R., Pringle, A. M., & Taylor, R. (1998). Effects of respective surgery for left-sided intracranial tunours on language function: A prospective study. *Lancet, 351,* 1014–1018.

Whitworth, A., Perkins, L., & Lesser, R. (1997). *Conversational Analysis Profile for People with Aphasia (CAPPA).* London: Whurr.

Whitworth, A., Webster, J., & Howard, D. (2005). *A cognitive neuropsychological approach to assessment and intervention in aphasia: A clinician's guide.* Hove, UK: Psychology Press.

WHOQOL Group. (1998). Development of the World Health Organization WHOQOL-BREF quality of life assessment. *Psychological Medicine, 28,* 551–558.

Wilcox, M. J., Davis, G. A., & Leonard, L. L. (1978). Aphasics' comprehension of contextually conveyed meaning. *Brain and Language, 6,* 362–377.

Wilkinson, R., Bryan, K., Lock, S., & Sage, K. (2010). Implementing and evaluating aphasia therapy targeted at couples' conversations: A single case study. *Aphasiology, 24,* 869–886.

Williams, B. W., Mack, W., & Henderson, V. W. (1989). Boston Naming Test in Alzheimer's disease. *Neuropsychologia, 27,* 1073–1079.

Williams, L. S., Weinberger, M., Harris, L. E., Clark, D. O., & Biller, J. (1999). Development of a stroke-specific quality of life scale. *Stroke, 30,* 1362–1369.

Williams, S. E., & Canter, G. J. (1982). The influence of situational context on naming performance in aphasic syndromes. *Brain and Language, 17,* 92–106.

Williams, S. E., & Canter, G. J. (1987). Action-naming performance in four syndromes of aphasia. *Brain and Language, 32,* 124–136.

Williams, S. E., & Seaver, E. J. (1986). A comparison of speech sound durations in three syndromes of aphasia. *Brain and Language, 29,* 171–182.

Willmes, K. (1995). Aphasia therapy research: Some psychometric considerations and statistical methods for the single-case study approach. In C. Code & D. J. Müller (Eds.), *The treatment of aphasia: From theory to practice* (pp. 286–308). San Diego, CA: Singular.

Wilshire, C. E. (2002). Where do aphasic phonological errors come from? Evidence from phoneme movement errors in picture naming. *Aphasiology, 16,* 169–197.

Wilshire, C. E. (2008). Cognitive neuropsychological approaches to word production in aphasia: Beyond boxes and arrows. *Aphasiology, 22,* 1019–1053.

Wilshire, C. E., & Fisher, C. A. (2004). "Phonological" dysphasia: A cross-modal phonological impairment affecting repetition, production, and comprehension. *Cognitive Neuropsychology, 21,* 187–210.

Wilson, B. A. (1987). *Rehabilitation of memory.* New York: Guilford Press.

Wilson, B. A. (2009). *Memory rehabilitation: Integrating theory and practice.* Youngsville, NC: Lash & Associates.

Wilson, B. A., Alderman, N., Burgess, P. W., Emslie, H. C., & Evans, J. J. (1996). *The Behavioural Assessment of the Dysexecutive Syndrome.* Reading, UK: Thames Valley Test Company.

Wilson, B. A., Baddeley, A. D., Cockburn, J., & Hiorns, R. (1989). The development and validation of a test battery for detecting and monitoring everyday memory problems. *Journal of Clinical and Experimental Neuropsychology, 11,* 855–870.

Wilson, B. A., Cockburn, J., & Baddeley, A. D. (1985). *The Rivermead Behavioural Memory Test.* Reading, UK: Thames Valley Test Company.

Wilson, B. A., Herbert, C. M., & Shiel, A. (2007). *Behavioural approaches in neuropsychological rehabilitation.* New York: Psychology Press.

Wilson, J. T. L., Pettigrew, L. E. L., & Teasdale, G. M. (1998). Structured interviews for the Glasgow Outcome Scale and the Extended Glasgow Outcome Scale: Guidelines for their use. *Journal of Neurotrauma, 15,* 573–585.

Winner, E., Brownell, H., Happé, F., Blum, A., & Pincus, D. (1998). Distinguishing lies from jokes: Theory of mind deficits and discourse interpretation in right hemisphere brain-damaged patients. *Brain and Language, 62,* 89–106.

Winner, E., & Gardner, H. (1977). Comprehension of metaphor in brain damaged patients. *Brain, 100,* 717–729.

Winner, E., & von Karolyi, C. (1998). Artistry and aphasia. In M. T. Sarno (Ed.), *Acquired aphasia* (3rd ed., pp. 375–411). New York: Academic Press.

Winslade, W. J. (1998). *Confronting traumatic brain injury: Devastation, hope, and healing.* New Haven, CT: Yale University Press.

Wisenburn, B., & Mahoney, K. (2009). A meta-analysis of word-finding treatments for aphasia. *Aphasiology, 23,* 1338–1352.

Wong, M. N., Murdoch, B., & Whelan, B.-M. (2010). Language disorders subsequent to mild traumatic brain injury (MTBI): Evidence from four cases. *Aphasiology, 24,* 1155–1169.

Woods, B., Spector, A. E., Jones, C. A., Orrell, M., & Davies, S. P. (2005). Reminiscence therapy for dementia. *Cochrane Database of Systematic Reviews* 2005, Issue 2. Art. No.: CD001120. DOI: 10.1002/14651858. CD001120.pub2.

World Health Organization (WHO). (1997). *ICIDH-2 International classification of impairments, activities, and participation.* Geneva, Switzerland: World Health Organization.

World Health Organization (WHO). (2001). *International classification for functioning, disability and health* (ICF). Geneva, Switzerland: World Health Organization.

Worrall, L., Brown, K., Cruice, M., Davidson, B., Hersh, D., Howe, T., & Sherratt, S. (2010). The evidence for a life-coaching approach to aphasia. *Aphasiology, 24,* 497–514.

Worrall, L., & Cruice, M. (2005). Why the WHO ICF and QOL constructs do not lend themselves to programmatic appraisal for planning therapy for aphasia: A commentary on Ross and Wertz, "Advancing appraisal: Aphasia and the WHO." *Aphasiology, 19,* 885–893.

Worrall, L., Sherratt, S., Rogers, P., Howe, T., Hersh, D., et al. (2011). What people with aphasia want: Their goals according to the ICF. *Aphasiology, 25,* 309–322.

Worrall, L. E., Rose, T., Howe, T., Brennan, A., Egan, J., et al. (2005). Access to information for people with aphasia. *Aphasiology, 19,* 923–929.

Worrall, L. E., Rose, T., Howe, T., McKenna, K., & Hickson, L. (2007). Developing an evidence-base for accessibility for people with aphasia. *Aphasiology, 21,* 124–136.

Wright, H. H., Downey, R. A., Gravier, M., Love, T., & Shapiro, L. P. (2007). Processing distinct linguistic information types in working memory in aphasia. *Aphasiology, 21,* 802–813.

Wright, H. H., & Shisler, R. J. (2005). Working memory in aphasia: Theory, measures, and clinical implications.

American Journal of Speech-Language Pathology, 14, 107–118

Wulf, H. H. (1979). *My world alone.* Detroit: Wayne State University Press.

Wulfeck, B., Bates, E., & Capasso, R. (1991). A cross-linguistic study of grammaticality judgments in Broca's aphasia. *Brain and Language, 41,* 311–336.

Wunderlich, A., & Ziegler, W. (2011). Facilitation of picture-naming in anomic subjects: Sound vs mouth shape. *Aphasiology, 25,* 202–220.

Yasuda, K., Nemoto, T., Takenaka, K., Mitachi, M., & Kuwabara, K. (2007). Effectiveness of a vocabulary data file, encyclopaedia, and Internet homepages on a conversation-support system for people with moderate-to-severe aphasia. *Aphasiology, 21,* 867–882.

Yedor, K. E., Conlon, C. P., & Kearns, K. P. (1993). Measurements predictive of generalization of response elaboration training. In M. L. Lemme (Ed.), *Clinical aphasiology* (Vol. 21, pp. 213–223). Austin, TX: Pro-Ed.

Ylvisaker, M., Szekeres, S. F., & Feeney, T. (2008). Communication disorders associated with traumatic brain injury. In R. Chapey (Ed.), *Language intervention strategies in aphasia and related neurogenic communication disorders* (5th ed., pp. 879–954). Philadelphia: Wolters Kluwer Health.

Yorkston, K. M., & Beukelman, D. R. (1980). An analysis of connected speech samples of aphasic and normal speakers. *Journal of Speech and Hearing Disorders, 45,* 27–36.

Youmans, G., & Bourgeois, M. (2010). Theory of mind in individuals with Alzheimer-type dementia. *Aphasiology, 24,* 515–534.

Youmans, G., Holland, A., Munoz, M. L., & Bourgeois, M. (2005). Script training and automaticity in two individuals with aphasia. *Aphasiology, 19,* 435–449.

Young, A. W., Newcombe, F., & Ellis, A. W. (1991). Different impairments contribute to neglect dyslexia. *Cognitive Neuropsychology, 8,* 177–192.

Youse, K. M., & Coelho, C. (2009). Treating underlying attention deficits as a means for improving conversational discourse: Preliminary study. *Neurorehabilitation, 24,* 355–364.

Youse, K. M., Coelho, C. A., Mozeiko, J. L., & Feinn, R. (2005). Discourse characteristics of closed-head-injured and non-brain-injured adults misclassified by discriminant function analyses. *Aphasiology, 19,* 297–313.

Youse, K. M., Gathof, M., Fields, R. D., Lobianco, T. F., Bush, H. M., et al. (2011). Conversational discourse analysis procedures: A comparison of two paradigms. *Aphasiology, 25,* 106–118.

Zaidel, E., Kasher, A., Soroker, N., & Batori, G. (2002). Effects of right and left hemisphere damage on performance of the "Right hemisphere communication battery." *Brain and Language, 80,* 510–535.

Zanetti, O., Zanieri, G., Di Giovanni, G., De Vreese, L. P., Pezzini, A., et al. (2001). Effectiveness of procedural memory stimulation in mild Alzheimer's disease patients: A controlled study. *Neuropsychological Rehabilitation, 11,* 263–272.

Zingeser, L. B., & Berndt, R. S. (1990). Retrieval of nouns and verbs in agrammatism and anomia. *Brain and Language, 39,* 14–32.

Zoccolotti, P., Scabini, D., & Violani, C. (1982). Electrodermal responses in patients with unilateral brain damage. *Journal of Clinical Neuropsychology, 4,* 143–150.

Zraick, R. I., & Boone, D. R. (1991). Spouse attitudes toward the person with aphasia. *Journal of Speech and Hearing Research, 34,* 123–128.

Zurif, E. B., Gardner, H., & Brownell, H. H. (1989). The case against the case against group studies. *Brain and Cognition, 10,* 237–255.

Zurif, E. B., Swinney, D., Prather, P., Soloman, J., & Bushell, C. (1993). An on-line analysis of syntactic processing in Broca's and Wernicke's aphasia. *Brain and Language, 45,* 448–464.

AUTHOR INDEX

SUBJECT INDEX